Tick-Borne Diseases of Humans

Tick-Borne Diseases of Humans

Edited by Jesse L. Goodman, David T. Dennis, and Daniel E. Sonenshine

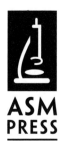

ASM
PRESS

Washington, D.C.

Copyright © 2005   ASM Press
American Society for Microbiology
1752 N St., N.W.
Washington, DC 20036-2904

Library of Congress Cataloging-in-Publication Data

Tick-borne diseases of humans / edited by Jesse L. Goodman, David T. Dennis, and Daniel E. Sonenshine.
    p. ; cm.
  Includes bibliographical references and index.
  ISBN 1-55581-238-4 (alk. paper)
  1. Tick-borne diseases.
  [DNLM: 1. Tick-Borne Diseases. 2. Arachnid Vectors. 3. Ticks. WC 600 T5556 2005] I. Goodman,
Jesse L. II. Dennis, David T. (David Tappen), 1939—III. Sonenshine, Daniel E.

RA641.T5T52 2005
616.9'68—dc22

                                                                                          2004022598

10 9 8 7 6 5 4 3 2 1

Address editorial correspondence to ASM Press, 1752 N St., N.W., Washington, DC 20036-2904, U.S.A.

Send orders to: ASM Press, P.O. Box 605, Herndon, VA 20172, U.S.A.
Phone: 800-546-2416; 703-661-1593
Fax: 703-661-1501
E-mail: books@asmusa.org
Online: www.asmpress.org

CONTENTS

CONTRIBUTORS

Abdu F. Azad
Department of Microbiology and Immunology, School of Medicine, University of Maryland, Baltimore, Baltimore, Maryland 21201

Alan G. Barbour
Departments of Medicine and Microbiology and Molecular Genetics, University of California, Irvine, Irvine, California 92697-4025

Richard N. Brown
Department of Wildlife, Humboldt State University, Arcata, California 95521-8222

Felicity J. Burt
Special Pathogens Unit, National Institute for Communicable Diseases, Sandringham 2131, Republic of South Africa

Grant L. Campbell
Division of Vector-Borne Infectious Diseases, National Center for Infectious Diseases, Centers for Disease Control and Prevention, Colorado State University, Foothills Campus, Fort Collins, Colorado 80521

J. E. Childs
Department of Biology, 2101 Rollins Basic Science Building, 1510 Clifton Road NE, Atlanta, Georgia 30602

Jenifer Coburn
Division of Geographic Medicine and Infectious Diseases, Tufts-New England Medical Center, Boston, Massachusetts 02111

Gregory A. Dasch
Viral and Rickettsial Zoonoses Branch, Centers for Disease Control and Prevention, 1600 Clifton Road, Atlanta, Georgia 30333

W. R. Davidson
Southeastern Cooperative Wildlife Disease Study, College of Veterinary Medicine, University of Georgia, Athens, Georgia 30602

J. E. Dawson
Chelan-Douglas Health District, 200 Valley Mall Parkway, East Wenatchee, Washington 98802

David T. Dennis
Division of Vector-Borne Infectious Diseases, National Center for Infectious Diseases, Centers for Disease Control and Prevention, P.O. Box 2087, Fort Collins, Colorado 80522

J. Stephen Dumler
Division of Medical Microbiology, Department of Pathology, The Johns Hopkins University School of Medicine, 720 Rutland Avenue, Baltimore, Maryland 21205

Lance A. Durden
Institute of Arthropodology and Parasitology, Georgia Southern University, Statesboro, Georgia 30460-8056

S. A. Ewing
224 Veterinary Medicine, Oklahoma State University, Stillwater, Oklahoma 74078

Pierre-Edouard Fournier
Unité des Rickettsies, CNRS UMR 6020, Faculté de Médecine, Université de la Méditerranée, 27 Boulevard Jean Moulin, 13385 Marseille Cédex 05, France

Howard S. Ginsberg
U.S. Geological Survey Patuxent Wildlife Research Center, Coastal Field Station, University of Rhode Island, Kingston, Rhode Island 02881

Lisa Glickstein
Center for Immunology and Inflammatory Diseases, Division of Rheumatology, Massachusetts General Hospital, Harvard Medical School, 55 Fruit Street, Boston, Massachusetts 02114

Jesse L. Goodman
Center for Biologics Evaluation and Research, U.S. Food and Drug Administration, 1401 Rockville Pike, Suite 200N, HFM-1, Rockville, Maryland 20852

Edward B. Hayes
Division of Vector-Borne Infectious Diseases, National Center for Infectious Diseases, Centers for Disease Control and Prevention, P.O. Box 2087, Fort Collins, Colorado 80522

Mary J. Homer
Infectious Disease Research Institute, Seattle Life Sciences Center, 1124 Columbia Street, Seattle, Washington 98104

Steven D. Jauron
Department of Entomology, University of Minnesota, 1980 Folwell Avenue, St. Paul, Minnesota 55108

James E. Keirans
Institute of Arthropodology and Parasitology, Georgia Southern University, Statesboro, Georgia 30460-8056

Timothy J. Kurtti
Department of Entomology, University of Minnesota, 1980 Folwell Avenue, St. Paul, Minnesota 55108

Milan Labuda
Institute of Zoology, Slovak Academy of Sciences, Dubravska cesta 9, 845 06 Bratislava, Slovakia

Robert S. Lane
Department of Environmental Science, Policy, and Management, Division of Insect Biology, University of California, Berkeley, California 94720

Allison M. Liddell
InfectiousCare, 8320 Walnut Hill Lane, Suite 300 LB3, Dallas, Texas 75231

S. E. Little
Department of Microbiology and Parasitology, College of Veterinary Medicine, University of Georgia, Athens, Georgia 30602

Kevin R. Macaluso
Department of Pathobiological Sciences, School of Veterinary Medicine, Louisiana State University, Skip Berman Drive, Baton Rouge, Louisiana 70803

Anthony A. Marfin
Division of Vector-Borne Infectious Diseases, National Center for Infectious Diseases, Centers for Disease Control and Prevention, Colorado State University, Foothills Campus, Fort Collins, Colorado 80521

Uwe U. Müller-Doblies
Center for Microbial Pathogenesis, School of Medicine, University of Connecticut Health Center, 263 Farmington Avenue, Farmington, Connecticut 06030

Ulrike G. Munderloh
Department of Entomology, University of Minnesota, 1980 Folwell Avenue, St. Paul, Minnesota 55108

Patricia A. Nuttall
Natural Environment Research Council (NERC) Centre for Ecology and Hydrology, Polaris House, North Star Avenue, Swindon SN2 1EU, United Kingdom

Christopher D. Paddock
Infectious Disease Pathology Activity, Centers for Disease Control and Prevention, 1600 Clifton Road, Atlanta, Georgia 30333

David H. Persing
Corixa Corporation, 1900 9th Avenue, Seattle, Washington 98101

Joseph F. Piesman
Division of Vector-Borne Infectious Diseases, National Center for Infectious Diseases, Centers for Disease Control and Prevention, P.O. Box 2087, Fort Collins, Colorado 80522

Didier Raoult
Unité des Rickettsies, CNRS UMR 6020, Faculté de Médecine, Université de la Méditerranée, 27 Boulevard Jean Moulin, 13385 Marseille Cédex 05, France

Daniel E. Sonenshine
Department of Biological Sciences, Old Dominion University, Norfolk, Virginia 23529

Kirby C. Stafford III
Connecticut Agricultural Experiment Station,
P.O. Box 1106, New Haven, Connecticut 06549

S. M. Standaert
3525 Ensign Rd., NE, Suite 02, Olympia,
Washington 98506

Allen C. Steere
Center for Immunology and Inflammatory Diseases,
Division of Rheumatology, Massachusetts General
Hospital, Harvard Medical School, 55 Fruit Street,
Boston, Massachusetts 02114

Gregory A. Storch
Department of Pediatrics, Washington University
School of Medicine, St. Louis, Missouri 63110

Robert Swanepoel
Special Pathogens Unit, National Institute
for Communicable Diseases, Sandringham 2131,
Republic of South Africa

Herbert A. Thompson
Viral and Rickettsial Zoonoses Branch, Centers for
Disease Control and Prevention, 1600 Clifton
Road, Atlanta, Georgia 30333

Stephen K. Wikel
Center for Microbial Pathogenesis,
School of Medicine, University of Connecticut
Health Center, 263 Farmington Avenue,
Farmington, Connecticut 06030

PREFACE

This book assembles in one place a comprehensive discussion of the tick-borne diseases that affect humans. Most sources that consider tick-borne diseases focus on either the vectors or the diseases, one usually being addressed at the expense of the other. We aim in the present work to address both perspectives, including state-of-the-art information on disease epidemiology, transmission, and ecology; clinical and laboratory findings; diagnosis; and treatment and prevention. Each contributor has specialized knowledge, and many have pioneered the discovery and understanding of these diseases, including their causative agents and the ticks that spread them. The reader can reap the benefits of hearing directly from experts who are not simply reviewing the literature but sharing their perspectives on continuing stories of discovery in which they themselves are engaged, often on clinical, laboratory, and population levels.

Almost everyone would agree that humans would be better off without ticks. Yet ticks and humans are increasingly in contact as people both spread into new environments and travel more for work or for pleasure. This contact has resulted in a striking increase in the incidence and subsequent awareness of a broad array of tick-borne diseases, with resultant medical, social, public health, and economic impacts. Some important tick-borne infections and their causative agents, such as Lyme borreliosis, have been recognized only recently, while others are being discovered at an increasing pace, and surveillance, diagnosis, treatment, prevention, and control of such infections have become high priorities. Most tick-borne infections of humans afflict domestic and wild animals also and thus can be important in agriculture and veterinary medicine. It is therefore not surprising that many tick-borne diseases were initially described in animals and that human medicine has benefited greatly from the contributions of our veterinary colleagues (and their patients).

Tick-borne illnesses are extremely diverse, both biologically and clinically. They can be due to toxic and allergic processes or to infectious agents, including viruses, bacteria (gram-positive, gram-negative, and spirochetal forms), and protozoa. They cause diseases that can be of acute onset and reapidly fatal (such as Rocky Mountain spotted fever), recurrent (relapsing fever), or multisystemic and chronic (Lyme borreliosis). Symptoms are often nonspecific, making recognition and appropriate treatment challenging, yet critical, in preventing adverse outcomes. For these reasons, especially in an age of widespread travel and migration, clinicians must be familiar with the major disease syndromes and their diagnosis, even for diseases that occur mostly outside their areas of practice.

There are three major sections in this book—and each one can be useful alone or in concert with the others. Section I synthesizes cross-cutting and diverse information that is relevant to the full spectrum of tick-borne diseases, most of which has not been presented previously in an integrated manner. It provides an overview of the ticks themselves, including their biology and identification, the distribution of the diseases that they transmit, and strategies for their control. Studies in recent years have shown that the tick-pathogen interaction is finely tuned and that pathogens may switch their gene expression and behavior as they cycle from tick to zoonotic host or human and vice versa. Understanding of both the general themes and the complexities of these interactions is critical for better, science-based, treatment and prevention of disease and is reviewed, as is the reaction to tick bites, which can range from local inflammation to paralysis. This section also provides a comprehensive review of the clinical approach to a patient with a possible tick-borne illness that includes the clinical history, geographic considerations, differential diagnosis based on clinical and laboratory findings, and guidelines for treatment of acutely ill patients. Section II includes a series of chapters that each comprehensively considers a specific disease, including history, biology, epidemiology, ecology, transmission, clinical manifestations, diagnosis, and treatment and prevention. Section III introduces original color illustrations, including maps of vector and disease distribution and an atlas of clinical and pathologic images with clear examples of diagnostically important skin lesions, blood smears, and other useful material, referenced in the text. Look for the color section in the body of the book.

Who should use this book, and how should it be used?

- Practitioners, trainees, and students of human and veterinary medicine should find especially useful the general chapters on clinical and epidemiologic aspects of tick-borne diseases, including the color section as well as the chapters dealing with specific diseases and with tick identification. Those interested in learning more about the biology of the organisms and about the ticks themselves will find this information readily accessible.
- Public health practitioners, scientists, and students—including epidemiologists, ecologists, and medical entomologists—can use this book

as both an introduction to the field and a ready reference source for complementing their specific areas of expertise, for example, with clinical information and with information about diseases occurring in other geographic areas.

- Microbiologists and other laboratory scientists who work on specific tick-borne pathogens or related organisms can learn more about ticks and about pathogen biology and disease pathogenesis, including interactions with tick, animal, and human hosts, and a broad array of infectious agents.
- Although much of this book is technical, the informed patient and the general public will find much of it accessible, including information about disease transmission, clinical and laboratory diagnosis and treatment, and the history of the infections of interest.

To all, welcome to what we trust will be an interesting and useful book! We look forward to your comments.

Jesse L. Goodman, Bethesda, Md.
David T. Dennis, Ft. Collins, Colo.
Daniel E. Sonenshine, Norfolk, Va.

ACKNOWLEDGMENTS

We thank our families, our mentors, and our colleagues for their inspiration and support. We thank Greg Payne of ASM Press, who first brought up the idea of a book, for his encouragement and patience.

We thank all of the contributors and all of those involved in the production of this book.

IMPORTANT NOTICE

I. TICKS, THEIR INTERACTIONS WITH HOSTS, AND THE DISEASES THEY TRANSMIT

Chapter 1

Overview of Tick-Borne Infections of Humans

DAVID T. DENNIS AND JOSEPH F. PIESMAN

HISTORY AND BACKGROUND

Tick-borne diseases, long known but historically underappreciated, are increasingly recognized as important threats to public health. Ticks are surpassed only by mosquitoes as arthropod vectors of disease. The diversity of human pathogens transmitted by ticks and mosquitoes is similar; for ticks, they span an array of bacteria (spirochetes, rickettsiae, *Francisella* spp.), viruses (flaviviruses, coltiviruses, and a nairovirus), and parasites (*Babesia* spp.) (Table 1). Previously unrecognized tick-borne agents and associated diseases are being discovered at a rapid pace, and many tick-borne diseases, old and new, are considered emergent or have that potential. With only one known exception (relapsing fever caused by *Borrelia duttonii*), tick-borne infections of humans are zooanthroponoses, or diseases of animals transmissible to humans in which humans are incidental, dead-end hosts. Tick bites are the sole or principal means by which most of these diseases are acquired by humans; some, however, may be transmitted by direct contact, ingestion, or aerosol exposure to infectious animal materials (tularemia and Q fever), by nosocomial exposures (Crimean-Congo hemorrhagic fever [CCHF]), by transfusion (babesiosis and Colorado tick fever), or by maternal transmission to the fetus. Usually, persons become infected with tick-borne diseases when they intrude into an established natural focus (biocenose) where the disease agent is quietly cycling between vertebrate reservoir hosts and their tick vectors. This intersection is increasingly frequent as human populations grow in number and mobility; as more persons reside, work, or recreate in tick-infested habitats; and as changing environments favor ticks and increase their range, density, and likelihood of human interaction. Further, evolving socioeconomic factors and human behaviors (e.g., suburbanization, increasing outdoor recreation, changing agricultural practices, reforestation, and pet ownership) can increase the risk that humans will come into contact with ticks and the disease agents they carry.

Ticks, which have been around in much the same form for approximately 200 million years, are among the oldest and most successful groups of arthropods. They were described as pests by the ancient Greeks and ever since have been treated in literature mostly with repugnance. Only scientists have much appreciation of them.

These primitive, obligate, blood-sucking parasites prey on every class of vertebrate in all parts of the world (32). They have diverse means of dispersion and are adaptable, and the range and population size of several important vector species are increasing (18). Long-term attempts to limit geographic expansion or to decrease the size of those populations responsible for human disease have been remarkably unsuccessful, with the possible exception of widespread use of dichlorodiphenyltrichloroethane (DDT) to control *Ixodes persulcatus* and tick-borne encephalitis (TBE) in the former Soviet Union from 1965 to 1971 (20).

Ticks were the first arthropods to be clearly established as vectors of infectious disease, owing to the discovery in 1893 by Smith and Kilbourne of the role of *Boophilus annulatus* as the vector of *Babesia bigemina*, the protozoal cause of Texas cattle fever (31). This discovery antedated by a decade or so the definitive reports of mosquitoes as vectors of malaria, yellow fever, and filariasis and of fleas as transmitters of the plague bacillus. In 1903, ticks were first proved as vectors of human disease, when J. E. Dutton, working in the Congo, discovered the principal cause of endemic relapsing fever (named *B. duttonii* in his honor) and its argasid (soft-tick) vector, *Ornithodoros moubata* (8). Unfortunately, Dutton became one of several early pioneers of tick-borne diseases of humans to die from experiments with the agents they studied. Shortly thereafter, H. T. Ricketts, after demonstrating that *Dermacentor* ticks were the vectors of Rocky Mountain spotted fever (RMSF), succumbed in the

David T. Dennis and Joseph F. Piesman • Division of Vector-Borne Infectious Diseases, National Center for Infectious Diseases, Centers for Disease Control and Prevention, P.O. Box 2087, Fort Collins, CO 80522.

Table 1. Principal tick-borne diseases of humans, agents, vectors, and reservoir hosts

Disease	Causative agent(s)	Primary tick vector(s)	Reservoir host(s)
TBE (Central European encephalitis, Russian spring summer encephalitis)	*Flavivirus*[a]	*I. ricinus, I. persulcatus*	Rodents, insectivores
Powassan encephalitis	*Flavivirus*[b]	*Ixodes, Dermacentor,* and *Haemaphysalis* spp.	Rodents, mustelids, lagomorphs
Kyasanur Forest disease	*Flavivirus*	*Haemaphysalis spinigera*	Monkeys, small mammals
Colorado tick fever	*Coltivirus*[b]	*D. andersoni*	Rodents
CCHF	*Nairovirus*[c]	*Hyalomma marginatum marginatum, Hyalomma marginatum rufipes,* others	Hares, hedgehogs, small mammals
RMSF	*R. rickettsii*	*D. variabilis, D. andersoni*	Rodents, lagomorphs
Boutonneuse fever, other widely distributed spotted fevers and/or tick typhuses worldwide	*Rickettsia conorii* complex, *Rickettsia sibirica, Rickettsia japonica, Rickettsia slovaca, Rickettsia africae, Rickettsia australis,* others	*Rhipicephalus sanguineus, Dermacentor marginatus, Amblyomma variegatum, Amblyomma hebraeum, D. reticulatus,* others	Small mammals, hedgehogs, dogs
Human anaplasmosis	*Anaplasma phagocytophilum*	*I. scapularis, I. pacificus, I. ricinus*	Rodents, other small mammals
Human monocytotropic ehrlichiosis	*Ehrlichia chaffeensis*	*Amblyomma americanum, D. variabilis*	Deer, dogs
Q fever	*Coxiella burnetii*	Many tick species	Domestic livestock
LB	*B. burgdorferi, Borrelia afzelii, Borrelia garinii*	*I. scapularis, I. pacificus, I. ricinus, I. persulcatus*	Rodents, birds
Tick-borne relapsing fever	*Borrelia* spp.	*Ornithodoros* spp.	Rodents, lagomorphs, humans (*B. duttonii*)
Tularemia	*F. tularensis*	*D. variabilis, D. andersoni, A. americanum, Ixodes apronophorus, D. reticulatus, I. ricinus* complex	Rodents, lagomorphs, others
Babesiosis	*Babesia microti, Babesia divergens,* others	*I. scapularis, I. ricinus,* others	Rodents, cattle, deer (?)

[a] Family *Flaviviridae*.
[b] Family *Reoviridae*.
[c] Family *Bunyaviridae*.

course of studies of the related epidemic typhus rickettsia. R. R. Parker, E. Francis, and other early workers first reported in the 1920s that ticks were important vectors of *Pasteurella* (later named *Francisella*) *tularensis*, an agent that also proved to be a dangerous, potentially fatal, laboratory hazard (11). Since those early and sometimes dangerous beginnings in tick-borne disease discovery, a growing list of other tick-borne infections has unfolded, including additional members of the large group of rickettsial spotted fevers; various viral encephalitides and hemorrhagic fevers; Colorado tick fever and Kyasanur Forest disease; and Q fever, ehrlichiosis, anaplasmosis, and babesiosis (27, 34).

The most remarkable recent tick-borne disease discovery, however, is that of Lyme borreliosis (LB), which, over the short period since its first comprehensive description in the 1970s, has come to be the most frequently reported vector-borne disease in temperate regions of the northern hemisphere (tens of thousands of cases are reported annually in both North America and Europe). LB is actually a complex of closely related syndromes, involving several genospecies of *Borrelia* vectored by various hard ticks in the *Ixodes ricinus* complex and spanning in range the entire holoarctic region (6, 9, 39). The emergence of LB as a major public health problem and the scientific challenges it poses have done much to revive interest and expertise in medical entomology and to spark a renaissance of research on tick-borne diseases in general.

PURPOSE OF THE BOOK

This book is intended first to be a ready resource for persons needing specific disease-oriented information immediately useful in the practice of medical and veterinary medicine and public health and second for entomologists, ecologists, students, and others needing a single source for reviews of specific tick-borne infections and their vectors. Although this book focuses on infectious diseases, ticks cause a number of problems other than infections for humans, including a diminished enjoyment of the outdoors along with the nuisance and cost of protecting against tick bites, allergic and toxic reactions to tick bites, an unreasonable fear of ticks and delusory parasitosis, and large agricultural and veterinary costs, including the cost of protecting pet dogs and cats. Of these noninfectious problems, only allergic and toxic reactions, including tick paralysis, are addressed specifically in this book, which is not intended to cover broad aspects of the impact of arthropods. These broader issues are dealt with elsewhere (10, 15, 17, 30, 33).

Although students of medicine and public health are usually taught the basics of the more important tick-borne diseases, the emphasis is on clinical diagnosis and management, with less attention paid to epidemiology and to ticks' fascinating but sometimes complex biology and ecology. Very little, if anything, is taught about tick vectors themselves. Biologists, on the other hand, may learn little about the medical and epidemiological aspects of vector-borne pathogens. This book attempts to give a more balanced view and to provide key information in an easy access format. To accomplish this, chapters in the first section provide general information on tick biology, interactions of pathogens with their tick vectors, the control and prevention of tick-borne diseases, clinical approaches to patients with tick exposure, and noninfectious complications of tick bites (such as allergic reactions and tick paralysis), as well as an overview of tick identification. The second section contains chapters encompassing all major tick-borne diseases in the world. The disease-specific chapters cover background, biology and life cycle, epidemiology, clinical features, diagnosis and treatment, and prevention and control and include comprehensive bibliographies. The book ends with a compendium of information on the global or regional geographic distributions of tick-borne diseases and their important vectors, with maps. (More specific descriptions and maps can be found in many individual disease chapters.) An atlas illustrating selected disease agents, some diagnostic clinical signs of infection, and principal vectors is also included for ready visual reference.

OVERVIEW OF TICK VECTORS AND THEIR NATURAL HISTORY

Tick Groupings

Tick vectors of human disease fall into two broad families, the Ixodidae, or hard ticks (so-called because

of the presence of a hard plate, or scutum, covering the dorsal body surface), and the Argasidae, or soft ticks, which lack a scutum and have a cuticle that exhibits a soft leathery appearance. Those Ixodidae transmitting disease to humans comprise members of five subfamilies and six genera; the most important of these are various *Ixodes*, *Dermacentor*, *Amblyomma*, *Haemaphysalis*, *Hyalomma*, and *Rhipicephalus* species (35). Of the Argasidae, only members of the genus *Ornithodoros* are known vectors of human pathogens (Table 2). For a more detailed review of tick systematics, see Chapter 7.

Tick Life Cycles

The life cycle of ixodid and argasid ticks includes the three stages of larva, nymph, and adult. Ixodid ticks have only one nymphal stage, whereas argasids have two or more nymphal stages. All ticks feed on blood during some or all stages of the life cycle. Larvae seek hosts, attach, feed, detach, and develop in sheltered microenvironments where they molt to nymphs; nymphs follow the same pattern and molt to adults (except argasids, which first molt into further nymphal stages); adults seek hosts, mate, feed, and in the case of engorged females, drop off to deposit eggs. Ticks are relatively long-lived; many can survive for 1 year or more without feeding. Host-seeking and -feeding tactics differ between species. *Ixodes* species quest in a stationary and mostly passive manner. Often, they wait in ambush on low-lying vegetation, extending and waving their barbed legs to snag prey as it brushes past. *Hyalomma* vectors of Crimean-Congo hemorrhagic fever (CCHF) are, on the other hand, hunters that may vigorously pursue their intended hosts, running rapidly across open space toward their prey, directed by sight and emitted CO_2. Ixodid ticks attach firmly to their hosts with embedded, barbed, and cemented mouthparts and usually take several days to complete the feeding process; most argasids, whose engorgement is not restricted by a rigid scutum, do not attach firmly and feed voraciously and quickly (within 35 to 70 min for adults) in the manner of bedbugs

Table 2. Groupings of principal tick vectors of disease to humans

Family	Subfamily (subgroup)	Genus (genera)
Ixodidae	Ixodinae	*Ixodes*
	Amblyomminae	*Amblyomma*
	Haemaphysalinae	*Haemaphysalis*
	Hyalomminae	*Hyalomma*
	Rhipicephalinae	*Dermacentor, Boophilus, Rhipicephalus*
Argasidae	Argasinae	*Ornithodoros*

before dropping off. *Ornithodoros hermsi*, the argasid vector of borrelial relapsing fever in mountainous areas of the western United States, is an example of a tick species that confines itself to a limited space (nidiculous), hiding in or near nests of its rodent hosts in such places as fallen logs and the recesses of rustic cabins. In the absence of its usual rodent hosts, *O. hermsi* emerges at night to actively seek and surreptitiously feed on sleeping humans or other suitable animals.

The life cycles of ixodid and argasid ticks differ considerably. During each stage of the ixodid life cycle, the tick takes a blood meal, except for the nonfeeding adult males of some species. When feeding occurs in each of the three parasitic stages and on different hosts, it is termed a three-host tick cycle, which is characteristic of more than 90% of ixodids. Two-host life cycles are those in which the larva and nymph feed on the same host, and the adult feeds on a different host, as occurs with some *Hyalomma* vectors of CCHF. Most argasid ticks have a multihost life cycle involving more than three hosts. In wet tropical climates, tick developmental times are relatively short, and several generations may occur in a single year, as occurs with *Amblyomma* vectors of African tick typhus. In regions with alternating and distinct dry and rainy seasons, ticks may cease seeking hosts in the driest period. Development is also delayed in temperate or subarctic climates, because ticks typically undergo diapause during the coldest months. This often results in a life cycle that may take 2 or more years, such as that of the *Ixodes* spp. vectors of LB, ehrlichiosis, and anaplasmosis. For a more detailed review of tick biology, see Chapter 2.

EPIDEMIOLOGY OF TICK-BORNE INFECTIONS

Epidemiology is, in simplest terms, the science of the distribution and determinants of disease in populations. It is the underpinning for determining the impact of diseases on the public's health and for developing rational strategies that will bring about the prevention and control of disease. In regard to tick-borne diseases, as with other infections, epidemiology identifies logical approaches for breaking links in the chains of transmission. Understanding the epidemiology of tick-borne diseases usually follows a pathway that begins with identifying a clinical syndrome, characterizing those affected by person, place, and time; finding an associated disease agent; determining its source in nature; and elucidating its mode(s) and dynamics of transmission, including those related to the sometimes complex ecology and biology of the ticks themselves. This pathway is superbly exemplified by the relatively recent elucidation of the principal features of LB in North America (6, 28, 36, 39), as detailed in Chapter 11.

Dynamics of Transmission (Transmission Cycles)

The cycles of tick-borne disease agents require a triad of events: (i) a vertebrate host that develops a level of infection that can be passed on to a feeding tick as it takes a blood meal; (ii) a tick that acquires infection with the pathogen (by blood feeding on a reservoir host, cofeeding transmission from one tick to another, or by passage from one stage of the tick to the next) and is able, in the same or later stage or generation, to pass the infection on to a vertebrate host; and (iii) adequate numbers of vertebrate hosts that are susceptible to tick-borne infection. In an anthroponosis, such as tick-borne relapsing fever caused by *B. duttonii*, the agent cycles solely between the tick vector and the human host. All other described tick-borne diseases of humans are zooanthroponoses in which human hosts do not contribute to the maintenance of the agent in nature.

As noted, a suitable vertebrate reservoir allows the agent to survive in the peripheral blood in sufficient density and duration to allow passage to feeding ticks. Tick-borne viruses and bacteria typically cause infections in which the organisms multiply to enormous numbers that circulate over relatively short periods and that either kill the host or engender a protective immunity. *F. tularensis*, the bacterial agent of tularemia, is an example of an agent that often kills its lagomorph (a rabbit or hare) or rodent reservoir hosts with overwhelming infection. *Rickettsia* spp., causing RMSF and other spotted fevers, on the other hand, do not usually kill their vertebrate reservoir hosts but engender a host immunity that limits their period of infectivity. In this circumstance, the tick vectors themselves are the important reservoirs of infection, often aided by the efficient maintenance of infection through stages or between generations. In a contrasting example, red blood cell parasites such as *Babesia* spp. (a malaria parasite-like protozoan) typically induce a vertebrate host tolerance that permits long duration of infectivity.

For a tick-borne disease to be sustained, a threshold level of potentially infective vertebrate hosts must be available. The epidemic threshold is the number or density of susceptible individuals required for epizootic or epidemic transmission to occur; the endemic threshold is the quantity of susceptible hosts needed to maintain persistent infection in a community of hosts. To effectively maintain cycles of transmission, vertebrate hosts must usually be abundant and either maintain susceptibility or have a high enough reproductive rate to ensure susceptible replacement. Similarly, in the usual case, an effective vector must be abundant, feed frequently on the reservoir host at a time when the infective agent is circulating in the peripheral blood, and survive long enough for the pathogen to multiply and/or develop to an infective stage. When vector ticks are diverted away from reservoir hosts and feed instead on nonsusceptible hosts, the force of transmission of the pathogen is dampened, and these hosts are termed zooprophylactic hosts. An important example of this is the feeding by immature stages of *Ixodes scapularis* and *Ixodes pacificus*, the principal vectors of LB in North America, on lizards rather than on susceptible rodents. Because lizards are incompetent hosts of *Borrelia burgdorferi* (complement in some lizard species lyses the borreliae), feeding by vector ticks on lizards is, from the standpoint of transmission, diversionary or zooprophylactic (37). In the southern United States, the ready availability of lizard hosts diverts immature *I. scapularis* to such an extent that the *B. burgdorferi* cycle has a difficult time maintaining itself, and infective risks to humans there are minimal.

The transmission of tick-borne pathogens follows several different pathways. Transfer from the tick to a susceptible host is termed horizontal transmission. Transmission from the enzootic cycle to dead-end hosts is termed tangential transmission. Passage from one generation of tick to another is called vertical transmission, achieved by transovarial transmission of infection from the female to her eggs and thence to the hatched larvae of the next generation, and furthered by transstadial transmission. Transstadial transmission is the passage of the pathogen from one tick life stage (instar) through a molt to the next instar (i.e., from larva to nymph or nymph to adult tick). Horizontal transmission is most efficiently accomplished through the inoculation of infective saliva (anterior station) at the time of tick feeding, which is the principal mode of transmission of tick-borne diseases. Occasionally, transmission can occur directly by the passage through breaks in the skin of infective tick coxal fluid (such as with some relapsing fever borreliae) or by inoculation or inhalation of aerosolized organisms from dried tick feces (posterior station), as rarely occurs with the agents of Q fever and tularemia.

Transstadial transmission is critical in maintaining a natural cycle of *B. burgdorferi*, the agent of LB. In this cycle, *Ixodes* spp. larvae in the northeastern and midwestern United States become infected during summer months while feeding on mice infected earlier in the year by nymphs, whose infection was acquired transstadially from a larva that had become infected in the previous year. The infective adult female feeds in the late autumn or early spring, having acquired its infection earlier in the fall by passage from a molting nymph. Although transovarial passage is insignificant

in the LB life cycle, it is important, for example, in maintaining the cycle of many of the viral and rickettsial pathogens. Sometimes there is more than one primary cycle in nature; cycles that markedly increase transmission are termed amplification cycles, and these may be important in reaching epidemic thresholds.

The different stages of ticks often have different host preferences and feeding patterns. *Ixodes* spp. generally have a low tolerance for desiccation; the immature stages, in particular, stay close to the soil in shaded niches, often covered by leaf litter, where the microclimate is moist and even. This places them in close contact with their preferred maintenance hosts, such as mice, shrews, other small mammals, and lizards. Adult ticks, however, having a greater environmental tolerance, can seek larger hosts that provide ample blood meals necessary for the female to develop her egg mass and serve as more efficient agents of dispersal. Hosts of adult stage ticks also serve as a convenient place for males and females of some species to meet and mate.

Tick vectors of human disease are true biological vectors, in which the pathogen either multiplies asexually without change from one developmental stage to another (e.g., bacteria, rickettsia, and viruses) or goes through development in stages, as occurs sexually with babesia or asexually in infections with agents of anaplasmosis and ehrlichiosis. Following ingestion by ticks, the agents of LB switch off the expression of some outer-surface proteins and newly express others to better adapt to their arthropod hosts and to prepare for their transfer to mammals. The tick-borne transmission to humans of a zoonotic infection generally requires a bridging vector, a tick species that feeds both on reservoir hosts and on humans; bridging vectors may or may not be the primary vectors maintaining the enzootic cycle.

Seasonality

Seasonal activity refers to the period of the year when ticks actively seek hosts, and patterns of seasonal activity can differ greatly between species and under differing climatologic and environmental conditions. Since blood meals are vital for supporting molts and egg production, the patterns of development of ticks are determined by their feeding behaviors. As well, the seasonal pattern of tick feeding determines the frequency distribution of disease onsets. Ixodid ticks in temperate or cold climates, which often experience diapause during the winter, typically begin feeding most actively in the spring and early summer months. Eggs are usually laid in the early spring, and they incubate and hatch into larvae in late spring and summer months. In the case of LB in the northeastern

United States, the nymphal stage of *I. scapularis* mostly feeds from mid-spring to midsummer, with a consequent peak in incidence of onsets of early-stage illness in humans in late spring and summer (6, 28). A much smaller and attenuated peak of incidence occurs in the period from late fall to early spring, a period associated with feeding on humans by infected adult female ticks. The spring-summer peak is less pronounced in the western United States and in Europe, where the periods of feeding of nymphs of the vector ticks *I. pacificus* and *I. ricinus*, respectively, are comparatively delayed and prolonged, and where feeding by infective adult ticks on humans may be more important in transmission (9, 13, 19).

Persons Affected

As far as is known, both sexes and all ages are equally susceptible to infection by the agents of tick-borne diseases. Differences in infection and disease rates by various demographic characteristics relate to differences in infective exposures based on geography, interface with vector habitat due to circumstances of residence, activities (occupational, leisure, and recreational), and personal behaviors. Innate and acquired host immunity may also be important.

SYNOPSIS OF CLINICAL SYNDROMES

Tick-borne diseases of humans are generally characterized by rapidly developing fever and other nonspecific symptoms of acute systemic infection, such as chills, sweats, headache, myalgias, arthralgias, lassitude, anorexia, nausea, and vomiting. Incubation periods are relatively short, generally less than 10 days and usually 3 to 7 days in duration (exceptions include Q fever, which averages 20 days, and LB and babesiosis, which may occasionally be weeks or months). Many early periods of illness are biphasic, with several days of illness followed by a few days of partial remission of symptoms; there may be a return of more severe acute illness, ending with convalescence, sometimes prolonged for weeks or months. Many of the illnesses are brief, mild, and self-limited; some are relapsing, some are protracted; some are associated with serious complications, which are sometimes fatal. The viral encephalitides are characterized by inflammation of the central nervous system and its coverings. CCHF, Omsk hemorrhagic fever, and Kyasanur forest disease are noted for severe gastrointestinal bleeding, other hemorrhagic manifestations, and a high case fatality ratio. The rickettsial spotted fevers and tick typhus infections variously exhibit a local cutaneous ulcer or eschar (tache noir) at the tick bite site, diffuse macular rashes, and petechiae and purpura in severe and complicated cases. Q fever and tularemia patients often develop pneumonia, and both diseases may lead to chronic illness if infection of a heart valve, anatomic defect, or implanted foreign device occurs. LB is a multistage (acute early stage and acute or chronic late stage) multisystem (cutaneous, cardiovascular, central and peripheral neurological, and musculoskeletal) illness. Tularemia has several distinct syndromes depending on the portal of entry and the consequences of systemic spread, e.g., an infective tick bite usually results in an ulcer at the site of inoculation and a regional afferent lymphadenitis (ulceroglandular form), but the ulcer may be absent (glandular form), and systemic spread frequently leads to pneumonia or a "typhoidal" illness. Babesiosis is often characterized by insidious onset, prolonged fevers, and a chronic progressive anemia. The onset of fever is sudden in Q fever and in tick-borne relapsing fever (TBRF). In Q fever, fever may be remittent. In TBRF, episodes of spirochetemia with high fever typically alternate with periods of spirochetal clearance and apyrexia.

MEDICAL AND PUBLIC HEALTH IMPORTANCE

Globally, tick-borne pathogens likely account for well over 100,000 cases of illness each year. Since humans are atypical hosts, tick-borne illness is usually acute and at times severe, disabling, or fatal. Disease surveillance and case reporting for tick-borne diseases are typically deficient, resulting in poor estimates of the true incidence of these diseases, their morbidity, mortality, and cost to society. LB in the United States is an excellent case in point. For the year 2002, more than 23,000 cases were reported to the Centers for Disease Control and Prevention. Yet, in the states in the northeastern region where LB is most endemic, underreporting of cases may range from three- to sixfold (4, 24). In contrast to the underreporting of cases in the northeastern region, many apparently misdiagnosed cases are reported from southern states, where transmission of *B. burgdorferi* to humans is probably rare (23). To further understand the true risk in the United States of exposure to ticks infected with *B. burgdorferi*, a county-by-county map of the principal vector species (*I. scapularis* and *I. pacificus*) was produced (7). This map was used as a basis for drawing a crude ecological risk map when developing recommendations for use of a vaccine against LB spirochetes (5). In the United States, a true ecological risk map should include knowledge of the density of nymphal *I. scapularis* and *I. pacificus*, the proportion of such ticks infected with *B. burgdorferi* sensu stricto, and the degree of human-tick contact on a local basis. The daunting task of putting together such a risk map would require the work of multidisciplinary teams with standardized techniques and a broad geographic coverage. A more cost-efficient approach is to use the large number of correlates of distribution available in the geographic information systems database to develop spatial models that can then be selectively validated by standard methods at specific sites. Extraordinary progress has been made in applying these computerized data management techniques to model, map, and better understand the distribution of LB in the United States and TBE in Europe (1, 14, 29).

Standard surveillance systems rarely collect data on reportable tick-borne diseases beyond monthly incidence by a patient's place of residence, age, and sex. Special studies are therefore required to understand the natural history of illness, the costs in terms of days of productive life lost, and the direct and indirect medical costs incurred. A few attempts have been made to estimate these costs for patients with LB in the United States (22, 25). It is the complications of disseminated infection that result in morbidity and high medical costs in LB, and potential fatality in some other antibiotic-susceptible diseases (e.g., RMSF and ehrlichiosis), highlighting the need for rapid diagnosis and timely treatment.

DISEASE CONTROL AND PREVENTION

Because the suppression and control of tick vectors of disease to humans have been largely unsuccessful, the principal means of primary prevention remain personal measures of avoidance of exposure, applying repellents, wearing protective clothing, and early detection and removal of ticks on clothing or skin. The only vaccines for the prevention of tick-borne diseases currently in use are those against TBE in Europe and Russia. The innovative and highly profiled recombinant vaccine against LB, developed by manufacturers in the United States and government-approved for targeted use, was withdrawn after only 2 years because of poor marketability (see Chapter 11). The enormous costs of product development and evaluation for vaccines that have only a limited market preclude the commercial manufacture of new tick-borne disease vaccines in the foreseeable future. With most bacterial and rickettsial diseases, such as LB, ehrlichiosis, tularemia, and the spotted fevers, early and effective antimicrobial treatment to prevent complications of infection is a highly cost-effective strategy. Environmental modifications that decrease tick density in limited areas show some promise in limiting exposures around homes and some recreational and occupational settings

(38). The strategy to kill ticks relies mostly on area-wide or host-targeted acaricides, and these have many environmental, operational, and cost-effectiveness hurdles to overcome. Biological control has much favorable potential, but various approaches are still in early stages of developmental research. For a more detailed review of methods and future developments in tick-borne disease control, see Chapter 4.

KNOWLEDGE GAPS AND RESEARCH DIRECTIONS

Changes in the epidemiology of several tick borne diseases have occurred during the 20th century. RMSF was so called because it was first recognized as a unique entity among pioneer ranchers in the northern Rocky Mountain region of North America. Later, a shift occurred in the distribution of this infection to the point where most of the cases are now reported from the southeastern and south-central United States. It is unknown why transmission of *Rickettsia rickettsii* by the western vector, *Dermacentor andersoni*, is now only rarely recognized, while transmission by the eastern vector, *Dermacentor variabilis*, is now dominant. Adding interest and complexity to this story is the recent description of *Rickettsia parkeri* as a newly recognized tick-borne spotted fever rickettsiosis in the southern United States (26). The epidemiology in the United States of tularemia has likewise changed. The first recognized outbreaks, occurring in arid far-western regions, were associated with bites by tabanid flies. As the disease was described and became better recognized, the numbers of reported cases increased, the epicenter shifting to midwestern, south-central, and southeastern states; cases were mostly linked to the handling of contaminated wild rabbit carcasses or to tick bites. Since the 1940s, there has been a marked fall in tularemia cases in the United States, from annual totals of more than 2,000 cases to less than 200, with rabbit exposures falling and tick bites increasing in importance as risk factors. In contrast, LB, first recognized in the United States in the 1970s as a rare disease occurring in limited foci along the New England coast, now exceeds 20,000 reported cases a year from 15 or so states in eastern, Midwestern, and Pacific coastal regions where the disease is endemic. Basic studies of the biology and ecology of these diseases are needed to better understand these large shifts.

A key challenge for the future of research in tick-borne diseases will be to harness the power of the new tools of molecular biology to identify potential new tick-borne pathogens, while keeping a focus on preventing the transmission of those we already know to be important. Until the early 1980s, *Borrelia* was thought to infect solely argasid ticks (with the possible exception of isolated reports of *Borrelia theileri* in some African tick species). Following the discovery by W. Burgdorfer that *B. burgdorfei* was carried in *I. scapularis* (2, 3), a whole diverse range of spirochete species or genospecies in these ticks has been described (21). With advanced molecular tools, these can be grouped either in the *B. burgdorfei* sensu lato group or in the hard tick relapsing fever group of spirochetes. In addition to the description of a diverse assemblage of spirochetes, genomic studies have identified a broad array of complex genes of *Borrelia*, and scientists are gradually assigning functions to the specific proteins expressed by these genes. The publication of the entire genome of *B. burgdorfei* has dramatically stimulated this field (12). But solutions to the public health challenge presented by tick-borne diseases will not be found only by studies in the most modern molecular biology laboratories. Entomologists capable of studying the biology and ecology of ticks and designing novel solutions to the prevention and control of tick-borne diseases are in ever-dwindling supply. Ideally, an amalgamation of molecular biologists working at the level of gene function, classical field biologists working with tick populations and their animal hosts, physicians, and epidemiologists would lead the charge to combat the ever-increasing public health threat of tick-borne disease. It is hoped that the information contained in this book will stimulate tick-borne disease researchers to take up the challenge, following in the footsteps of such pioneering giants as R. R. Parker, W. Burgdorfer, and H. Hoogstraal (16), who set the highest standards for their principal passion, tick-borne disease research.

REFERENCES

1. **Brownstein, J. S., T. R. Holford, and D. Fish.** 2003. A climate-based model predicts the spatial distribution of the Lyme disease vector *Ixodes scapularis* in the United States. *Environ. Health Perspect.* 111:1152–1157.
2. **Burgdorfer, W., A. G. Barbour, S. F. Hayes, J. L. Benach, E. Grunwaldt, and J. P. Davis.** 1982. Lyme disease—a tick-borne spirochetosis. *Science* 216:1317–1319.
3. **Burgdorfer, W., A. G. Barbour, S. F. Hayes, O. Peter, and A. Aeschlimann.** 1983. Erythema chronicum migrans—a tick-borne spirochetosis. *Acta Trop.* 40:79–83.
4. **Campbell, G. L., C. L. Fritz, D. Fish, J. Nowakowski, R. B. Nadelman, and G. P. Wormser.** 1998. Estimation of the incidence of Lyme disease. *Am. J. Epidemiol.* 148:1018–1026.
5. **Centers for Disease Control and Prevention.** 1999. Recommendations for the use of Lyme disease vaccine: recommendations of the Advisory Committee on Immunization Practices (ACIP). *Morb. Mortal. Wkly. Rep.* 48:1–25.
6. **Dennis, D. T., and E. B. Hayes.** 2002. Epidemiology of Lyme borreliosis, p. 251–280. *In* J. Gray, O. Kahl, R. S. Lane, and G. Stanek (ed.), *Lyme Borreliosis: Biology, Epidemiology and Control.* CAB International, New York, N.Y.
7. **Dennis, D. T., T. S. Nekomoto, J. C. Victor, W. S. Paul, and J. Piesman.** 1998. Reported distribution of *Ixodes scapularis* and *Ixodes pacificus* (Acari: Ixodidae) in the United States. *J. Med. Entomol.* 35:629–638.
8. **Dutton, J. E., and J. L. Todd.** 1905. The nature of tick fever in the eastern part of the Congo Free State, with notes on the distribution and bionomics of the tick. *Br. Med. J.* 2:1259–1260.
9. **Eisen, L., and R. S. Lane.** 2002. Vectors of *Borrelia burgdorferi* sensu lato, p. 91–116. *In* J. Gray, O. Kahl, R. S. Lane, and G. Stanek (ed.), *Lyme Borreliosis: Biology, Epidemiology and Control.* CAB International, New York, N.Y.
10. **Eldridge, B. F., and J. D. Edman (ed.).** 2000. *Medical Entomology: A Textbook on Public Health and Veterinary Problems Caused by Arthropods.* Kluwer Academic, Dordrecht, The Netherlands.
11. **Francis, E.** 1929. A summary of the present knowledge of tularemia. *Medicine* (Baltimore). 7:411–432.
12. **Fraser, C. M., S. Casjens, W. M. Huang, G. G. Sutton, R. Clayton, R. Lathigra, O. White, K. A. Ketchum, R. Dodson, E. K. Hickey, M. Gwinn, B. Dougherty, J. F. Tomb, R. D. Fleischmann, D. Richardson, J. Peterson, A. R. Kerlavage, J. Quackenbush, S. Salzberg, M. Hanson, R. van Vugt, N. Palmer, M. D. Adams, J. Gocayne, J. Weidman, T. Utterback, L. Watthey, L. McDonald, P. Artiach, C. Bowman, S. Graland, C. Fujii, M. D. Cotton, K. Horst, K. Roberts, B. Hatch, H. O. Smith, and J. C. Venter.** 1997. Genomic sequence of a Lyme disease spirochaete. *Nature* 390:580–586.
13. **Gern, L., and P. F. Humair.** 2002. Ecology of *Borrelia burgdorferi* sensu lato in Europe, p. 149–174. *In* J. Gray, O. Kahl, R. S. Lane, and G. Stanek (ed.), *Lyme Borreliosis: Biology, Epidemiology and Control.* CAB International, New York, N.Y.
14. **Guerra, M., E. Walker, C. Jones, S. Paskewitz, M. R. Cortinas, A. Stancil, L. Beck, M. Bobo, and U. Kitron.** 2002. Predicting the risk of Lyme disease: habitat suitability for *Ixodes scapularis* in the north central United States. *Emerg. Infect. Dis.* 8:289–297.
15. **Harwood, R. F., and M. T. James (ed.).** 1979. *Entomology in Human and Animal Health*, 7th ed. Macmillan Co., New York, N.Y.
16. **Hoogstraal, H.** 1981. Changing patterns of tickborne disease in a modern society. *Annu. Rev. Entomol.* 26:75–99.
17. **Kettle, D. S.** 1995. *Medical and Veterinary Entomology*, 2nd ed. CAB International, Wallingford, United Kingdom.
18. **Korch, G. W., Jr.** 1991. Geographic dissemination of tick-borne zoonoses, p. 139–197. *In* D. E. Sonenshine (ed.), *Biology of Ticks*, vol. 1. Oxford University Press, New York, N.Y.
19. **Korenberg, E. I., N. B. Gorelova, and Y. V. Kovalevskii.** 2002. Ecology of *Borrelia burgdorferi* sensu lato in Russia, p. 175–200. *In* J. Gray, O. Kahl, R. S. Lane, and G. Stanek (ed.), *Lyme Borreliosis: Biology, Epidemiology and Control.* CAB International, New York, N.Y.
20. **Korenberg, E. I., and Y. V. Kovalevskii.** 1999. Main features of tick-borne encephalitis eco-epidemiology in Russia. *Zentralbl. Bakteriol.* 289:525–539.
21. **Kurtenbach, K., S. M. Schäfer, S. Michelis, S. Etti, and H. S. Sewell.** 2002. *Borrelia burgdorferi* sensu lato in the vertebrate host, p. 117–148. *In* J. Gray, O. Kahl, R. S. Lane, and G. Stanek (ed.), *Lyme Borreliosis: Biology, Epidemiology and Control.* CAB International, New York, N.Y.
22. **Maes, E., P. Lecompte, and N. Ray.** 1998. Cost-of-illness study of Lyme disease in the United States. *Clin. Ther.* 20:993–1008.
23. **Mathiesen, D. A., J. H. Oliver, Jr., C. P. Kolbert, E. D. Tullson, B. J. Johnson, G. L. Campbell, P. D. Mitchell, K. D. Reed, S. R. Telford III, J. F. Anderson, R. S. Lane, and D. H. Persing.** 1997. Genetic heterogeneity of *Borrelia burgdorferi* in the United States. *J. Infect. Dis.* 175:98–107.

24. Meek, J. I., C. L. Roberts, E. V. Smith, Jr., and M. L. Cartter. 1996. Underreporting of Lyme disease by Connecticut physicians, 1992. *J. Public Health Manag. Pract.* **2:**61–65.

25. Meltzer, M. J., D. T. Dennis, and K. A. Orloski. 1999. The cost-effectiveness of vaccinating against Lyme disease. *Emerg. Infect. Dis.* **5:**321–328.

26. Paddock, C. D., J. W. Summer, J. A. Comer, S. R. Zaki, C. S. Goldsmith, J. Goddard, S. L. F. McLellan, C. L. Tamminga, and C. A. Ohl. 2004. *Rickettsia parkeri*: a newly recognized cause of spotted fever rickettsiosis in the United States. *Clin. Infect. Dis.* **38:**805–811.

27. Parola, P., and D. Raoult. 2001. Ticks and tickborne bacterial diseases in humans: an emerging infectious threat. *Clin. Infect. Dis.* **32:**897–928.

28. Piesman, J. 2002. Ecology of *Borrelia burgdorferi* sensu lato in North America, p. 223–250. *In* J. Gray, O. Kahl, R. S. Lane, and G. Stanek, (ed.), *Lyme Borreliosis: Biology, Epidemiology and Control.* CAB International, New York, N.Y.

29. Randolph, S. E. 2001.The shifting landscape of tick-borne zoonoses: tick-borne encephalitis and Lyme borreliosis in Europe. *Philos. Trans R. Soc. Lond. B* **356:**1045–1056.

30. Service, M. W. 2000. *Medical Entomology for Students*, 2nd ed. Cambridge University Press, Cambridge, United Kingdom.

31. Smith, T., and F. L. Kilbourne. 1893. Investigations into the nature, causation, and prevention of Texas or southern cattle fever. *Bull. Bur. Anim. Ind.* **1:**177–304.

32. Sonenshine, D. E. 1991. Introduction, p. 3–12. *In* D. E. Sonenshine (ed.), *Biology of Ticks*, vol. 1. Oxford University Press, New York, N.Y.

33. Sonenshine, D. E. (ed.). 1993. *Biology of Ticks*, vol. 2. Oxford University Press, New York, N.Y.

34. Sonenshine, D. E. 1993. Tick-borne and tick-caused diseases, p. 107–319. *In* D. E. Sonenshine (ed.), *Biology of Ticks*, vol. 2. Oxford University Press, New York, N.Y.

35. Sonenshine, D. E., R. S. Lane, and W. L. Nicholson. 2002. Ticks (*Ixodida*), p. 517–558. *In* G. Mullen and L. Durden (ed.), *Medical and Veterinary Entomology.* Academic Press, New York, N.Y.

36. Spielman, A. 1976. Lyme disease and human babesiosis on Nantucket Island: transmission by nymphal *Ixodes* ticks. *Am. J. Trop. Med. Hyg.* **25:**784–787.

37. Spielman, A., J. F. Levine, and M. L. Wilson. 1984. Vectorial capacity of North American *Ixodes* ticks. *Yale J. Biol. Med.* **57:**507–513.

38. Stafford, K. C., and U. Kitron. 2002. Environmental management for Lyme borreliosis control, p. 301–334. *In* J. Gray, O. Kahl, R. S. Lane, and G. Stanek (ed.), *Lyme Borreliosis: Biology, Epidemiology and Control.* CAB International, New York, N.Y.

39. Steere, A. C. 2001. Lyme disease. *N. Engl. J. Med.* **321:**586–596.

Chapter 2

The Biology of Tick Vectors of Human Disease

DANIEL E. SONENSHINE

INTRODUCTION

Ticks are among the most important vectors of disease to humans throughout the world. Among the diverse microbes transmitted by ticks to humans are several protozoan, viral, and bacterial (including rickettsial) pathogens. Important examples include Lyme disease (the most important vector-borne disease in North America and Europe), tularemia, Rocky Mountain spotted fever, ehrlichiosis, tick-borne encephalitis, and Crimean-Congo hemorrhagic fever. Tick bites can cause severe allergic reactions, irritation, various types of tick toxicoses, and tick paralysis. The last is frequently fatal if the tick causing the paralysis is not promptly removed. Frequently, the wounds caused by tick bites may be painful and in some cases can lead to secondary infection with skin surface microbes. In addition, ticks are important as pests. Heavy tick infestations can degrade the recreational value of parks and other natural areas, as well as add a significant financial burden to property owners. The presence of tick-borne diseases such as babesiosis, theileriosis, heartwater, and others, as well as the damaging effects of tick infestations, has made it difficult or impossible to raise domestic animals in many tropical and subtropical regions of the world.

Most ticks fall into two families: the hard ticks, or Ixodidae, and the soft ticks, or Argasidae. This chapter describes the biological attributes of ticks, thereby providing a basis for understanding how ticks feed and survive in their natural environment and the physiological and biochemical factors that facilitate the transmission of disease-causing pathogens. More detailed descriptions of tick biology and evolution can be found in other references (for example, see references 20, 37, and 38).

MORPHOLOGY

External Anatomy

Unfed adult ticks are visible to the naked eye, ranging in size from only 2 to 3 mm in the smallest species to more than 20 mm in some *Amblyomma* or *Ornithodoros* species. The flattened body is elongated and noticeably longer than it is wide. There are four pairs of legs. Nymphs and larvae resemble the adults, only smaller, although the larvae have only three pairs of legs. The body shape becomes distorted following engorgement, especially among females of the hard ticks. When fully engorged, the enormously swollen females may increase to more than 25 mm in length and weigh up to 100 times their unfed body weight.

The major external regions of ticks are the capitulum (gnathosoma), body (idiosoma), and legs (see Chapter 7, Fig. 1). The capitulum contains the mouthparts, including the palps, chelicerae, the hypostome, and the posterior basis capituli. The palps are segmented, leglike structures with four distinct segments, although the distal segment is much smaller than the others and often recessed in a cavity of the third segment. The distal end of this tiny segment bears numerous chemosensory sensilla known to function in host chemical recognition. The chelicerae protrude from the anterior end of the basis capituli, with the cheliceral shafts situated medially between the palps. At their terminal ends, each chelicera bears two movable digits with sharp pointed teeth oriented laterally. These are the structures that are used to cut into the host's skin during feeding. The large toothed hypostome is situated medially between the palps, ventral to the chelicerae, and it is obscured by the latter structures when viewed dorsally. Therefore, the hypostome is visible only when viewed from the ventral aspect. The hypostome serves as both an anchor for attachment to the host skin and the food channel that directs blood into the tick's mouth or saliva into the wound during blood feeding. A narrow food canal visible in the midline of the dorsal surface accommodates the uptake of blood and outflow of saliva. The posterior region of the capitulum contains the basis capituli. This structure encloses the mouth, the pharynx, and the spinose shaft and expanded base of each chelicera.

Daniel E. Sonenshine • Department of Biological Sciences, Old Dominion University, Norfolk, VA 23529.

The posterior end of the basis capituli articulates with the body, allowing it to bend up or down.

In ixodid ticks, the capitulum is located at the anterior end of the body and is readily visible when the tick is viewed from the dorsal aspect (Fig. 1). In females, a pair of pore clusters, the porose areas, occur on the dorsal surface of the basis capituli. The porose areas are believed to secrete antioxidants that inhibit degradation of the waxy compounds in the secretions of Gené's organ (4), and possibly facilitate the smooth movements of this organ. The hypostome with its numerous recurved teeth is readily visible from the ventral aspect. Also visible are the tiny recessed terminal segments of the palps with a field of small chemosensory sensilla useful for detecting specific compounds on the host skin (Fig. 1). This is described further in the context of tick feeding behavior (see "Behavior," below).

In argasid ticks, the capitulum is similar, but it is located on the ventral side of the body. It is obscured by a cone-like extension of the body, the hood, and consequently it is not visible dorsally in nymphs or adults. In the larvae, however, the capitulum is located anteriorly, as in the ixodid ticks. The structure of the palps, chelicerae, and hypostome is similar to these same structures in the ixodid ticks. However, the segments of the palps are subequal in size, and there is no recessed terminal segment. In many argasids, especially in the genus *Ornithodoros*, small flaps known as cheeks occur alongside the capitulum. These flaplike structures can be folded to cover the delicate mouthparts when not in use.

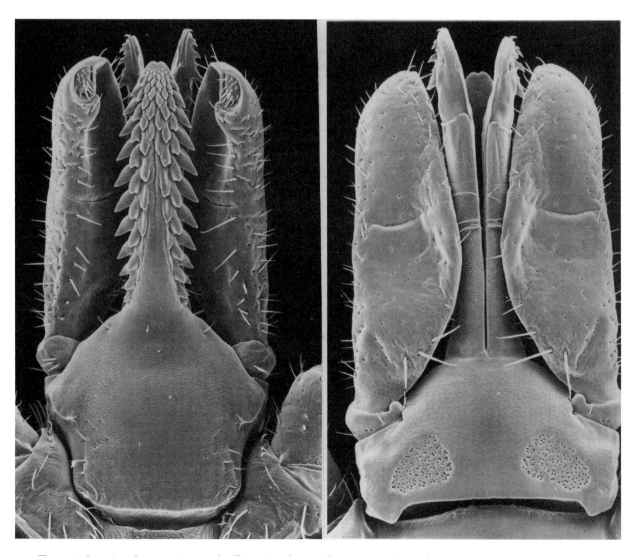

Figure 1. Scanning electron micrographs illustrating the mouthparts (capitulum) of a representative female ixodid tick, *I. scapularis*. (Left) Ventral aspect; (right) dorsal aspect.

The body posterior to the capitulum is divided into two parts, an anterior region that bears the legs and the genital pore, and a posterior region behind the legs that bears the spiracles and the anal aperture. In ixodid ticks, the body is covered with a relatively tough cuticle that contains sclerotized plates (sclerites) in certain locations. The most prominent plate is the scutum, a hard, relatively smooth structure that covers the anterior half of the dorsal surface in females and in juvenile stages and the entire dorsal surface in males. A pair of simple eyes occur on the dorsal surface of the body in most ixodid ticks but are absent in ticks of the genus *Ixodes*. The tough, dense cuticle serves to protect the animal from desiccation and injury, as well as acting as the site of muscle attachment. The cuticle bears numerous sensory setae, as well as various pores representing the openings of dermal glands or sensilla. Except for the hard, sclerotized scutum, the cuticle is relatively flexible and expands during feeding. Additional sclerites occur on the ventral side of the body of males in the genus *Ixodes*. Other important structures on the ventral side of the body are the genital pore, anus, and spiracles situated within the spiracular plates. The body structure of argasid ticks is generally similar to that of the ixodids, but argasids lack a scutum or other sclerites and the flexible body cuticle is leathery (hence the term "soft ticks"). The cuticle is covered with innumerable tiny protuberances—the mammillae, or disks which provide its leathery appearance.

The legs are jointed appendages used for locomotion. The forelegs also function in odor detection in a manner resembling that of insect antennae. There are four pairs of legs in nymphs and adults but only three pairs in larvae. The legs are attached to the body by the large coxal joints. Leg structure is similar in members of both the Ixodidae and Argasidae. There are six segments, termed the coxa, trochanter, femur, patella (genu), tibia, and tarsus. Although the coxae may have limited lateral movement, the other segments can be flexed or extended as a result of internal muscles that extend between the segments. When not used for walking, the legs are tightly folded against the body. At its terminal end, the tarsal segment of each leg has a prominent pair of claws. In addition, ixodid ticks have a pad-like pulvillus underneath the claws, a structure that facilitates walking on smooth surfaces. However, the pulvillus is absent in argasid nymphs and adults. All ticks have a unique sensory organ, the Haller's organ, on the dorsal surface of the tarsus of the first leg (leg I). This organ is present in all species and all life stages. Haller's organ is a complex structure comprising two parts, an anterior pit and a posterior capsule. Different hair-like sensilla in the different parts of the organ detect odors and chemicals on the host skin as well as changes in temperature and air currents.

Ixodidae

This family comprises the hard ticks, so called because of the hard, shell-like scutum on the dorsal surface. When the ticks are examined from the dorsal aspect, they are immediately recognizable by the presence of this unique structure. In males, the scutum covers the entire dorsal surface of the body (see Chapter 7, Fig. 1). In females, as well as in the nymphal and larval stages, the scutum only covers the anterior half of the dorsal body surface (see Chapter 7, Fig. 1). The body region posterior to the scutum is termed the alloscutum. In this region of the body, the cuticle is more flexible than the hard scutum. It is also highly folded, giving it a fingerprint-like appearance. In males, the full scutum minimizes expansion during feeding. However, in females and juveniles, the body expands enormously during blood feeding. The dorsal body surface is also covered with numerous small hair-like setae that serve as touch receptors. Also present on the alloscutum are a pair of foveal pores (absent in ticks of the genus *Ixodes*) from which site the volatile sex pheromone 2,6-dichlorophenol is emitted. Another important organ is Gené's organ, which is found only in females. This bifurcated sac usually is found retracted into the capitular foramen, a cavity between the scutum and the capitulum. During oviposition, the finger-like ends of Gené's organ are extended and protrude, to apply wax to each newly deposited egg.

When ixodid ticks are examined on their ventral surface, most are found to be devoid of hard plates (see Chapter 7, Fig. 1). An important exception occurs in the genus *Ixodes*, where hard sclerotized plates cover the ventral body surface in the males (see Chapter 7, Fig. 19). In the anterior region of the body, a prominent genital pore is evident between the first and second pairs of coxae. In most species, the genital pore is a U- or V-shaped opening. In males, the genital pore occurs in the same location, but it is covered by a movable plate. Also present on the ventral surface in both males and females are a pair of prominent spiracular plates immediately posterior to the fourth pair of coxae. Each irregularly shaped plate contains numerous tiny depressions and a small ostium, the opening to the respiratory system. In the midline behind the legs is the anal aperture, covered by movable plates. The ventral body surface contains numerous small hair-like setae and tiny sensory pores, the sensilla auriformia. In the larvae, the number of setae is greatly reduced, but their location is useful for distinguishing the species and different genera of these ticks.

The immature stages, the nymphs and larvae, are similar to the adults but are much smaller. Nymphs are similar but lack the genital aperture. Larvae also lack the genital aperture and have only three pairs of walking legs (see Chapter 7, Fig. 3).

Argasidae

Argasid ticks, or soft ticks, generally resemble the ixodid ticks, but the body lacks a scutum. The absence of a scutum is the major distinguishing feature between the two families. In the adults and the nymphal stages, the dorsal body margin protrudes anteriorly beyond the capitulum, obscuring that structure when the tick is viewed from the dorsal aspect. Examples of soft ticks are illustrated in Chapter 7, Fig. 8 to 11. Most species, especially in the genus *Ornithodoros*, have a leathery cuticle; the body margins are rounded and covered by numerous small elevations known as mammillae. Soft ticks of the genus *Argas* also have a leathery, folded cuticle, but they have a flattened body margin, the sutural line. The many small integumental folds usually have a button-like appearance, each with a pit at the top. A pair of tiny coxal pores occur between coxae I and II on each side of the body. These pores serve as openings for the coxal glands that eliminate excess water and salts from the digestive tract during rapid blood feeding. Also present on the ventral marginal folds are a pair of small spiracular plates, located between coxae III and IV. In some species, a pair of tiny eyes also occur along the marginal folds. In the midline of the ventral body surface is the prominent genital pore. The genital pore appears as a horizontal slit surrounded by a prominent fold in the females; it appears as a subtriangular or suboval structure covered by a genital apron in males. Nymphal ticks that mature into females have an inconspicuous depression in the same location where the genital pore will develop after the final molt. Other differences between the nymphs and the adult females include the absence of foveal pores on the dorsum and the lack of porose areas on the capitulum.

In the larval stage, the capitulum is situated at the anterior end of the body, in the same location as in the ixodid ticks. In addition, a sclerotized plate occurs in the middle of the dorsal body surface. The dorsal plate should not be confused with the scutum in ixodid ticks.

Internal Anatomy, Physiology, and Innate Immunity

The interior of the tick body consists of an open cavity, the hemocoel, containing the vital organs, including the midgut, salivary glands, synganglion, peripheral nerves, reproductive organs, and the Malpighian tubules, all bathed in a circulating fluid known as the hemolymph (Fig. 2 and 3). Although frequently mislabeled as blood, the hemolymph does not contain hemoglobin and has no role in oxygen transport. The hemolymph contains an unusually high concentration of proteins, especially the so-called common protein (13) believed to remove harmful heme from the body tissues, antimicrobial peptides that combat microbial invasion, and numerous other unidentified proteins (Fig. 4). It is also rich in other soluble proteins, salts, amino acids, lipids, and other dissolved substances. Hemolymph contains a large population of phagocytic cells (plasmatocytes and granulocytes) as well as other types of hemocytes (Fig. 5). Hemocytes play an important role in the tick's immune defenses against microbial invasion. Hemolymph circulation is accomplished by contractions of the body muscles and is also aided by a simple heart located in the middorsal region of the body. The heart is surrounded by a delicate membrane that filters hemolymph prior to its entry into the heart chambers, several ostia for inflow of filtered hemolymph, and an anterior vessel that directs hemolymph towards the synganglion.

Ticks have an innate immune system similar to that found in other invertebrates that enables them to combat invasion by a variety of ubiquitous gram-positive or gram-negative bacteria, fungi, and other organisms. When challenged with bacteria or other microbes, defensins, lysozyme, lectins, and possibly other antimicrobial peptides are secreted into the hemolymph plasma where they act selectively to disrupt the peptidoglycan layer of gram-positive bacteria and kill these organisms (17, 18, 19, 22, 23, 28, 29). Some invading bacteria, e.g., *Escherichia coli*, provoke a type of encapsulation response known as nodulation, wherein the cells adhere to one another, forming clumps that prevent further multiplication of these microbes. These sticky clumps are gradually surrounded by masses of granular hemocytes in nonmelanotic capsules, which effectively wall them off from the body tissues (8). Although the precise mode of action is unknown, the clumping reaction is believed to be mediated by secretion of lectins, molecules known to occur in the soft tick *Ornithodoros moubata* and presumably in other species as well (23). Defensin, lysozyme, and lectins are believed to be stored in the granules of the granular hemocytes and secreted following challenge with foreign organisms. Antimicrobial peptides, e.g., defensin (21, 22) and lysozyme (22), and presumably lectins, are also expressed in the midgut when this organ is stimulated by blood feeding, even in the absence of microbial challenge. Digestion of α-chain hemoglobin in the midgut also liberates peptides that are antimicrobial, at least against *Staphylococcus aureus*, contributing to midgut defense against some microbes (30). These peptides are cleaved as a result of digestive

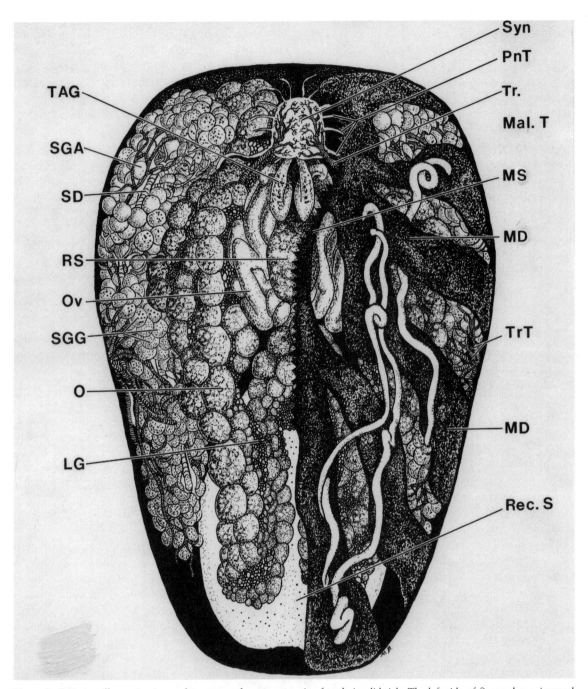

Figure 2. Drawing illustrating internal anatomy of a representative female ixodid tick. The left side of figure shows internal organs minus the midgut. The right side of figure shows the midgut overlaying the internal organs. LG, longitudinal groove of the ovary; Mal. T, malpighian tubules; MD, midgut diverticulum; MS, midgut stomach; O, ovary; OV, oviduct; PnT, pedal nerve trunks; Rec. S, rectal sac; SGA, salivary gland zone of granular acini; SGG, salivary gland zone of granular acini; SD, salivary gland duct; Syn, synganglion; TAG, tubular accessory gland; TrT, tracheal trunks. Figure (illustration by M. Bloomfield) from *Biology of Ticks*, vol. 1, by Daniel E. Sonenshine, ©1991 by Oxford University Press, Inc. Used by permission of Oxford University Press, Inc.

activity in the midgut, i.e., their antimicrobial activity is the result of the tick's digestive enzymes. In addition, it is likely that receptors that recognize pathogen-associated molecular patterns such as those described for insects (26, 48) may also trigger the expression and/or secretion of these antimicrobial peptides in the tick gut, although none have been reported yet for

these arthropods. Phagocytosis also plays an important role in controlling the spread and multiplication of invading microbes (49). Nevertheless, some infectious microbes, including *Borrelia burgdorferi* and *Rickettsia rickettsii*, elude these immune defenses and survive in the tick's body tissues where they can be transferred to vertebrates and cause disease. An im-

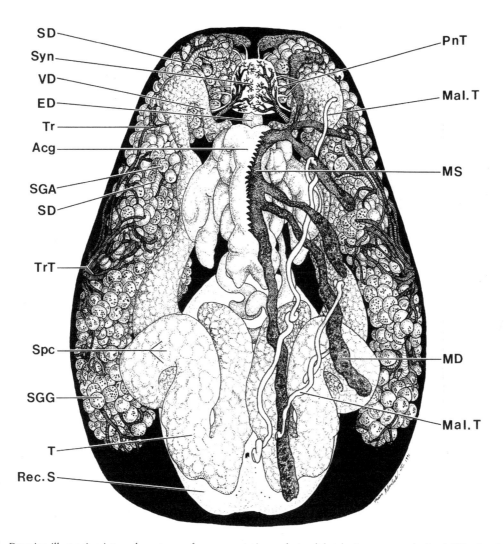

Figure 3. Drawing illustrating internal anatomy of a representative male ixodid tick. Acg, accessory gland; ED, ejaculatory duct; Mal. T, Malphighian tubule; MD, midgut diverticulum; MS, midgut stomach region; PnT, peripheral nerve trunks; Rec.S, rectal sac; SD, salivary gland duct; SGA, salivary gland alveolar acini; SGG, salivary gland granular acini; Spc, spermatogonial zone of testis; Syn, synganglion; T, testis; Tr, trachea; TrT, tracheal trunks; VD, vas deferens. Figure (illustration by M. Bloomfield) from *Biology of Ticks*, vol. 1, by Daniel E. Sonenshine, ©1991 by Oxford University Press, Inc. Used by permission of Oxford University Press, Inc.

portant factor contributing to the invasive success of the infectious microbes is their expression of specific surface proteins that bind to receptors on the host cell membrane, e.g., outer surface protein A (OspA) of the Lyme disease spirochete *B. burgdorferi*, that binds to a receptor on the midgut epithelium of its natural vector, *Ixodes scapularis* (33). Spirochetes that invade the tick's hemolymph during nymphal or adult blood feeding do not provoke secretion of antimicrobial peptides, and many of these bacteria are able to invade the salivary glands and other tissues. In contrast, spirochetes injected into the hemocoel of *Dermacentor variabilis*, a noncompetent vector, provoke the release of defensin, lysozyme, and perhaps other antimicrobial peptides that result in the spirochetes' rapid destruction (19). Vector competency—the ability of different ticks to

harbor and transmit specific disease-causing microbes—appears to be dependent upon these differences in the tick's receptor composition and ability to recognize and destroy invading microbes. Blood feeding also provokes secretion of antimicrobial peptides by the midgut epithelium, even in the absence of microbial infection (40).

The largest organ in the body cavity is the midgut, a large sac-like structure with numerous lateral diverticuli that appear small and narrow in unfed ticks (Fig. 2 and 3). During blood feeding, the diverticuli enlarge greatly and occupy most of the interior of the body cavity. Histological sections of the midgut of feeding ticks show the presence of enormously enlarged digestive cells, many filled with masses of hematin deposits near the luminal edge. Other, smaller cells in varying stages of differentiation, or undifferentiated stem cells,

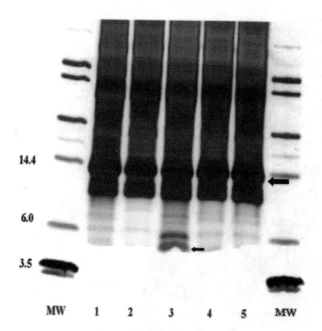

Figure 4. Antimicrobial peptides in *D. variabilis* hemolymph challenged with three different bacteria. Hemolymph collected 1 h after inoculation. Lanes: MW, molecular weight markers; 1, challenged with *B. subtilis*, 2.1×10^4 cells; 2, challenged with *E. coli*, 3×10^6 cells; 3, challenged with *B. burgdorferi*, 3.5×10^4 cells; 4, unstimulated; 5, sham inoculated with 3 µl of tick saline; 6, molecular weight markers. Lanes 1 to 5 were loaded with 200 µg of protein. Arrows indicate proteins expressed following challenge with different microbes: in lane 3, the arrow indicates defensin; in lane 5, the arrow indicates α/β-chain hemoglobin and putative lysozyme.

occur between the giant digestive cells (Fig. 6). Electron micrographs of the feeding midgut show the presence of numerous microvilli along the luminal edge of the giant digestive cells, as well as numerous inclusions (Fig. 7). Blood digestion in ticks is almost entirely intracellular. Blood cells, especially erythrocytes, are digested in the midgut lumen, releasing hemoglobin. Hemoglobin binds to clathrin-coated pits in the luminal surfaces of the epithelial cells lining the midgut, a process known as receptor-mediated endocytosis (10). Tiny pseudopod-like processes are extruded around the coated pits (a process known as pinocytosis), and the cell membrane folds around the pit, forming a vesicle within the digestive cell. Fusion with lysosomes results in the formation of enzyme-filled phagolysosomes, where intracellular digestion takes place, liberating amino acids and ending in iron-rich indigestible residues. Gradually, the distal portions of the enormously enlarged digestive cells fill with black droplets (Fig. 6). Eventually, the waste-filled cells detach from the basal lamina into the lumen. Although the proteinaceous portion of the hemoglobin molecule is digested, releasing abundant amino acids, most of the heme moiety is converted to nontoxic hematin and stored in the cell for later dis-

posal. Amino acids, monosaccharides, free fatty acids, and large amounts of water and salts may be absorbed directly from the lumen. Little else in the massive blood meal, e.g., serum proteins, is digested.

Also evident throughout the tick's body cavity are the numerous branches of the tracheal system that spread out over the surfaces of the midgut diverticuli and the other internal organs (Fig. 2 and 3). Air is carried via these branching tracheae directly to the cells and tissues of the internal organs. The tracheae are connected to the exterior via the paired spiracles on the ventrolateral margins of the body. Periodic opening and closing of the spiracles facilitate ventilation of the tracheal system and the elimination of the CO_2, as well as entry of fresh air. Larvae, however, lack a tracheal system and evidently carry out gaseous exchange directly through the thin body cuticle.

In the anterior region of the body are the paired salivary glands (Fig. 2 and 3). Each large multilobular gland is connected to the mouthparts by means of a ribbed salivary duct. The saliva secreted by these glands contains an impressive variety of proteins that facilitate wound formation, suppress inflammatory activity, dilate blood vessels, counteract the activity of host histamine, and even combat host immunoglobulins. Included are immunoglobulin-binding proteins that protect the feeding tick against host immunoglobulins (46). These potent effector molecules facilitate successful invasion of tick-borne pathogens, as well as aid in blood feeding. In several cases, the secretions of the salivary glands have been demonstrated to facilitate pathogen survival in the vector tick. An example is the anti-complement protein secreted by *I. scapularis* nymphs that inactivates host anti-spirochetal antibodies, thereby facilitating survival of *B. burgdorferi* in the tick's midgut (44). In ixodid ticks, compounds also are secreted that harden into a tough cement that binds the tick's mouthparts to the skin, a phenomenon familiar to anyone who has attempted to remove an attached tick. As feeding progresses, certain parts of the salivary glands are transformed into water-secreting compartments that effectively eliminate most of the excess water from the blood meal. The fast-feeding argasid ticks do not secrete cement and eliminate excess blood meal water via the coxal glands instead of using their salivary glands.

The reproductive organs are prominent structures that occupy much of the interior of the tick's body (Fig. 2 and 3). These organs increase in size during feeding, especially in females.

The male reproductive system comprises the testes that extend horizontally across the posterior region of the body, the paired vasa deferentia, the single seminal vesicle, and the cuticle-lined ejaculatory duct that carries that sperm to the genital pore (Fig. 3). A large,

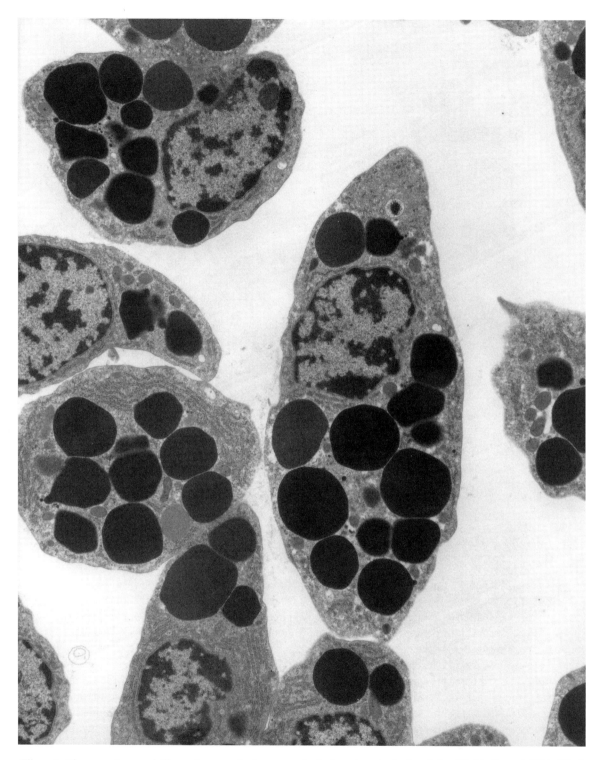

Figure 5. Electron micrograph illustrating granular hemocytes in the hemolymph of a female ixodid tick (*D. variabilis*). All of the hemocytes shown are granulocytes. Magnification, ×16,800. Figure from *Biology of Ticks*, vol. 1, by Daniel E. Sonenshine, ©1991 by Oxford University Press, Inc. Used by permission of Oxford University Press, Inc.

white accessory gland containing multiple lobes surrounds the ejaculatory duct. Aside from the salivary glands, the accessory gland is the largest organ in the anterior region of the male's body. During mating, this organ secretes the proteinaceous components that combine to form the spermatophore, a sac that contains and transports the immature spermiophores. During copulation, the male uses its chelicerae to seize

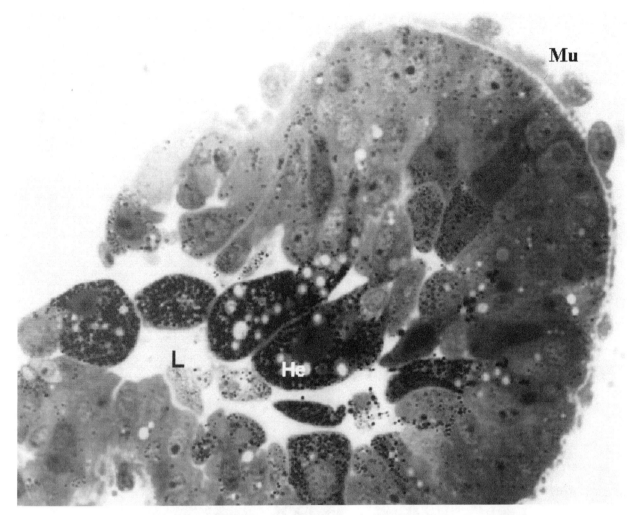

Figure 6. Photomicrograph illustrating the histological structure of the midgut from a feeding female tick (*D. variabilis*). He, hematin-filled digestive cells; L, lumen; Mu, muscle layer on external surface of midgut. Magnification, ×400.

the emerging spermatophore and insert it into the female's genital pore.

The female reproductive system comprises the ovary, situated horizontally in the posterior region of the body, the paired tubular oviducts, the uterus, the vagina, and the seminal receptacle. Tiny paired tubular accessory glands extend from the vagina near its junction with the seminal receptacle. Although small and inconspicuous in unfed ticks, the ovary begins to expand during feeding and reaches its maximum size in fully engorged, mated females. As it increases in size, numerous amber-colored, yolk-filled eggs in various stages of development protrude from its sides and into the adjacent oviducts. In the anterior region of the female body, the eggs pass via the oviducts into the vagina. The posterior part of this organ contains masses of circular muscles that propel the eggs anteriorly, while the narrow, cuticle-lined vestibular vagina enlarges and protrudes into the genital aperture to facilitate egg passage. Lobular accessory glands of unknown

function surrounding the vestibular vagina are believed to secrete a sex pheromone that enables the male's chelicerae to recognize the conspecific identity of the female and complete copulation (2).

In contrast to insects and most other arthropods, ticks have a highly centralized central nervous system. The entire central nervous system is concentrated into a fused, whitish structure termed the synganglion, which is located in the anterior region of the body above the genital pore. The synganglion is often mislabeled the brain, but this term is inappropriate because there is no separate ventral nerve cord, as occurs in insects. Along the synganglion's lateral margins, large pedal nerves extend to the legs. Smaller nerves protrude from its anterior edge and extend anteriorly to innervate the palps, chelicerae, and other parts of the capitulum. Other nerves extend posteriorly and ventrally to innervate the major internal body organs. The synganglion is surrounded by a periganglionic membrane, enclosing a small periganglionic

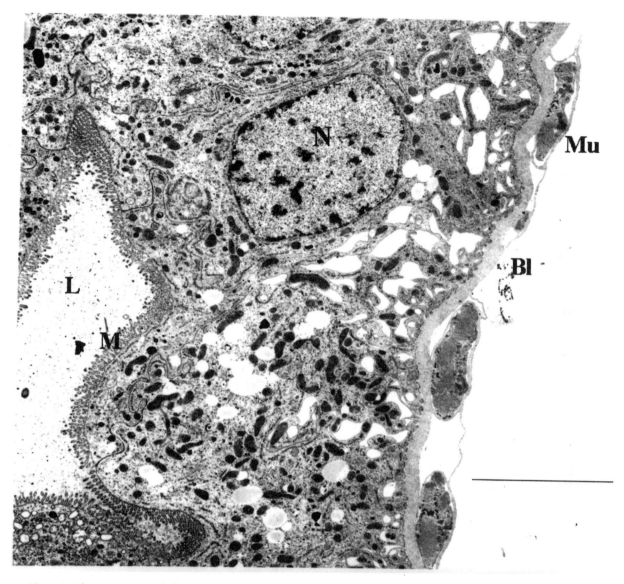

Figure 7. Electron micrograph illustrating the ultrastructure of the midgut of a feeding female tick (*D. variabilis*). Magnification, ×11,400. Bl, basal lamina; L, lumen; M, microvilli bordering the luminal surface of the epithelial cells; Mu, muscle cell on external surface of midgut; N, nucleus. Bar, 2.5 μm.

sinus that is filled with fresh, filtered hemolymph from the heart.

The excretory system in ticks consists of a pair of long coiled Malpighian tubules that extend throughout almost all regions of the tick's body. These tiny thin tubules are connected to the lateral sides of the rectal sac located in the posterior midsection of the body. The tubules appear white, due to the presence of numerous guanine crystals, the predominant form of nitrogenous waste removal in these arthropods. The rectal sac can be identified readily by its whitish color, especially when filled with large masses of guanine crystals. The rectal sac is also the repository for the black hematin and other undigested residues from the midgut. The contents of the rectal sac are evacuated via the anal aperture, usually during or after feeding. Argasid ticks also have an unusual set of excretory organs, the coxal glands. These sac-like structures are located in the anterior region of the body immediately above the coxae, each connected by a duct to the tiny coxal pore between the coxae of legs I and II. During or immediately after rapid blood feeding, these organs extract excess water and accompanying salts and excrete this watery waste via the coxal pores. The emission of copious quantities of this watery coxal fluid enables the fast-feeding argasid ticks to concentrate the large volumes of blood they imbibe without compromising their internal water balance. Each gland consists of a membranous sac that serves as a filtration chamber and a coiled tubule that selectively reabsorbs small, soluble molecules and ions as needed. In some soft-tick species, spirochetes that cause relapsing fever in humans, e.g., *Borrelia hermsii*, can be passed from the tick's body during blood feeding and be transmitted by accidental wound contamination.

LIFE HISTORY

Ticks have a hemimetabolous life cycle, a life cycle pattern in which the immature stages resemble the adults. Ticks are ectoparasites of vertebrates, i.e., they can survive only by feeding on a vertebrate host. Blood is their only food source, and blood feeding initiates development to the next life stage or reproductive activity. Similar life cycle patterns are found in certain groups of insects, such as the true bugs (order Hemiptera). In all tick species, the life cycle consists of the egg and three active stages (known as instars), namely, the larva, the nymph, and the adult. Ixodid ticks have only a single nymphal instar, whereas most argasid species have two or more nymphal instars. Most ixodid species are three-host ticks, i.e., each life stage engorges and drops off its host to develop in the natural environment and then emerges in the subsequent life stage to attack new hosts, feed, and drop off again. In the adult stage, feeding and mating also take place on the host, after which engorged females drop off to lay their eggs. Argasid ticks have a multihost life cycle, with the precise number of hosts dependent upon the number of nymphal stages. The number of hosts attacked is also increased by the fact that female argasid ticks can lay eggs several times after feeding instead of only once, as in the ixodid ticks. As a result of the frequent intervals of feeding and development and the ability of most ticks to survive for long periods between blood meals, the tick life cycle can extend over several years. In this highly secretive family of ticks, records of life cycles lasting up to 20 years have been reported (5).

Ixodid Ticks

Hard ticks generally require several days to complete their blood meals. During blood feeding, new cuticle is synthesized to accommodate the influx of blood, a process that requires several days for the immature stages and even longer to make room for the enormous blood meals of the mated females. Males feed for brief periods of several days and detach to mate if sexually active females are located nearby. Following mating, males often reattach, feed for brief periods, and mate again. If no females are present, the males remain attached and wait until females become available. In some tick species, males do not feed, and

mating takes place in the nests or burrows of the vertebrate hosts.

Following successful host finding, the ticks crawl about in the hair coat of the host until they select a suitable location for attachment. Feeding site selection is determined by sensory information, particularly body odors and heat from the skin, acquired by sensilla on the palps and forelegs (Haller's organ). Among the most important are CO_2 and NH_3, found in host breath and urine; butyric acid and lactic acid, commonly found in sweat and other body fluids; and possibly even squalene, commonly found in fecal waste. Body heat also excites the ticks and probably acts synergistically with host odors to foster attachment behavior. Once a suitable site is selected, each tick begins the attachment process by cutting into the skin with its chelicerae. Next, the hypostome with its multiple recurved barbs is inserted into the wound created by the chelicerae. The palps are spread horizontally and remain on the outside surface of the skin. With the anterior end of the capitulum now fully inserted into the host skin, the tick begins to secrete saliva from its salivary glands. The salivary fluid contains proteins that form a cement layer, solidifying around the delicate mouthparts, oozing out onto the skin surface, and forming a tight bond that anchors the tick in this position. Thus, ticks do not "bite" their hosts but rather attach in the manner described above. Once the tick is firmly attached, it can commence sucking blood from the wound. Attachment takes many hours or even a day or more but once it is completed, the tick is very difficult to remove. Cement secretion is an energy-expensive process, and occasionally some ticks, especially older or exhausted individuals, die while attempting to blood feed even though they have succeeded in acquiring a suitable host.

Blood feeding over a period of days or weeks is a strategy for consuming enormous quantities of blood in a single meal, but it entails the risk of host rejection. No other blood-feeding arthropods have succeeded in adapting this strategy as well as ticks. To accomplish blood feeding, the ticks secrete a veritable pharmacopoeia of bioactive compounds that compromise the ability of the host to maintain hemostasis and counteract damage to its tissues. These compounds may include potent anticoagulants and anti-inflammatory proteins that inhibit platelet aggregation, facilitate blood flow (vasodilation), inhibit the coagulation pathway, and suppress host wound healing and inflammation. Immunoglobulin-binding proteins suppress the ability of the host's antibodies to reject repeated tick attacks. Among the most important proteins are enzymes that cleave complement, disrupting the complement cascade and producing byproducts that attract neutrophils in large numbers. Neutrophil degranulation liberates host proteins that damage adjacent tissue, expanding the feeding pool below the tick's mouthparts. In some species, e.g., *I. scapularis*, salivary enzymes destroy host complement, thereby facilitating the survival of pathogens such as *B. burgdorferi* (44). Indeed, researchers have often found that it is much easier to infect animals by allowing pathogen-infected ticks to feed on a susceptible host than by needle inoculation, even with massive numbers of infectious microbes. Antihistamines secreted in the saliva function as vasodilators, increasing blood flow while anticoagulants prevent coagulation as the blood is withdrawn slowly into the mouthparts. One of the most potent anticoagulants is apyrase, an enzyme that mediates platelet aggregation by hydrolyzing ADP (9). Other enzymes, e.g., anaphylatoxins, minimize inflammation, which reduces pain and irritation. Thus, tick feeding proceeds largely unnoticed, at least in tick-naïve hosts (i.e., hosts that have never experienced a previous tick bite). The secretion of complement-binding proteins acts to minimize the host immune response, even in hosts attacked a second time. However, repeated feeding on the same host generally induces a vigorous immune rejection of attempted feeding (47).

Having established a suitable feeding pool, ticks begin sucking blood. Blood meal digestion generates needed proteins and other nutrients to facilitate new cuticle synthesis, which proceeds rapidly (except in males). Feeding larvae and nymphs increase in weight by as much as 10 times their unfed weights, while females may expand as much as 100-fold after they have mated. To concentrate the blood meals, certain cells in the salivary glands gradually become transformed into water-secreting cells. Salivary gland lobes rich in these cells extract water and excess salts from the hemolymph and secrete the watery solution into the salivary ducts, where it is transferred into the feeding pool in the host. This method of water elimination, along with limited transpiration via the cuticle, allows the tick to concentrate the blood meal to such an extent that the true volume of blood consumed is often two to three times the final body weight of the engorged tick.

Most ixodid tick species are three-host ticks and must seek new hosts for their blood meals in each life stage (see Fig. 11). Males, however, may remain attached following mating; after a brief period of further feeding, they will seek females to mate again. Following the completion of feeding in each life stage, the ticks drop from their hosts to continue development in the natural environment. This is the process of ecdysis, in which the ticks increase in size and shed their cuticles (molting) to accommodate the expanded body. Fed larvae and nymphs develop in their hosts' habitat,

e.g., in rotting vegetation, leaf litter, cracks or crevices, or soil. In some cases, especially the nidicolous species of the genus *Ixodes*, this development takes place in the nest or burrow of the vertebrate host (this is described more fully in "Ecology: Adaptations for Survival," below). Developmental success (ecdysis) is dependent upon the presence of sufficient moisture in these microenvironments to prevent dessication. The rate at which ecdysis proceeds is dependent upon ground temperature. The ecdysial process is under hormonal control. Feeding initiates increases in the concentration of the molting hormone, 20-hydroxy-ecdysone, in the hemolymph. In response, new cuticle is synthesized, old cuticle dissolves and is resorbed in the molting fluid, and the old cuticle begins to separate (apolysis). When completed, a thin remnant of the old cuticle, the epicuticle, splits and the enlarged nymph escapes from the castoff skin. After molting, the emerging nymphs must seek another host and feed. This process is repeated following nymphal engorgement and molting to the adult stage. As a result of the lengthy developmental periods characteristic of most ticks, more than 90% of the life cycle is spent off the host.

Some species are two-host ticks, in which the larvae remain attached after completing their blood meals and molt in situ, and the emerging nymphs reattach to the same host, e.g., the camel tick (*Hyalomma dromedarii*). Others are one-host ticks, in which all three life stages feed and molt on the same host, e.g., the cattle tick (*Boophilus annulatus*) or the winter tick (*Dermacentor albipictus*). Such unusual adaptations facilitate successful parasitism by reducing the risks of starvation while waiting for hosts, but at the cost of increased dependence on a more limited variety of vertebrate species as hosts.

Reproductive activity in ixodid ticks is absolutely dependent upon blood feeding. In the metastriate ticks, i.e., all of the ixodid species except those of the genus *Ixodes*, mating always takes place on the host. Within a few days after the commencement of feeding, females secrete the volatile sex pheromone 2,6-dichlorophenol, which attracts male ticks feeding nearby. Following contact with a pheromone-secreting female, the males identify their partners by the presence of a specific mixture of nonvolatile cholesteryl esters on the female body and commence copulation. In a few species, a genital sex pheromone is also needed to stimulate copulation (a more detailed description of pheromone-mediated regulation of mating behavior is given elsewhere; see "Mating Behavior," below). Females accelerate feeding after mating, swelling enormously to as much as 100 times their prefeeding body weight, and drop from their hosts. Once on the ground, the replete (i.e., fully engorged and mated) female seeks a sheltered location such as a crack or crevice in the soil or leaf litter in the forest and begins ovipositioning. Oviposition takes many days and results in the deposition of thousands of eggs. Following oviposition, the spent female dies. Ticks that adopt this reproductive strategy are said to have a single gonotrophic cycle.

Argasid Ticks

These ticks specialize in rapid feeding, often completing their blood-feeding activity in less than 1 h. Attachment to the skin begins in a manner similar to that seen in the ixodid ticks. The ticks use their chelicerae to cut through the epidermis into the dermis, lacerate tiny blood vessels, and embed their barbed hypostomes. However, these ticks do not secrete cement, and they can withdraw their mouthparts quickly if disturbed. The ticks swell rapidly, using their powerful pharyngeal muscles to pump blood from the feeding pool into their digestive diverticuli. Examination of a feeding argasid tick with a stereoscopic microscope reveals the rapid alternating pulsations of the pharynx and spurts of red blood along the hypostomal food canal, interspersed with pulses of salivary secretion. As the ticks fill with blood, drops of clear, colorless fluid (the coxal fluid) begin to appear in the vicinity of the coxal pores, tiny openings between the coxae of legs I and II. This secretion contains water and salts, thereby allowing the ticks to concentrate their blood meals and adjust their internal water balance. The quantity of coxal fluid increases until as much as 50% or more of the weight of imbibed blood is eliminated (some individuals delay coxal fluid secretion until they drop off and run away to find a suitable shelter). Records that my graduate students collected during one of our experiments with *Ornithodoros parkeri* showed increases in tick body weight to 7.32 ± 10.76 times their prefed weight. During or after feeding, the ticks eliminated as much as $39.26\% \pm 13.38\%$ of their engorged body weight as coxal fluid. Further expansion is limited by the ability of the cuticle to stretch. No new cuticle is created during this period of rapid blood feeding, as occurs in the ixodid ticks; hence, the argasid ticks can only imbibe blood until the cuticle is fully stretched. Nevertheless, this is sufficient for a huge increase in body weight, often 10 times the prefeeding weight. Once they have fed, the ticks run from the host and seek shelter for further development. Given the opportunity, engorged ticks will bury themselves in sand, dust, litter, or leaf litter or hide in cracks and crevices in their habitats. In these sheltered locations, the larval and nymphal ticks undergo ecdysis. Nymphal ticks feed and molt several times, i.e., there are multiple nymphal stages. Thus, most argasid

ticks are multihost ticks. Often, three to five nymphal stages occur in the life cycle, with males emerging earlier than females. Hormonal regulation of larval and nymphal ecdysis is similar to that of ixodid ticks. Argasid ticks can survive for long periods between blood meals during each nymphal stage, which accounts for their unusual longevity. As a result, the entire life cycle may span 10 to 20 years. Variation in the life cycle pattern within the same species is common, which facilitates survival of nidicolous species that may have to wait for long periods before new hosts invade their shelters (14).

Mating and reproduction also differ markedly from these functions in ixodid ticks. Mating usually occurs away from the host and is not dependent upon blood feeding. Adults become sexually mature soon after emergence from the nymphal molt and may mate at any time. Argasid females frequently feed several times and can mate multiple times. The mated females lay small numbers of eggs after each feeding (multiple gonotrophic cycles) with up to 500 eggs in each egg batch.

Several exceptions to the typical argasid developmental strategy are known. In many of the species of the genus *Ornithodoros* that attack birds and bats, larvae remain attached for several days and feed in a manner similar to that of their ixodid relatives. Following feeding, the bloated larvae molt twice without an additional meal. Host seeking and feeding begin again with the second nymphal stage, after which the remainder of the life cycle is similar to that of other multihost argasid ticks. In contrast, the African tampans, *Ornithodoros savignyi* and *O. moubata* (sensu latu), bypass the larval stage during their development, emerging from the eggs as first-stage nymphs. Another unusual pattern occurs in the life cycle of the spinose ear tick (*Otobius megnini*), an important pest of ungulates and other livestock. In this species, there is only one nymphal stage. Neither the males nor the females feed, mating occurs away from the host, and the females metabolize the enormous blood meal consumed during their nymphal phase for egg production. Oviposition without feeding is known as autogeny.

BEHAVIOR

Except when feeding on vertebrate hosts, most ticks survive in the vegetation of their natural habitats or shelter in the nests, burrows, and caves used by their host animals. When ready to feed, the ticks engage in host-seeking behavior, which enables them to make contact with prospective hosts. For the free-living, nonnidicolous ticks, host-seeking activity is dependent upon changes in environmental conditions. In the temperate and subarctic regions of the world, host-seeking behavior is initiated in response to increasing air and ground temperatures and increasing day length. The gradual warming trend that occurs during spring or early summer in such regions favors development and reproduction. However, in tropical regions close to the equator where there are periods of dryness interspersed with rainy seasons, ticks such as the brown ear tick (*Rhipicephalus appendiculatus*) or the tropical bont tick (*Amblyomma variegatum*) shelter in the soil or rotting vegetative mat in rangelands or bushlands during the hot, dry season. Host-seeking behavior begins with the transition from the dry to the rainy season.

Strategies for Finding Hosts

Host-seeking ticks exhibit at least two strategies for locating potential targets for their blood meals, namely, ambush and hunter strategies.

Ticks employing the ambush strategy climb onto weeds, grasses, bushes, or other leafy vegetation to wait for passing hosts. The height to which the ticks climb depends upon many factors. In many species, larvae remain closest to the ground layer where they are most likely to encounter small mammals, ground-feeding birds, and other small vertebrate hosts. The later stages, especially the adults, climb higher in the vegetation where they are more likely to encounter larger animals such as deer, carnivores, and humans. Clinging to vegetation, the ticks remain on the undersides of leaves or other protective cover with their legs folded. Here they can remain for many hours until increasing desiccation initiates a descent to the cooler, humid ground layer where they can replenish lost body water (see below, "Adaptations for survival"). Regaining water via direct sorption of atmospheric moisture (21), they can climb again and continue waiting for passing hosts (see also "Adaptations for survival," below). This behavior is termed questing, in which the ticks remain at rest but nevertheless alert to any passing animals. Host-seeking ticks of many species respond to shadows, vibrations, odors, tactile cues, and other stimuli indicating the presence of a host, whereupon they extend their forelegs anterolaterally and cling to the hair or clothing of the passing host. For example, vibrating the grass stems on which ticks are perched can elicit questing behavior almost immediately. Because of this questing behavior, ambush ticks are easily captured by dragging a cloth (known as the tick drag) through the tick-infested habitat, since they cling to the cloth and do not immediately distinguish it from a living host. Even sound can attract ticks. The sounds produced by barking dogs have been reported to attract the brown dog tick (*Rhipicephalus sanguineus*), while sounds in the range emitted by cattle are known to attract larvae of the cattle tick (*Boophilus microplus*) (45). The raucous sounds emitted by nesting cliff swallows have been reported to attract the argasid ticks (*Ornithodoros concanensis*) from their shelters under rock ledges to attack the birds in nearby nests (38).

The hunter strategy is the method used by several species that parasitize large mammals such as the desert-inhabiting, xerophilic camel tick (*H. dromedarii*) or the southern African veld-inhabiting bont tick (*Amblyomma hebraeum*). These hunter ticks remain buried in soil, sand, or duff where they are protected from extreme heat and desiccation. However, when excited by host odors, the ticks emerge and run rapidly across the ground to attack these hosts, often up to 2 or 3 m away. Hunter ticks such as the bont tick can discriminate dark shapes against the bright background of the sky. They are easily excited by carbon dioxide, such as that emitted from a block of dry ice. CO_2 in high concentrations is believed to act as a general excitant but may not facilitate identification of the source. In addition, tick pheromones and possibly host odors can provide the directional information that leads the ticks to cattle or other ungulate hosts (32). Odorants are detected by olfactory sensilla, especially the prominent multiporose sensillum in the Haller's organ on the tarsus of leg I (Fig. 8).

Diapause

In the temperate, subarctic, and arctic regions of the world, many tick species exhibit diapause, a behavior that enables them to survive adverse environmental conditions and conserve energy until conditions improve. Ticks in diapause exhibit reduced metabolic rates and reduced physical activity, and they may refuse to feed even when offered suitable hosts. Several reports suggest that the physiological basis for this phenomenon involves changes in the activity of several neurosecretory centers in the tick synganglion (16). Two types of diapause behavior are known, host-seeking diapause and morphogenetic diapause. In the first type, host-seeking activity declines or stops completely in response to changing photoperiod and ambient temperatures in the microhabitat where the ticks quest for hosts. An example is seen in the case of the American dog tick (*D. variabilis*). In this species, larvae emerging in late summer or early fall are exposed to declining day lengths and gradually declining air temperatures. In response, these ticks shelter in soil, leaf litter, or rotting vegetation instead of climbing to commence seeking hosts, i.e., they express host-seeking diapause. The same phenomenon occurs in

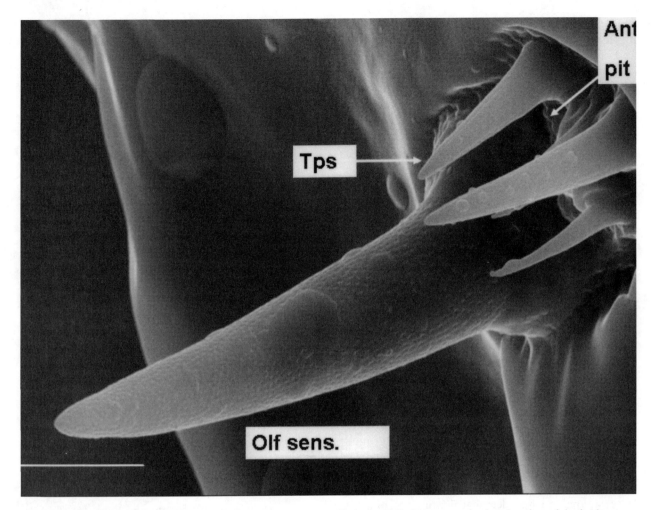

Figure 8. Scanning electron micrograph illustrating sensory sensilla in the Haller's organ on the dorsal surface of the foreleg of a female ixodid tick (*D. variabilis*). Ant. pit, anterior pit; Olf. sens., multiporose olfactosensory sensillum; Tps, tip of pore sensillum. Bar, 1 μm.

adult ticks of this species emerging in late summer or fall. Host-seeking activity resumes in the spring, in response to increasing photoperiod (day length), increasing amounts of solar radiation, and gradually warming soil and air temperatures. This pattern of interrupted host-seeking behavior enables *D. variabilis* larvae and adults to survive the cold winter conditions throughout most of their geographic range, conditions that would be unsuitable for population expansion. The effect of diapause is not only to extend the life cycle but also to synchronize feeding with those periods of the year when hosts are most likely to be available and when climatic conditions are optimal for development and reproduction. Another example is found in the black-legged tick (*I. scapularis*), where diapause delays activity by the recently molted nymphs so that they do not commence host seeking until the following spring or early summer. As a result, nymphal ticks that acquired the Lyme disease agent, *B. burgdorferi*, from reservoir hosts during their larval blood

meal retain the infectious microbes over the winter (38). Subsequently, when the nymphs emerge from their winter diapause, they commence host-seeking activity and transmit the bacteria to new hosts. This pattern of nymphal diapause allows transmission of the Lyme disease organisms to susceptible vertebrate hosts, thereby facilitating the spread of the infection to the larvae that emerge and feed on the same hosts soon afterwards. This strategy for nymphal survival is essential for perpetuating the infection in the natural environment, since *I. scapularis* females cannot transovarially transmit *B. burgdorferi* to their embryos. Diapause also delays host-seeking activity by adults until the fall, often several months after molting from nymphs fed in the spring.

The second type of diapause involves ovipositional or development delay, hence the term morphogenetic diapause (38). An example is found in the life cycle of the palearctic tick *Dermacentor marginatus*, a species that is widely distributed in northern Europe and northwestern Asia. Adults are active throughout the spring, summer, and early fall and feed readily on available hosts. However, the day length and ambient temperatures that the ticks experience prior to feeding determine the ovipositional response. Females that seek hosts and feed during periods of increasing day length, i.e., in spring or early summer, will lay their eggs almost immediately. In contrast, females exposed to declining day length prior to feeding delay oviposition until the following spring. Morphogenetic diapause also occurs in the life cycles of many species of argasid ticks, particularly nidicolous ticks that parasitize migratory birds and bats. In this case, the tick-infested nests or other shelters used by these hosts are abandoned during the migratory period. To avoid population expansion during this starving period, the females delay oviposition so that hatching occurs at about the time the hosts return. An example is seen in the case of the heron tick (*Argas arboreus*), which infests heron rookeries in Egypt and elsewhere in northern Africa. The bird hosts of these ticks abandon their rookeries while they migrate to their northern feeding grounds, often not returning for 5 or 6 months. While female ticks that feed on the returning birds oviposit soon afterwards, others that fed the previous year also begin ovipositing, leading to hordes of new larvae to exploit the expanding breeding colonies of bird hosts. A similar phenomenon occurs in the bat tick (*Ornithodoros kelleyi*), which infests bat roosts in buildings and other habitations in the eastern United States. The bats inhabit these shelters in the spring and summer, during which time they mate and produce their offspring. Ticks that engorge on bats in the spring commence oviposition almost immediately after blood feeding. However, those that feed in fall delay oviposition until the following spring. Just what determines this behavior is unknown. Nevertheless, the biological advantages for these highly host-specific ticks are obvious. Ovipositional delay by fall-feeding ticks avoids the risk that larvae will emerge at a time when their bat hosts have migrated to the cold caves and caverns where they survive the winter (38).

Attachment and feeding behavior

Hungry ticks respond to an impressive array of stimuli that enable them to recognize their hosts and facilitate feeding. Included are numerous different odors, body heat, and mechanical stimuli such as vibrations, air movements, sound, and visual cues such as shadows. Chemical cues that facilitate host recognition are known as kairomones, i.e., compounds or mixtures of compounds that the ticks use to identify their hosts. Examples include CO_2, ammonia, and H_2S (41, 42), which act primarily as long-range attractants,

and oily substances from the tarsal glands of white-tailed deer (*Odocoileus virginianus*) or rubbings from the fur of carnivores deposited on vegetation that act as arrestment pheromones. Similar responses were observed with the South African tick (*Ixodes neitzi*), when this tick encountered vegetation contaminated by substances from the klipspringer antelope. The tick clusters on vegetation marked with emanations of the animal's preorbital glands, thereby enhancing opportunities for finding hosts (34). *D. variabilis* will even cluster around carcasses of dead animals, attracted presumably by CO_2, NH_3, and other odorants emanating from the rotting body tissues (25).

Arrestment pheromones containing compounds originating from the tick body fluids and excreta (12) facilitate host finding by inducing clustering behavior in locations frequented by vertebrate animals, e.g., deer trails. In this behavior, the ticks remain in a non-ambulatory posture but are easily aroused by host stimuli. Arrestment leads to formation of clusters of ticks where they are likely to contact hosts (1). Host-originated compounds deposited on vegetation or objects left by hosts also attract ticks but do not necessarily lead to arrestment behavior. I personally have found numerous ticks crawling about sweat-covered instruments left in the field on hot summer days. Carroll and Grasela described other examples where up to 200 ticks were found surrounding the carcasses of dead deer (6).

Attracted to their hosts (or to locations frequented by hosts) by the odors and physical stimuli noted above, ticks cling to the hair or skin of the animal they have contacted. However, additional stimuli are required to identify the animal as a suitable host for feeding. Different species of ticks are highly selective in their response to odors from different vertebrate animals. For example, the cattle tick (*B. microplus*) responds aggressively to odors from extracts of cattle skin but less to odors in human breath and not at all to dry air. Compounds on the skin surface or in sweat, e.g., butyric acid, lactic acid, urea, and even squalene, often act as short-range attractants that provide selective information. These low-volatility compounds are believed to be detected primarily by single-pore contact chemosensilla in the sensory fields on the terminal segments of the palps and possibly also in the Haller's organ on the foreleg tarsi (Fig. 8). Small increases in radiant heat excite ticks and act synergistically with host odors. In addition, tactile stimuli received from hair, feathers, or the skin surface when ticks contact their hosts help to determine the selection of suitable feeding sites. These stimuli often induce ticks to wander over the host body surface in search of the most suitable feeding site. Ticks will not attach to a host unless this mixture of chemical and physical stimuli is received in the appropriate sequence.

Stimulated by the odorants and physical stimuli described above, the tick or ticks commence the attachment process that is the prelude to actual feeding. Frequently, this will not occur until the ticks find sheltered locations on the body where they are protected from grooming, e.g., by inserting themselves under the hair coat or by being partially compressed between adjoining body parts. On the relatively hairless bodies of humans, this often occurs under or adjacent to pressure points created by sites where clothing adheres to the skin. In ixodid ticks, attachment begins when the chelicerae begin cutting through the skin into the dermis. This is quickly followed by the secretion of cement that infiltrates into the wound site and spreads out onto the adjacent skin surrounding the mouthparts. The cement is a proteinaceous material of unknown composition elaborated primarily by the type I acini of the salivary glands. Rapid hardening of the cement serves to secure the ticks to the wound site. However, cement secretion continues for many hours, often requiring 1 to 2 days for completion; attached ticks are easily removed if pulled off the skin before secretion is completed. Following cement secretion, blood sucking begins, and different acini of the salivary glands commence production of anticoagulants, antihistamine, apyrase, and other enzymes that facilitate successful bloodsucking activity. Tissue damage caused by the ripping and tearing activities of the cheliceral digits and salivary enzymes attracts a massive influx of leukocytes, primarily neutrophils, that enlarges the feeding pool. Tick feeding is a gradual process, with brief periods of bloodsucking alternating with salivation. Ixodid ticks must first create new cuticle to accommodate the relatively massive blood meal that they will consume. As a result, ixodid ticks remain attached for many days, from as few as 2 or 3 days for larvae to as long as 13 days for females. To concentrate the hypotonic blood meal (tick body fluids typically have a higher osmotic pressure than vertebrate blood), they must eliminate as much of the excess water as possible. This is accomplished by certain acini of the salivary glands, especially the granular acini that contain groups of cells that are gradually transformed during the feeding process for water secretion. Excess water and salts are secreted from these cells into the salivary ducts and back into the host. Salivation alternates with periods of feeding, so that growth in body size continues to occur gradually during the lengthy feeding period. When completed, the engorged tick is found to weigh about 10 to 20 times the prefeeding weight of the larval or nymphal stage and as much as 100 to 120 times the prefeeding weight in engorged, mated females. However, since so much excess water is secreted back into the host during feeding, the engorged weight of the postfeeding tick is not

an accurate measure of the blood and tissue fluid volume consumed. This volume is actually much greater, often two to three times the engorged postfeeding weight, as determined by measurement of radioactive water or salts (37). For large ticks such as *Hyalomma asiaticum*, volumes as great as 8.9 ml were found to have been consumed by a single female tick (5).

In many tick species, completion of engorgement and drop-off from their hosts is correlated with the rhythms of host activity and environmental conditions. An example is found in the cattle tick (*B. microplus*), where replete females frequently drop in large numbers soon after dawn, when the animals commence grazing activity in the pastures. In contrast, immature *D. variabilis* ticks typically drop off their small mammal hosts during the night, coincident with the nocturnal behavior of these hosts (3). Synchronizing drop-off patterns with host behavior offers important ecological advantages for nonnidicolous ticks, since this synchronization tends to disperse fed ticks in optimal habitats where they are likely to find new hosts (see also "Adaptations for Survival," below). Studies by George (11) showed that the photoperiod appears to be the dominant exogenous factor affecting drop-off patterns in the rabbit tick (*Haemaphysalis leporispalustris*). Immature feeding ticks exhibited an endogenous drop-off rhythm entrained by the scotophase (dark period), which facilitated drop-off during daylight hours when their lagomorph hosts were confined in their forms or warrens. This probably contributes to the observation that adults of this tick are found solely on lagomorphs. Photoperiod entrainment is partially reversible, and detachment can also be coordinated with the periods of maximum host activity, leading to dispersal of these ticks into the natural environment where the larvae may attack ground-feeding birds as well as rabbits or hares.

In contrast to the lengthy feeding periods seen with ixodid ticks, argasid ticks attach for only brief periods. In many cases, this can be as little as 20 min for larvae or early stage nymphal ticks and only 35 to 70 min for adults. Soft ticks cut into the host skin with their mouthparts but, in contrast to hard ticks, they do not secrete cement. Instead, they commence bloodsucking almost immediately. Although sufficiently well embedded to imbibe blood, they can quickly withdraw if the host becomes active or attempts to dislodge them, facilitating their escape to feed again (see also "Life History, Argasid Ticks," above). Another reason that feeding is so rapid is that excess blood meal water is eliminated rapidly via the coxal pores, often while the tick is feeding. In addition, the body wall stretches to accommodate the influx of fresh fluid, enabling the feeding tick to swell to a volume many times its original, unfed weight. No new cuticle is secreted during feeding as it is in ixodid ticks (see also "Life History, Argasid Ticks," above).

Mating behavior

Mate-finding behavior is a highly regulated process mediated, at least in part, by pheromones. In prostriate Ixodidae ticks and in ticks of the family Argasidae, mate-finding behavior begins soon after the adults emerge from the nymphal molt and become sexually mature. Free-ranging, nonnidicolous ticks such as *Ixodes ricinus* or *I. scapularis* often mate in vegetation, although they are capable of mating while feeding on their hosts (Fig. 9). Others mate in the nests of their hosts. However, little is known about the mate-finding processes. The occurrence of arrestment pheromones described previously in this chapter (see "Attachment and Feeding Behavior," above) may facilitate mating by bringing males and females together. However, it is likely that some signal is needed for mate recognition. In the case of the argasid tick *Ornithodoros tholozani*, an unidentified compound (or compounds) in the coxal fluid was reported to serve as the female sex pheromone that attracted males for mating (27).

In contrast to the prostriate and argasid ticks, mating in the metastriate Ixodidae is highly regulated. Mating in these ticks occurs only during feeding. In all metastriate ticks, adults emerge from the nymphal molt with immature gonads, which remain undeveloped so long as the ticks remain unfed. Thus, males and females do not recognize one another as mates. However, feeding stimulates gametogenesis and initiates the secretion of sex pheromones by the females. Developmental periods for these processes vary in the different tick species. In the American dog tick (*D. variabilis*), females commence pheromone secretion within as little as 24 to 48 h after attachment, and males become responsive to this volatile sex attractant within 2 to 3 days of continuous blood feeding. Mate-finding behavior is mediated by two or, rarely, three pheromones, in accordance with a complex, hierarchical pattern of responses (Fig. 10). The first in this complex hierarchy is the sex attractant pheromone, 2,6-dichlorophenol, secreted by the foveal glands via the foveae dorsales on the female's dorsal surface. Perception of this volatile compound excites males feeding nearby, inducing them to detach and seek the females. As the males crawl over the host body surface, they compare the intensity of the response they perceive with the Haller's organ receptors on their forelegs until they approach the female (or clusters of females) emitting the pheromone. If the mate-searching male contacts the female, it recognizes her by means of a second pheromone, the mounting sex pheromone, a mixture of cholesteryl esters on the female's body surface. As described by Sonenshine (37), the precise identity of the specific cholesterol esters and their proportion in relation to one another determine the extent to which the male will commence mounting behavior or depart in search of another female. Thus, the cholesteryl ester composition provides, at least to a limited extent, species-specific discrimination. In the case of *D. variabilis*, the specific compound that must be recognized is cholesteryl oleate, and this is sufficient to trigger the mounting response. In other, even more closely related species, a more complex mixture of cholesteryl esters must be recognized for mounting to occur. If the male perceives the appropriate chemical compounds, it climbs onto the female's dorsal body surface, probes with tiny chemosensory hairs on its foreleg tarsi, and then turns to the female's ventral body surface. After turning onto the underside, the male advances anteriorly and probes for the gonopore. When the male locates the gonopore, it extrudes a spermatophore, a specialized sperm-filled sac, and it implants the spermatophore into the female's vulva with its chelicerae. In some species, e.g., *D. variabilis* and *Dermacentor andersoni*, formation of the spermatophore is dependent upon the detection of the genital sex pheromone found in the vestibular vagina of the female's reproductive tract (2). The pheromone is detected by gustatory sensilla on the digits of the chelicerae. If these structures are excised, the males carry out the first stages of mating behavior but are unable to copulate (39). The signals detected by the cheliceral digits are essential for stimulating spermatophore production, which occurs in the large accessory gland of the sexually mature male during the mating process. Following copulation, the male reattaches to the host skin near the mated female and, after several days of feeding, is ready to mate again. Whether the genital sex pheromone is a specialized requirement for ensuring species-specific mating in only a few species such as *D. variabilis* and *D. andersoni* or is more widespread is unknown.

Reproduction

Ovipositioning occurs after the completion of blood feeding. A blood meal is essential for oviposition, although examples of egg laying without blood feeding (autogeny) have been recorded in some argasid species. In the Ixodidae, oviposition may begin within a few days or may be delayed for many weeks or months in ticks that feed in the fall or winter (morphogenetic diapause). Oviposition occurs gradually over a period of several weeks. Hundreds of eggs may be deposited each day, especially during the first few days, leading to the accumulation of a huge egg mass comprising thousands of eggs. As the eggs exit the

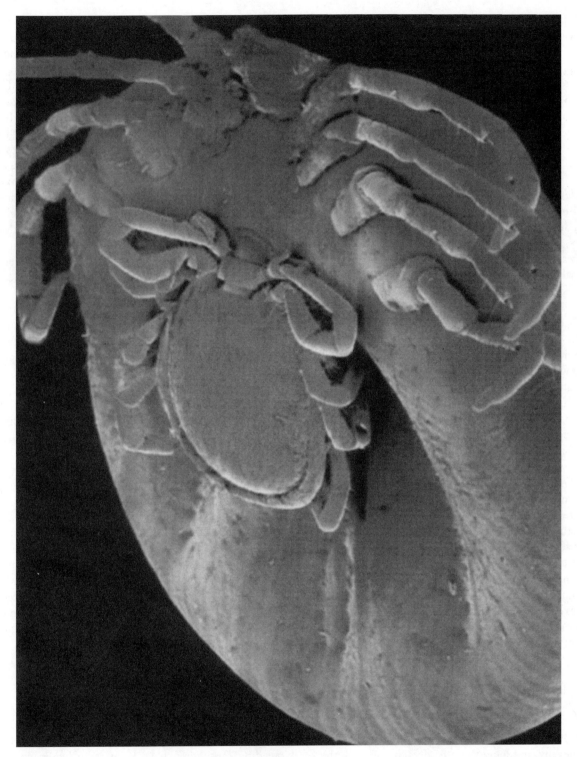

Figure 9. Scanning electron micrograph showing a mating pair of ixodid ticks (*I. ricinus*). The mouthparts of the smaller male are inserted into the vulva of the greatly swollen, engorged female. Measurement bar, 1 mm. Image kindly provided by Volker Steger, Munich, Germany.

gonopore, the female bends its capitulum, capturing each egg with its mouthparts and passing it over onto the dorsal surface, where it is waxed by the finger-like extensions of the Gené's organ. All of the numerous eggs produced by each mated female are deposited during a single, continuous period, after which the female dies (single gonotrophic cycle). Argasid ticks, however, may feed and lay eggs on several occasions

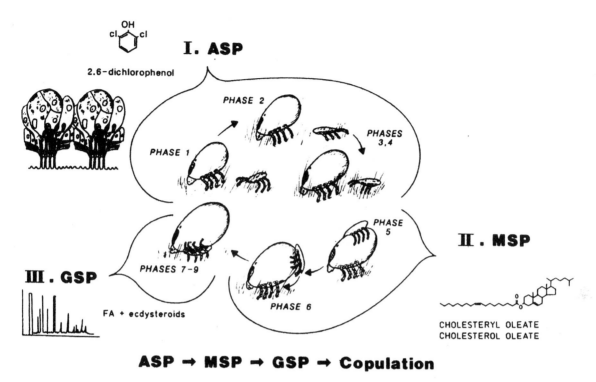

Figure 10. Drawing illustrating a hypothetical model of mating behavior in ixodid ticks. From D. E. Sonenshine, 1985, *Annu. Rev. Entomol.* 30:1–28, with permission from Annual Reviews, Inc.

over many months or even years, depending upon the interval between blood feeding. Thus, argasid ticks have multiple gonotrophic cycles. Argasid females produce relatively small egg clutches containing only a few hundred eggs, after which the females are ready to feed and oviposit again. As many as eight gonotrophic cycles have been reported in some species. However, egg mass size and egg viability tend to be reduced in the later cycles. The occurrence of mating is independent of feeding. This process of frequent feeding and oviposition enables these ticks to survive for many years. As a result, disease-causing organisms transmitted by these vectors also may persist for long periods.

ECOLOGY

The approximately 850 known species of ticks occur on every continent, with the possible exception of Antarctica, reflecting a remarkable range of adaptation to the many varied habitats present throughout these different regions. The tick species that occur in these varied localities can be divided into two major categories, namely, (i) nonnidicolous species, also known as exophiles, that live exposed in the open environment rather than in shelters and disperse throughout the variety of habitats where they encounter pass-

ing hosts and (ii) nidicolous ticks that infest the nests, burrows, or other shelters used by their hosts or hide nearby. Most exophiles are species of the metastriate Ixodidae. In contrast, most nidicoles are species of the Argasidae and prostriate Ixodidae.

Nonnidicolous ticks are the most widespread, occurring in virtually all regions, from the northern tundras and arboreal forests to the equatorial rain forests. They occur in dense forests, second-growth areas of scrub and brush, savannahs, and grassy meadows where they shelter in leaf litter, duff, and rotting vegetation at the floor of woods and grasslands. They emerge from these microenvironments and climb on stems and branches to await passing hosts. Others survive in deserts or semideserts, where they remain buried in sand or sandy soils, under stones, and in crevices, from whence they emerge when attracted by hosts that arrive nearby.

Adaptations for Survival While Waiting or Searching for Hosts

Nidicolous ticks such as the nest- or burrow-inhabiting argasids typically show more limited tolerances than the nonnidicolous species. These ticks frequently survive in dark enclosures such as caves, burrows, basements, or similar locations where conditions are more uniform throughout the year than in the external macroenvironment. Usually, the relative humidity is higher and air temperatures are cooler than the external atmosphere, even when hosts are absent. Colonization by vertebrate hosts raises the humidity and temperature considerably, creating yet more favorable conditions for the ticks. Nidicolous ticks exhibit behavioral patterns that restrict their distribution to these cryptic microhabitats, avoiding bright sunlight and low humidity. Under these conditions, nidicolous ticks can wait for months or even years until hosts arrive and take up residence in these shelters.

For the nonnidicolous ticks, survival in the open environment depends upon many factors, among the most important of which is tolerance to desiccation. Ticks adapted to the cool, humid arboreal and deciduous forests of northern Europe and North America typically have only limited tolerance of desiccation. After brief periods of questing on vegetation for passing hosts where they are exposed to subsaturated air, the loss of body water overwhelms their hunger and induces them to retreat to saturated atmospheres in rotting meadow vegetation or damp leaf litter on the forest floor. Often cooler as well as much more humid, these favorable microclimatic conditions enable the ticks to restore their lost body water. Some ticks, e.g., *I. ricinus* and *I. scapularis*, secrete a salt-rich saliva onto the exposed region of the food canal in the hypostome. This salty solution is highly hygroscopic, resulting in droplets of water condensing on the tick's hypostome. When sufficient water has accumulated, the tick sucks this dilute solution back into its body. Over a period of several hours, with repeated cycles of secretion and ingestion of the collected water, the tick is able to restore its internal body water balance. This process, known as direct sorption from saturated and mildly subsaturated atmospheres, has been described for many species of ticks and insects (21, 31). *I. ricinus* ticks questing in meadows and at the ecotones of brush or wooded areas extend the duration of their host-seeking behavior by periodic descent to the saturated microenvironments for rehydration. However, this energy-exhausting process becomes increasingly difficult as the unfed ticks age. In other, more desiccation-tolerant, species such as *D. variabilis*, the ticks are able to sorb atmospheric moisture during the cool (<15°C) humid nighttime periods and thus rehydrate without having to abandon their questing activity (24). Moreover, larvae and nymphs of this tick quest for their small mammal hosts close to the ground, near the base of the vegetative mat in meadows, or in the thick vine and leafy vegetation along the ecotone between forests and meadows. This dense vegetation affords them shade and increased availability of mois-

ture. In contrast, the adult ticks tend to quest much higher onto taller stems and branches, dispersing further into the grassy meadows as well as on the vegetation along roadsides and woodland trails.

Ticks adapted to arid habitats such as deserts, semideserts, or dry grasslands are the most desiccation tolerant of the different species. The waxy coating found on their cuticles allows them to tolerate relatively high temperatures, ensuring adequate water-proofing even when the ticks are exposed to intense sunlight. Some species, e.g., the camel tick *H. dromedarii* or the central Asian tick *H. asiaticum*, bury themselves in the sand or duff of the ground where hosts frequently pass or congregate, such as caravan-series, cattle barns, corrals, or similar shelters. When stimulated by host odors, the ticks emerge and run towards these animals, thereby minimizing their exposure to the extreme xeric conditions of these environments. Larvae and nymphs survive in rodent burrows or tunnels such as those built underground by gerbils. *H. dromedarii* is common in the steppes and semidesert habitats found in large areas of North Africa and the Middle East, while *H. asiaticum* occurs in the dry grassy steppes and semideserts of central Asia.

Host Specificity

Most tick species feed only on a limited variety of vertebrate hosts, i.e., they are host specific. Examples include ticks that feed only on large ruminants, others that feed only on bats, birds, and so on. Although some tick species are generalists, with little or no limits on their choice of hosts, the vast majority are specialists that exhibit relatively strict host specificity (15). Host specificity is especially pronounced among the nidicolous ticks. An example is *Amblyomma tuberculatum*, which parasitizes the gopher tortoise. The ticks survive in the burrows utilized by these reptiles. Many argasid ticks live in cracks or crevices of trees near the nests of their bird hosts, e.g., the heron tick *A. arboreus*. Others hide in cracked plaster, stone, or brick work of old buildings colonized by bats, e.g., the bat tick *O. kelleyi*, found in the eastern United States. In contrast, ticks such as the European sheep tick, *I. ricinus*, or the North American deer tick, *I. scapularis*, have a much more catholic host range. In both cases, the larvae and nymphs will feed on virtually any available vertebrate, including lizards, birds, small mammals, and larger mammals such as dogs, sheep, and even humans. Adults, however, restrict their host range to medium-sized or larger mammals, especially deer or other ungulates. More than 300 species of vertebrates have been recorded as hosts for *I. ricinus* and more than 120 species for *I. scapularis*.

The determinants of host specificity are not well understood. However, several factors are believed to be especially important. One such factor is the ability of the tick to evade or suppress host homeostatic systems and avoid rejection (35, 36). Tick feeding introduces an array of immunologically challenging proteins which would be expected to cause inflammation, pain, and irritation. Just such an effect can occur when ticks are induced to feed on abnormal hosts (43) but not when they are allowed to feed on hosts frequently encountered in their natural environment, i.e., so-called normal hosts. For example, the saliva of the black-legged tick *I. scapularis* contains pharmacologically active compounds that suppress host mediators of edema and inflammation such as anaphylatoxins, bradykinin, and other kinins. Other salivary components prevent the release of host inflammatory agents from leukocytes while enhancing vasodilation, which brings more blood to the mouthparts. *I. scapularis* saliva also contains a complement-inactivating enzyme, preventing or minimizing the development of natural immunity in white-footed mice and other small mammals that are the usual hosts of the immature stages of these ticks. Complement inactivation also facilitates the survival of pathogens such as *B. burgdorferi* ingested during blood feeding (44). Notably lacking is antihistamine, an enzyme common in the saliva of other tick species and other blood-feeding arthropods. White-footed mice and other natural hosts that lack histamine-containing basophils in their blood tolerate repeated feeding by *I. scapularis* with little if any evidence of immune rejection. However, if ticks are allowed to feed on abnormal hosts such as guinea pigs, animals with blood rich in histamine-containing basophils, cutaneous basophil hypersensitivity develops rapidly; further tick feeding is contained or aborted (36). The extent to which immune rejection has influenced the evolution of host specificity is poorly understood and certainly merits further study.

Host specificity is also strongly influenced by the habitats in which ticks occur. Ticks adapted to a specific habitat type (e.g., grassland) are most likely to encounter those vertebrates adapted to the same habitat. However, ticks that have somewhat broader tolerances and can survive at the boundaries (ecotones) between adjacent habitats will be exposed to a much greater range of potential hosts. *D. variabilis* is an example of an ecotonal species. These ticks are most abundant at the forest boundary adjacent to trails, roadsides, and old fields (38) where they encounter both woodland- and meadow-inhabiting mammals. For ticks that quest on vegetation while searching for hosts (ambush method), the height to which ticks climb is also important. Ticks, e.g., unfed adults, that climb up to or near the tops of grassy or woody stems will encounter large or medium-sized mammals, whereas juvenile ticks that quest on or near the ground will be exposed almost entirely to small mammals as well as lizards or ground-feeding birds.

Odors constitute another factor that influences host specificity. Although some host odors, e.g., NH_3 and CO_2, act as nonspecific attractants, other odors are peculiar to particular hosts. The ability of ticks to recognize and respond to specific host odors has been documented in several species. One example is the cattle tick, *B. microplus*, which can distinguish and respond to odors from cattle. Electrophysiological recordings made from the tarsi of these ticks show that the neurons detect distinctive odors in the washings from cattle skin but not from human skin (45).

Seasonal Activity

Most nonnidicolous ticks seek hosts only during specific periods of the year. This pattern of seasonal activity enables them to avoid adverse environmental conditions, especially freezing during the winter season. These ticks often diapause during the cooler months of the year. An example of this pattern is seen in the black-legged tick (*I. scapularis*). Each life stage is active at different periods of the year. The seasonal peak for larvae occurs in July or August, depending upon the geographic region. In the northern part of its range, e.g., New York and New England, where the larval activity peak occurs in late summer, those nymphs that molted from fed larvae do not emerge until late summer or early fall. Exposed to declining day length and reduced amounts of solar radiation, the newly emerging nymphs diapause until the following spring. Nymphs that feed in the spring molt in summer, but the young adults delay host seeking until fall, often for as long as 3 to 4 months. This pattern results in a 2-year life cycle. This pattern also facilitates the overwinter survival of the spirochete *B. burgdorferi*, from one year to the next. Emerging adults commence activity in the fall, typically in October, and remain active until interrupted by freezing conditions. These ticks reemerge from the ground layers when temperatures climb above freezing, even on occasional warm days in winter. Surviving adults continue host-seeking activity into spring, until they find hosts or die of exhaustion. In the southernmost part of its range, e.g., Florida and Georgia, *I. scapularis* seasonal activity commences much earlier in the year. As a result, these southern populations may complete their life cycle in just 1 year.

The American dog tick, *D. variabilis*, is an example of a seasonally active tick, but in contrast to *I. scapularis*, all activity occurs in the spring and summer. In this species, larvae and adults overwinter, sheltering in the forest or meadow soils just below the

Life cycle *Dermacentor variabilis*

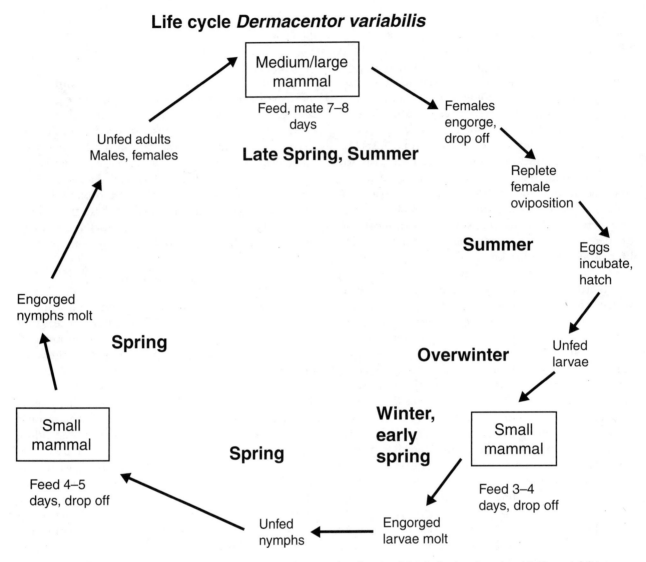

Figure 11. Diagram illustrating the life cycle of a representative three-host ixodid tick, the American dog tick (*D. variabilis*).

frost level where they are protected by the dense mat of rotting vegetation. As the ground warms with the onset of warmer spring temperatures, *D. variabilis* larvae emerge from winter diapause to feed on small mammals, especially mice and voles. As daytime temperatures increase, ever greater numbers of larvae emerge to attack these hosts, culminating within a few weeks in the seasonal activity peak. This usually occurs in mid-April in the southeastern United States but not until mid-May or early June in the northern United States or southern Canada. Following molting of the fed larvae, nymphal ticks appear in increasing numbers while the numbers of host-seeking larvae decline. The nymphal peak follows the larval peak within a few weeks. Surviving unfed adults also begin to emerge, seeking medium-sized mammals and larger hosts. Their numbers begin to increase as newly molted young adults join the year-old survivors, reaching peak abundance in June or early July. In the southern parts of their range, overwintering *D. variabilis* adults emerge early and soon overlap with those that develop from nymphs fed in the spring. As a result, most adults that find hosts experience increasing day length and intense solar radiation, conditions that foster rapid oviposition and hatching of the next larval population. This allows the entire life cycle to be completed in 1 year in this region. In the northern part of its range, however, tick activity is delayed due to cooler spring temperatures and shorter day lengths. Although larvae and nymphs feed and molt during the late spring and summer, adult emergence is delayed until August or September when day length and solar radiation are declining. Rather than commencing questing activity, these adults undergo diapause and emerge the following spring. This pattern of feeding and diapause results in a 2-year life cycle (Fig. 11).

A few tick species are active during the cooler months of the year, especially fall and winter, and diapause during the hottest months of the year. In the winter tick, *D. albipictus*, larvae commence host-seeking activity on deer, moose, cattle, and other un-gulates only in late summer or early fall. In this one-host species, larvae and nymphs feed and molt on the same hosts, and the resulting adults reattach, feed, and mate. Replete females drop off the host and oviposit in the soil. In the northernmost parts of its range, adults usually do not appear until late winter, with peak occurrence in April. Subsequent oviposi-tion and hatching occur in late spring, when the emerging larvae diapause and do not emerge to com-mence host seeking until after an extended period of declining photoperiod. As in the previous examples, development proceeds faster in the southernmost parts of the tick's range.

REFERENCES

1. Allan, S. A., and D. E. Sonenshine. 2002. Evidence of an as-sembly pheromone in the black-legged deer tick, *Ixodes scapu-laris*. *J. Chem. Ecol.* **28**:15–27.

2. Allan, S. A., J. S. Phillips, and D. E. Sonenshine. 1989. Species recognition elicited by differences in composition of the genital sex pheromone in *Dermacentor variabilis* and *Dermacentor andersoni* (Acari: Ixodidae). *J. Med. Entomol.* **26**:539–546.

3. Amin, O. 1970. The circadian rhythm of dropping of en-gorged larvae and nymphs of the American dog tick *Derma-centor variabilis* (Say). *J. Med. Entomol.* **7**:251–255.

4. Atkinson, P.W., and K. C. Binington. 1973. New evidence on the function of the porose areas of ixodid ticks. *Experientia* **29**:799–800.

5. Balashov, Yu S. 1972. Bloodsucking ticks (Ixodoidea)—vectors of disease of man and animals. *Misc. Publ. Entomol. Soc. Am.* **8**:163–376. (In Russian.)

6. Carroll, J. F., and J. J. Grasela. 1986. Occurrence of adult American dog tick, *Dermacentor variabilis* (Say), around small animal traps and vertebrate carcasses. *Proc. Entomol. Soc. Wash.* **88**:77–82.

7. Carroll, J. F., G. D. Mills, and E. T. Schmidmann. 1996. Field and laboratory responses of adult *Ixodes scapularis* (Acari: Ixodidae) to kairomones produced by white-tailed deer. *J. Med. Entomol.* **33**:640–644.

8. Ceraul, S. M., D. E. Sonenshine, and W. L. Hynes. 2002. Investigations into the resistance of the tick, *Dermacentor variabilis* (Say) (Acari: Ixodidae) following challenge with the bacterium, *Escherichia coli* (Enterobacteriales: Enterobacteri-aceae). *J. Med. Entomol.* **39**:376–383.

9. Champagne, D. E., and J. G. Valenzuela. 1996. Pharmacology of haematophagus arthropod saliva, p. 85–106. *In* S. K. Wikel (ed.), *The Immunology of Host-Ectoparasitic Arthropod Rela-tionships*. CAB International, Wallingford, United Kingdom.

10. Coons, L. B., R. Rosell-Davis, and B. I. Tarnovski. 1986. Bloodmeal digestion in ticks, p. 248–279. *In* J. R. Sauer and J. A. Hair (ed.), *Morphology, Physiology, and Behavioral Bi-ology of Ticks*. Ellis Horwood, Chichester, United Kingdom.

11. George, J. E. 1971. Drop-off rhythms of engorged rabbit ticks, *Haemaphysalis leporispalustris* (Packard, 1896) (Acari: Ixodi-dae). *J. Med. Entomol.* **8**:461–479.

12. Grenacher, S., T. Kröber, P. M. Guerin, and M. Vlimant. 2001. Behavioral and chemoreceptor cell responses of the tick, *Ixodes ricinus*, to its own faeces and faecal constituents. *Exp. Appl. Acarol.* **25**:641–660.

13. Gudderra, N. P., P. A. Neese, D. E. Sonenshine, C. S. Apper-son, and R. M. Roe. 2001. Developmental profile, isolation, and biochemical characterization of a novel carrier protein from the American dog tick, *Dermacentor variabilis*, and ob-servations on a similar protein in the soft tick, *Ornithodoros parkeri* (Acari: Ixodidae). *Insect Biochem. Mol. Biol.* **31**:299–311.

14. Hoogstraal, H. 1985. Argasid and nuttalliellid ticks as para-sites and vectors. *Adv. Parasitol.* **24**:135–238.

15. Hoogstraal, H., and A. Aeschlimann. 1982. Tick host speci-ficity. *Bull. Soc. Entomol. Suisse* **55**:5–32.

16. Ioffe, I. D. 1964. Seasonal changes in neurosecretion contents of neurosecretory cells in *Dermacentor pictus* Herm. ticks (Ixodoidea: Acarina). *Med. Parazitol. (Moscow)* **34**:57–63. (In Russian.)

17. Johns, R., D. E. Sonenshine, and W. L. Hynes. 1998. Control of bacterial infections in the hard tick *Dermacentor variabilis* (Acari: Ixodidae): evidence for the existence of antimicrobial proteins in tick hemolymph. *J. Med. Entomol.* **35**:458–464.

18. Johns, R., J. Onishi, A. Broadwater, D. E. Sonenshine, A. deSilva, and W. L. Hynes. 2001. Contrasts in tick innate im-mune responses to *Borrelia burgdorferi* challenge: immunotol-erance in *Ixodes scapularis* versus immunocompetence in *Der-macentor variabilis* (Acari: Ixodidae). *J. Med. Entomol.* **38**: 99–107.

19. Johns, R., D. E. Sonenshine, and W. L. Hynes. 2001. Identifi-cation of a defensin from the hemolymph of the American dog tick, *Dermacentor variabilis*. *Insect Biochem. Mol. Biol.* **31**: 857–865.

20. Klompen, J. H. S., W. C. Black IV, J. E. Keirans, and J. H. Oliver, Jr. 1996. Evolution of ticks. *Ann. Rev. Entomol.* **41**: 141–161.

21. Knülle, W., and D. Rudolph. 1982. Humidity relationships and water balance of ticks, p. 43–70. *In* F. D. Obenchain and R. Galun (ed.), *Physiology of Ticks*. Pergamon Press, Oxford, United Kingdom.

22. Kopacek, P., R. Vogt, L. Jindrak, C. Weise, and I. Safarik. 1999. Purification and characterization of the lysozyme from the gut of the soft tick *Ornithodoros moubata*. *Insect Biochem. Mol. Biol.* **29**:989–997.

23. Kovar, V., P. Kopacek, and I. Grubhoffer. 2000. Isolation and characterization of Dorin M, a lectin from plasma of the soft tick *Ornithodoros moubata*. *Insect Biochem. Mol. Biol.* **30**: 195–205.

24. McEnroe, W. D. 1974. The regulation of adult American dog tick, *Dermacentor variabilis* (Say), seasonal activity and breed-ing potential (Acarina: Ixodidae). *Acarologia* **17**:651–663.

25. McNemee, R. B., Jr., W. J. Sames IV, and F. A. Maloney, Jr. 2003. Occurrence of *Dermacentor variabilis* (Acari: Ixodidae) around a porcupine (Rodentia: Erthethizontidae) carcass at Camp Ripley, Minnesota. *J. Med. Entomol.* **40**:108–111.

26. Medzhitov, R., and C. A. Janeway. 1997. Innate immunity: the virtues of a nonclonal system of recognition. *Cell* **91**:295–298.

27. Mohamed, F. S. A., G. M. Khalil, A. S. Marzouk, and M. A. Roshdy. 1990. Sex pheromone recognition of mating behavior in the tick *Ornithodoros (Ornithodoros) savignyi* (Audouin) (Acari: Argasidae). *J. Med. Entomol.* **27**:288–294.

28. Nakajima, Y., A. van der Goes Naters-Yasui, D. Taylor, and M. Yamakawa. 2001. Two isoforms of a member of the arthro-pod defensin family from the soft tick, *Ornithodoros moubata* (Acari: Ixodidae). *Insect Biochem. Mol. Biol.* **31**:747–751.

29. Nakajima, Y., A. van der Goes Naters-Yasui, D. Taylor, and M. Yamakawa. 2002. Antibacterial peptide defensin is involved in midgut immunity of the soft tick, *Ornithodoros moubata*. *Insect Mol. Biol.* **11**:611–618.

30. Nakajima, Y., K. Oghara, D. Taylor, and M. Yamakawa. 2003. Antibacterial hemoglobin fragments from the midgut of the soft tick *Ornithodoros moubata* (Acari: Ixodidae). *J. Med. Entomol.* **40**:78–81.

31. Needham, G. R., and P. D. Teel. 1991. Off-host physiological ecology of ixodid ticks. *Annu. Rev. Entomol.* **36**:659–681.

32. Norval, R. A. I., D. E. Sonenshine, S. A. Allan, and M. J. Burridge. 1996. Efficacy of pheromone-acaricide-impregnated tail-tag decoys for control of the bont tick, *Amblyomma hebraeum* (Acari: Ixodidae), on cattle in Zimbabwe. *Exper. Appl. Acarol.* **20**:31–46.

33. Pal, U., A. M. deSilva, R. R. Montgomery, D. Fish, J. Anguita, J. F. Anderson, Y. Lobert, and E. Fikrig. 2000. Attachment of *Borrelia burgdorferi* within *Ixodes scapularis* mediated by outer surface protein A. *J. Clin. Investig.* **106**:561–569.

34. Rechav, Y., and G. B. Whitehead. 1978. Field trials with pheromone-acaricide mixtures for control of *Amblyomma hebraeum*. *J. Econ. Entomol.* **71**:149–151.

35. Ribeiro, J. M. C. 1987. Role of saliva in blood feeding by arthropods. *Annu. Rev. Entomol.* **32**:463–478.

36. Ribeiro, J. M. C. 1989. Role of saliva in tick/host interactions. *Exp. Appl. Acarol.* **7**:15–20.

37. Sonenshine, D. E. 1991. *Biology of Ticks*, vol. 1. Oxford University Press, New York, N.Y.

38. Sonenshine, D. E. 1993. *Biology of Ticks*, vol. 2. Oxford University Press, New York, N.Y.

39. Sonenshine, D. E., P. J. Homsher, and K. A. Carson. 1984. Evidence of the role of the cheliceral digits in the perception of genital sex pheromones during mating of the American dog tick, *Dermacentor variabilis* (Say) (Acari: Ixodidae). *J. Med. Entomol.* **21**:296–306.

40. Sonenshine, D. E., S. M. Ceraul, W. L. Hynes, K. Macaluso, and A. F. Azad. 2003. Innate immunity in ticks: midgut and hemolymph expression of antimicrobial peptides and their contribution to vector competency. *Exp. Appl. Acarol.* **28**:127–134.

41. Steullet, P., and P. M. Guerin. 1992. Perception of breath components by the tropical bont tick *Amblyomma variegatum* Fabricius (Ixodidae). I. CO_2-excited and CO_2-inhibited receptors. *J. Comp. Physiol. A* **170**:665–676.

42. Steullet, P., and P. M. Guerin. 1992. Perception of breath components by the tropical bont tick *Amblyomma variegatum* Fabricius (Ixodidae). II. Sulfide receptors. *J. Comp. Physiol. A* **170**:677–685.

43. Trager, W. 1939. Acquired immunity to ticks. *J. Parasitol.* **25**:57–81.

44. Valenzuela, J. G., R. Charlab, T. N. Mather, and J. M. C. Ribeiro. 2000. Purification, cloning and expression of a novel salivary anticomplement protein from the tick, *Ixodes scapularis*. *J. Biol. Chem.* **275**:18717–18723.

45. Waladde, S. M., and M. J. Rice. 1982. The sensory basis of tick feeding behavior, p. 71–118. *In* F. D. Obenchain and R. Galun, (ed.), *Physiology of Ticks*. Pergamon Press, Oxford, United Kingdom.

46. Wang, H., G. C. Paesen, P. A. Nuttall, and A. G. Barbour. 1998. Male ticks help their mates to feed. *Nature* **391**:753–754.

47. Wikel, S. K. 1996. Immunology of the tick-host interface, p. 204–231. *In* S. K. Wikel, (ed.), *The Immunology of Host-Ectoparasitic Arthropod Relationships*. CAB International, Wallingford, United Kingdom.

48. Yu, X.-Q., Y. F. Zhu, C. Ma, J. A. Fabrick, and M. R. Kanost. 2002. Pattern recognition proteins in *Manduca sexta* plasma. *Insect Biochem. Mol. Biol.* **32**:1287–1293.

49. Zhioiua, E., R. A. Lebrun, P. W. Johnson, and H. S. Ginsberg. 1996. Ultrastructure of the haemocytes of *Ixodes scapularis* (Acari: Ixodidae). *Acarologia* **37**:173–179.

Chapter 3

The Tick: a Different Kind of Host for Human Pathogens

ULRIKE G. MUNDERLOH, STEVEN D. JAURON, AND TIMOTHY J. KURTTI

INTRODUCTION

Tick-borne pathogens, especially the ehrlichias, anaplasmas, and spirochetes, are recognized as causing a growing spectrum of diseases in domestic and feral animals and humans. Originally, these pathogens were classified according to vertebrate host species and target cells, which obscured their relationship. But as our knowledge of the molecular interrelatedness of known and newly discovered microbes expands, traditional phylogenetic assignments are broken down and species concepts are redrawn. At the same time, novel and surprising strategies of immune evasion or modulation and host-specific adaptive mechanisms that are used by these pathogens are emerging. One of the underlying principles governing the life cycle of tick-borne pathogens is their ability to survive and thrive in two extremely different environments—one presented by the homeostatic environment of the mammal, and the other presented by the vector tick, under conditions that change dramatically with activity and feeding status. The microbes must be able to sense pathophysiological changes in their hosts, distinguish the multitude of signals received, and react appropriately. Differential expression of specific antigens (DESA) mediates transition to the new host. This chapter will highlight what is known about the response of these microbes to host cues and how they manage existence in and passage between the divergent environments of mammalian host and vector tick. We focus on the human pathogenic rickettsiae and spirochetes as they prepare to leave the ticks and invade the mammalian host. Also covered are the basic features of the tick as a microbial environment and how the tick environment differs from that of the vertebrate host and how ticks recognize and respond to microbial invaders. For details on the structure and function of tick physiological systems and host-parasite interactions, the reader is referred to the comprehensive two-volume treatise of Sonenshine, *Biology of Ticks* (217a, 218).

HISTORICAL PERSPECTIVE

At the end of the 19th century, Theobald Smith and Frederick L. Kilbourne reported for the first time that ticks transmit agents of disease. Stimulated by the discoveries of the preeminent microbiologists Robert Koch and Paul Ehrlich, Smith and Kilbourne experimentally demonstrated that the cattle tick transmitted the causative agent of Texas fever of cattle, a protozoan, *Babesia bigemina*. This work set the foundation for later discoveries demonstrating that ticks also transmit pathogens that cause human disease (7). Based on the findings of Smith and Kilbourne, at the dawn of the 20th century it was generally presumed that ticks did not transmit any bacterial pathogens to humans. However, in 1907 Ricketts determined that the Rocky Mountain wood tick, *Dermacentor andersoni*, carried and transmitted the spotted fever agent and that the Rocky Mountain spotted fever agent had bacterial, not protozoal, characteristics. However, he was unable to culture it to satisfy Koch's postulates. Wolbach is credited with identifying the causative bacterium, later classified as *Rickettsia rickettsii*, in the tick and demonstrating that the cultivation of this "wholly new type of microorganism" (84) was dependent on living cells. It is now recognized that ticks transmit the widest diversity of pathogenic microbes of humans of any of the arthropods.

DIVERSITY OF BACTERIA ASSOCIATED WITH TICKS

The phylogenetic relationships, inferred from 16S ribosomal RNA gene sequences, of bacteria associated with ticks are presented in Fig. 1. Most belong to the alpha and gamma subdivisions of the *Proteobacteria* and the class *Spirochaetes* (175). Members of the low-G+C gram-positive bacteria (136, 206) and the

Ulrike G. Munderloh, Steven D. Jauron, and Timothy J. Kurtti • Department of Entomology, University of Minnesota, St. Paul, MN 55108.

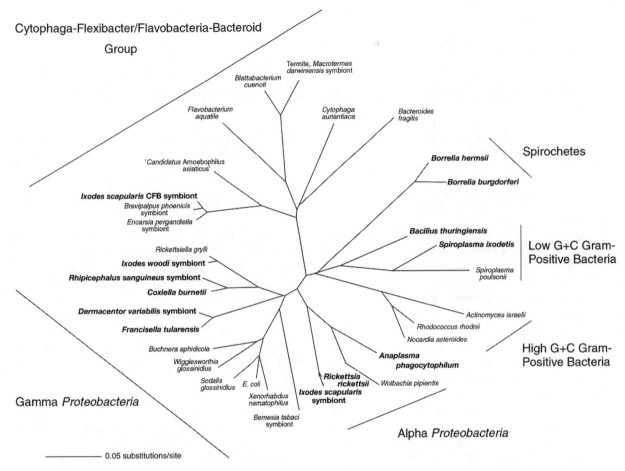

Figure 1. Phylogenetic relationship of bacteria associated with ticks. Endosymbionts and pathogens transmitted by ticks are shown in boldface type. The relationships between major bacterial groups are somewhat uncertain, and those shown in this unrooted tree are inferred from 16S rDNA sequences available in GenBank with the neighbor-joining method with PAUP*. The number of nucleotides being compared is 791. A list of the sequences used to construct this tree is available on request.

Cytophaga-Flexibacter/Flavobacteria-Bacteroid group (121) are also present, but less is known about their interaction with ticks.

The interaction between bacteria and ticks is a continuum between parasitism and mutualism. In addition to human and animal pathogens, ticks harbor bacterial endosymbionts maintained in nature via transovarial transmission. Tick-associated bacteria form distinct monophyletic groupings, and bacterial pathogens and endosymbionts cluster together. Endosymbionts appear to be nonpathogenic and are thought to provide essential nutrients to arthropods such as ticks that feed on a single nutritionally incomplete food source such as blood during all postembryonic life stages (28). Although the bacterial flora of ticks appears somewhat limited, combinations of endosymbionts and pathogens are often detected by microscopic and molecular diagnostic tests. These most frequently comprise phylogenetically unrelated bacteria, as there is evidence for interference between closely related species (see

"Rickettsiae," below). The ovaries of the wood tick *D. andersoni* can harbor a rickettsial endosymbiont, *Rickettsia peacockii*, and the DAS symbiont closely related to *Francisella tularensis* (Fig. 2) (157, 159). Often ticks are coinfected with symbiotic and pathogenic bacteria, and the challenge is to distinguish the risk for transmission of a pathogen during a tick bite. For example, the black-legged tick *Ixodes scapularis* can harbor both a rickettsial endosymbiont (237) that is not transmitted (Fig. 3) and the Lyme disease spirochete *Borrelia burgdorferi*. Less common, but of greater concern, is the coinfection and simultaneous transmission of two pathogens by the same tick. Several reports demonstrate that *Ixodes* ticks can harbor the human gran-ulocytic agent *Anaplasma phagocytophilum* and *B. burgdorferi* (70, 117, 123). The possible simultaneous infection and transmission of two or more pathogens have important clinical diagnostic and treatment implications that physicians need to be aware of (127, 141).

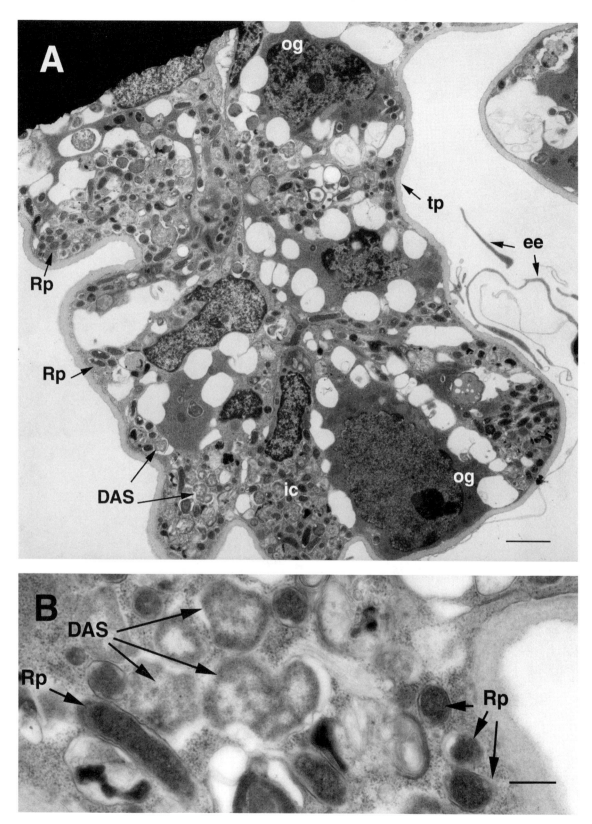

Figure 2. Transmission electron micrographs of ovarian tissues from unfed female *D. andersoni* ticks. This female was from the colony of ticks used to isolate cell line DAE100 chronically infected with *R. peacockii*. Ovarian tissues are coinfected with *R. peacockii* and the *Francisella*-related DAS bacterium. (A) Low magnification view of section of ovary with oogonia (og) and interstitial cells (ic). The ovary is surrounded by the tunica propria (tp) and external epithelium (ee). Note that interstitial cells (ic) are heavily infected with *R. peacockii* (Rp) and the DAS bacterium (DAS). Bar, 2 μm. (B) Cytoplasmic region of an interstitial cell containing aggregates of DAS bacterium and *R. peacockii*. Bar, 1 μm.

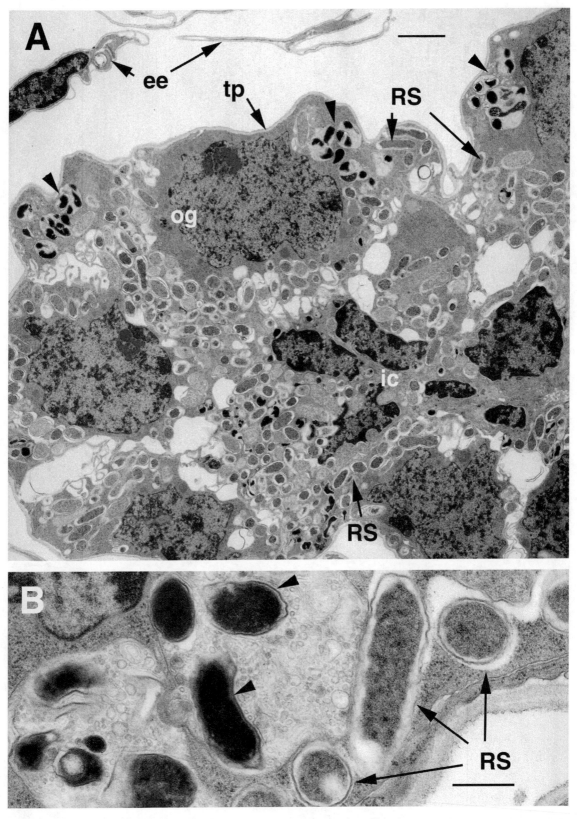

Figure 3. Transmission electron micrographs of *I. scapularis* ovarian tissues. This unfed female was from a laboratory colony persistently infected with a rickettsial organism (RS) closely related to *Rickettsia monacensis*, isolated from *I. ricinus* (215). Ovarian tissues are heavily infected with rickettsiae free in the cytoplasm (arrows) or within vacuoles (arrowheads). (A) Low-magnification view of section of ovary with oogonia (og) and interstitial cells (ic). Ovary is surrounded by the tunica propria (tp) and external epithelium (ee). Bar, 2 μm. (B) Cytoplasm of interstitial cell containing rickettsiae free in the cytoplasm (arrows) and being digested within phagolysosomes (arrowheads). Bar, 0.5 μm.

A NEW AND DIFFERENT KIND OF HOST—THE TICK

During their sojourn in the tick, pathogens experience drastic fluctuations in temperature, hemolymph osmotic pressure (values of 350 mosmol/liter may increase to >450 in unfed ticks), pH (varying from 6.8 in the gut to 9.5 in saliva), O_2 and CO_2 tensions in tissues (17 to 18% O_2 and 3% CO_2 in active feeding [F] ticks versus O_2 levels as low as 3% and CO_2 levels as high as 6% in unfed ticks), and nutrient flow (129, 148, 155). These changes, which are correlated with the physiological status of ticks, provide cues that induce DESA in pathogens and likely mediate transition from one host to the other at the appropriate time. A temperature increase and the beginning of engorgement are signals that have been shown to activate multiplication and release of tick-borne pathogens into the tick salivary duct, e.g., *Ehrlichia canis* (217) and *Anaplasma marginale* (224).

Digestive System and Saliva

Ticks feed exclusively on blood during all of their postembryonic life stages, which determines the microbes they are likely to contact. Ingested blood is taken into the midgut lumen, causing a drop in temperature to 30 to 34°C, depending on mammalian species and the tick attachment site. Concomitantly, loss of CO_2 from the blood meal causes the pH to change significantly. The midgut contents in hard ticks are weakly alkaline, and pH declines during the blood meal (11, 193, 240). Uptake of blood induces secretion of a peritrophic membrane that envelops the blood meal and serves as a potential microbial barrier (202). Digestion involves the lysis of erythrocytes within the gut lumen, ingestion of hemolysate by the digestive cells, and intracellular digestion of protein and lipids (45). Hemolysin activity in the midgut lumen (193) prepares the ingested blood for uptake by the midgut epithelial cells and intracellular digestion. Digestive cells are connected together at the apical borders by intercellular junctions that seal off the microbes in the lumen from the hemocoel and lateral spaces between the gut cells, but during the blood meal the gut barrier becomes penetrable by microbes such as spirochetes. The blood is concentrated as excess water, and ions are transported to the hemocoel and excreted back into the host as salivary secretions (208), providing an ideal transmission vehicle for tick-borne, salivarian pathogens. Blood-borne pathogens may take advantage of these mechanisms to enter and cross the midgut to infect other tissues and eventually be transferred back to the vertebrate via saliva. Tick saliva is alkaline at pH 9.5, hypertonic relative to hemolymph for sodium, and isotonic for potassium and chloride (11, 208, 240). During the blood meal, the size and protein content levels of the glands increase, and numerous genes are upregulated (21, 124, 156, 230) to overcome the host's hemostatic and immune responses at the bite site.

Blood is digested intracellularly by digestive cells that ingest the hemolysate by phagocytosis and receptor-mediated endocytosis (45). The subcellular compartments involved with intracellular digestion are hostile to most microbes. Digestive cells have lysosomes containing aspartic and cyteine proteinases (cathepsin L) with acidic pH optima of 3.0, similar to the enzymes within mammalian lysosomes (140). The activity of these lysosomal enzymes is influenced by the environmental pH of the cell, and an alkaline environment can make the lysosomes "sleepy" (66). Within lysosomes, hemoglobin is broken down into heme and globin.

Ticks and their microbes need to contend with an excess of heme, which can be toxic. Heme, a catalyst for the formation of reactive oxygen species (ROS), damages membrane lipids susceptible to peroxidation. Ticks have evolved mechanisms to address this excess of heme. The primary route of heme elimination is the conversion of heme to hematin by the digestive cells of the midgut. Hematin is liberated into the gut lumen by exocytosis and by digestive cell detachment and disruption (1, 45, 218). *Boophilus microplus* does not have an operative heme biosynthetic pathway (26) and relies on the salvage of the heme prosthetic group, a tetrapyrrole ring that chelates Fe^{2+} from the host blood meal. Hard and soft ticks have lipoglycoheme carrier proteins that sequester heme and have transferrin-like functions (81, 138). Tick vitellogenins and vitellins also function as heme carrier proteins and to sequester iron (130). Heme in tick tissues is stored by ferritin, which is cytosolic, as it is in vertebrates (113). Transferrin also has antimicrobial functions in that it sequesters iron away from pathogenic microbes that might need it. The recent findings about heme utilization and iron manipulation by ticks have implications for tick-microbe interactions that remain to be defined.

Tick Immunity

Ticks do not have the highly sophisticated and specific immune system of vertebrates (98), relying instead on small peptides (e.g., lysozyme and defensins) that attack microbial cell walls (153). Antigens that are strongly expressed in response to the mammalian immune defense are downregulated in the tick (67, 201, 212). Moreover, tick hemolymph contains lectins that are specific for glycoproteins bearing sialic acid residues, among others (80), and which act as receptors on the surfaces of mammalian cells for many pathogens. It seems unlikely, therefore, that tick-borne pathogens would utilize those same receptor components to spread through tick tissues as they do in vertebrates.

Hemocytes mediate the cellular defense response of ticks to microbes. In hard and soft ticks, coagulation of hemolymph is slow and the hemolymph does not darken when exposed to air (56). The basic types of hemocytes are prohemocytes, plasmatocytes, and granular hemocytes (granulocytes) (56, 75, 93, 119, 176, 250). The granular hemocytes have strong protease activity (93), and the lysosomal compartments contain acid phosphatase while lysozyme is present in the endoplasmic reticular cisternae and in primary lysosomes (119). The hemocyte composition of hemolymph is dynamic and influenced by microbial infection. The total hemocyte count in ticks is typically 10^3 to 10^4 hemocytes per μl and increases in response to a bacterial challenge, indicating that the hemocytes play a role in the phagocytosis of bacteria and yeasts (40, 99, 118, 132). Plasmatocytes phagocytize bacteria but not latex beads, while the granulocytes phagocytize both (119). The encapsulation of inanimate particles by granulocytes and plasmatocytes is biphasic: granulocytes degranulate to deposit a nonmelanized matrix around the implants, and plasmatocytes attach to and encapsulate the coated particle (60). Little is known about the role of opsonizing factors on the process of phagocytosis by tick hemocytes, but serum components from the host may play a role (93). There is selectivity in the hemocytic response of ticks to bacteria (40, 99). Hemocytes of *B. microplus* produce ROS during the phagocytosis of bacteria and yeasts (176), and since the protein kinase C activator induces this ROS production, the oxidative burst probably involves protein kinase C modulation, similar to what occurs with vertebrate phagocytes.

The tick's innate immune system includes lectins, phenoloxidase, lysozyme, and defensin. In terms of molecular structure, the innate immune system of ticks appears to be phylogenetically more closely related to that of lower arthropods than that of insects. Lectins are associated with the gut and hemolymph and participate in the recognition, opsonization, phagocytosis, and destruction of microbes by tick cells (80). A lectin (Dorin M) with hemagglutinating activity and specificity for sialic acid and *N*-acetylglucosamine moieties has been purified from the hemolymph of *Ornithodoros moubata* (115). The role that phenoloxidase and the production of melanin, a microbicide, play in the innate immune response of ticks is equivocal. Phenoloxidase activity could not be detected in hemolymph or whole-body homogenates of *Dermacentor variabilis*, *I. scapularis*, or *Amblyomma americanum* (251). Phenoloxidase activity in soft ticks is influenced by the molting cycle but is at lower levels than in insects (110). An α-2 macroglobulin-like glycoprotein with protease-inhibiting properties has been identified in the plasma and may play a role in phenoloxidase activity (112). Proteolytic cascades are involved in invertebrate clot formation, prophenoloxidase activation, and expression of antimicrobial peptides. This protease inhibitor is active against a broad spectrum of proteases and may be involved in the regulation of immune proteolytic cascades in ticks. Lysozyme, an enzyme that degrades the peptidoglycan in bacterial cell walls, is present in soft and hard ticks (182). The lysozymes from ticks are active against gram-positive bacteria but not the gram-negative *Escherichia coli*. The *O. moubata* lysozyme, a 14-kDa protein with a pH optima of 6, is found mainly with the gut. Its activity is highest after a blood meal (111).

Defensins are cationic peptides active against gram-positive bacteria. These peptides are found in soft and hard ticks. A family of defensins in *O. moubata* gut and hemolymph is primarily involved with midgut immunity against microbes in the blood meal (152, 153, 231). The isoforms A and B are expressed constitutively and inducible in response to bacteria and the blood meal. Isoforms C and D are upregulated during feeding and are at highest levels in the gut 5 to 15 days after feeding. All four defensins, coded as preprodefensins, have four exons and three introns, similar to the gene organization seen in mussels but not in insects (152). They comprised 73 amino acids with putative signal sequences. Another defensin-like protein has been isolated from *D. variabilis* (101). Host blood also contributes elements of the host's innate and adaptive immune system to the tick. Two blood proteins from the host that provide antimicrobial activity (transferrin and immunoglobulin G) are present in the hemolymph after feeding. A peptide with antibacterial (against gram-positive organisms) and antifungal activity is processed from hemoglobin by *B. microplus* (72).

The life cycle of ticks and their microbes can be subdivided into two phases: feast and famine. Dynamic physiological changes occur in ticks during the blood meal and prior to molting, a time of water and nutrient availability. After molting and until the next blood meal, ticks and their associated microbes persist under conditions of nutrient depletion. Tick-transmitted pathogens have evolved small genomes that limit their biosynthetic capabilities but still enable them to survive periods of nutrient starvation and respond quickly to environmental changes. Differential gene expression ensures that only those genes that are necessary for survival and transmission are expressed when needed. The environmental cues to which tick-transmitted pathogens respond include temperature, pH, nutrient availability, microbial numbers, and osmotic pressure.

Borrelia

Dynamics of *B. burgdorferi* development in *I. scapularis*

I. scapularis acquires *B. burgdorferi* when larvae or nymphs feed on a spirochetemic host. Transovarial transmission is rare, and its role in the epidemiology of Lyme disease is uncertain (178). The number of borreliae per larva increases during and after the blood meal; replete larvae harbor up to 3,000 spirochetes. But shortly before and during the molt to the nymph stage, the number of spirochetes declines to a few hundred (181). During the first 36 h after nymphal attachment, spirochetes multiply and fill the gut with several thousand spirochetes. During the next 12 h, spirochetes continue to multiply and penetrate the spaces between the gut epithelial cells to invade the hemocoel and salivary glands (52, 252). At this time, spirochetes in the gut become "wolves in sheep's clothing" by coating themselves with plasminogen from the blood of the tick's host. In the presence of urokinase (also from the blood), plasminogen is converted to plasmin, a disseminating factor that enhances the ability of the spirochetes to penetrate between the midgut cells and invade the hemocoel (44). By the time the spirochetes are in the salivary gland and infectious spirochetes are likely to be transmitted to a mammalian host (48 to 72 h postattachment), the nymph can harbor up to 100,000 spirochetes (52). Spirochetes continue to increase after the replete nymph has dropped off the host but, for unknown reasons, decline again during the molt to the adult (181).

The variable Osp expression paradigm

Variable expression of the outer surface lipoproteins (Osps), especially the two major immunogenic lipoproteins OspA and OspC, is hypothesized to be involved in spirochetal survival and transmission (210). OspA and OspC are two major immunogenic lipoproteins that are variably expressed in ticks (68, 212). Spirochetes upregulate OspA expression during their colonization of the larval gut (54) and continue to express OspA until the next blood meal. At the time of the nymphal blood meal, spirochetes downregulate OspA expression and upregulate OspC (68, 69, 211, 212).

Antibodies to OspA are borreliacidal and block spirochetal colonization of the tick. If larvae feed on spirochetemic animals passively immunized with OspA antibodies, spirochetes fail to colonize the larvae (54).

OspA promotes spirochetal adherence to the gut cells, and antibodies to OspA inhibit this binding (169, 170). Recombinant OspA- and OspA-expressing spirochetes selectively bind to tick gut extracts and tissues but not to the salivary gland. OspA also binds plasminogen from the blood, and the presence of this proteolytic enzyme on the outer surface enhances the spirochetes' ability to penetrate the gut and invade the salivary glands (44). The OspA epitopes involved with adhesion and borreliacidal activity are distinct from each other. During the blood meal, OspA is cleared from the surfaces of most (80%) of the spirochetes (167). Elimination of OspA facilitates the release of the spirochetes from the gut cells and migration to the salivary glands. Spirochetes that do not express OspA are resistant to OspA antibodies (53, 55). The receptor(s) for OspA in the gut remains to be fully characterized, but a putative receptor with a molecular mass of more than 100 kDa has been identified (169). The surface proteins responsible for the selective adherence and invasion of the salivary glands have not been identified.

The expression of OspC by spirochetes during the blood meal correlates with their acquisition of spirochetal infectivity for the mammalian host. The addition of tick hemolymph to culture medium induces the expression of OspC, an effect independent of temperature (100). Similarly, the cocultivation of spirochetes with *I. scapularis* cells at 37°C induces a decline in OspA and an induction of OspC expression (163). These results indicate that tick factors are involved with the induction of changes in the Osp composition of spirochetes, making them a research subject well worth studying.

Borrelia burgdorferi populations in feeding nymphs are heterogeneous

During the blood meal, spirochete populations become genetically and antigenically heterogeneous. The hypotheses that OspA mediates *B. burgdorferi* adherence to gut epithelial cells and that OspC is involved with dissemination and salivary gland invasion lead to the prediction that OspA-expressing spirochetes will remain confined to the gut, while those expressing OspC will move to the salivary glands (167). Indeed, spirochete populations in the guts of unfed ticks are relatively homogenous and most (85%) express only OspA, whereas the remainder express neither OspA nor OspC. In feeding ticks, spirochetes expressing only OspA decline, and the proportion that expresses OspC or neither Osp increases. At the time when spirochetes acquire infectivity (48 to 72 h) (179, 180), the great majority (80 to 90%) do not express either OspA or OspC (167). During the blood meal, spirochetes in the midgut and salivary glands express many of the OspE/F/Elp paralogs, whereas those spirochetes in the salivary glands that express these antigens express neither OspA nor OspC (86, 87). In UF ticks, the *vlsE* locus is stable, but during the blood meal multiple *vlsE* alleles are observed (167).

Differential gene expression by spirochetes in ticks

Numerous genes, in addition to those that code for Osps, are also differentially expressed and play a role in the survival and transmission of spirochetes (77, 154). Spirochetes use two basic mechanisms to regulate the expression of genes that code for surface lipoproteins. Genes, such as *ospA* and *ospC*, are under transcriptional control. Others such as the *vlsE* locus, a postulated virulence factor and antigenic variation protein, are under genetic control involving the unidirectional recombination between silent cassettes and the *vlsE* gene (247). The differential expression with customized amplification library (DECAL) approach has identified 48 genes differentially expressed in ticks: 16 in spirochetes within unfed ticks and 32 within fed ticks (154). The genes, most of which are located on the chromosome, are upregulated as spirochetes prepare to invade the mammalian host; the genes are also involved in several different cellular processes: DNA synthesis, energy (glycerol) metabolism, and nutrient uptake. Also activated are genes for putative lipoproteins and the periplasmic proteins, components of signaling circuits, and an integrin receptor. A gene that encodes N-acetylglucosamine-6-phosphate deacetylase is also upregulated, supporting the hypothesis that the spirochetes use N-acetylglucosamine as a source of energy and/or cell wall biosynthesis.

Environmental cues that impact B. burgdorferi gene activity

The interacting effects of environmental parameters on *B. burgdorferi* gene expression in the vector can be examined with controlled in vitro conditions. The use of an in vitro model is subject to the caveat that the results need to be compared with those obtained with ticks, as not all genes upregulated by an increase in temperature are upregulated in the tick at the time of the blood meal (82). *B. burgdorferi* grown axenically in Barbour-Stoenner-Kelly (BSK) medium is quite homogeneous and its protein expression profile is said to most closely resemble that of spirochetes in the gut of a questing tick (51, 212). Nevertheless, gene expression and antigen profiles of cultured spirochetes differ from spirochetes directly purified from infected ticks (187). Fundamental to determining the environmental cues that impact gene expression is the

determination of the physiological extremes that spirochetes are exposed to within *Ixodes* ticks. The pH of the midgut of an unfed *I. scapularis* is alkaline (pH 7.4) and declines to near neutral (pH 6.8) as the tick feeds. Hemolymph pH has been measured as 6.8, but during periods of hypoxia (discontinuous respiration) and hypercapnia (increased CO_2) (129) this value remains to be determined. Infection with spirochetes does not appear to disrupt the pH of nymphal or adult body fluids (240).

The reciprocal expression of OspA and OspC is regulated by the interaction of pH and temperature. The expression of more than 37 genes is modulated by pH of the culture medium within a pH range of 6 to 8, but not the OspE-related proteins (Erps) (38, 39). At 23°C, pH has no effect on *ospA*, *ospB*, or *ospC* expression (240). Spirochetes exposed to a decline in medium pH (pH 7.4 to pH 6.8) or an increase in temperature (to ≥34°C) express OspC when the culture reaches a high population density, while expression of OspA is downregulated (240). Expression is not affected by an alkaline pH similar to that of saliva (i.e., pH 9.7). These results agree with the studies noted above that the *ospC* gene is upregulated while spirochetes are still in the gut at a pH of 6.8 during the blood meal (167). Other genes are also regulated in a reciprocal manner and show either the *ospC* (*ospF*, *mlp8*, *dbpA*, and *rpoS*) or *ospA* (*relA/spoT*, *lp6.6*, and *p22*) patterns. A putative global regulator, the *rpoS* gene that encodes the transcription sigma^S (σ^S) factor also shows the *ospC* pattern, suggesting that genes upregulated during the blood meal are under the control of σ^S (240). Microarray analyses also demonstrate that a significant proportion of the genome is differentially expressed when spirochetes are exposed to changes in culture conditions that simulate those in unfed (UF) and feeding (F) nymphs (191, 200). Comparing spirochetes cultured in BSK medium at 37°C and pH 6.8 with those incubated at 23°C and pH 7.5 demonstrates that 150, or 9%, of the genes are differentially expressed at the higher temperature and that most genes encode proteins that are exported (191). Under the restrictive unfed conditions, there is a stringent response, as well as an induction of factors that restrict spirochete division. Most of the genes expressed in the fed condition are transiently active and associated with energy metabolism, spirochetal mobility, transport proteins, and synthesis of proteins and the cell wall. Members of the *bdr* gene family, paralogous genes encoding the highly polymorphic inner membrane proteins, also respond selectively and differentially to changes in culture temperature and serum deprivation and correlate with conditions prevalent in fed ticks (200). Deletion of serum from BSK medium simulates conditions in unfed ticks. Serum provides essential lipids and fatty acids that spirochetes cannot synthesize de novo, and deprivation induces at least 20 spirochetal proteins. The effects are selective in that only subsets of the Bdr paralogs are affected (2). In addition, OspA and a VlsE homolog are upregulated during serum deprivation but not OspC or GroEl. Spirochetes grown under serum deprivation conditions transform into nonmotile cyst forms, similar to those forms observed with ticks and tick cell culture (34, 122).

Regulatory mechanisms of spirochetal gene expression

Pathogenic bacteria use quorum-sensing mechanisms to regulate gene expression within a population and coordinate their biological activities (209). Key components of this intracellular signal transduction mechanism are the autoinducer molecule autoinducer-2 (AI-2) and the enzyme LuxS. *B. burgdorferi* uses the LuxS-autoinducer to regulate protein synthesis at the population level (154, 222). It is hypothesized that *B. burgdorferi* uses the autoinducer to regulate protein synthesis during the tick-to-mammal transmission step.

Peptide transporters (signaling oligopeptide permeases) play a role in the bacterial response to environmental changes. Oligopeptide permeases are especially crucial to bacteria, such as *B. burgdorferi* (73), that lack genes for the synthesis of amino acids. Spirochetes are hypothesized to use peptides as pheromones to trigger an adaptive response to a change in their environment as they cycle between the tick and the mammalian host. The genes that encode putative oligopeptide permeases include a chromosomal *opp* operon, which encodes three substrate-binding lipoproteins, and two additional plasmid genes (23). The permease promoters are responsive to pertinent environmental signals, and each gene has its own upstream promoter region and is independently regulated and transcribed (23, 234). All five *oppA* genes appear to be functional and active in *B. burgdorferi*, and temperature has varied effects on the promoter activity of these genes. The OppA homologs are differentially expressed in the tick (154, 234). Medium temperature and changes in nutrient availability affect gene expression, but pH does not (234).

The global response of *B. burgdorferi* to environmental change in cultured spirochetes has been examined (29, 61). A stringent response in bacteria is a global response triggered by nutritional or environmental stress, during which cellular metabolism, macromolecular synthesis, and growth decline. The stringent response is mediated by the alarmones ppGpp and (p)ppGp that are generated by the sigma factors RelA (a synthase) and SpoT (a hydrolase), respectively.

B. burgdorferi has an active *relA/spoT* homolog that generates a stringent response in BSK culture that is dampened when spirochetes are grown with tick cells (29). The proteins RpoS and RpoN control the expression of OspC and DbpA in BSK-cultured *B. burgdorferi* (91a). RpoN controls the transcription of *rpoS*, *ospC*, and *dbpA* genes, and RpoS is involved with the resistance of *B. burgdorferi* to osmotic stress (e.g., exposure to 1 M NaCl) (61). The stringent response of spirochetes in starved and fed ticks needs to be examined in order to evaluate the significance of these findings.

Ehrlichia and *Anaplasma*

Organisms in the genus *Ehrlichia* have stirred the imagination and interest of researchers in the biomedical sciences because of their complex life history, particularly since their recognition as human pathogens (3, 46). Previous publications have reviewed in detail the clinicopathological features of the ehrlichioses (9, 168, 188, 198, 243), and we do not intend to repeat this significant body of information. On the other hand, insights gained from studies with the animal-pathogenic *Anaplasma*, *Cowdria*, and *Ehrlichia* have contributed importantly to our understanding about mechanisms of immune evasion used by these microbes (15, 189) and their development in the tick (107, 108, 217). Even if by name not all are classified as *Ehrlichia* species at the time this review is written, the recent reexamination of their phylogenetic placement warrants their inclusion here (27). The members of the tribe *Ehrlichieae* have recently been transferred to the family *Anaplasmataceae*, and the genus *Anaplasma* has been emended to include *Anaplasma* (*Ehrlichia*) *phagocytophilum* (*phagocytophila*), the genus *Ehrlichia* has been emended to include *Ehrlichia* (*Cowdria*) *ruminantium*, and the genus *Neorickettsia* has been emended to include *Neorickettsia* (*Ehrlichia*) *risticii* (58). The latter genus will not be considered in this review.

The family *Anaplasmataceae* includes animal disease agents known for many years as well as emerging pathogens of humans. All share the characteristics of an obligate intracellular existence and are contained in a membrane-lined vacuole primarily within blood cells, cells associated with blood vessels, and the reticuloendothelial system (3, 10, 57, 186, 199). The type species of the genus *Ehrlichia* is the etiologic agent of tropical canine pancytopenia, *E. canis* (62, 92, 196). Until quite recently, no species of *Ehrlichia* were thought to infect humans, but at least three species— *Ehrlichia chaffeensis*, the human monocytic ehrlichiosis agent (3, 47, 64); the human granulocytic anaplasmosis (HGA) agent (10, 14, 42, 79, 232); and

Ehrlichia ewingii (4, 30)—are now recognized among emerging tick-borne zoonotic agents with animal reservoirs. Humans are likely an incidental, dead-end host, becoming infected when the vector tick habitat is entered (91), and may suffer a life-threatening illness (59, 79). Humans do not play a role in the maintenance of the ehrlichias in nature. Unlike ehrlichias' natural hosts (e.g., cattle for the bovine pathogen, *Anaplasma marginale* [172], deer for *E. chaffeensis* [47], or canines for *Ehrlichia canis* [94]), there is to date no evidence that humans become persistently infected. The illness in humans is typically an acute, febrile condition accompanied by myalgias and general malaise. Laboratory findings are characterized by leukopenia, thrombocytopenia, and elevated serum transaminase levels (10, 59, 79). In contrast, natural reservoir hosts either recover from an initial acute infection and go on to become carriers, as in bovine anaplasmosis (15), or do not suffer outward signs of illness, as in *E. chaffeensis* infections of white-tailed deer (47, 64). The animal species that serve as reservoirs for the HGA agent have not unequivocally been identified. While a number of feral small animals have been found to be naturally infected, including white-footed mice (232), these animals seem to become immune and clear the infection within a few weeks (228). Nevertheless, long-term infection in animals is not necessarily a prerequisite for their function as pathogen reservoirs. Animals need only to be parasitemic and available to vectors for a time sufficient to allow infection of the vector. This time period depends in part on the efficiency with which the vector is able to acquire the organism. Studies to determine these parameters remain to be done for most ehrlichias and anaplasmas.

The classification of pathogens considered ehrlichias has undergone a revision that is important to our understanding of their biology (58). Originally, taxonomic assignment relied largely on identification of the mammalian host species (as for *E. canis*), the target cells recognized by microscopy (as for the monocytic versus granulocytic species), and the presence of these pathogens in an intracellular endosomal compartment. This meant that quite closely related pathogens, such as *A. marginale*, parasitizing bovine erythrocytes, and the former *E. phagocytophilum/Ehrlichia equi/*human granulocytic ehrichiosis (HGE) group (now *A. phagocytophilum*), infecting neutrophil granulocytes (43), were considered different genera. On the other hand, phylogenetically much more distant microbes, such as *N. risticii* (formerly *E. risticii*), were included in the same genus. The use of molecular techniques, notably sequence analysis of the gene for the highly conserved 16S ribosomal subunit (27) and the *groESL* genes, has reconfirmed some but dismantled other groupings (58). As these genes have changed little over evolutionary time, these techniques allowed resolution of the major branches in the family tree of ehrlichias, and it became apparent that *N. risticii*, the causative agent of Potomac horse fever, is not an ehrlichia. Grouping *N. risticii* with the neorickettsiae that also include the agent of salmon poisoning, *Neorickettsia helminthoeca*, and of Sennetsu fever caused by *N. sennetsu* (17, 185) has led researchers to reconsider the idea that Potomac horse fever must be transmitted by ticks or other bloodsucking arthropods (31, 83). Indeed, as for *N. helminthoeca*, trematodes infesting fresh-water snails have recently been incriminated (17, 190). This neatly leaves a much more coherent group of tick-borne *Anaplasma* and *Ehrlichia* species that are pathogenic for humans and animals and which are the subject of this review.

Development in the tick and potential relevance to parasite evolution and pathogenesis

For a tick-borne pathogen, passage from the mammal to the vector is a required step for its maintenance in nature and is therefore obligatory. The organisms have to be present in the blood, enter the tick bite site in sufficient numbers, and be biologically fit to infect the tick productively, so that they can eventually be transferred to and survive in a new vertebrate host when the tick takes its next blood meal. Gametocytes, which are specific, morphologically distinct developmental stages, infectious only for ticks, have been identified in *Babesia microti* (202), a protozoan blood parasite that causes a disease similar to malaria. Given the drastic physiological changes experienced by ehrlichiae when ingested by the tick during its blood meal, it is conceivable that ehrlichiae produce tick-infectious organisms in response to some cue from the mammal or are able to rapidly respond to signals from their new host, the tick. Neither of these strategies has been shown to be utilized by anaplasmas or ehrlichias, although their constant low-level presence in circulating blood may expressly serve this function, while other sites in the body are the primary locations of replication. In support of this hypothesis is the finding that those ehrlichial pathogens for which data are available are known to infect and often persist in tissues such as the bone marrow (e.g., the HGA agent) (79), endocardium and capillary endothelium (e.g., *E. ruminantium*) (186), and spleen, kidney, lymph nodes, and liver (e.g., *E. canis* and *E. chaffeensis*) (71, 94).

Anaplasma marginale as a model for development in the tick

As noted above, the life phase of the cattle pathogen *A. marginale* in one of its vectors, the Rocky Mountain wood tick, *D. andersoni*, has been studied rather extensively by light and transmission electron microscopy. This pathogen is unique and differs from others in the genogroup in that it is capable of infecting and being biologically transmitted by many tick species (63, 177). Moreover, it invades and replicates profusely in most tissues of the tick, starting with the midgut epithelium and eventually spreads to the salivary glands via hemocytes, muscle, nervous tissue, and subcutis (107, 221, 224). Even so, transovarial transmission does not occur. However, *Anaplasma* takes unique advantage of the male *Dermacentor* tick's habit of feeding intermittently while seeking out females for mating. In crowded herd situations where animals are in close contact, male ticks may switch hosts repeatedly. In males that have ingested infected blood, the anaplasmas multiply rapidly and progress to infectious particles within salivary glands in about a week (109). Thus, adult male ticks serve as highly efficient vectors capable of quickly disseminating bovine anaplasmosis throughout a herd (244). Development in nymphs is more protracted than in males, continuing throughout an intermolt period that lasts weeks (107).

During their development in tick tissues, *Anaplasma* show much greater morphological diversity and complexity than in bovine erythrocytes. Still, the blood meal that remains in the midgut interferes with light and electron microscopic observation of *Anaplasma* development for the first week or more after tick attachment, leaving the initial phases of invasion and spread obscure. By day 10, membrane-bound colonies of *A. marginale* are found in tissues and organs throughout the tick's body. They contain either pale, relatively large (up to 1.2 μm in diameter) organisms with recognizable threads of DNA, reticulate bodies that are thought to be the actively replicating form, or smaller (<1 mm in diameter) more condensed individuals thought to be the infectious form (22). Single cells may contain colonies of different morphological types.

Anaplasma and *Ehrlichia* in vector cell culture

Anaplasmas and ehrlichias are difficult to study in ticks, because with the exception of *A. marginale* (107) and *E. ruminantium* (108, 186), only very few colonies have been found in *E. canis*-infected brown dog ticks (217), and none in lone star ticks or black-legged ticks infected with *E. chaffeensis* or *A. phagocytophilum*, respectively. It appears that in ticks, these organisms either are very rare and do not multiply significantly or are in an obscure state. In addition, until recently, there were no suitable vector cell culture systems to study their development in vitro (147, 149). Consequently, very little was known about the molec-

ular, cellular, and immune biology of members of the family *Anaplasmataceae* during their sojourn in the tick, an area critical to understanding pathogenesis as well as providing key data to potentially allow control of the disease through immune prophylaxis or prevention of transmission. The ability to study the anaplasmas and ehrlichias in vector cell cultures has opened new avenues to circumvent such obstacles. Once they became available, established tick cell lines from the primitive genus *Ixodes* proved to be susceptible to a wide range of tick-associated rickettsial organisms, symbiotic nonpathogenic (8, 216) as well as pathogenic (19, 22, 144, 146, 151). For some, e.g., *A. marginale*, whose only known target cell in cattle appears to be the mature, nonreplicating erythrocyte, tick cell culture offers a self-replicating in vitro system (144). Curiously, earlier attempts to culture *A. marginale* in tick cell lines from vector ticks (90, 205) did not result in establishment and continuous replication of cattle-infectious organisms. It is likely that these culture systems failed to provide the other, additionally important cues that signal commencement of tick feeding and a chance for transmission to the bovine. *E. canis* was most infectious when partially fed and ground-up ticks were used to inoculate dogs (217). Similarly, the successful isolation and continuous cultivation of vertebrate-infectious *A. marginale*, *A. phagocytophilum*, and *E. canis* all required simulation of an "activated tick" environment. Features included incubation at an elevated temperature of 34°C, addition of bicarbonate as a CO_2 source (shown to be essential for spotted fever rickettsiae) (114), use of a medium (L-15B) that mirrors the feeding tick internal biochemical environment (147), a medium pH of 7.5 or higher, and for *A. phagocytophilum*, reduction of the osmotic pressure to 300 mosmol/liter. These are some of the stimuli that in concert signal tick-borne pathogens to resume growth after a period of dormancy and prepare for transmission to the vertebrate host (102). In this context, it is of interest to note that *E. ruminantium* grows slowly in IDE8 cells cultured at 30°C in medium of about 400 mosmol/liter and is not infectious for sheep (19).

The individual *A. marginale* organisms and the types of colonies that form inside *I. scapularis* cell line IDE8 or ISE6 (Fig. 4) (22, 144) closely resemble those found in the tick *D. andersoni* (107), and are unlike the tiny inclusions seen in erythrocytes, supporting the validity of this system to study the vector phase of ehrlichiae in vitro. These morphological changes are accompanied by quantitative or qualitative changes in antigen expression (95, 96, 171). Comparison of *Anaplasma* antigens derived from cattle erythrocytes and ticks (144, 171) demonstrated that major surface proteins (MSPs) were expressed in the agent from

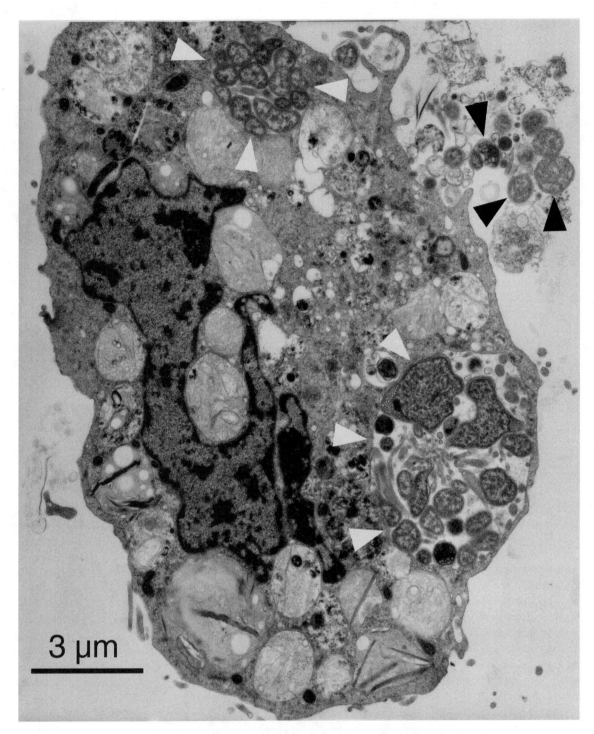

Figure 4. Electron micrograph of *A. marginale* in the *I. scapularis* tick cell line ISE6. Note the considerable degree of pleomorphism of individual organisms in an endosome. Note a convoluted network of excess membranes at one pole of some microbes, long, tail-like extensions arising from several of the anaplasmas within intracellular inclusions (white arrowheads). Black arrowheads indicate extracellular organisms. Bar, 3 μm.

either source. However, blood-derived *Anaplasma* appeared to preferentially express MSP2 (36 kDa), MSP3 (86 kDa), and an antigen of about 55 kDa (12, 144) when probed with antiserum raised against purified erythrocytic stages of *A. marginale*, while those from tick salivary glands and tick cell cultures expressed MSP4 more strongly. Nevertheless, monoclonal antibodies (MAbs) detected the presence of MSP1 to MSP5 in tick cell-cultured *Anaplasma* (12), indicating the stability of these antigens in the cultured organisms. The meaning of these qualitative differences in antigen expression of *Anaplasma* from infected cattle versus tick salivary glands or tick cell culture is not known but hints at adaptive differential expression in response to unique host environments.

E. canis isolated from dog blood became established and continuously grew in IDE8 cells as well. Electron microscopy identified large intracellular inclusions like those seen in ticks (217), which were recognized by immunofluorescence assays of infected dog sera. These ehrlichiae remained infective and pathogenic for dogs for at least five in vitro passages (65), in contrast to *E. canis* cultured in the dog macrophage cell line DH82 (48, 238), which does not retain infectivity for dogs (137). Western blot patterns of *E. canis* from IDE8 tick cells were quite different from those of the same isolate from DH82 cells. In this study, dogs infected by inoculation of infected IDE8 cells became blood-smear positive 10 to 16 days postinoculation (p.i.), much sooner than after tick bite. When reacted with *E. canis* from DH82 cells, sera from these dogs recognized primarily low-molecular-mass antigens of approximately 18 to 25 and 30 to 32 kDa. The latter were probably P28 (major antigenic protein 1 [MAP1]) (139, 164, 189, 225) surface antigens expressed by an immune-dominant gene family conserved in this ehrlichia genogroup (i.e., comprising *E. canis*, *E. chaffeensis*, and *E. ruminantium*). Larger molecular mass bands of 38, 45, and 55 kDa were found, but not consistently. In tick cell-cultured *E. canis*, antigen bands were sharper and more numerous than those from DH82 cultures, although bands in the 30- to 32-kDa mass range were less well recognized. Apparently, survival of *E. canis* in the dog macrophage cell line requires enhanced expression of the MAP1 homologs, which appeared downregulated in tick cell culture.

A. phagocytophilum likewise can be cultured in *I. scapularis* cell lines (146, 151). These organisms have not been demonstrated morphologically in vivo in ticks, but their presence in *I. scapularis*, *Ixodes pacificus*, and the European *Ixodes ricinus* has been confirmed by PCR and transmission studies of susceptible animals (16, 70, 173, 174, 197, 228). In cultures of cell lines IDE8 and ISE6 of the biological vector *I. scapularis*, the organisms undergo striking morphological changes after transfer from equine or dog blood neutrophils to tick cells (146, 151). A similar transformation is observed when infected HL60 cells are used as the inoculum (79, 146). Notably, ehrlichial inclusions (colonies) within tick cells can become very large, and individual ehrlichiae are much more pleomorphic than in peripheral blood granulocytes or the human leukemia cell line HL60. These changes occurred rapidly; after only 1 week, *I. scapularis* IDE8 or ISE6 cultures contained only those ehrlichial colonies

typically found in tick cell culture. Presumably, they represent the ehrlichial stages specific to the tick. Time sequence-of-infection studies using a human *A. phagocytophilum* isolate (79) showed that the ehrlichiae attached rapidly and were taken into tick cells via phagocytosis within 4 h. Areas of cell-ehrlichial membrane adhesion appeared to slide around the bacteria until they were totally enclosed in a host endosome, suggesting a specific, receptor-mediated process. Organisms seen enclosed inside endosomes started to divide as early as 8 to 12 h p.i., leading to formation of large endosomes filled with numerous mostly electron-lucent ehrlichiae, including a few electron-dense forms by 48 h (146).

Like *E. canis*, *A. phagocytophilum* grown in tick cell culture remained infectious and severely pathogenic for the horse and could be reisolated in tick cell culture from a horse inoculated with such material (151). Laboratory hamsters and mice inoculated intraperitoneally with the HGA agent from ISE6 cells seroconverted and developed an immune response similar to that seen with humans (96). Again, the antigen pattern in Western blots observed with tick cell-cultured *A. phagocytophilum* was distinct from that obtained from HL60 culture. Notably, the intensity and number of bands in the 40- to 45-kDa molecular mass range was much reduced. Like the MAP1 family of the genogroup that includes *E. canis*, the p44 proteins are immune dominant proteins that are structurally and antigenically conserved among the anaplasmas and thought to be involved in immune evasion (248). Their reduced expression in tick cells would seem to support that role.

Immune evasion and antigenic variation

Anaplasmas and ehrlichias express specific sets of immune-reactive proteins on their surfaces that can be used in clinical applications to diagnose the species causing an infection (41). It was soon noticed that there were certain dominant antigens that showed variability in size and number of bands on Western blots when different isolates of the same species were compared (6) and that certain antigens showed significant cross-reactivity among different species and genera (41, 48, 135, 225). Tick-borne anaplasmas and ehrlichias express variable, immunodominant outer membrane proteins (OMPs) that are encoded by multigene families and which are related by nucleotide sequence and amino acid composition. They have a central hypervariable region flanked by highly conserved sequences. These sequences appear to function in immune evasion to allow the pathogen to persist in animals through successive generations of antigenically variant strains (74). In *E. ruminantium*, *E. canis*, and *E. chaffeensis*, these are arranged in tandem (135, 165–167); in *A. phagocytophilum* and *A. marginale*, they are not clustered (13, 248). Chronic, persistent anaplasma and ehrlichia infections have been well documented in some animals that presumably are the natural reservoirs for the respective pathogen, e.g., cattle infected with anaplasmosis (74) and dogs suffering from tropical pancytopenia due to *E. canis* (94). Such persistent infections have, however, not been documented in humans.

In bovine *A. marginale* infections, five MSPs have been identified that give rise to neutralizing antibodies, termed MSP1 to MSP5. MSP1 is a large heterodimer composed of two units linked by disulfide bonds. The larger MSP1a is encoded by a single-copy gene and shows significant variation among isolates. MSP1b, on the other hand, is coded for by a multicopy gene and is stable among strains. Indeed, MSP1a appears stable over as long as 2 years, as only a single genotype was identified in a herd after a recent outbreak in an area where *A. marginale* infection was not endemic. By contrast, in an endemic situation, many different genotypes of *msp1α* were detected in a herd of persistently infected reservoir animals. It is possible that over time, new isolates may be introduced by the acquisition of carrier cows from distant regions. MSP2 and MSP3 are also encoded by multicopy genes, while MSP4 and MSP5 have single-copy genes. One of the characteristics of chronic anaplasmosis of cattle is the cyclic recurrence of rickettsemic peaks at intervals of 1 to 2 months. Each population representing a new wave of rickettsiae expresses a novel MSP2 antigenic type, characterized by changes in the central hypervariable region of the protein. During the course of a disease that can persist for years, numerous variants are generated through combinatorial recombination into a polymorphic expression site, representing the only complete and functional gene, involving polycistronic mRNA. This mechanism, which is similar to the function of the *vls* genes of *B. burgdorferi*, utilizes an estimated 20 silent genes, or pseudogenes, that are recombined into the expression site to generate the large number of *msp2* variants expressed during each wave of rickettsemia (13). The pseudogenes possess a central hypervariable region that is flanked by highly conserved sequences that are truncated with respect to the complete gene, such that they are nonfunctional and silent until recombined into the expression site. Additional variants arise through a mechanism of gene conversion, creating the potential to generate far in excess of the 500 variants needed for *A. marginale* to persist during the life of an infected bovine (25). Even so, only a small number of variant *msp2* genes are detected and expressed in tick salivary glands, supporting the notion that immune pressure in the bovine host is the force driving generation of the many variants seen there. Sequence analysis of transcripts from ticks infected with the South Idaho strains showed only two expressed variants, SGV1 and SGV2, independent of the variants present in the bovine blood at the time when the ticks fed. Moreover, only these two variants were expressed during the acute rickettsemia that resulted from tick bite transmission (203). Different isolates of *A. marginale* similarly demonstrate a restricted pattern of variants expressed in the tick, although not the same ones as in the South Idaho isolate. Moreover, tick vector species may influence the types of MSP2 variants that they transmit, overall resulting in a heterogeneous array of MSP2 variants causing the initial rickettsemic wave after infection. This implies that ticks represent a strong selective force in the epidemiology of anaplasmosis and that vaccines based on or incorporating MSP2 must be designed with this in mind (204). Three additional open reading frames (ORFs), *opag1* to *opag3*, are located within the 3.5-kb operon containing *msp2*, upstream of the *msp2* ORF. In contrast to *msp2*, these MSP2 operon-associated proteins are well conserved among isolates. Although *opag1* mRNA was detectable, no corresponding protein could be found, suggesting that mRNA is subject to posttranscriptional modification and that *opag1* may be in the process of deletion from the *A. marginale* genome. On the other hand, OpAG2 and OpAG3 are surface proteins that are expressed in the bovine host, whereas only OpAG2 is expressed in ticks. This tick-specific variant arises in the midgut early during transmission feeding, which suggests that salivary gland factors are unlikely to play a role in their generation or selection. The role of the OpAG proteins has not been determined, but their differential expression in the tick and the mammal and their being well conserved indicate that they play an important role during transfer between the two host systems (131).

Interestingly, a pseudogene for another variable MSP, *msp3*, was found located on the DNA strand opposite to the one holding the *msp2* pseudogenes, separated by an identical sequence stretch of 321 bp. Moreover, the 5′ region of the *msp2* and *msp3* pseudogenes was identified as a highly conserved region of about 600 nucleotides. Presumably, MSP3, which is also variant and encoded by a multigene family, uses the same mechanism as MSP2 to generate intrastrain diversity, at the same time maximizing use of a small genome of only about 1.2 Mbp (24).

A. phagocytophilum, the HGA (formerly known as HGE) agent, is the closest genetic relative to *A. marginale*. Although an animal reservoir capable of supporting a months-long persistent infection has not been identified for this pathogen, it might be expected to use similar mechanisms of antigenic variation and immune evasion. In HL60 cell culture, the HGA agent abundantly expresses immunodominant proteins in a mass range of about 38 to 47 kDa that are encoded by a multigene family, *p44*, and are considered to be homologous to MSP2 (248). Multiple copies of the corresponding proteins expressed by different isolates, even if from the same geographic area, can vary (249), suggesting that they are subject to immune selection and possibly play a role in immune evasion or modulation. At least 18 copies of *p44* were identified in the HZ isolate of *A. phagocytophilum*, and a monospecific mouse serum against recombinant p44 recognized two to six p44 homologs in different isolates (248). The homologs' structure resembled that of MSP2 of *A. marginale*, with highly conserved regions flanking a hypervariable, 94-amino-acid central portion. The encoding genes were not arranged in a cluster but were dispersed throughout the chromosome. Whether p44 functions like MSP2 of *A. marginale* has not been determined because an animal model that experiences the recurrent waves of rickettsemia seen in anaplasmosis has not been identified. Nevertheless, mice vaccinated with HL60 culture-derived *A. phagocytophilum* antigen were only partially protected against homologous challenge, despite a vigorous response to p44 (226), suggestive of antigenic variation. Moreover, the genomic expression site for p44 in *A. phagocytophilum* is organized in much the same way as the MSP2 expression site of *A. marginale*, suggesting it functions in a similar manner to generate antigenic variants of p44. As in *A. marginale*, truncated pseudogenes characterized by a central, hypervariable region flanked by conserved sequences are utilized to generate an array of antigenic variants by segmental gene conversion of the polycistronic *p44* expression site. This was demonstrated by examining *A. phagocytophilum* DNA and mRNA of organisms cultured alternatingly in tick and human cells. Of interest, transfer between host cell types caused a shift in p44 variants expressed by *A. phagocytophilum* culture populations, with certain variant types being preferentially expressed in tick versus human cells (14). As an alternative explanation, the dominant expression of the p44 proteins in HL60 culture could reflect their important role in protection of the HGA agent from destruction by its host cell, the neutrophil granulocyte. Conceivably, the p44 proteins might function to modify normal endocytic pathways to prevent lysosomal fusion (143).

In the cluster of ehrlichial pathogens that include *E. canis*, *E. chaffeensis*, and *E. ruminantium*, antigenically variable, cross-reactive proteins have been identified as well. These proteins have been referred to as OMPs for *E. chaffeensis* and *E. canis*, and MAPs for *E. ruminantium*, but in this chapter, the term MAP is used for all of them. MAP1 and its homologs are pro-

teins of about 28 to 30 kDa that are capable of inducing protective immunity. The structure of their genes and organization in the genome differs from the *msp2/p44* multigene family in that they are tandemly arranged instead of being dispersed throughout the genome. *E. ruminantium* and *E. canis* possess multiple copies of the *map1* genes placed in tandem; in *E. chaffeensis*, one expressed and four or five silent, nonidentical genes have been identified (135, 165, 189, 225). Sequence analysis of the two gene members of *E. ruminantium* from African and Caribbean isolates demonstrated that the first, upstream gene was well conserved while the second comprised variable as well as nonvariable regions. Of interest, the variable regions of the downstream *E. ruminantium map1* gene were related to the corresponding genes of *E. chaffeensis* and *E. canis*. The *E. canis* MAP1 homolog corresponds to the 30-kDa protein, expressed by a multigene family present in the genome in multiple copies that encodes proteins having one semivariable and three hypervariable regions. In contrast to the expression of polycistronic mRNA for *msp2* of *A. marginale*, the genes of the *p28/p30* multigene locus of *E. canis* appear to be transcribed as monocistronic messages (139). The five-gene locus identified in this study encoded proteins with 51 to 74% amino acid homology, but within the sequences analyzed, two geographically separate *E. canis* isolates were identical. Recently, 22 paralogs were identified downstream from what is likely a transcriptional regulator in the *map1* gene family of both *E. canis* and *E chaffeensis*. Together, these form transcriptionally active gene clusters in which paralogs, separated by short intergenic spacers, were cotranscribed with adjacent genes (164). The authors suggest that these gene clusters likely are involved in adaptive responses of both ehrlichial species to their changing environment when switching from the mammalian to the tick host.

Specific *Ehrlichia*-host cell interaction

The pathogens that comprise the tick-borne anaplasmas and ehrlichias target surprisingly different cellular elements of the mammalian bloodstream, including platelets (*Anaplasma platys*), erythrocytes (*A. marginale*), monocytes (*E. canis* and *E. chaffeensis*), and granulocytes (*A. phagocytophilum* and *E. ewingii*). Not surprisingly, this diversity in host cell targets was one of the reasons for the early taxonomic confusion. Intuitively, one might think that closely related pathogens in a genogroup would evolve to utilize similar mechanisms of host cell entry, but insufficient data are available to draw this conclusion. The least studied among the group that can be cultured in vitro is *A. marginale*, for which a continuous culture method has only recently been developed (144). Because this system utilizes tick cells, it may be less useful in helping to unravel pathways of adhesion and invasion into mammalian cells. Nevertheless, the *A. marginale* MSP1, a heterodimer composed of MSP1a and MSP1b and encoded by two separate genes, *msp1α* and *msp1β*, was shown to be an adhesin by separately cloning the genes for the two subunits into *E. coli*. Expression of MSP1a caused *E. coli* to adhere to erythrocytes as well as to cultured *I. scapularis* and isolated *D. andersoni* gut cells, whereas expression of MSP1b resulted in adherence only to erythrocytes (50). The reason for this differential property of the two MSP1 subunits is unknown but might reflect unavailability of the MSP1b ligand on tick cells. It would be of great interest to determine if MSP1a binds to the same or a different ligand in each host system.

The monocytic and granulocytic anaplasmosis-ehrlichiosis agents have evolved to survive in the normally extremely hostile environment of the most efficient professional phagocytes found in the cellular arsenal of the mammalian immune system. In fact, *A. phagocytophilum*, *E. ewingii*, and *E. ruminantium* are the only known pathogens not only to survive but to actively replicate in neutrophil granulocytes. To disable the killing machinery of these cells, the ehrlichias must interact and bind to them in a fashion that does not trigger the normal phagocytic chain of events. To learn how they accomplish this trick requires knowledge of the cell surface receptors they bind to and how they manipulate subsequent cell signaling pathways to prevent maturation of their endosome into a mature, fully functional phagolysosome. There is evidence to suggest that a large (120-kDa) OMP of *E. chaffeensis* may be the adhesin that mediates binding to mammalian cells, but additional confirmatory data for this or other *Anaplasma* and *Ehrlichia* species have not been obtained (184, 242).

A. phagocytophilum may avoid being killed by its neutrophil host cell by utilizing ligands that are involved in cell-cell adherence rather than phagocytosis. A molecule that interacts with activated capillary endothelium, platelets, and others through the cells' selectin is sialylated Lewis x (CD15s), expressed richly on neutrophils and bone marrow cells found susceptible to infection with *A. phagocytophilum* (104, 106). Indeed, a MAb to CD15s prevented entry of *A. phagocytophilum* into these cells but did not inhibit its binding, suggesting that the CD15s molecule was but one component of a receptor complex (78). Further research targeting the neutrophil mechanism of binding to selectins of tissue cells identified the leukocyte P-selectin ligand, PSGL-1, as the main site to which the organisms adhere on the granulocyte surface (89). Utilizing a molecule that is involved in cell-

cell interaction may allow *A. phagocytophilum* access into the granulocyte without setting in motion the events that trigger phagocytosis, lysosomal fusion, and killing. This conclusion is supported by the finding that *A. phagocytophilum* resides in an intracellular compartment that lacks endosomal markers, while *E. chaffeensis* appears to localize into an early endosome that accumulates transferrin receptor molecules (18, 142). Apparently, *A. phagocytophilum* is taken into a cellular compartment that is not targeted for lysosomal fusion, which obviates the need for the bacteria to inhibit this activity, whereas *E. chaffeensis* is taken up into an endosome, suggesting that it binds to a different cell surface receptor.

Infection and survival in immune cells is a delicate balancing act for the intracellular pathogen and involves trade-offs between suppressing and activating the immune system. Also, the response of a naïve host is likely very different from one that has circulating antibody at the time of infection. In addition, *A. phagocytophilum* infects the neutrophil granulocyte as its major known host cell and vehicle for infection of and transfer to the tick vector. These cells normally have a short life span of only hours in the peripheral blood, potentially limiting anaplasma survival and availability to the vector. This disadvantage is partially overcome by a unique ability of the HGA agent to prolong survival time of peripheral blood neutrophils about fourfold (241). We recently obtained evidence suggesting that endothelial cells of the microvasculature are a station in the process of pathogenesis of human and bovine anaplasmosis. Both bovine and primate endothelial cell lines are highly susceptible to and support replication of *A. marginale* and *A. phagocytophilum* (150) (Fig. 5). The skin microvascular endothelium near the tick bite site would be an ideal intermediate host site for development of *A. phagocytophilum* while waiting to be transferred to and carried into the peripheral blood by neutrophils (as in *A. phagocytophilum*) or erythrocytes (as in *A. marginale*).

Production of messenger molecules is one of many ways in which leukocytes signal to other cells, stimulating or repressing their activities. Promyelocytic HL60 cells produce myelosuppressive chemokines upon contact with either live or killed anaplasmas, which could be responsible for the pancytopenia characteristic of HGA (105). On the other hand, the immune-dominant p44 proteins (226, 248) of *A. phagocytophilum* themselves have been reported to result in the induction of proinflammatory cytokines in monocytes (interleukin-1β [IL-1β], IL-6, and tumor necrosis factor alpha [TNF-α]), but only IL-1β in granulocytes (103). Still, leukocytes can be induced to kill *A. phagocytophilum*, even after infection has been established. Thus, HL60 cells, when treated with 12-O-

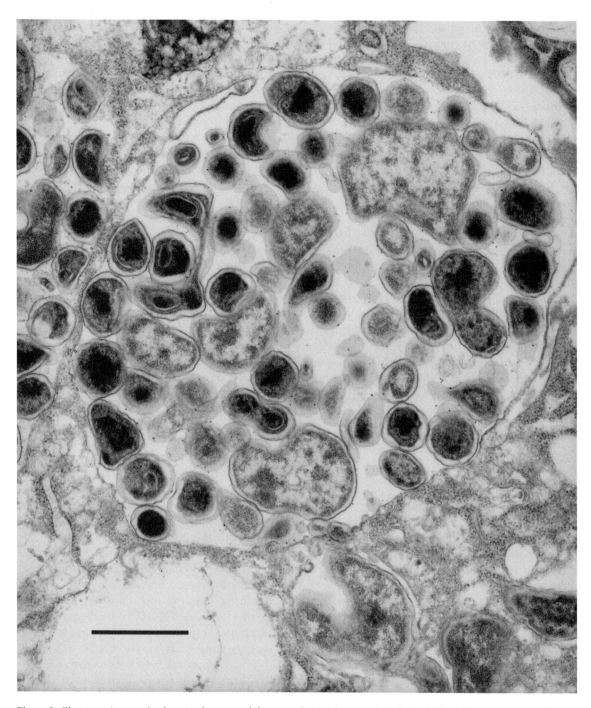

Figure 5. Electron micrograph of an *A. phagocytophilum* morula in a rhesus endothelial cell. The inclusion contains a heterogeneous mixture of reticulate and dense forms. Bar, 1 μm.

tetradecanoylphorbol-13-acetate, differentiated towards a monocytic cell lineage and were capable of killing *A. phagocytophilum* after its successful entry. Importantly, gamma interferon (IFN-γ), a cytokine that plays an important role in cell-mediated immunity, had a similar if less potent effect. IFN-γ is also likely to be involved in resistance to *E. chaffeensis* and apparently acts to restrict the availability of iron to

the pathogen (18). Interestingly, *E. chaffeensis* has developed the ability to interfere with IFN-γ-mediated resistance of the host cell by blocking signal transduction pathways that would otherwise lead to activation of IFN-γ-responsive nuclear genes (126). Peripheral blood monocytes from cattle immunized with *E. ruminantium* responded in a similar fashion when stimulated in vitro with live ehrlichia or major antigens. In particular, CD4$^+$ and $\gamma\delta$T cells expressing high levels of IFN-γ, TNF-α, TNF-β, and IL-2 were detected after autologous stimulation. Effective clearance of intracellular pathogens relies on the stimulation of these factors, and their induction in vitro is an important, measurable parameter of immunity.

Humans and animals visiting or living in tick-infested areas are likely exposed to tick-borne pathogens on repeated occasions, generating an antibody response that influences the outcome of a subsequent encounter. Pathogenesis studies with human patient material and specific breeds of mice (126) indicate that inflammatory responses to E. chaffeensis or an ehrlichia infection from Ixodes ovatus in Japan (219) may be major mediators of tissue damage. Granulomatous inflammation was present in several organs, most notably the liver. Human monocytes exposed to E. chaffensis responded by production with a number of cytokines (IL-1β, IL-8, and IL-10), but only complexes of specific antibody and the ehrlichias caused expression of genes for major cytokines implicated in generating a proinflammatory response (TNF-α, IL-6, and enhanced levels of IL-1β). This indicates that antibody-ehrlichia complexes may play an important part in the pathogenesis and general outcome of an ehrlichial infection (125).

Rickettsiae

In comparison with the Borrelia species, the interaction between spotted fever group-rickettsiae and vector ticks is less well understood. Attention has been focused on factors that influence rickettsial infectivity and interference with transovarial transmission.

R. rickettsii acquires infectivity for the mammalian host during the tick's blood meal. R. rickettsii in unfed D. andersoni ticks loses infectivity for guinea pigs, but if the ticks are warmed to 37°C for 3 days the rickettsiae reacquire infectivity (220). Reacquisition of infectivity correlates with reappearance of the microcapsular and slime layers of the rickettsial outer surface (85) that may be involved with actin polymerization and rickettsial mobility in tick cells (145, 215). The induction of R. rickettsii protein expression has been examined in tick cell cultures but not in ticks (183). Both rickettsial OMPs A (rOmpA) and B (rOmpB) are expressed in vitro, and the rickettsiae have prominent electron-lucent layers separating the outer membrane from the host cytoplasm. Cultivation of R. rickettsii in tick cells at 34°C induces several unidentified low-molecular-weight antigens that are not expressed at 28°C.

Ticks are refractory to superinfection by more than one closely related rickettsial species. Viral interference is defined as the "inhibition (partial or complete) of virus replication by another virus" (37), and this definition can be extended to include rickettsiae. Ticks are candidates for the manifestation of interference because of their possible exposure to multiple rickettsial species by feeding on multiple hosts. Interference is of epidemiological significance when nonpathogenic or less-pathogenic rickettsiae block or interfere with the tick's ability to support replication or transmission of a pathogenic species. Ticks are more likely to harbor nonpathogenic and symbiotic rickettsia than pathogenic ones. Symbiotic rickettsiae are highly adapted to living in the host tick where they are transmitted transstadially and transovarially but not horizontally. The high prevalence of these bacteria indicates that ticks benefit from their presence. A corollary to the aforementioned viral interference is the phenomenon of homologous interference, where the presence of a bacterial symbiont renders the tick refractory to superinfection or interferes with the transmission of a closely related pathogen. This phenomenon has been established for Rickettsia species associated with ticks. Rickettsial species that appear to be nonpathogenic and that can induce interference include R. peacockii (the East Side Agent [ESA]) (159), Rickettsia montanensis, and Rickettsia rhipicephali (32, 134). Ticks infected with these rickettsiae still acquire a secondary infection but transovarially transmit only one species, the primary one, because the ovarian tissues appear to be refractory to a secondary infection. Thus, unfed field-collected ticks are likely to be infected with a single rickettsial species, as only the original primary infection species is transovarially transmitted. Nevertheless, the evidence that R. peacockii interferes with R. rickettsii establishment in D. andersoni is equivocal. Ticks harboring the ESA still acquire and transmit R. rickettsii transstadially and horizontally, but transovarial transmission of R. rickettsii to the progeny is reduced (36, 159). It is hypothesized that R. rickettsii is unable to invade oocytes harboring the ESA. R. peacockii has been isolated in tick cell culture (216), offering an experimental system to test the hypothesis that nonpathogenic symbiotic rickettsiae can interfere with the stable maintenance of a pathogenic species. In another system, cultured I. scapularis cells infected with one genotype (strain) of A. marginale excluded superinfection with another genotype (49). On the other hand, unrelated microbes do not interfere with each other's maintenance in ticks. For example, there is no interaction between A. phagocytophilum and B. burgdorferi in I. scapularis. Neither pathogen interfered with the ability of the tick to acquire or transmit the other (127). Dually infected ticks cotransmitted both pathogens as efficiently as ticks infected with just one pathogen. However, these results are in contrast with those of an earlier study indicating that the primary infection by either agent interfered with the transmission of the second agent (128), possibly the result of a heavy primary pathogen load that adversely affected the vectorial fitness of *I. scapularis*.

TICK-BORNE PATHOGENS AS TICK PATHOGENS

Interference aside, virulence of a pathogen for the vector is a major factor influencing the prevalence and maintenance of arthropod-borne pathogens in nature. Several pathogenic bacteria and protozoa have deleterious impacts on ticks. The negative effects include increased mortality, reduced fecundity and feeding, and increased time to engorge. Developmental abnormalities can also result including the disruption of the molting process and abnormal development of the appendages. *R. rickettsii* causes high mortality in *D. andersoni* larvae and nymphs, and ticks infected during the previous instar die after the next blood meal and prior to molting (158). The few females that survive to the adult stage feed poorly and are less fecund. These effects offer an additional explanation for the low prevalence of *R. rickettsii*-infected ticks in the field. Similar results have been reported for *R. montanensis*, *Rickettsia bellii*, and *R. rhipicephali* (133). Spirochetes also cause pathologic changes in ticks. *B. burgdorferi* generally remains localized within the gut of infected *I. scapularis* ticks but can become systemically dispersed during and after the blood meal. Once systemic, the spirochetes invade oocytes, disrupt oogenesis, and reduce fecundity (35). Babesial and theilerial pathogens of cattle are also pathogenic for the vector. The protozoan cattle pathogen *Theileria parva* causes pathologic changes in salivary gland and gut tissue in *Rhipicephalus appendiculatus* that include formation of pycnotic nuclei, disruption of tissue integrity, and vacuolization (235). It is of interest that in *D. andersoni* the DAS, which is closely related to *Francisella tularensis* subsp. *tularensis* (157), is restricted to the ovaries; animals fed on by ticks harboring the endosymbiont do not seroconvert or display any disease. However, guinea pigs inoculated parenterally with DAS strongly seroconvert, the symbiont replicates in chick embryo yolk sac tissues, and the cultured forms are highly pathogenic for both ticks and rodents upon needle inoculation (33, 157). Therefore, the tick is able to control the microbe by an unknown mechanism, perhaps one that is related to its antimicrobial immunity.

The tick's immune system is in part a determinant of vector competency. Even in a competent vector, the transmitted microbe induces an immune response but one that is less severe than that in a nonvector tick. The immune reaction of *D. variabilis* to *B. burgdorferi*

is more stringent than that of *I. scapularis*, a competent vector (97). Spirochetes inoculated parenterally into the hemocoel of *D. variabilis* are rapidly cleared from the hemocoel within 24 h due to hemocyte, lysozyme, and defensin activity, while in *I. scapularis* viable borreliae can be reisolated from the hemolymph. Spirochetes incubated in *I. scapularis* hemolymph or plasma remain viable and motile, but those in *D. variabilis* hemolymph are killed within 45 min. The innate immunity of the adult brown ear tick, *R. appendiculatus*, is active against bacteria (*Micrococcus luteus*) and modestly increased in ticks needle pricked with *M. luteus*. However, activation of the innate immune response had no negative impact on the ability of the ticks to acquire *T. parva* or on the ability of the parasite to develop in the ticks (236). Further studies of activity of the tick innate immunity against the acquisition and development of tick-transmitted pathogenic microbes are needed, but evidence indicates that ticks are immunotolerant of the pathogens they transmit while incompetent vectors are highly immunocompetent.

RETURN TO AND SURVIVAL IN THE MAMMALIAN HOST: THE TICK-PATHOGEN CONSPIRACY

Many factors come into play to favor transmission of tick-borne pathogens to the mammal. It might be argued that the center piece of the arrangement between the three organisms involved is the ability of ixodid ticks to remain attached to their host and feed for days, ingesting several milliliters of blood that are concentrated by secretion of copious amounts of saliva into the host (207, 208). This makes it necessary for the tick to overcome the responses of its host, to avoid being detached by grooming as well as overcoming the immunological, inflammatory, and hemostatic defenses of the mammal (160, 195). During the entire period of attachment and cyclic feeding-salivation activity, the intracutaneous bite site must be maintained for continuous blood inflow, prevention of sensitization to tick saliva, inhibition of the function of immune-mediator cells such as neutrophil granulocytes and T cells, and removal or inactivation of antibody. Salivary gland proteins disrupt a wide array of immunological functions, including interference with antigen presentation by the macrophages, NK cells, T- and B-lymphocyte functions, and the complement cascade (239).

The salivary glands of ixodid ticks are complex structures combining clusters of specialized cells, called acini, with different functions, many of which are not completely understood. The pharmacopoeia of tick saliva includes antihemostatic, anti-inflammatory, and immunomodulatory molecules (161) and disrupts the three main branches of the host hemostatic system: platelet aggregation, coagulation, and vasoconstriction. Tick saliva contains several immunomodulators: prostaglandins, immunoglobulin-binding proteins (IGBPs), and complement inhibitors (5, 124, 192, 230). This array of pharmacologically active compounds interacts directly and indirectly with the host's defense systems. These include an activity that directly inhibits the function of neutrophil granulocytes, which are professional phagocytes that tend to infiltrate the feeding lesion (196). Also present is a protein that binds IL-2, thereby preventing T-cell proliferation and stimulation of other immune cells, as well as causing upregulation of IL-10 (76). Saliva also contains a small (18.5-kDa) protein that inhibits C3b, a component of the alternative complement cascade (162, 229). A particularly striking feature of tick saliva composition is the extraordinarily high levels of prostaglandin E2, sufficient to induce vasodilation and in turn stimulate secretion (162, 194, 195, 207, 229). Moreover, IGBPs, small proteins in tick saliva, interfere with antibody activity by binding immunoglobulins (20). Host immunoglobulin taken up with the blood meal can pass intact into the hemocoel, and IGBPs are found in the hemolymph and salivary glands. The resultant complexes are transferred through the gut wall into the hemocoel, taken into the salivary glands, and excreted back into the host, preventing them from binding to their target in the tick or the feeding lesion (233). The IGBPs provide the tick with a mechanism to escape the detrimental effects of anti-tick-directed immunoglobulins and transport them to the salivary glands where they are excreted (161). Saliva-activated transmission (SAT) is the ability of saliva or salivary gland extracts to promote the transmission of pathogenic microbes by arthropods (161) and is mediated by the sum of the pharmacological effects of saliva that turn the feeding lesion into an immune-compromised site.

Ehrlichias and other tick-borne pathogens that require more than a day of growth and/or development after tick attachment to be transferred to their new host benefit directly and indirectly from the immune-modulatory activity of tick saliva. They are released into a site protected from immune effector cells, particularly Th1 cells, steering the immune system toward a Th2 response (214). This causes a delayed, altered, and inefficient host immune response to anaplasma and ehrlichia and essentially impacts pathogenesis and pathogen persistence. In addition, any specific antibody already circulating in the peripheral bloodstream that enters the bite site is likely to be bound up and made ineffective. Thus, several of the animal anaplasmoses and ehrlichioses, notably bovine anaplasmosis, heartwater of cattle, and probably canine tropical pancytopenia caused by E. canis, are characterized by

an inability of the animal host to mount a vigorous immune response and develop sterile immunity, resulting in carrier status (94, 213, 227), i.e., animals that become pathogen reservoirs for the vector ticks (172).

Disruption of host hemostatic and immune systems at the bite site also enhances the transmission and establishment of tick-borne spirochetes in the mammalian host; passive reconstitution of the host's immune system with cytokines restores host immunity to tick-transmitted pathogens (245). Members of the OspE and OspF family facilitate spirochete survival and transmission during the blood meal. OspE/OspF/Elp paralogs are upregulated in the tick during the blood meal and in response to a shift up in temperature (86, 223). OspE and the complement regulatory-acquiring surface proteins are surface ligands that bind the complement control proteins factor H and factor H-like protein-1/reconectin (88, 116, 120). The joint activity of salivary proteins that inhibit complement deposition by the host (192) and the spirochetal proteins that bind complement regulatory proteins help spirochetes evade complement attack and phagocytosis. It is hypothesized that the diversification of the Borrelia species is a result of complement-mediated selection and not the tick species per se (120). SAT enhances the transmission of spirochetes. For example, transmission of the European spirochete Borrelia lusitaniae is enhanced significantly when it is coinoculated with saliva from its natural vector I. ricinus. Similarly, coinoculation of B. burgdorferi with saliva from the North American species I. scapularis enhances its transmission (246). Reciprocal coinoculations do not display this enhancement, leading to the speculation that tick-transmitted pathogens have specifically adapted to the milieu of the salivary gland components of their vector (246).

Acknowledgments. The research described in this chapter was supported by grants (AI49424 and AI42792 to U.G.M., AI37909 to T.J.K., and AI40952 to Jesse Goodman) from the U.S. Public Health Service.

We gratefully acknowledge Ann Palmer for the electron micrographs presented in this chapter.

REFERENCES

1. **Agbede, R. I. S.** 1986. Scanning electron microscopy of digest cells in the midgut epithelium of *Boophilus microplus*. *Exp. Appl. Acarol.* **2:**329–335.
2. **Alban, P. S., P. W. Johnson, and D. R. Nelson.** 2000. Serum-starvation-induced changes in protein synthesis and morphology of *Borrelia burgdorferi*. *Microbiology* **146:**119–127.
3. **Anderson, B. E., J. E. Dawson, D. C. Jones, and K. C. Wilson.** 1991. *Ehrlichia chaffeensis*, a new species associated with human ehrlichiosis. *J. Clin. Microbiol.* **29:**2838–2842.
4. **Anderson, B. E., C. E. Greene, D. C. Jones, and J. E. Dawson.** 1992. *Ehrlichia ewingii* sp. nov., the etiologic agent of canine granulocytic ehrlichiosis. *Int. J. Syst. Bacteriol.* **41:**299–302.

5. Anguita, J., N. Ramamoorthi, J. W. R. Hovius, S. Das, V. Thomas, R. Persinski, D. Conze, P. W. Akenase, M. Rincón, F. S. Kantor, and E. Fikrig. 2002. Salp15, an *Ixodes scapularis* salivary protein, inhibits CD4$^+$ T cell activation. *Cell* 16:1–20.

6. Asanovich, K. M., J. S. Bakken, J. E. Madigan, M. Aguero-rosenfeld, G. P. Wormser, and J. S. Dumler. 1997. Antigenic diversity of granulocytic ehrlichia isolates from humans in Wisconsin and New York and a horse in California. *J. Infect. Dis.* 176:1029–1034.

7. Assadian, O., and G. Stanek. 2002. Theobald Smith—the discoverer of ticks as vectors of disease. *Wien. Klin. Wochenschr.* 114:479–481.

8. Attoui, H., J. M. Stirling, U. G. Munderloh, F. Billoir, S. M. Brookes, J. N. Burroughs, P. de Micco, P. P. C. Mertens, and X. de Lamballerie. 2001. Complete sequence characterization of the genome of the St Croix River virus, a new orbivirus isolated from cells of *Ixodes scapularis. J. Gen. Virol.* 82:795–804.

9. Bakken, J. S., and J. S. Dumler. 2000. Human granulocytic ehrlichiosis. *Clin. Infect. Dis.* 31:554–560.

10. Bakken, J. S., J. S. Dumler, S.-M. Chen, M. R. Eckman, L. L. Van Etta, and D. H. Walker. 1994. Human granulocytic ehrlichiosis in the upper midwest United States: a new species emerging? *JAMA* 272:212–218.

11. Balashov, Y. S. 1972. Bloodsucking ticks (Ixodoidea)—vectors of diseases of man and animals. *Miscell. Publ. Entomol. Soc. Am.* 8:161–376.

12. Barbet, A. F., R. Blentkinger, A. M. Lundgren, J. Yi, E. Blouin, and K. M. Kocan. 1999. Comparison of surface proteins of *Anaplasma marginale* grown in tick cell culture, tick salivary glands, and cattle. *Infect. Immun.* 67:102–107.

13. Barbet, A. F., A. Lundgren, J. Yi, F. R. Rurangirwa, and G. H. Palmer. 2000. Antigenic variation of *Anaplasma marginale* by expression of MSP2 mosaics. *Infect. Immun.* 68:6133–6138.

14. Barbet, A. F., P. F. M. Meeus, M. Bélanger, M. V. Bowie, J. Yi, A. M. Lundgren, A. R. Alleman, S. J. Wong, F. K. Chu, U. G. Munderloh, and S. D. Jauron. 2003. Expression of multiple outer membrane protein sequence variants from a single genomic locus *Anaplasma phagocytophilum. Infect. Immun.* 71:1706–1718.

15. Barbet, A. F., J. Yi, B. R. McEwen, E. Blouin, and K. M. Kocan. 2001. Antigenic variation of *Anaplasma marginale* major surface protein 2 diversity during cyclic transmission between ticks and cattle. *Infect. Immun.* 69:3057–3066.

16. Barlough, J. E., J. E. Madigan, E. DeRock, and L. Bigornia. 1996. Nested polymerase chain reaction for detection of *Ehrlichia equi* genomic DNA in horses and ticks (*Ixodes pacificus*). *Vet. Parasitol.* 63:319–329.

17. Barlough, J. E., G. H. Reubel, J. E. Madigan, L. K. Vredevoe, P. E. Miller, and Y. Rikihisa. 1998. Detection of *Ehrlichia risticii*, the agent of Potomac horse fever, in freshwater stream snails (Pleuroceridae: *Juga* spp.) from northern California. *Appl. Environ. Microbiol.* 64:2888–2893.

18. Barnewall, R. E., and Y. Rikihisa. 1994. Abrogation of gamma interferon-induced inhibition of *Ehrlichia chaffeensis* infection in human monocytes with iron transferrin. *Infect. Immun.* 62:4804–4810.

19. Bell-Sakyi, L., E. A. Paxton, U. G. Munderloh, and K. J. Sumption. 2000. Growth of *Cowdria ruminantium*, the causative agent of heartwater, in a tick cell line. *J. Clin. Microbiol.* 38:1238–1240.

20. Bergman, D. K., R. N. Ramachandra, and S. K. Wikel. 1998. Characterization of an immunosuppressant protein from *Dermacentor andersoni* (Acari: Ixodidae) salivary glands. *J. Med. Entomol.* 35:505–509.

21. Bior, A. D., R. C. Essenberg, and J. R. Sauer. 2002. Comparison of differentially expressed genes in the salivary glands of male ticks, *Amblyomma americanum* and *Dermacentor andersoni. Insect Biochem. Mol. Biol.* 32:645–655.

22. Blouin, E. F., and K. M. Kocan. 1998. Morphology and development of *Anaplasma marginale* (Rickettsiales: Anaplasmataceae) in cultured *Ixodes scapularis* (Acari: Ixodidae) cells. *J. Med. Entomol.* 35:788–797.

23. Bono, J. L., K. Tilly, B. Stevenson, D. Hogan, and P. Rosa. 1998. Oligopeptide permease in *Borrelia burgdorferi*: putative peptide-binding components encoded by both chromosomal and plasmid loci. *Microbiology* 144:1033–1044.

24. Brayton, K. A., D. P. Knowles, T. C. McGuire, and G. H. Palmer. 2001. Efficient use of a small genome to generate antigenic diversity in tick-borne ehrlichial pathogens. *Proc. Natl. Acad. Sci. USA* 98:4130–4135.

25. Brayton, K. A., G. H. Palmer, A. Lundgren, J. Yi, and A. F. Barbet. 2002. Antigenic variation of *Anaplasma marginale* msp2 occurs by combinatorial gene conversion. *Mol. Microbiol.* 43:1151–1159.

26. Braz, G. R. C., H. S. L. Coelho, H. Masuda, and P. L. Oliveira. 1999. A missing metabolic pathway in the cattle tick *Boophilus microplus. Curr. Biol.* 9:703–706.

27. Brenner, D. J., S. P. O'Connor, H. H. Winkler, and A. G. Steigerwalt. 1993. Proposals to unify the genera *Bartonella* and *Rochalimaea*, with descriptions of *Bartonella quintana* comb. nov., *Bartonella vinsonii* comb. nov., *Bartonella henselae* comb. nov., and *Bartonella elizabethae* comb. nov., and to remove the family *Bartonellaceae* from the order *Rickettsiales. Int. J. Syst. Bacteriol.* 43:777–786.

28. Brooks, M. A. 1964. Symbiotes and the nutrition of medically important insects. *Bull. W. H. O.* 31:555–559.

29. Bugrysheva, J., E. Y. Dobrikova, H. P. Godfrey, M. L. Sartakova, and F. C. Cabello. 2002. Modulation of *Borrelia burgdorferi* stringent response and gene expression during extracellular growth with tick cells. *Infect. Immun.* 70:3061–3067.

30. Buller, R. S., M. Arens, S. P. Hmiel, C. D. Paddock, J. W. Sumner, Y. Rikihisa, A. Unver, M. Gaudreault-Keener, F. A. Manian, A. M. Liddell, N. Schulewitz, and G. A. Storch. 1999. *Ehrlichia ewingii*, a newly recognized agent of human ehrlichiosis. *New Engl. J. Med.* 15:148–155.

31. Burg, J. G., A. W. Roberts, N. M. Williams, D. G. Powell, and F. W. Knapp. 1990. Attempted transmission of *Ehrlichia risticii* (Rickettsiaceae) with *Stomoxys calcitrans* (Diptera: Muscidae). *J. Med. Entomol.* 27:874–877.

32. Burgdorfer, W. 1988. Ecological and epidemiological considerations of Rocky Mountain spotted fever and scrub typhus, p. 33–50. *In* D. H. Walker (ed.), *Biology of Rickettsial Diseases.* CRC Press, Inc., Boca Raton, Fla.

33. Burgdorfer, W., L. P. Brinto, and L. E. Hughes. 1973. Isolation and characterization of symbiotes from the Rocky Mountain wood tick, *Dermacentor andersoni. J. Invertebr. Pathol.* 22:424–434.

34. Burgdorfer, W., and S. F. Hayes. 1989. Vector-spirochete relationship in louse-borne and tick-borne borrelioses with emphasis on Lyme disease, p. 127–150. *In* K. F. Harris (ed.), *Advances in Disease Vector Research*, vol. 6. Springer Verlag, New York, N.Y.

35. Burgdorfer, W., S. F. Hayes, and D. Corwin. 1989. Pathophysiology of the Lyme disease spirochete, *Borrelia burgdorferi*, in ixodid ticks. *Rev. Infect. Dis.* 11:S1442–S1450.

36. Burgdorfer, W., S. F. Hayes, and A. J. Mavros. 1981. Nonpathogenic rickettsiae in *Dermacentor andersoni*: a limiting factor for the distribution of *Rickettsia rickettsii*, p. 585–594.

In W. Burgdorfer and R. L. Anacker (ed.), *Rickettsiae and Rickettsial Diseases*. Academic Press, New York, N.Y.

37. **Cann, A. J.** 1997. *Principles of Molecular Virology*. Academic Press, San Diego, Calif.

38. **Carroll, J. A., R. M. Cordova, and C. F. Garon.** 2000. Identification of 11 pH-regulated genes in *Borrelia burgdorferi* localizing to linear plasmids. *Infect. Immun.* **68**:6677–6684.

39. **Carroll, J. A., C. F. Garon, and T. G. Schwan.** 1999. Effects of environmental pH on membrane proteins in *Borrelia burgdorferi*. *Infect. Immun.* **67**:3181–3187.

40. **Ceraul, S. M., D. E. Sonenshine, and W. L. Hynes.** 2002. Resistance of the tick *Dermacentor variabilis* (Acari: Ixodidae) following challenge with the bacterium *Escherichia coli* (Enterobacteriales: Enterobacteriaceae). *J. Med. Entomol.* **39**:376–383.

41. **Chen, S.-M., L. C. Cullman, and D. H. Walker.** 1997. Western immunoblotting analysis of the antibody responses of patients with human monocytotropic ehrlichiosis to different strains of *Ehrlichia chaffeensis* and *Ehrlichia canis*. *Clin. Diag. Lab. Immunol.* **4**:731–735.

42. **Chen, S.-M., J. S. Dumler, J. S. Bakken, and D. H. Walker.** 1994. Identification of a granulocytotropic *Ehrlichia* species as the etiologic agent of human disease. *J. Clin. Microbiol.* **32**:589–595.

43. **Chen, S.-M., J. S. Dumler, H.-M. Feng, and D. H. Walker.** 1994. Identification of the antigenic constituents of *Ehrlichia chaffeensis*. *Am. J. Trop. Med. Hyg.* **50**:52–58.

44. **Coleman, J. L., J. A. Gebbia, J. Piesman, J. L. Degen, T. H. Bugge, and J. L. Benach.** 1997. Plasminogen is required for efficient dissemination of *B. burgdorferi* in ticks and for enhancement of spirochetemia in mice. *Cell* **89**:1111–1119.

45. **Coons, L. B., R. Rosell-Davis, and B. I. Tarnowski.** 1986. Bloodmeal digestion in ticks, p. 248–279. *In* J. R. Sauer and J. A. Hair (ed.), *Morphology, Physiology, and Behavioral Biology of Ticks*. Ellis Horwood Limited, Chichester, United Kingdom.

46. **Dawson, J. E., B. E. Anderson, D. B. Fishbein, J. L. Sanchez, C. S. Goldsmith, K. H. Wilson, and C. W. Duntley.** 1991. Isolation and identification of an *Ehrlichia* sp. from a patient diagnosed with human ehrlichiosis. *J. Clin. Microbiol.* **29**:2741–2745.

47. **Dawson, J. E., J. E. Childs, K. L. Biggie, C. Moore, D. Stallknecht, J. Shaddock, J. Bouseman, E. Hofmeister, and J. G. Olson.** 1994. White-tailed deer as a potential reservoir of *Ehrlichia* spp. *J. Wildlife Dis.* **30**:162–168.

48. **Dawson, J. E., Y. Rikihisa, S. A. Ewing, and D. B. Fishbein.** 1991. Serologic diagnosis of human ehrlichiosis using two *Ehrlichia canis* isolates. *J. Infect. Dis.* **163**:91–95.

49. **de la Fuente, J., J. C. Garcia-Garcia, E. Blouin, J. T. Saliki, and K. M. Kocan.** 2002. Infection of tick cells and bovine erythrocytes with one genotype of the intracellular ehrlichia *Anaplasma marginale* excludes infection with other genotypes. *Clin. Diag. Lab. Immunol.* **9**:658–668.

50. **de la Fuente, J., J. C. Garcia-Garcia, E. F. Blouin, and K. M. Kocan.** 2001. Differential adhesion of major surface proteins 1a and 1b of the ehrlichial cattle pathogen *Anaplasma marginale* to bovine erythrocytes and tick cells. *Int. J. Parasitol.* **31**:145–153.

51. **de Silva, A. M., and E. Fikrig.** 1997. *Borrelia burgdorferi* genes selectively expressed in ticks and mammals. *Parasitol. Today* **1997**:267–270.

52. **de Silva, A. M., and E. Fikrig.** 1995. Growth and migration of *Borrelia burgdorferi* in *Ixodes* ticks during blood feeding. *Am. J. Trop. Med. Hyg.* **53**:397–404.

53. **de Silva, A. M., E. Fikrig, E. Hodzic, F. S. Kantor, S. R. Telford III, and S. W. Barthold.** 1998. Immune evasion by tickborne and host-adapted *Borrelia burgdorferi*. *J. Infect. Dis.* **177**:395–400.

54. **de Silva, A. M., D. Fish, T. R. Burkot, Y. Zhang, and E. Fikrig.** 1997. OspA antibodies inhibit the acquisition of *Borrelia burgdorferi* by *Ixodes* ticks. *Infect. Immun.* **65**:3146–3150.

55. **de Silva, A. M., S. R. Telford III, L. R. Brunet, S. W. Barthold, and E. Fikrig.** 1996. *Borrelia burgdorferi* OspA is an arthropod-specific transmission-blocking Lyme disease vaccine. *J. Exp. Med.* **183**:271–275.

56. **Dolp, R. M.** 1970. Biochemical and physiological studies of certain ticks (Ixodoidea). Qualitative and quantitative studies of hemocytes. *J. Med. Entomol.* **7**:277–288.

57. **Donatien, A., and F. Lestoquard.** 1935. Existence en Algérie d'une Rickettsia du chien. *Bull. Soc. Pathol. Exot.* **28**:418–419.

58. **Dumler, J. S., A. F. Barbet, C. P. J. Bekker, G. Dasch, G. H. Palmer, S. C. Ray, Y. Rikihisa, and F. R. Rurangirwa.** 2001. Reorganization of genera in the families *Rickettsiaceae* and *Anaplasmataceae* in the order *Rickettsiales*; unification of some species of *Ehrlichia* with *Anaplasma*, *Cowdria* with *Ehrlichia* and *Ehrlichia* with *Neorickettsia*, descriptions of six new species combinations and designation of *Ehrlichia equi* and 'HGE agent' as subjective synonyms of *Ehrlichia phagocytophila*. *Int. J. Syst. Evol. Microbiol.* **51**:2145–2165.

59. **Dumler, J. S., S.-M. Chen, K. Asanovich, E. Trigiani, V. L. Popov, and D. H. Walker.** 1995. Isolation and characterization of a new strain of *Ehrlichia chaffeensis* from a patient with nearly fatal monocytic ehrlichiosis. *J. Clin. Microbiol.* **33**:1704–1711.

60. **Eggenberger, L. R., W. J. Lamoreaux, and L. B. Coons.** 1990. Hemocytic encapsulation of implants in the tick *Dermacentor variabilis*. *Exp. Appl. Acarol.* **9**:279–287.

61. **Elias, A. F., J. L. Bono, J. A. Carroll, P. Stewart, K. Tilly, and P. Rosa.** 2000. Altered stationary-phase response in a *Borrelia burgdorferi rpoS* mutant. *J. Bacteriol.* **182**:2909–2918.

62. **Ewing, S. A.** 1969. Canine ehrlichiosis, p. 331–353. *In* C. A. Brandley and C. E. Cornelius (ed.), *Advances in Veterinary Science and Comparative Medicine*, vol. 13. Academic Press, New York, N.Y.

63. **Ewing, S. A.** 1981. Transmission of *Anaplasma marginale* by arthropods, p. 395–423. *In* R. J. Hidalgo and E. W. Jones (ed.), *Proceedings of the 7th National Anaplasma Conference*. Mississippi State University Press, Mississippi State, Miss.

64. **Ewing, S. A., J. E. Dawson, A. A. Kocan, R. W. Barker, C. K. Warner, R. J. Panciera, J. C. Fox, K. M. Kocan, and E. F. Blouin.** 1995. Experimental transmission of *Ehrlichia chaffeensis* (Rickettsiales: Ehrlichieae) among white-tailed deer by *Amblyomma americanum* (Acari: Ixodidae). *J. Med. Entomol.* **32**:368–374.

65. **Ewing, S. A., U. G. Munderloh, and S. D. Jauron.** Unpublished.

66. **Fagotto, F.** 1995. Regulation of yolk degradation, or how to make sleepy lysosomes. *J. Cell Sci.* **108**:3645–3647.

67. **Fikrig, E., S. R. Telford III, S. W. Barthold, F. S. Kantor, A. Spielman, and R. A. Flavell.** 1992. Elimination of *Borrelia burgdorferi* from vector ticks feeding on OspA-immunized mice. *Proc. Natl. Acad. Sci. USA* **89**:5418–5421.

68. **Fingerle, V., U. Hauser, G. Liegl, B. Petko, V. Preac-Mursic, and B. Wilske.** 1995. Expression of outer surface proteins A and C of *Borrelia burgdorferi* in *Ixodes ricinus*. *J. Clin. Microbiol.* **33**:1867–1869.

69. **Fingerle, V., H. Laux, U. G. Munderloh, U. Schulte-Spechtel, and B. Wilske.** 2000. Differential expression of outer surface proteins A and C by individual *B. burgdorferi* in different genospecies. *Med. Microbiol. Immunol.* **189**:59–66.

70. Fingerle, V., U. G. Munderloh, G. Liegl, and B. Wilske. 1999. Coexistence of ehrlichiae of the phagocytophila group with Borrelia burgdorferi in Ixodes ricinus from southern Germany. Med. Microbiol. Immunol. 188:145–149.

71. Fishbein, D. B., J. E. Dawson, and L. E. Robinson. 1994. Human ehrlichiosis in the United States, 1985 to 1990. Ann. Internal Med. 120:736–743.

72. Fogaca, A., P. J. da Silva, M. T. M. Miranda, A. G. Bianchi, A. Miranda, P. E. M. Ribolla, and S. Daffre. 1999. Antimicrobial activity of a bovine hemoglobin fragment in the tick Boophilus microplus. J. Biol. Chem. 274:25330–25334.

73. Fraser, C. M., S. Casjens, W. M. Huang, G. G. Sutton, R. Clayton, R. Lathigra, O. White, K. A. Ketchum, R. Dodson, E. K. Hickey, M. Gwinn, B. Dougherty, J.-F. Tomb, R. D. Fleischmann, D. Richardson, J. Peterson, A. R. Kerlavage, J. Quackenbush, S. Salzburg, M. Hanson, R. van Vugt, N. Palmer, M. D. Adams, J. Gocayne, J. Weidman, T. Utterback, L. Watthey, L. McDonald, P. Artiach, C. Bowman, S. Garland, C. Fujii, M. D. Cotton, K. Horst, K. Roberts, B. Hatch, H. O. Smith, and J. C. Venter. 1997. Genomic sequence of a Lyme disease spirochaete, Borrelia burgdorferi. Nature 390:580–586.

74. French, D. M., T. F. McElwain, T. C. McGuire, and G. H. Palmer. 1998. Expression of Anaplasma marginale major surface protein 2 variants during persistent cyclic rickettsemia. Infect. Immun. 66:1200–1207 (Erratum, 1266:2400.)

75. Fujisaki, K., S. Kitaoka, and T. Morii. 1975. Hemocyte types and their primary cultures in the argasid tick, Ornithodoros moubata Murray (Ixodoidea). Appl. Ent. Zool. 10:30–39.

76. Gillespie, R. D., M. C. Dolan, J. Piesman, and R. G. Titus. 2001. Identification of an IL-2 binding protein in the saliva of the Lyme-disease vector tick, Ixodes scapularis. J. Immunol. 166:4319–4326.

77. Glimore, R. D., Jr., M. L. Mbow, and B. Stevenson. 2001. Analysis of Borrelia burgdorferi gene expression during life cycle phases of the tick vector Ixodes scapularis. Microbes Infect. 3:799–808.

78. Goodman, J. L., C. M. Nelson, M. B. Klein, S. F. Hayes, and B. W. Weston. 1999. Leukocyte infection by the granulocytic ehrlichiosis agent is linked to expression of a selectin ligand. J. Clin. Investig. 103:407–412.

79. Goodman, J. L., C. M. Nelson, B. Vitale, J. E. Madigan, J. S. Dumler, T. J. Kurtti, and U. G. Munderloh. 1996. Direct cultivation of the causative agent from patients with human granulocytic ehrlichiosis. New Engl. J. Med. 334:209–215.

80. Grubhoffer, L., J. Veres, and F. Dusbábek. 1991. Lectins as the molecular factor of recognition and defence reaction of ticks, p. 381–388. In F. Dusbábek and V. Bukva (ed.), Modern Acarology. SFB Academic Publishing, Prague, Czech Republic.

81. Gudderra, N. P., P. A. Neese, D. E. Sonenshine, C. S. Apperson, and R. M. Roe. 2001. Developmental profile, isolation, and biochemical characterization of a novel lipoglycohemecarrier protein from the American dog tick, Dermacentor variabilis (Acari: Ixodidae) and observation on a similar protein in the soft tick, Ornithodoros parkeri (Acari: Argasidae). Insect Biochem. Mol. Biol. 31:299–311.

82. Hagman, K. E., X. Yang, S. K. Wikel, G. B. Schoeler, M. J. Caimano, J. D. Radolf, and M. V. Norgard. 2000. Decorinbinding protein A (DbpA) of Borrelia burgdorferi is not protective when immunized mice are challenged via tick infestation and correlates with the lack of DbpA expression by B. burgdorferi in ticks. Infect. Immun. 68:4759–4764.

83. Hahn, N. E., M. Fletcher, R. M. Rice, K. M. Kocan, J. W. Hansen, J. A. Hair, R. W. Barker, and B. D. Perry. 1990. Attempted transmission of Ehrlichia risticii, causative agent of Potomac horse fever, by the ticks, Dermacentor variabilis,

Rhipicephalus sanguineus, Ixodes scapularis and Amblyomma americanum. Exp. Appl. Acarol. 8:41–50.

84. Harden, V. A. 1990. Rocky Mountain Spotted Fever: History of a Twentieth Century Disease. The Johns Hopkins University Press, Baltimore, Md.

85. Hayes, S. F., and W. Burgdorfer. 1982. Reactivation of Rickettsia rickettsii in Dermacentor andersoni ticks: an ultrastructural analysis. Infect. Immun. 37:779–785.

86. Hefty, P. S., S. E. Jolliff, M. J. Caimano, S. K. Wikel, and D. R. Akins. 2002. Changes in temporal and spatial patterns of outer surface lipoprotein expression generate population heterogeneity and antigenic diversity in the Lyme disease spirochete Borrelia burgdorferi. Infect. Immun. 70:3468–3478.

87. Hefty, P. S., S. E. Jolliff, M. J. Caimano, S. K. Wikel, J. D. Radolf, and D. R. Akins. 2001. Regulation of OspE-related, OspF-related, and Elp lipoproteins of Borrelia burgdorferi strain 297 by mammalian host-specific signals. Infect. Immun. 69:3618–3627.

88. Hellwage, J., T. Meri, T. Heikkilä, A. Alitalo, J. Panelius, P. Lahdenne, I. J. T. Seppälä, and S. Meri. 2001. The complement regulator factor H binds to the surface protein OspE of Borrelia burgdorferi. J. Biol. Chem. 276:8427–8435.

89. Herron, M. J., C. M. Nelson, J. Larson, K. R. Snapp, G. S. Kansas, and J. L. Goodman. 2000. Intracellular parasitism by the human granulocytic ehrlichiosis bacterium through the P-selectin ligand, PSGL-1. Science 288:1653–1656.

90. Hidalgo, R. J., G. H. Palmer, E. W. Jones, J. E. Brown, and A. J. Ainsworth. 1989. Infectivity and antigenicity of Anaplasma marginale from tick cell culture. Am. J. Vet. Res. 50:2033–2036.

91. Hoogstraal, H. 1981. Changing patterns of tick-borne diseases in modern society. Ann. Rev. Entomol. 26:75–99.

91a. Hübner, A., X. Yang, D. M. Nolen, T. G. Popova, F. C. Cabello, and M. V. Norgard. 2001. Expression of Borrelia burgdorferi OspC and DbpA is controlled by a RpoN-RpoS regulatory pathway. Proc. Natl. Acad. Sci. USA 98:12724–12729.

92. Huxsoll, D. L., P. K. Hildebrandt, R. M. Nims, J. A. Ferguson, and J. S. Walker. 1969. Ehrlichia canis, the causative agent of a hemorrhagic disease of dogs? Vet. Rec. 85:857.

93. Inoue, N., K. Hanada, N. Tsuji, I. Igarashi, H. Nagasawa, T. Mikami, and K. Fujisaki. 2001. Characterization of phagocytic hemocytes in Ornithodoros moubata (Acari: Ixodidae). J. Med. Entomol. 38:514–519.

94. Iqbal, Z., and Y. Rikihisa. 1994. Application of the polymerase chain-reaction for the detection of Ehrlichia canis in tissues of dogs. Vet. Microbiol. 42:281–287.

95. Jauron, S. D., S. A. Ewing, J. E. Dawson, K. M. Kocan, and U. G. Munderloh. 1999. Reactivity of dog sera with Ehrlichia canis antigen from dog or tick cell culture, abstr. 144. In Proceedings of the 80th Conference of Research Workers in Animal Diseases, Chicago, Ill.

96. Jauron, S. D., C. M. Nelson, V. Fingerle, M. D. Ravyn, J. L. Goodman, R. C. Johnson, R. Lobentanzer, B. Wilske, and U. G. Munderloh. 2001. Host cell specific expression of a p44 epitope by the human granulocytic ehrlichiosis agent. J. Infect. Dis. 184:1445–1450.

97. Johns, R., J. Ohnishi, A. H. Broadwater, D. E. Sonenshine, A. M. De Silva, and W. L. Hynes. 2001. Contrasts in tick innate immune responses to Borrelia burgdorferi challenge: immunotolerance in Ixodes scapularis versus immunocompetence in Dermacentor variabilis (Acari: Ixodidae). J. Med. Entomol. 38:99–107.

98. Johns, R., D. Sonenshine, and W. L. Hynes. 2000. Response of the tick Dermacentor variabilis (Acari: Ixodidae) to hemo-

coelic inoculation of *Borrelia burgdorferi* (Spirochetales). *J. Med. Entomol.* **37**:265–270.

99. Johns, R., D. E. Sonenshine, and W. L. Hynes. 1998. Control of bacterial infection in the hard tick *Dermacentor variabilis* (Acari: Ixodidae): evidence for the existence of antimicrobial proteins in tick hemolymph. *J. Med. Entomol.* **35**:458–464.

100. Johns, R., D. E. Sonenshine, and W. L. Hynes. 2000. Enhancement of OspC expression by *Borrelia burgdorferi* in the presence of tick hemolymph. *FEMS Microbiol. Lett.* **193**:137–141.

101. Johns, R., D. E. Sonenshine, and W. L. Hynes. 2001. Identification of a defensin from the hemolymph of the American dog tick, *Dermacentor variabilis*. *Insect Biochem. Mol. Biol.* **31**:857–865.

102. Katavolos, P., P. M. Armstrong, J. E. Dawson, and S. R. Telford III. 1998. Duration of tick attachment required for transmission of granulocytic ehrlichiosis. *J. Infect. Dis.* **177**:1422–1425.

103. Kim, H. Y., and Y. Rikihisa. 2000. Expression of interleukin-1β, tumor necrosis factor alpha, and interleukin-6 in human peripheral blood leukocytes exposed to human granulocytic ehrlichiosis agent or recombinant major surface protein P44. *Infect. Immun.* **68**:3394–3402.

104. Klein, M. B., S. F. Hayes, and J. L. Goodman. 1998. Monocytic differentiation inhibits infection and granulocytic differentiation potentiates infection by the agent of human granulocytic ehrlichiosis. *Infect. Immun.* **66**:3410–3415.

105. Klein, M. B., S. Hu, C. C. Chao, and J. L. Goodman. 2000. The agent of human granulocytic ehrlichiosis induces the production of myelosuppressing chemokines without induction of proinflammatory cytokines. *J. Infect. Dis.* **182**:200–205.

106. Klein, M. B., J. S. Miller, C. M. Nelson, and J. L. Goodman. 1997. Primary bone marrow progenitors of both granulocytic and monocytic lineages are susceptible to infection with the agent of human granulocytic ehrlichiosis. *J. Infect. Dis.* **176**:1405–1409.

107. Kocan, K. M. 1986. Development of Anaplasma marginale Theiler in ixodid ticks: coordinated development of a rickettsial organism and its tick host, p. 472–505. *In* J. R. Sauer and J. A. Hair (ed.), *Morphology, Physiology, and Behavioral Biology of Ticks*. Ellis Horwood, Chichester, United Kingdom.

108. Kocan, K. M., and J. D. Bezuidenhout. 1987. Morphology and development of *Cowdria ruminantium* in *Amblyomma* ticks. *Onderstepoort J. Vet. Res.* **54**:177–182.

109. Kocan, K. M., D. Stiller, W. L. Goff, P. L. Claypool, W. Edwards, S. A. Ewing, T. C. McGuire, J. A. Hair, and S. J. Barron. 1992. Development of *Anaplasma marginale* in male *Dermacentor andersoni* transferred from parasitemic to susceptible cattle. *Am. J. Vet. Res.* **53**:499–507.

110. Kodata, K., E. Satoh, M. Ochiai, N. Inoue, N. Tsuji, I. Igarashi, H. Nagasawa, T. Mikami, F. G. Claveria, and K. Fujisaki. 2002. Existence of phenol oxidase in the argasid tick *Ornithodoros moubata*. *Parasitol. Res.* **88**:781–784.

111. Kopácek, P., R. Vogt, L. Jindrák, C. Weise, and I. Safarik. 1999. Purification and characterization of the lysozyme from the gut of the soft tick *Ornithodoros moubata*. *Insect Biochem. Mol. Biol.* **29**:989–997.

112. Kopáček, P., C. Weise, T. Saravanan, K. Vítová, and L. Grubhoffer. 2000. Characterization of an α-macroglobulin-like glycoprotein from the plasma of the soft tick *Ornithodoros moubata*. *Eur. J. Biochem.* **267**:465–475.

113. Kopáček, P., J. Ždychová, T. Yoshiga, C. Weise, N. Rudenko, and J. H. Law. 2002. Molecular cloning, expression and isolation of ferritins from two tick species—*Ornithodoros moubata* and *Ixodes ricinus*. *Insect Biochem. Mol. Biol.* **33**:103–113.

114. Kopmans-Gargantiel, A. I., and J. C. L. Wisseman. 1981. Differential requirements for enriched atmospheric carbon dioxide content for intracellular growth in cell culture among selected members of the genus *Rickettsia*. *Infect. Immun.* **31**:1277–1280.

115. Kovár, V., P. Kopáček, and L. Grubhoffer. 2000. Isolation and characterization of Dorin M, a lectin from plasma of the soft tick *Ornithodoros moubata*. *Insect Biochem. Mol. Biol.* **30**:195–205.

116. Kraiczy, P., C. Skerka, V. Brade, and P. F. Zipfel. 2001. Further characterization of complement regulator-acquiring surface proteins of *Borrelia burgdorferi*. *Infect. Immun.* **69**:7800–7809.

117. Krause, P. J., K. McKay, C. D. Thompson, V. K. Sikand, R. Lentz, T. Lepore, L. Closter, D. Christianson, S. Telford, D. Persing, J. D. Radolf, A. Spielman, and the Deer-Associated Infection Study Group. 2002. Disease-specific diagnosis of coinfecting tickborne zoonoses: babesiosis, human granulocytic ehrlichiosis, and Lyme disease. *Clin. Infect. Dis.* **34**:1184–1191.

118. Kryochechnikov, V. N. 1991. Protective responses of Ixodoidea hemocytes, p. 331–334. *In* F. Dusbábek and V. Bukva (ed.), *Modern Acarology*, vol. 1. Academia SPB Academic Publishing bv, Prague, Czech Republic.

119. Kuhn, K. H., and T. Haug. 1994. Ultrastructural, cytochemical, and immunocytochemical characterization of haemocytes of the hard tick *Ixodes ricinus* (Acari: Chelicerata). *Cell Tissue Res.* **277**:493–504.

120. Kurtenbach, K., S. De Michelis, S. Etti, S. M. Schäfer, H.-S. Sewell, V. Brade, and P. Kraiczy. 2002. Host association of *Borrelia burgdorferi* sensu lato—the key role of host complement. *Trends Microbiol.* **10**:74–79.

121. Kurtti, T. J., U. G. Munderloh, T. G. Andreadis, L. A. Magnarelli, and T. N. Mather. 1996. Tick cell isolation of an intracellular prokaryote from the tick *Ixodes scapularis*. *J. Invertebr. Pathol.* **67**:318–321.

122. Kurtti, T. J., U. G. Munderloh, S. F. Hayes, D. E. Krueger, and G. G. Ahlstrand. 1994. Ultrastructural analysis of the invasion of tick cells by Lyme disease spirochetes (*Borrelia burgdorferi*) in vitro. *Can. J. Zool.* **72**:977–994.

123. Layfield, D., and P. Guilfoile. 2002. The prevalence of *Borrelia burgdorferi* (Spirochaetales: Spirochaetaceae) and the agent of human granulocytic ehrlichiosis (Rickettsiaceae: Ehrlichieae) in *Ixodes scapularis* (Acari: Ixodidae) collected during 1998 and 1999 from Minnesota. *J. Med. Entomol.* **39**:218–220.

124. Leboulle, G., C. Rochez, J. Louahed, B. Rutti, M. Brossard, A. Bollen, and E. Godfroid. 2002. Isolation of *Ixodes ricinus* salivary gland mRNA encoding factors induced during blood feeding. *Am. J. Trop. Med. Hyg.* **66**:225–233.

125. Lee, E. H., and Y. Rikihisa. 1997. Anti-*Ehrlichia chaffeensis* antibody complexed with *E. chaffeensis* induces potent proinflammatory cytokine mRNA expression in human monocytes through sustained reduction of I κB-a and activation of NF-κB. *Infect. Immun.* **65**:2890–2897.

126. Lee, E. H., and Y. Rikihisa. 1998. Protein kinase A-mediated inhibition of gamma interferon-induced tyrosine phosphorylation of Janus kinases and latent cytoplasmic transcription factors in human monocytes by *Ehrlichia chaffeensis*. *Infect. Immun.* **66**:2514–2520.

127. Levin, M. L., and D. Fish. 2000. Acquisition of coinfection and simultaneous transmission of *Borrelia burgdorferi* and *Ehrlichia phagocytophila* by *Ixodes scapularis* ticks. *Infect. Immun.* **68**:2183–2186.

128. Levin, M. L., and D. Fish. 2001. Interference between the agents of Lyme disease and human granulocytic ehrlichiosis in a natural reservoir host. *Vector Borne Zoonotic Dis.* **1**:139–148.

129. Lighton, J. R. B., L. J. Fielden, and Y. Rechav. 1993. Discontinuous ventilation in a non-insect, the tick *Amblyomma marmoreum* (Acari: Ixodidae): characterization and metabolic modulation. *J. Exp. Zool.* 180:229–245.

130. Logullo, C., J. Moraes, M. Dansa-Petretski, I. S. Vaz, Jr., A. Masuda, M. H. F. Sorgine, G. R. Braz, H. Masuda, and P. L. Oliveira. 2002. Binding and storage of heme by vitellin from the cattle tick, *Boophilus microplus*. *Insect Biochem. Mol. Biol.* 32:1805–1811.

131. Löhr, C. V., F. R. Rurangirwa, T. F. McElwain, D. Stiller, and G. H. Palmer. 2002. Specific expression of *Anaplasma marginale* major surface protein 2 salivary gland variants occurs in the midgut and is an early event during tick transmission. *Infect. Immun.* 70:114–120.

132. Loosová, G., L. Jindrák, and P. Kopácek. 2001. Mortality caused by experimental infection with the yeast *Candida haemulonii* in the adults of *Ornithodoros moubata* (Acarina: Argasidae). *Folia Parasitol.* 48:149–153.

133. Macaluso, K. R., D. E. Sonenshine, S. M. Ceraul, and A. F. Azad. 2001. Infection and transovarial transmission of rickettsiae in *Dermacentor variabilis* ticks acquired by artificial feeding. *Vector Borne Zoonotic Dis.* 1:45–53.

134. Macaluso, K. R., D. E. Sonenshine, S. M. Ceraul, and A. F. Azad. 2002. Rickettsial infection in *Dermacentor variabilis* (Acari: Ixodidae) inhibits transovarial transmission of a second *Rickettsia*. *J. Med. Entomol.* 39:809–813.

135. Mahan, S. M., B. Allsopp, K. M. Kocan, G. H. Palmer, and F. Jongejan. 1999. Vaccine strategies for *Cowdria ruminantium* infections and their application to other ehrlichial infections. *Parasitol. Today* 15:290–294.

136. Martin, P. A. W., and E. T. Schmidtmann. 1998. Isolation of aerobic microbes from *Ixodes scapularis* (Acari: Ixodidae), the vector of Lyme disease in eastern United States. *J. Med. Entomol.* 91:864–868.

137. Mathew, J. S., S. A. Ewing, R. W. Barker, J. C. Fox, J. E. Dawson, C. K. Warner, G. L. Murphy, and K. M. Kocan. 1996. Attempted transmission of *Ehrlichia canis* by *Rhipicephalus sanguineus* after passage in cell culture. *Am. J. Vet. Res.* 57:1594–1598.

138. Maya-Monteiro, C. M., S. Daffre, C. Logullo, F. A. Lara, E. W. Alves, M. L. Capurro, R. Zingali, I. C. Almeida, and P. L. Oliveira. 2000. HeLp, a heme lipoprotein from the hemolymph of the cattle tick, *Boophilus microplus*. *J. Biol. Chem.* 275:36584–36589.

139. McBride, J. W., X. J. Yu, and D. H. Walker. 2000. A conserved, transcriptionally active p28 multigene locus of *Ehrlichia canis*. *Gene* 254:245–252.

140. Mendiola, J., M. Alonso, M. C. Marquetti, and C. Finlay. 1996. *Boophilus microplus*: multiple proteolytic activities in the midgut. *Exp. Parasitol.* 82:27–33.

141. Moss, W. J., and J. S. Dumler. 2003. Simultaneous infection with *Borrelia burgdorferi* and human granulocytic ehrlichiosis. *Pediatr. Infect. Dis. J.* 22:91–92.

142. Mott, J., R. E. Barnewall, and Y. Rikihisa. 1999. Human granulocytic ehrlichiosis agent and *Ehrlichia chaffeensis* reside in different cytoplasmic compartments in HL-60 cells. *Infect. Immun.* 67:1368–1378.

143. Mott, J., and Y. Rikihisa. 2000. Human granulocytic ehrlichiosis agent inhibits superoxide anion generation by human neutrophils. *Infect. Immun.* 68:6697–6703.

144. Munderloh, U. G., E. F. Blouin, K. M. Kocan, N.-L. Ge, W. L. Edwards, and T. J. Kurtti. 1996. Establishment of the tick (Acari: Ixodidae)-borne cattle pathogen *Anaplasma marginale* (Rickettsiales: Anaplasmataceae) in tick cell culture. *J. Med. Entomol.* 33:656–664.

145. Munderloh, U. G., S. F. Hayes, J. Cummings, and T. J. Kurtti. 1998. Microscopy of spotted fever rickettsia movement through tick cells. *Microsc. Microanal.* 4:115–121.

146. Munderloh, U. G., S. D. Jauron, V. Fingerle, L. Leitritz, S. F. Hayes, J. M. Hautman, C. M. Nelson, B. W. Huberty, T. J. Kurtti, G. G. Ahlstrand, B. Greig, M. A. Mellencamp, and J. L. Goodman. 1999. Invasion and intracellular development of the human granulocytic ehrlichiosis agent in tick cell culture. *J. Clin. Microbiol.* 37:2518–2524.

147. Munderloh, U. G., and T. J. Kurtti. 1989. Formulation of medium for tick cell culture. *Exp. Appl. Acarol.* 7:219–229.

148. Munderloh, U. G., and T. J. Kurtti. 1995. Cellular and molecular interrelationships between ticks and prokaryotic tick-borne pathogens. *Annu. Rev. Entomol.* 40:221–243.

149. Munderloh, U. G., Y. Liu, M. Wang, C. Chen, and T. J. Kurtti. 1994. Establishment, maintenance and description of cell lines from the tick *Ixodes scapularis*. *J. Parasitol.* 80:533–543.

150. Munderloh, U. G., M. J. Lynch, and A. T. Palmer. 2002. Infection of endothelial cells with human and bovine *Anaplasma* species, abstr. O-11. In *IX International Conference on Lyme Borreliosis and Other Tick-Borne Diseases, New York, N.Y.*

151. Munderloh, U. G., J. E. Madigan, J. S. Dumler, J. L. Goodman, S. F. Hayes, J. E. Barlough, C. M. Nelson, and T. J. Kurtti. 1996. Isolation of the equine granulocytic ehrlichiosis agent, *Ehrlichia equi*, in tick cell culture. *J. Clin. Microbiol.* 34:664–670.

152. Nakajima, Y., A. van der Goes van Naters-Yasui, D. Taylor, and M. Yamakawa. 2002. Antibacterial peptide defensin is involved in midgut immunity of the soft tick, *Ornithodoros moubata*. *Insect Mol. Biol.* 11:611–618.

153. Nakajima, Y., A. van der Goes van Naters-Yasui, D. Taylor, and M. Yamakawa. 2001. Two isoforms of a member of the arthropod defensin family from the soft tick, *Ornithodoros moubata* (Acari: Argasidae). *Insect Biochem. Mol. Biol.* 31:747–751.

154. Narasimhan, S., F. Santiago, R. A. Koski, B. Brei, J. F. Anderson, D. Fish, and E. Fikrig. 2002. Examination of the *Borrelia burgdorferi* transcriptome in *Ixodes scapularis* during feeding. *J. Bacteriol.* 184:3122–3125.

155. Needham, G. R., and P. D. Teel. 1986. Water balance by ticks between bloodmeals, p. 100–151. In J. R. Sauer and J. A. Hair (ed.), *Morphology, Physiology, and Behavioral Biology of Ticks*. Ellis Horwood Limited, Chichester, United Kingdom.

156. Nene, V. L. D., J. Quackenbush, R. Skilton, S. Mwaura, M. J. Gardner, and R. Bishop. 2002. AvGI, an index of gene transcribed in the salivary glands of the ixodid tick *Amblyomma variegatum*. *Int. J. Parasitol.* 32:1447–1456.

157. Niebylski, M. L., M. G. Peacock, E. R. Fischer, S. F. Porcella, and T. G. Schwan. 1997. Characterization of an endosymbiont infecting wood ticks, *Dermacentor andersoni*, as a member of the genus *Francisella*. *Appl. Environ. Microbiol.* 63:3933–3940.

158. Niebylski, M. L., M. G. Peacock, and T. G. Schwan. 1999. Lethal effect of *Rickettsia rickettsii* on its tick vector (*Dermacentor andersoni*). *Appl. Environ. Microbiol.* 65:773–778.

159. Niebylski, M. L., M. E. Schrumpf, W. Burgdorfer, E. R. Fischer, K. L. Gage, and T. G. Schwan. 1997. *Rickettsia peacockii* sp. nov., a new species infecting wood ticks, *Dermacentor andersoni*, in western Montana. *Int. J. Syst. Bacteriol.* 47:446–452.

160. Nuttall, P. A. 1998. Displaced tick-parasite interactions at the host interface. *Parasitology* 116:S65–S72.

161. Nuttall, P. A., G. C. Paesen, C. H. Lawrie, V. Hajnická, N. Fuchsberger, and H. Wang. 2001. Tick-host interactions in spirochete transmission, p. 53–60. In J. M. H. Saier and J. García-Lara (ed.), *The Spirochetes: Molecular and Cellular Biology*. Horizon Press, Oxford, United Kingdom.

162. Nuttall, P. A., G. C. Paesen, C. H. Lawrie, and H. Wang. 2000. Vector-host interactions in disease transmission. *J. Mol. Microbiol. Technol.* **2**:381–386.

163. Obonyo, M., U. G. Munderloh, V. Fingerle, B. Wilske, and T. J. Kurtti. 1999. *Borrelia burgdorferi* in tick cell culture modulates expression of outer surface proteins A and C in response to temperature. *J. Clin. Microbiol.* **37**:2137–2141.

164. Ohashi, N., Y. Rikihisa, and A. Unver. 2001. Analysis of transcriptionally active gene clusters of major outer membrane protein multigene family in *Ehrlichia canis* and *E. chaffeensis*. *Infect. Immun.* **69**:2083–2091.

165. Ohashi, N., A. Unver, N. Zhi, and Y. Rikihisa. 1998. Cloning and characterization of multigenes encoding the immunodominant 30-kilodalton major outer membrane proteins of *Ehrlichia canis* and application of the recombinant protein for serodiagnosis. *J. Clin. Microbiol.* **36**:2671–2680.

166. Ohashi, N., N. Zhi, Y. Zhang, and Y. Rikihisa. 1998. Immunodominant major outer membrane proteins of *Ehrlichia chaffeensis* are encoded by a polymorphic multigene family. *Infect. Immun.* **66**:132–139.

167. Ohnishi, J., J. Piesman, and A. M. De Silva. 2001. Antigenic and genetic heterogeneity of *Borrelia burgdorferi* populations transmitted by ticks. *Proc. Natl. Acad. Sci. USA* **98**:670–675.

168. Paddock, C. D., S. M. Folk, G. M. Shore, L. J. Machado, M. M. Huycke, L. N. Slater, A. M. Liddell, R. S. Buller, G. A. Storch, T. P. Monson, D. Rimland, J. W. Sumner, J. Singleton, K. C. Bloch, Y. W. Tang, S. M. Standaert, and J. E. Childs. 2001. Infections with Ehrlichia chaffeensis and Ehrlichia ewingii in persons coinfected with human immunodeficiency virus. *Clin. Infect. Dis.* **33**:1586–1594.

169. Pal, U., A. M. de Silva, R. R. Montgomery, D. Fish, J. Anguita, J. F. Anderson, Y. Lobet, and E. Fikrig. 2000. Attachment of *Borrelia burgdorferi* within *Ixodes scapularis* mediated by outer surface protein A. *J. Clin. Investig.* **106**:561–569.

170. Pal, U., R. R. Montgomery, D. Lusitani, P. Voet, V. Weynants, S. E. Malawista, Y. Lobet, and E. Fikrig. 2001. Inhibition of *Borrelia burgdorferi*-tick interactions in vivo by outer surface protein A antibody. *J. Immunol.* **166**:7398–7403.

171. Palmer, G. H., K. M. Kocan, S. J. Barron, J. A. Hair, A. F. Barbet, W. C. Davis, and T. C. McGuire. 1985. Presence of common antigens, including major surface protein epitopes, between the cattle (intraerythrocytic) and tick stages of *Anaplasma marginale*. *Infect. Immun.* **50**:881–886.

172. Palmer, G. H., F. R. Rurangirwa, and T. F. McElwain. 2001. Strain composition of the ehrlichia *Anaplasma marginale* within persistently infected cattle, a mammalian reservoir for tick transmission. *J. Clin. Microbiol.* **39**:631–635.

173. Pancholi, P., C. P. Kolbert, P. D. Mitchell, K. D. Reed, J. S. Dumler, J. S. Bakken, S. R. Telford III, and D. H. Persing. 1995. *Ixodes dammini* as a potential vector of human granulocytic ehrlichiosis. *J. Infect. Dis.* **172**:1007–1012.

174. Parola, P., L. Beati, M. Cambon, P. Brouqui, and D. Raoult. 1998. Ehrlichial DNA amplified from *Ixodes ricinus* (Acari: Ixodidae) in France. *J. Med. Entomol.* **35**:180–183.

175. Paster, B. J., and F. E. Dewhirst. 2001. Phylogenetic foundation of spirochetes, p. 5–9. *In* J. M. H. Saier and J. García-Lara (ed.), *The Spirochetes: Molecular and Cellular Biology*. Horizon Press, Oxford, United Kingdom.

176. Pereira, L. S., P. L. Oliveira, C. Barja-Fidalgo, and S. Daffre. 2001. Production of reactive oxygen species by hemocytes from the cattle tick *Boophilus microplus*. *Exp. Parasitol.* **99**:66–72.

177. Peterson, K. J., R. J. Raleigh, R. K. Stroud, and R. L. Goulding. 1977. Bovine anaplasmosis transmission studies conducted under controlled natural exposure in a *Dermacentor andersoni* (*venustus*) indigenous area of eastern Oregon. *Am. J. Vet. Res.* **38**:351–354.

178. Piesman, J., J. G. Donahue, T. N. Mather, and A. Spielman. 1986. Transovarially acquired Lyme disease spirochetes (*Borrelia burgdorferi*) in field-collected larval *Ixodes dammini* (Acari: Ixodidae). *J. Med. Entomol.* **23**:219.

179. Piesman, J., T. N. Mather, R. J. Sinsky, and A. Spielman. 1987. Duration of tick attachment and *Borrelia burgdorferi* transmission. *J. Clin. Microbiol.* **25**:557–558.

180. Piesman, J., G. O. Maupin, E. G. Campos, and C. M. Happ. 1991. Duration of adult female *Ixodes dammini* attachment and transmission of *Borrelia burgdorferi*, with description of a needle aspiration isolation method. *J. Infect. Dis.* **163**: 895–897.

181. Piesman, J., J. R. Oliver, and R. J. Sinsky. 1990. Growth kinetics of the Lyme disease spirochete (*Borrelia burgdorferi*) in vector ticks (*Ixodes dammini*). *Am. J. Trop. Med. Hyg.* **42**:352–357.

182. Podboronov, V. M., and A. M. Podboronov. 1997. Immunity of ticks. *Acarina* **5**:87–89.

183. Policastro, P., U. G. Munderloh, E. R. Fischer, and T. Hackstadt. 1997. *Rickettsia rickettsii* growth and temperature-inducible protein expression in embryonic tick cell lines. *J. Med. Microbiol.* **46**:839–845.

184. Popov, V. L., X.-J. Yu, and D. H. Walker. 2000. The 120 kDa outer membrane protein of *Ehrlichia chaffeensis*: preferential expression on dense-core cells and gene expression in *Escherichia coli* associated with attachment and entry. *Microb. Pathog.* **28**:71–80.

185. Pretzman, C., D. Ralph, D. R. Stothard, P. A. Fuerst, and Y. Rikihisa. 1995. 16S rRNA gene sequence of *Neorickettsia helminthoeca* and its phylogenetic alignment with members of the genus *Ehrlichia*. *Int. J. Syst. Bacteriol.* **45**:207–211.

186. Prozesky, L., and J. L. Du Plessis. 1987. Heartwater. The development and life sycle of *Cowdria ruminantium* in the vertebrate host, ticks and cultured endothelial cells. *Onderstepoort J. Vet. Res.* **54**:193–196.

187. Rathinavelu, S., and A. M. De Silva. 2001. Purification and characterization of *Borrelia burgdorferi* from feeding nymphal ticks (*Ixodes scapularis*). *Infect. Immun.* **69**:3536–3541.

188. Ratnasamy, N., E. D. Everett, W. E. Roland, G. McDonald, and C. W. Caldwell. 1996. Central nervous system manifestations of human ehrlichiosis. *Clin. Infect. Dis.* **23**:314–319.

189. Reddy, G. R., C. R. Sulsona, A. F. Barbet, S. M. Mahan, M. J. Burridge, and A. R. Alleman. 1998. Molecular characterization of a 28 kDa surface antigen gene family of the tribe Ehrlichiae. *Biochem. Biophys. Res. Commun.* **247**: 636–643.

190. Reubel, G. H., J. E. Barlough, and J. E. Madigan. 1998. Production and characterization of *Ehrlichia risticii*, the agent of Potomac horse fever, from snails (Pleuroceridae: *Juga* spp.) in aquarium culture and genetic comparison to equine strains. *J. Clin. Microbiol.* **36**:1501–1511.

191. Revel, A. T., A. M. Talaat, and M. V. Norgard. 2002. DNA microarray analysis of differential gene expression in *Borrelia burgdorferi*, the Lyme disease spirochete. *Proc. Natl. Acad. Sci. USA* **99**:1562–1567.

192. Ribeiro, J. M. C. 1987. *Ixodes dammini* salivary anti-complement activity. *Exp. Parasitol.* **64**:347–353.

193. Ribeiro, J. M. C. 1988. The midgut hemolysin of *Ixodes dammini* (Acari: Ixodidae). *J. Parasitol.* **74**:532–537.

194. Ribeiro, J. M. C., P. M. Evans, J. L. MacSwain, and J. R. Sauer. 1992. *Amblyomma americanum*: characterization of salivary prostaglandins E2 and F2 alpha by RP-HPLC/bioassay and gas chromatography-mass spectrometry. *Exp. Parasitol.* **74**:112–116.

195. Ribeiro, J. M. C., G. T. Makoul, J. Levine, D. R. Robinson, and A. Spielman. 1985. Antihemostatic, antiinflammatory,

and immunosuppressive properties of the saliva of a tick, *Ixodes dammini. J. Exp. Med.* **161:**332–344.

196. Ribeiro, J. M. C., J. J. Weis, and S. R. Telford III. 1990. Saliva of the tick *Ixodes dammini* inhibits neutrophil function. *Exp. Parasitol.* **70:**382–388.

197. Richter, P. J., Jr., R. B. Kimsey, J. E. Madigan, J. E. Barlough, J. S. Dumler, and D. L. Brooks. 1996. *Ixodes pacificus* (Acari: Ixodidae) as a vector of *Ehrlichia equi* (Rickettsiales: Ehrlichieae). *J. Med. Entomol.* **33:**1–5.

198. Rikihisa, Y. 1999. Clinical and biological aspects of infection caused by *Ehrlichia chaffeensis. Microbes Infect.* **1:**367–376.

199. Ristic, M., and A. M. Watrach. 1963. Anaplasmosis IV. Studies and a hypothesis concerning the cycle of development of the causative agent. *Am. J. Vet. Res.* **24:**267–276.

200. Roberts, D. M., M. Caimano, J. McDowell, M. Theisen, A. Holm, E. Orff, D. Nelson, S. K. Wikel, J. D. Radolf, and R. T. Marconi. 2002. Environmental regulation and differential production of members of the Bdr protein family of *Borrelia burgdorferi. Infect. Immun.* **70:**7033–7041.

201. Roehrig, J. T., J. Piesman, A. R. Hunt, M. G. Keen, C. M. Happ, and B. J. B. Johnson. 1992. The hamster immune response to tick-transmitted *Borrelia burgdorferi* differs from the response to needle-inoculated, cultured organisms. *J. Immunol.* **149:**3648–3653.

202. Rudzinska, M. A., A. Spielman, S. Lewengrub, J. Piesman, and S. Karakashian. 1982. Penetration of the peritrophic membrane of the tick by *Babesia microti. Cell Tissue Res.* **221:**471–481.

203. Rurangirwa, F. R., D. Stiller, D. M. French, and G. H. Palmer. 1999. Restriction of major surface protein 2 (MSP2) variants during tick transmission of the ehrlichia *Anaplasma marginale. Proc. Natl. Acad. Sci. USA* **96:**3171–3176.

204. Rurangirwa, F. R., D. Stiller, and G. H. Palmer. 2000. Strain diversity in major surface protein 2 expression during tick transmission of *Anaplasma marginale. Infect. Immun.* **68:**3023–3027.

205. Samish, M., E. Pipano, and B. Hana. 1989. Cultivation of *Anaplasma marginale* from cattle in a *Dermacentor* cell line. *Am. J. Vet. Res.* **49:**254–256.

206. Samish, M., and J. Rehacek. 1999. Pathogens and predators of ticks and their potential in biological control. *Annu. Rev. Entomol.* **44:**159–182.

207. Sauer, J. R., R. C. Essenberg, and A. S. Bowman. 2000. Salivary glands in ixodid ticks: control and mechanism of secretion. *J. Insect Physiol.* **46:**1069–1078.

208. Sauer, J. R., J. L. McSwain, A. S. Bowman, and R. C. Essenberg. 1995. Tick salivary gland physiology. *Ann. Rev. Entomol.* **40:**245–267.

209. Schauder, S., K. Shokat, M. G. Surette, and B. L. Bassler. 2001. The LuxS family of bacterial autoinducers: biosynthesis of a novel quorum-sensing signal molecule. *Mol. Microbiol.* **41:**463–476.

210. Schwan, T. G. 1996. Ticks and *Borrelia*: model systems for investigating pathogen-arthropod interactions. *Infect. Agents Dis.* **5:**167–181.

211. Schwan, T. G., and J. Piesman. 2000. Temporal changes in outer surface proteins A and C of the Lyme disease-associated spirochete, *Borrelia burgdorferi*, during the chain of infection in ticks and mice. *J. Clin. Microbiol.* **38:**382–388.

212. Schwan, T. G., J. Piesman, W. T. Golde, M. C. Dolan, and P. A. Rosa. 1995. Induction of an outer surface protein on *Borrelia burgdorferi* during tick feeding. *Proc. Natl. Acad. Sci. USA* **92:**2909–2913.

213. Semu, S. M., T. F. Peter, D. Mukwedeya, A. F. Barbet, F. Jongejan, and S. M. Mahan. 2001. Antibody responses to MAP 1B and other *Cowdria ruminantium* antigens are down

regulated in cattle challenged with tick-transmitted heartwater. *Clin. Diagn. Lab. Immunol.* **8:**388–396.

214. Shaw, S. E., M. J. Day, R. J. Birtles, and E. B. Breitschwerdt. 2001. Tick-borne infectious diseases of dogs. *Trends Parasitol.* **17:**74–80.

215. Simser, J. A., A. T. Palmer, V. Fingerle, B. Wilske, T. J. Kurtti, and U. G. Munderloh. 2002. *Rickettsia monacensis* sp. nov., a spotted fever group rickettsia, from ticks (*Ixodes ricinus*) collected in a European city park. *Appl. Environ. Microbiol.* **68:**4559–4566.

216. Simser, J. A., A. T. Palmer, U. G. Munderloh, and T. J. Kurtti. 2001. Isolation of a spotted fever group rickettsia, *Rickettsia peacockii*, in a Rocky Mountain wood tick, *Dermacentor andersoni*, cell line. *Appl. Environ. Microbiol.* **67:**546–552.

217. Smith, R. D., D. M. Sells, E. H. Stephenson, M. Ristic, and D. L. Huxsoll. 1976. Development of *Ehrlichia canis*, causative agent of canine ehrlichiosis, in the tick *Rhipicephalus sanguineus* and its differentiation from a symbiotic rickettsia. *Am. J. Vet. Res.* **37:**119–126.

217a. Sonenshine, D. E. 1991. *Biology of Ticks*, vol. 1. Oxford University Press, New York, N.Y.

218. Sonenshine, D. E. 1993. *Biology of Ticks*, vol. 2. Oxford University Press, New York, N.Y.

219. Sotomayor, E. A., V. L. Popov, H.-M. Feng, D. H. Walker, and J. P. Olano. 2001. Animal model of fatal human monocytotropic ehrlichiosis. *Am. J. Pathol.* **158:**757–769.

220. Spencer, R. R., and R. R. Parker. 1923. Rocky mountain spotted fever: infectivity of fasting and recently fed ticks. *Public Health Rep.* **38:**333–339.

221. Stackebrandt, E., R. G. E. Murray, and H. G. Trüper. 1988. Proteobacteria classis nov., a name for the phylogenetic taxon that includes the "purple bacteria and their relatives." *Int. J. Syst. Bacteriol.* **38:**321–325.

222. Stevenson, B., and K. Babb. 2002. LuxS-mediated quorum sensing in *Borrelia burgdorferi*, the Lyme disease spirochete. *Infect. Immun.* **70:**4099–4105.

223. Stevenson, B., T. Schwan, and P. A. Rosa. 1995. Temperature-related differential expression of antigens in the Lyme disease spirochete, *Borrelia burgdorferi. Infect. Immun.* **63:**4535–4539.

224. Stich, R. W., J. R. Sauer, J. A. Bantle, and K. M. Kocan. 1993. Detection of *Anaplasma marginale* (Rickettsiales: Anaplasmataceae) in secretagogue-induced oral secretions of *Dermacentor andersoni* (Acari: Ixodidae) with the polymerase chain reaction. *J. Med. Entomol.* **30:**789–794.

225. Sulsona, C. R., S. F. Mahan, and A. F. Barbet. 1999. The *map1* gene of *Cowdria ruminantium* is a member of a multigene family containing both conserved and variable genes. *Biochem. Biophys. Res. Commun.* **257:**300–305.

226. Sun, W., J. W. IJdo, S. R. Telford III, E. Hodzic, Y. Zhang, S. W. Barthold, and E. Fikrig. 1997. Immunization against the agent of human granulocytic ehrlichiosis in a murine model. *J. Clin. Investig.* **100:**3014–3018.

227. Swift, B. L., and G. M. Thomas. 1983. Bovine anaplasmosis: elimination of the carrier state with injectable long-acting oxytetracycline. *J. Am. Vet. Med. Assoc.* **183:**63–65.

228. Telford, S. R., III, J. E. Dawson, P. Katavolos, C. K. Warner, C. P. Kolbert, and D. H. Persing. 1996. Perpetuation of the agent of human granulocytic ehrlichiosis in a deer tick-rodent cycle. *Proc. Natl. Acad. Sci. USA* **9:**6209–6214.

229. Valenzuela, J. G., R. Charlab, T. N. Mather, and J. M. C. Ribeiro. 2000. Purification, cloning, and expression of a novel salivary anticomplement protein from the tick, *Ixodes scapularis. J. Biol. Chem.* **275:**18717–18723.

230. Valenzuela, J. G., I. M. B. Francischetti, V. M. Pham, M. K. Garfield, T. N. Mather, and J. M. C. Ribeiro. 2002. Explor-

ing the sialome of the tick *Ixodes scapularis*. *J. Exp. Biol.* **205:**2843–2864.

231. **van der Goes van Naters-Yasui, A., D. Taylor, T. Shono, and M. Yamakawa.** 2000. Purification and partial amino acid sequence of antibacterial peptides from the hemolymph of the soft tick, *Ornithodoros moubata* (Acari: Argasidae), p. 189–194. *In* M. L. M. Kazimirová and P.A. Nuttall (ed.), *Proceedings of the 3rd International Conference "Ticks and Tick-borne Pathogens: into the 21st Century."* Institute of Zoology, Slovak Academy of Sciences, Bratislava, Slovakia.

232. **Walls, J. J., B. Greig, D. F. Neitzel, and J. S. Dumler.** 1997. Natural infection of small mammal species in Minnesota with the agent of human granulocytic ehrlichiosis. *J. Clin. Microbiol.* **35:**853–855.

233. **Wang, H., and P. A. Nuttall.** 1999. Immunoglobulin-binding proteins in ticks: new target for vaccine development against a blood-feeding parasite. *Cell. Mol. Life Sci.* **56:**286–295.

234. **Wang, X.-G., B. Lin, M. Kidder, S. Telford, and L. T. Hu.** 2002. Effects of environmental changes on expression of the oligopeptide permease (*opp*) genes of *Borrelia burgdorferi*. *J. Bacteriol.* **184:**6198–6206.

235. **Watt, D. M., and A. R. Walker.** 2000. Pathological effects and reduced survival in *Rhipicephalus appendiculatus* ticks infected with *Theileria parva* protozoa. *Parasitol. Res.* **86:**207–214.

236. **Watt, D. M., A. R. Walker, K. A. Lamza, and N. C. Ambrose.** 2001. Tick-*Theileria* interactions in response to immune activation of the vector. *Exp. Parasitol.* **97:**89–94.

237. **Weller, S. J., G. D. Baldridge, U. G. Munderloh, H. Noda, J. Simser, and T. J. Kurtti.** 1998. Phylogenetic placement of rickettsiae from the ticks *Amblyomma americanum* and *Ixodes scapularis*. *J. Clin. Microbiol.* **36:**1305–1317.

238. **Wellman, M. L., S. Krakowa, R. M. Jacobs, and G. J. Kociba.** 1988. A macrophage-monocyte cell line from a dog with malignant histiocytosis. *In Vitro Cell Dev. Biol.* **24:**223–229.

239. **Wikel, S. K.** 1999. Tick modulation of host immunity: an important factor in pathogen transmission. *Int. J. Parasitol.* **29:**851–859.

240. **Yang, X., M. S. Goldberg, T. G. Popova, G. B. Schoeler, S. K. Wikel, K. E. Hagman, and M. V. Norgard.** 2000. Interdependence of environmental factors influencing reciprocal patterns of gene expression in virulent *Borrelia burgdorferi*. *Mol. Microbiol.* **37:**1470–1479.

241. **Yoshiie, K., H.-Y. Kim, J. Mott, and Y. Rikihisa.** 2000. Intracellular infection by the human granulocytosis agent inhibits human neutrophil apoptosis. *Infect. Immun.* **68:**1125–1133.

242. **Yu, X. J., P. Crocquetvaldes, and D. H. Walker.** 1997. Cloning and sequencing of the gene for a 120-kDA immunodominant protein of *Ehrlichia chaffeensis*. *Gene* **184:**149–154.

243. **Zaidi, S. A., and C. Singer.** 2002. Gastrointestinal and hepatic manifestations of tickborne diseases in the United States. *Clin. Infect. Dis.* **34:**1206–1212.

244. **Zaugg, J. L., D. Stiller, M. E. Caan, and S. D. Lincoln.** 1986. Transmission of *Anaplasma marginale* Theiler by males of *Dermacentor andersoni* Stiles fed on an Idaho field-infected, chronic carrier cow. *Am. J. Vet. Res.* **47:**2269–2271.

245. **Zeidner, N. S., M. Dreitz, D. Belasco, and D. Fish.** 1996. Suppression of acute *Ixodes scapularis*-induced *Borrelia burgdorferi* infection using tumor necrosis factor-alpha, interleukin-2, and interferon-gamma. *J. Infect. Dis.* **173:**187–195.

246. **Zeidner, N. S., B. S. Schneider, M. S. Nuncio, L. Gern, and J. Piesman.** 2002. Coinoculation of *Borrelia* spp. with tick salivary gland lysate enhances spirochete load in mice and is tick species-specific. *J. Parasitol.* **88:**1276–1278.

247. **Zhang, J.-R., J. M. Hardham, A. G. Barbour, and S. J. Norris.** 1997. Antigenic variation in Lyme disease borreliae by promiscuous recombination of VMP-like sequence cassettes. *Cell* **89:**275–285.

248. **Zhi, N., N. Ohashi, and Y. Rikihisa.** 1999. Multiple p44 genes encoding major outer membrane proteins are expressed in the human granulocytic ehrlichiosis agent. *J. Biol. Chem.* **274:**17828–17836.

249. **Zhi, N., N. Ohashi, Y. Rikihisa, H. W. Horowitz, G. P. Wormser, and K. Hechemy.** 1998. Cloning and expression of the 44-kilodalton major outer membrane protein gene of the human granulocytic ehrlichiosis agent and application of the recombinant protein to serodiagnosis. *J. Clin. Microbiol.* **36:**1666–1673.

250. **Zhioua, E., R. A. Lebrun, P. W. Johnson, and H. S. Ginsberg.** 1996. Ultrastructure of the haemocytes of *Ixodes scapularis* (Acari: Ixodidae). *Acarologia* **37:**173–179.

251. **Zhioua, E., M. T. Yeh, and R. A. Lebrun.** 1997. Assay for phenoloxidase activity in *Amblyomma americanum*, *Dermacentor variabilis*, and *Ixodes scapularis*. *J. Parasitol.* **83:**553–554.

252. **Zung, J. L., S. Lewengrub, M. A. Rudzinska, A. Spielman, S. R. Telford, and J. Piesman.** 1989. Fine structural evidence for the penetration of the Lyme disease spirochete *Borrelia burgdorferi* through the gut and salivary tissues of *Ixodes dammini*. *Can. J. Zool.* **67:**1737–1748.

Tick-Borne Diseases of Humans
Edited by Jesse L. Goodman et al.
© 2005 ASM Press, Washington, D.C.

Chapter 4

Management of Ticks and Tick-Borne Diseases

HOWARD S. GINSBERG AND KIRBY C. STAFFORD III

INTRODUCTION

Ticks cause substantial problems, both as nuisance pests and as vectors of human disease. They are also responsible for enormous economic losses resulting from decreased vigor in infested farm animals and transmission of diseases to domestic and agricultural animals. As such, a great deal of effort has been devoted to controlling ticks, and a great variety of techniques are currently available. Traditionally, most effort has focused on ways to kill ticks or to avoid tick attachment to humans and cattle, with relatively little effort devoted to integrated pest management (IPM) as applied to tick control.

In this chapter, we first review tick control techniques, including both traditional and novel approaches. Additional treatment of these methods can be found in several recent reviews (184, 198, 215). We then examine the decision-making process in tick management, both in the traditional agricultural setting and in the context of prevention of human disease. We hope, in this way, to foster a debate about the goals and principles of tick and tick-borne disease management that will result in a more robust, efficient, theory-driven, science-based practice of IPM for tick control.

TICK MANAGEMENT METHODS

Self-Protection

Precautions for self-protection from tick bites have the advantage of universal applicability to humans and domestic animals, with essentially no adverse environmental effects. The major difficulty is that in areas with dense tick populations and/or high pathogen prevalence in ticks, considerable diligence is required, sometimes to the point where self-protection is impractical.

Avoidance of ticks

Tick avoidance requires detailed knowledge of tick distribution and behavior. Surveys of distribution are available for ticks of economic or medical importance on worldwide, continental, national, state, county, and local scales (22, 39, 59, 89, 107, 129). The advent of geographic information systems (GIS) technology has greatly increased our capacity to map these distributions and quantify trends. However, the ability of GIS programs to interpolate between data points can result in misleading risk maps. Even in areas with high tick densities, for example, local tick abundance depends heavily on distribution of appropriate habitats (63) and hosts (216). Therefore, sites with little risk are often contiguous with high-risk sites. Avoidance of behaviors that put people or domestic animals at risk for exposure to ticks requires public education about tick distribution at the local level, as well as information about geographical distribution and seasonal activity. Investigators have developed protocols that can be used to assess risk of tick exposure based on site characteristics (65, 69, 174), some using satellite data (31). Nevertheless, geographical distributions of tick species can change through time (60, 205), and local populations often vary seasonally and from year to year (195), so active surveillance programs provide the best estimates of risk of exposure to ticks or tick-borne diseases.

Precautions

Commonly cited precautions to avoid tick bites include tucking pants into socks (to keep ticks outside clothing), taping to seal the junctions, wearing light-colored pants (to see dark ticks on the light background), spraying the clothing with repellents (e.g., *N,N*-diethyl-*m*-toluamide [DEET]) and/or acaricide (e.g., permethrin), and frequently pausing to find and remove ticks. Tick-transmitted pathogens generally

Howard S. Ginsberg • USGS Patuxent Wildlife Research Center, Coastal Field Station, Woodward Hall-PLS, University of Rhode Island, Kingston, RI 02881. **Kirby C. Stafford III** • Connecticut Agricultural Experiment Station, P.O. Box 1106, New Haven, CT 06549.

require a considerable period of tick attachment to be transmitted to the host, so careful self-inspection and rapid removal of ticks after returning from a tick habitat is an important method of preventing exposure to tick-borne pathogens (139). The most effective means of tick removal is to grasp the tick near the mouthparts with fine forceps or a similar device, and to slowly pull the tick straight out (126).

While these precautions can collectively reduce human exposure to tick-borne diseases substantially, conscientious application is required. Studies of compliance suggest that few individuals maintain diligent compliance with precautions over long periods, even when they are knowledgeable about tick behavior and disease risks (142). Public education programs using signage and informational displays that are targeted to high-risk areas can foster use of precautions when they are most needed.

Manipulation of Tick Habitat

The majority of the life cycle of free-living ixodid ticks is spent off host, where ticks are subject to macro- and microenvironmental conditions that can impact their survival and reproduction. The availability of a suitable microhabitat is crucial to seeking a host, molting, and laying eggs. A balance between energy use and body water homeostasis dictates off-host survival (127, 128). Subadult stages of ticks have a small water mass and relatively permeable cuticle and, therefore, are very susceptible to lower relative humidities (RHs) (30, 192, 219). Stafford (192) found that maximal survival of *Ixodes scapularis* larvae dropped rapidly from 24 to only 3 days as RH went from only 85 to 75%. Nymphs survived longer, but maximum survival dropped from 162 to only 8 days as the RH declined from 85 to 65%. Nymphal mortality increased at lower temperatures only when RH was reduced to 75% (30). Observations of lower densities of *I. scapularis* on manicured lawns with relatively little shade despite high tick densities in adjacent woodlots (25, 107, 199) and of higher tick survival in woods than in open habitats (63) suggest that modifications or alterations to the landscape may be particularly effective against the hydrophilic subadult stages of many tick species.

Manipulation of tick habitat to reduce RH and soil moisture and, consequently, tick survival has been examined as a management tool for a number of tick species, particularly the lone star tick, *Amblyomma americanum* (11, 14, 26, 77, 110, 118). Methods for manipulating the vegetation include mechanical clearing of vegetation, use of herbicides, removal of leaf litter, and controlled burns. Early work in England found that removing accumulated lower vegetative layers in sheep pastures could reduce *Ixodes ricinus*

numbers (114). Tick reductions were attributed to reduced cover and, consequently, lower humidity. Mowing and burning produced a dramatic decline (70 to 80%) in adult *I. scapularis* abundance on Great Island, Mass., but the effect was temporary as no effect on adult numbers was detected 1.5 years later (214). Several other studies have documented limited or temporary reductions in the abundance of *I. scapularis* following vegetative burns. Rogers (157) noted significantly lower numbers of *I. scapularis* in pine palmetto flatwoods burned 1 to 2 years prior to sampling than in an area burned 14 years previously. An area on Shelter Island, N.Y., that received a single light burn produced 49% fewer nymphs than an unburned tract (100). Stafford (194) found that a moderate to severe burn in a northeastern deciduous forest resulted in a 97% reduction of nymphs, while a single light to moderate controlled spring burn reduced nymphal ticks by 74%. Again, the effect was temporary, judging by the comparable number of adult *I. scapularis* ticks recovered in the burned and unburned tracts the following autumn. However, the prospects for use of controlled burns for the control of *I. scapularis* are probably limited because many Lyme disease foci are located in relatively densely populated residential areas.

Nevertheless, landscape management could be a useful strategy in reducing tick abundance in residential settings and public parks where exposure to ticks is high, particularly along the lawn-woodland ecotone. Most ticks on manicured lawns are within a few meters of edge with woodlands, ornamental plantings, or stone walls (25, 107, 199). Mowing and clearing brush, leaf litter, and other vegetative cover could reduce habitat suitability for both tick and small mammalian hosts. Removal of leaf litter in wooded residential plots or at lawn perimeters has been shown to significantly reduce the abundance of *I. scapularis* nymphs (reference 168 and K. C. Stafford, unpublished data). Xeric barriers such as untreated landscape stones and pine bark woodchips deter the movement of *I. scapularis* in the laboratory (135), and a wood chip border at the edge of residential lawns (Fig. 1b) has been found to reduce tick populations along the lawn perimeter by approximately 50% on average (Stafford, unpublished). Habitat or vegetative modifications for managing *I. scapularis* could become an important and environmentally acceptable component of an integrated tick management program in residential settings. They could be incorporated into current landscape practices and plans by landscape architects.

Host-Centered Approaches

Tick management methods that are directed specifically at tick hosts can be divided into methods that

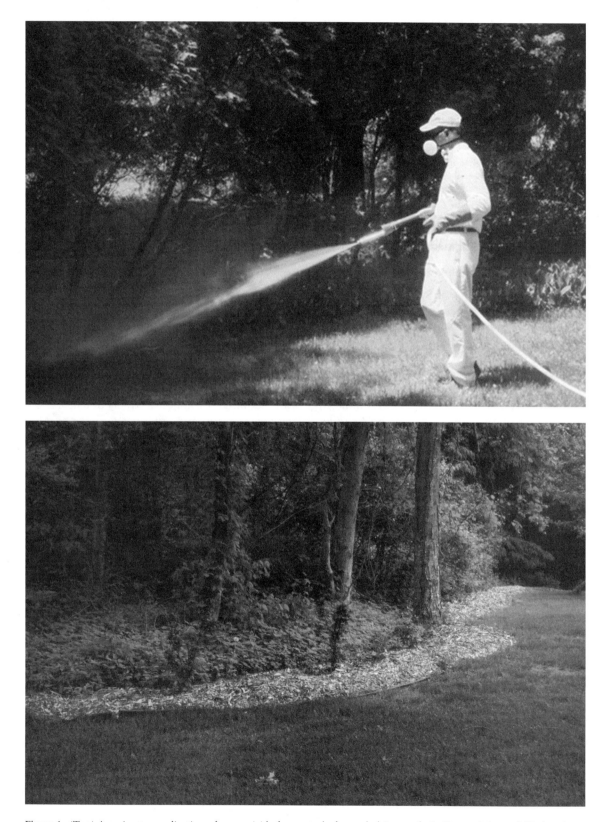

Figure 1. (Top) A perimeter application of an acaricide for control of nymphal *I. scapularis*. (Bottom) A woodchip barrier at the woodland-residential lawn interface to reduce movement of ticks into the lawn. Photographs by K. C. Stafford.

are designed to protect the targeted host and methods that target natural tick hosts to protect humans or domestic animals from tick-borne diseases. Techniques directed at the target host include development of tick-resistant breeds of cattle, and anti-tick vaccines. Host-centered methods that protect humans from tick-borne diseases include manipulation of host populations, vaccination of reservoir host species, and management of natural communities to minimize disease transmission. Host-targeted pesticides are discussed in the pesticide section.

Tick-resistant cattle

It has long been recognized that certain breeds of cattle were able to acquire resistance to tick infestations (53, 81). This naturally acquired resistance has been an important approach in managing cattle ticks and cattle babesiosis because of the development of resistance to acaricides by many tick species on livestock. Immunologically mediated, acquired resistance is associated with cutaneous hypersensitivity reactions, which result in reduced tick weight, tick detachment, fewer engorged ticks, reduced tick fecundity, increased feeding times, impaired disease transmission, and tick death. Some types of cattle (e.g., *Bos indicus*) develop greater resistance than others (e.g., *Bos taurus* varieties) to feeding by cattle ticks (*Boophilus microplus*). Thus, breeding for resistant strains can be applied to agricultural tick management (2, 16, 42), where it can reduce the number of acaricide treatments needed for livestock.

Vaccination

Tick feeding and host immune response. Ixodid ticks attach and feed on their hosts for many days and introduce through the saliva a variety of pharmacologically active compounds that aid the feeding process (i.e., to modulate hemostatis, inhibit blood clotting and pain, and cause vasodilation), improve engorgement success, limit host detection, and impact pathogen transmission (18). Tick feeding modulates both innate and acquired host immunity. Consequently, there is a balance between immune-mediated resistance by the host and strategies employed by the tick to circumvent host-acquired resistance mechanisms. The expression of acquired resistance includes antibodies, complement, cell-mediated immunity, cytokines, and other inflammatory response mediators. Ticks can inhibit complement activation, cytokine elaboration, antibody production, and T-cell response (206). *I. scapularis* secretes a potent platelet aggregation inhibitor and vasodilator (prostaglandins), an inhibitor of the alternative complement pathway, and

inhibitors of immune and inflammatory responses (151, 153–156). Because salivary gland extracts suppress immune function, the administration of several cytokines to mice was found to inhibit *Borrelia burgdorferi* infection (220).

Vaccination against tick bite. The induction of resistance in guinea pigs to *Dermacentor variabilis* larvae by the injection of an extract of whole larval ticks first demonstrated the concept of vaccine-induced resistance for arthropod control (202). Acquired resistance to feeding ticks is not developed by all hosts. The expression of resistance to *I. scapularis* following multiple feedings is subtle in white-footed mice (4, 101), affecting only the percentage of blood-engorged larvae and duration of feeding. By contrast, dogs develop acquired resistance to adult *I. scapularis* with successive exposure (52). The bank vole, *Clethrionomys glareolus*, but not the yellow-necked mouse, *Apodemus flavicollis*, becomes resistant to infestations of *I. ricinus* (41).

Elements in the saliva function as antigens or immunogens that stimulate the host immune response (3), and vaccination with salivary gland derived or other antigens can induce resistance similar to naturally acquired resistance. Extracts of entire ticks, salivary glands, gut, and other tissues have been used to induce immunity and have potential as vaccine immunogens (209, 213). Concealed or novel antigens, like those in the gut that are not displayed to the host during the normal course of feeding, have been successful in inducing anti-tick immunity. The recombinant form of the gut cell protein Bm86 from *B. microplus* is the basis for a commercial anti-*B. microplus* vaccine (213). Because these antigens are not exposed to the host during normal tick infestations (they remain in the tick midgut), booster vaccinations are required, but vaccination of cattle reduces the number, weight, and fecundity of engorging female *B. microplus* ticks. The Bm86 vaccine is also highly effective against *Boophilus annulatus* with some cross-protection against *Hyalomma* and *Rhipicephalus* species, but there are strains of *B. microplus* that are vaccine resistant (49). Another *B. microplus* gut antigen, Bm95, offers protection against Bm86-resistant tick strains (37, 51). However, in areas where cattle ticks have been eradicated or are quarantined and there is a zero tolerance for the presence of the tick on imported livestock (e.g., in the south Texas border region), the vaccine would have little utility. Nevertheless, vaccination against ticks is a proven and promising strategy for the control of ticks and transmission of babesiosis in livestock and offers the potential to limit transmission of tick-borne infections in reservoir hosts or the prevention of disease in human hosts. While there have been major advances in understanding immunology of the tick/host interface at the cellular and molecular levels, little is known about the processes leading to reduced tick engorgement and fecundity, and few antigens have been characterized.

Vaccination against tick-borne diseases. The immunological response in natural hosts to feeding ticks or to tick-borne pathogens is complex, and it regulates feeding success and pathogen transmission cycles (93, 95, 152). Vaccines have been developed for selected tick-borne diseases of cattle such as East Coast fever (204) and anaplasmosis (91) and diseases of humans such as tick-borne encephalitis (12) and Lyme borreliosis (179, 200) (although the Lyme vaccine, LYMErix, produced by GlaxoSmithKline, was withdrawn from the market in 2002). These vaccines offer the potential for effective management of tick-borne diseases with minimal if any environmental effects. However, they do not lower tick numbers and are commercially feasible only for widespread diseases with large populations requiring vaccination.

Wikel et al. (211) found that BALB/c mice infested repeatedly with pathogen-free *I. scapularis* developed resistance to transmission of *B. burgdorferi*. Apparently, proteins in the saliva of some tick species interact with features of the host immune system, including host complement (218) and cytokines (207) to determine vector competence for selected pathogens. This interaction offers the possibility of developing broad-based vaccines against tick-borne diseases by targeting the constituents of tick saliva responsible for modification of the host immune response (166, 208). Such vaccines could potentially have broad applicability, and thus commercial viability.

Vaccination or treatment of wild reservoir hosts. Vaccination or treatment of wild animal reservoirs with antimicrobials may also have potential to reduce transmission of zoonotic pathogens and subsequently the risk of human disease. The vaccination of *B. burgdorferi*-infected *Peromyscus leucopus* with recombinant OspA reduced transmission of spirochetes to ticks fed upon vaccinated animals. Prevalence of infection in xenodiagnostic *I. scapularis* larval ticks was reduced by 48, 92, or 99% and the number of spirochetes was reduced by 84, 98, or 99%, with one, two, or three doses of OspA, respectively (203). Similarly, immunization of the yellow-necked mouse in Europe with the OspA vaccine prevented infection by *B. burgdorferi* (94). A parenteral vaccine with multiple dosing of wild rodent reservoirs would not be practical in the field, and an oral vaccine would be desirable. The oral delivery of purified OspA to mice generated an antibody response, and

immunized animals were protected against needle challenge with *B. burgdorferi* (98). Another possibility is the oral treatment of reservoir hosts with an antibiotic such as tetracycline, although this may raise concerns about the development of resistance in pathogens.

Host management

Manipulation of hosts has been an important part of managing populations of several tick species. For example, pasture spelling in conjunction with acaricidal dips has been important in managing cattle ticks (*Boophilus* spp.) by denying a primary host to free-living larvae of this one-host tick (212). The *Ixodes* complex are three-host ticks with a broad host range, attacking many avian and mammalian hosts. However, adult *Ixodes* ticks often have a narrower host range than the immature stages, with a principal host that can be targeted in host management approaches. Milne (115) estimated that sheep fed 94 to 99% of adult *I. ricinus* ticks in northern England pastures, so pasture spelling can be effective in controlling *I. ricinus* by denying this host to the tick (149). Similarly, significantly lower densities of *I. ricinus* are found in areas where fallow deer, *Dama dama*, are excluded (67). Although adult *I. scapularis* ticks attack a variety of other medium- to large-animal hosts (47), white-tailed deer (*Odocoileus virginianus*) are the preferred host for the adult stage of this species. Wilson et al. (216) estimated that over 90% of these ticks feed on deer. Consequently, deer have been linked to the abundance and distribution of this tick and, indirectly, the increasing incidence of Lyme disease.

Host management for *Ixodes* can take two basic approaches. The first approach focuses on the principal host for the adult tick and the reproductive success of the tick, while the second focuses on reservoir-competent hosts for the Lyme disease spirochetes in an attempt to reduce or break the pathogen transmission cycle. A number of birds and rodents are reservoirs for *B. burgdorferi* sensu lato, especially the white-footed mouse, *P. leucopus*. Management of small rodent host populations or habitat for the control of *I. scapularis* and *B. burgdorferi* has not been well studied, and control strategies with these animals have focused on acaricidal treatment to kill host-feeding ticks. Most research has focused on either managing deer population densities or treatment of these animals with acaricides.

Lowering host populations

A number of studies have examined the impact of white-tailed deer reductions on the abundance of *I. scapularis*. The virtual elimination of deer from the

240-ha Great Island near Cape Cod, Mass., produced a dramatic reduction in the subadult population of the tick (217). The incremental removal of deer over a 7-year period at a 567-ha site in Ipswich, Mass., reduced the abundance of *I. scapularis* larvae and nymphs on white-footed mice by roughly one-half (36). Similarly, the reduction of deer from over 90 per km^2 to as low as 10.4 per km^2 over a 10-year period at two forested tracts in Connecticut resulted in approximately a 5- to 10-fold decline in nymphal tick abundance (196). Apparently, tick numbers fluctuate around a mean level determined by deer density, but these fluctuations are so large that in some years ticks can be as common after as they were before deer reduction (36). These fluctuations can result from local factors, such as movement of hosts into oak forests during high mast years (82, 134), but overall fluctuations tend to be synchronized over large geographical areas (61), suggesting that the responsible factors operate on a regional scale (e.g., weather).

It remains unclear how far a deer population must be reduced to impact the transmission dynamics of Lyme disease and tick-human transmission of disease. A density of only 8 deer/mi^2 was suggested by ongoing evaluation of the Great Island study (201). The computer simulation model LYMESIM, developed to assess the population dynamics of *I. scapularis*, indicated there was a curvilinear relationship between deer and tick density with a reduction in tick abundance with each decrease in deer density (120). A 10-year simulation of deer reduction on tick density with this model predicted that when an initial deer density of 25 animals/km^2 was reduced by 70, 90, and finally 99%, infected nymphs declined by 74% by year 3 and 98% by year 10 at the lowest deer density of only 0.25 deer/km^2 (121). Risk of disease may increase in the short term with moderate decreases in deer density. Host-seeking or deer-feeding adult tick abundance and prevalence of infection by *B. burgdorferi* increased immediately following the reduction of deer in the deer reduction studies, although adult tick densities eventually decline after deer are removed. As fewer deer remove adult ticks from the environment, apparent host-seeking activity will increase (64) and more subadult ticks may feed on alternative, reservoir-competent hosts. In the model, infection rates initially increased with moderate deer reductions, then dropped with less than 0.75 deer per km^2 and went to zero at 0.3 deer/km^2. A density of *I. scapularis* below a threshold of 87 nymphs/ha did not maintain *B. burgdorferi* in the ecosystem.

The published studies and the computer model demonstrate that a substantial reduction in the white-tailed deer population can potentially reduce vector abundance and impact the dynamics of disease transmission. As evident on several islands and tracts along the New England coast, unmanaged or inadequately managed high deer populations can result in super-abundant tick populations. However, it may be difficult to reduce deer sufficiently to affect tick populations or the dynamics of disease transmission except on islands or other geographically isolated tracts. Wildlife managers have traditionally relied on regulated seasonal hunting or controlled hunts to manage deer populations. Deer reductions or implementation of controlled hunts can be controversial, particularly on public lands (88), and the drastic reductions needed to achieve satisfactory tick control mean that this strategy may be unrealistic in most areas.

Host exclusion

An alternative approach is the exclusion of these hosts from areas by fencing. A substantial reduction in the population of *A. americanum* larvae (98%) and nymphs (53%) was observed within a 2.4-ha deer exclosure at the Land Between the Lakes recreational area in Tennessee (14, 15). On Fire Island, N.Y., deer exclusion from two 1-ha plots reduced nymphal *A. americanum* ticks by an average of 48.4% (58). The exclusion of deer by a seven-strand, high-tensile electric fence from two areas of approximately 3.5 and 7.4 ha reduced the abundance of *I. scapularis* larvae, nymphs, and adults in areas >70 m from the fence line by 100, 83.8, and 74.1%, respectively (191). Similarly, Daniels et al. (34) reported that exclusion of deer from five areas with traditional fencing resulted in 83% fewer *I. scapularis* nymphs and 90% fewer larvae inside the exclosures. The size of the fenced area appears to be the primary factor in the impact of exclusion on the tick population as small- and medium-sized mammals and birds may passively reintroduce ticks within the fenced tract (15, 32, 191). Other strategies to reduce the frequency or number of deer visiting residential properties such as repellents and browse-resistant plantings could also conceivably reduce the prevalence of ticks in the residential landscape, although their effectiveness is strongly dependent upon deer densities and availability of alternate food sources. Nevertheless, the exclusion of deer from relatively small tracts, residences, or group of residences and managing deer on the property could notably reduce tick abundance and the risk of tick-borne disease, especially when combined with other tick management strategies.

Managing host diversity

Epizootiology of tick-borne zoonoses depends, in part, on the relative abundances and degrees of reservoir competence of the various tick host species at a site (101). Higher biodiversity can potentially lower infection rates in ticks (thus lowering risk of human disease) by diluting infection among a diversity of tick hosts with moderate reservoir competence (97). The ultimate effect of increased diversity, as opposed to increased dominance of tick hosts, depends on the reservoir competence of the dominant host. If the dominant host is a highly competent reservoir (like *P. leucopus* for *B. burgdorferi*), then higher host diversity will lower disease transmission. If the dominant host is a poor reservoir, then greater diversity can theoretically increase disease risk.

Biological Control

Tick natural enemies and potential biological control methods have been reviewed by several authors (80, 122, 158, 163). However, effective and widely applicable biological control of ticks has not yet been achieved. In natural populations, ticks are attacked by predators, parasites, and diseases. Unfortunately, few (with the exception of some birds and some parasitoid wasps) are specific to ticks, and the importance of these organisms in natural regulation of tick populations is unknown.

Predators

The primary vertebrate predators of ticks are birds, and the only birds that are specific to ticks are the oxpeckers (*Buphagus africanus* and *Buphagus erythrorhynchus*), which are native to Africa (163). These birds eat ticks from both wild and domestic ungulates and have been successfully introduced into natural areas (68). Oxpecker density depends to a large extent on tick density, which often remains high even when the birds are present. Nevertheless, evidence of beneficial effects of oxpeckers on mammals in tick-infested areas has been reported (163). Domestic fowl, including chickens and helmeted guinea fowl, readily consume ticks and have been proposed as biocontrol agents. Field trials have sometimes shown modest declines in tick abundance associated with the presence of these birds (44, 73), but consistent effects useful for routine biocontrol have not been demonstrated.

The primary arthropod predators of ticks are ants, beetles, and spiders (158), but these are nonspecific feeders and their effects on tick populations have not been studied.

Parasitoids

The parasitoid wasp genus *Ixodiphagus* (Encyrtidae) includes seven species, all of which are parasitic on ticks (124). The most widely distributed species, *Ixodiphagus hookeri*, has been released for tick control and has been successfully established but generally has not lowered tick numbers (96, 180). Mather et al. (103) found that wasp-infested *I. scapularis* at their study site did not carry *B. burgdorferi*, the etiologic agent of Lyme borreliosis, while uninfested ticks often did, suggesting that wasp infestation might lower pathogen prevalence in ticks. However, this might have resulted from wasps using deer, the tick host, to find ticks to parasitize, resulting in parasitization of ticks on a host that is not a competent reservoir of *B. burgdorferi*. This question requires further study.

In southern New York and New England in the United States, *I. hookeri* is found only where ticks are highly abundant and is often absent from nearby sites with only moderate tick densities (64, 79, 197). Therefore, the wasps might require high tick densities to survive and might thus be unlikely to provide tick control under natural conditions. Stafford et al. (196) found that the prevalence of *I. hookeri* declined to extremely low levels or disappeared as superabundant deer and tick densities were reduced to moderate densities. Nevertheless, an inundative release on a small farm in Kenya lowered tick numbers significantly (123), so inundative releases at appropriate sites might successfully control *I. scapularis* (90). Additional field trials are needed under varied conditions to assess the eventual utility of this approach. For such control programs to be feasible, it will be necessary to develop methods to inexpensively raise large numbers of *I. hookeri* for release.

Nematodes

Several taxa of entomopathogenic nematodes are also pathogenic to ticks, including members of the families Mermithidae, Heterorhabditidae, and Steinernematidae (162). Upon entering the host, infective juvenile heterorhabditids and steinernematids release bacteria of the genus *Xenorhabdus*, which kill the host (1). Pathogenicity has been demonstrated in laboratory trials with such important tick species as *B. annulatus* and *I. scapularis* (161, 224), but effectiveness varies among tick species and nematode strains (76, 92, 105). Infective juveniles, which live in the upper soil layer, can potentially attack ticks in the same habitat. However, nematodes are minimally effective against immature ticks and flat ticks of all stages and are highly pathogenic only to engorged female ticks (163). This results, in part, from the fact that nematodes often enter the tick through the genital pore, which is everted in the engorged female (224), even though entry by other routes also occurs (162).

Nematode pathogenicity to ticks has been demonstrated repeatedly in the laboratory, but field application remains problematic. Environmental conditions, including low moisture, presence of animal manure, and low temperatures, can compromise pathogenicity (159, 224). Furthermore, the nematodes do not complete their life cycles in the ticks (163), so repeated applications would be necessary. Nevertheless, the susceptibility of engorged female ticks to nematodes that dwell in the same soil environments suggests that selected nematode strains can effectively manage ticks under appropriate conditions. Study of factors that influence pathogenicity in the field and possibly selection of improved nematode strains will be necessary to develop nematodes as biological control agents for ticks.

Fungi

Entomopathogenic fungi, including species of *Beauveria* and *Verticillium*, are commonly found infecting ticks and might influence tick populations in nature (85, 164, 222). Lab trials have shown that both *Beauveria bassiana* and *Metarhizium anisopliae* are pathogenic to several species of ticks (84, 160, 221). Fungi have the advantage that they attack all tick stages and can penetrate the cuticle, so they have considerable potential as tick biocontrol agents.

The primary difficulties with use of entomopathogenic fungi for tick control have to do with delivery systems. Inappropriate environmental conditions (e.g., insufficient moisture) can reduce spore germination and adversely affect pathogenicity (17, 116, 147). Field trials with fungi have generally produced only modest tick control (13), but the finding that fungal applications in oil-based carriers resulted in greater tick mortality than in water-based carriers (83) suggests that improved delivery systems can lead to effective control. Therefore, development of improved delivery systems has great potential to provide effective fungal products for tick management. Another potential problem with entomopathogenic fungi (and nematodes) as tick biocontrol agents is that they affect diverse arthropod species and can potentially affect nontarget species. Flexner et al. (48) reviewed the effects of microbial pesticides on nontarget arthropods and found only modest effects. However, pathogenicity of entomogenous fungi has been reported for numerous arthropod taxa (225), and horizontal transmission in laboratory trials (62) suggests that inappropriate application can lead to epizootics in nontarget species. It is important to note that pathogenicity is often far lower in the field than in laboratory trials where conditions are optimal for fungal growth (70). Furthermore, applications of fungal spores can be targeted at ticks on host animals or conducted at times of the year when other arthropods are not active to minimize the likelihood of nontarget effects.

Bacteria

Numerous species of bacteria have been isolated from ticks caught in the wild, including some that are known to be entomopathogenic (99, 130). Pathogenicity of several species of bacteria against ticks has been described in the laboratory (20, 21, 74). Individual strains of *Bacillus thuringiensis*, which are narrowly pathogenic to specific taxa of insects, are nevertheless pathogenic to ticks in laboratory trials (74). For example, "*Bacillus thuringiensis* subsp. *kurstaki*," a subspecies that is primarily pathogenic to Lepidoptera and commonly used to control gypsy moths and other lepidopterous pests, is also pathogenic to *I. scapularis* in the laboratory (223). This raises the question of mode of pathogenicity because *B. thuringiensis* generally needs to be ingested to be effective; it produces endotoxins that disrupt the arthropod midgut cells. Since ticks ingest little other than host blood, it is not clear how the ticks are killed. They might incidentally ingest enough material to be affected when dipped in or sprayed with spore solutions, but other modes of pathogenicity (e.g., other toxins, bacterial reproduction in the tick, or physical blocking of tick structures by spores) might also play a role. This is a worthwhile area for future research because *B. thuringiensis* products are already available, production methods are well established, and the bacteria display some degree of host specificity (thus potentially minimizing nontarget effects). Further research is needed to determine the mode of pathogenicity to ticks and whether bacterial formulations can be effective under field conditions.

Area-Wide Use of Pesticides

Acaricides (pesticides that kill mites and ticks) have been and continue to be a major tool in the control or management of ticks and tick-associated diseases. These chemicals are commonly used for short-term control of *I. scapularis* around private residences and other localized high-risk areas (193). Environmental and safety concerns continue to restrict the availability, wide-scale use, and public acceptability of these chemicals in tick management programs. Synthetic pyrethroid insecticides, particularly cyfluthrin, are increasingly becoming the chemicals of choice for tick control in the residential landscape. Residential use of two broad-spectrum organophosphate insecticides (i.e., chlorpyrifos and diazinon) that are used for tick control has been phased out by the U.S. Environmental Protection Agency (EPA), largely because of safety and exposure concerns for children (www.epa. gov). A survey of licensed commercial applicators in 1996 found that cyfluthrin and chlorpyrifos, followed by carbaryl, were the principal chemicals used for tick control (193). A smaller follow-up survey in 1999 found that cyfluthrin was being used by over half of the commercial applicators (Stafford, unpublished). Although pyrethroids offer a better environmental and safety profile than the chemicals they replace (86), newer, less-toxic alternatives and the integration of these materials with other approaches are needed. Least-toxic pesticide strategies (i.e., lower toxic materials, selective applications to high-risk areas, combinations with tick attractants, and biopesticides) and host-targeted applications are alternative approaches currently being studied, especially within an overall integrated management approach.

Acaricides, both conventional liquid and granular formulations, have been shown to provide relatively consistent, highly effective short-term suppression of ticks. In the case of nymphal *I. scapularis* (45, 195), acaricide effectiveness depends, in part, upon contact with the litter layer, depth of the leaf litter, and penetration of vegetation and the leaf litter with the chemical (167). Single applications of carbaryl, diazinion, and chlorpyrifos to residential properties (Fig. 1a) or forest have provided roughly 86 to 96% control of *I. scapularis* nymphs or adults for up to 2 months (29, 172, 188). Similar reductions of adult *Ixodes pacificus* with applications of chlorpyrifos and carbaryl were obtained by Monsen et al. (117) in northern California. Granular formulations of diazinon, chlorpyrifos, and carbaryl also provide effective control of *I. scapularis* (169, 171, 173). A single application of the synthetic pyrethroid cyfluthrin is particularly effective against *I. scapularis* nymphs at application rates up to 45 times lower than organophosphate and carbamate applications. Solberg et al. (182) and Curran et al. (29) reported liquid or granular formulations of cyfluthrin could provide >90% control of *I. scapularis* nymphs. The pyrethroid deltamethrin, applied as a granule at woodland edges, was also effective in reducing the abundance of *I. scapularis* nymphs in residential settings (reference 170 and Stafford, unpublished). While tick control with a single acaricide application in these studies was generally effective for a couple of months after application, reintroduction of ticks into the treated areas by infested hosts will require that chemical applications for nymphal or adult ticks be performed on an annual basis. Targeting annual acaricide applications to high-risk areas and as a barrier treatment around the home could help reduce the amount of material applied, degree of exposure to the chemicals, and acceptability of their use to reduce the risk of tick-borne disease.

Public acceptance of area applications of synthetic chemicals for tick control appears relatively low, although tick control in Connecticut by licensed commercial pesticide applicators has increased with the rise in the incidence of Lyme disease (193). Use of commercial applicators may further increase as older acaricides are withdrawn from residential use and fewer materials are available for homeowner use. A survey of residents in two communities in southwestern Connecticut found only 22.5% of 402 respondents had applied acaricides for the control of *I. scapularis* and that most (79%) respondents indicated that the likelihood of future pesticide use was low (Connecticut Department of Public Health, unpublished data). However, of those who did treat for ticks, most (75.6%) used a commercial service for the acaricide application and only 16.9% made the application themselves. Nonresidual chemical control products such as desiccants, insecticidal soaps, and natural pyrethrins are alternatives to synthetic pesticides. These materials have been found to significantly reduce nymphal and adult *I. scapularis* in laboratory and small field trials (7, 135, 136). Larger trials on residential properties with various combinations of pyrethrin, the synergist piperonyl butoxide, diatomaceous earth, and insecticidal soap found synergized pyrethrin with insecticidal soap to be the most effective combination of these least-toxic products (Stafford, unpublished).

Host-Targeted Acaricide Control

Acaricides have long been the principal method for controlling ticks on domestic livestock (43). A more recent approach, however, is the application of acaricides to large wild-animal hosts for the control of free-living ticks. White-tailed deer serve as the principal hosts for the adult stage of both *I. scapularis* and the lone star tick, *A. americanum*. Depending on the compound, the acaricide can be delivered orally (a systemic) or topically. Ivermectin, a broad-spectrum systemic parasiticide derived from the soil bacterium *Streptomyces avermitilis*, has been shown to control lone star ticks on deer (111, 146). Similarly, the use of ivermectin-treated corn with free-ranging deer on an isolated island in Maine provided >90% control of *I. scapularis* on adequately treated animals (148), although no reduction in free-living tick abundance was obtained, presumably because of underestimates of the deer population and inadequate treatment of the population. The use of a systemic agent in the United States for the control of ticks on deer is unlikely because of the withdrawal period required for clearance of a drug in food animals prior to human consumption and the correspondence of adult tick activity and the deer-hunting season.

Several devices have been developed for the topical application of an acaricide to deer. Sonenshine et al. (185) developed a self-application device for the control of ticks on deer. Another topical self-application system was developed by the U.S. Department of Agriculture, Agricultural Research Service (USDA-ARS) at their Livestock Insects Research Laboratory in Kerrville, Tex. (143). The USDA-ARS device, termed the 4-poster (Fig. 2a), consists of a central bin that contains bait to attract deer with one trough and two vertical pesticide-impregnated rollers on each end (145). Deer contact one of the acaricide-treated rollers as they feed, treating the head, neck, and ears. The application of 2% amitraz to deer during the tick season over 3 consecutive years provided 92 and 94% control of lone star ticks on the animals (144). The efficacy of the 4-poster in controlling free-living populations of *I. scapularis* was evaluated in restricted and unrestricted forested, suburban settings in several states in the northeastern United States from 1997 to 2002. Although there was competition from acorns during some years of the study and some adjustments had to be made to ensure sufficient delivery of the material to northern deer, the treatment of deer has reduced populations of the black-legged tick in comparison with untreated communities. Nymphal tick abundance was down by 68 to 71% after the third year of treatment in Maryland, with similar results in Connecticut (69%) and the other project sites after 4 to 6 years (reference 108 and Stafford, unpublished). Higher levels of tick control, 91 to 100% reduction of questing *I. scapularis*, were obtained by year 3 with the application of 10% permethrin to a fenced, nonhunted deer population (181). Although the treatment of free-ranging deer has a number of technical issues (concerning delivery, pesticide efficacy, and residues) and potential issues associated with excessive feeding of wildlife, the application of acaricides to white-tailed deer is a promising approach that can conceivably reduce ticks and impact Lyme borreliosis on a community-wide scale with minimal environmental concerns and minimal participation by most residents. At the time of this writing, a 10% permethrin formulation (Y-TEX 4-Poster Tickicide, Y-TEX Corporation, Cody, Wyo.) has been registered for use on deer by the EPA and by numerous state pesticide agencies. State wildlife agency reviews are pending, and the 4-poster device is in commercial development. By contrast, the treatment of small mammalian hosts with their smaller home ranges would require the active participation of most residents to reduce the risk of tick bite and disease but would still offer the environmental and safety benefits of a host-targeted approach.

An approach used originally for the control of plague vectors (87), the application of acaricides to small mammalian hosts through a baited box, has the potential to not only impact tick abundance, but also disrupt the enzootic cycle of pathogens in reservoir hosts. An acaricide bait-box treatment station reduced infestations of immature American dog ticks, *D. vari-*

abilis, on rodents by >90% (186). In several studies, the application of cardboard tubes containing permethrin-treated cotton balls produced varying reductions in infestations of immature *I. scapularis* on white-footed mice (*P. leucopus*), which collect the cotton as nesting material, and in Sweden, *I. ricinus* on bank voles (35, 54, 104, 109, 189). However, no reductions in infected, host-seeking *I. scapularis* nymphs were observed over a 3-year period at treated woodland and residential areas of about 1.6 ha or less (33, 189, 190). Although one large-scale Massachusetts study reported reductions in the abundance of both *I. scapularis* on mice and in host-seeking nymphs with the treatment of one 7.3-ha site (35), the failure of permethrin-treated cotton to significantly affect the tick population in smaller areas may be due to the availability of alternative nesting materials, alternative tick hosts that do not collect the nesting material, and immigration of untreated tick-infested hosts.

A more recent application of the classic rodent bait box approach uses fipronil as the acaricide (Fig. 2b). Fipronil has been commercially available for over a decade for the control of fleas and ticks on dogs and cats. Discovered in 1987, fipronil belongs to a new class of insecticides, the phenyl pyrazoles, and is a reversible inhibitor of the gamma-aminobutyric-regulated chloride channel that displays selectively tighter binding in insects than in mammals (10). The compound concentrates in the epidermis, hair follicle, and sebaceous glands of dogs (27), and tick control can last up to a month with a single application. On a mouse, a single topical application of fipronil can kill ticks on the animal for up to 42 days in the laboratory (106), reducing the need for frequent reapplication and providing continued tick control as the mouse forages in the environment. Treatment of white-footed mice in an island community in Connecticut with fipronil (one bait box ≈ every 10 m at lawn woodland edge, stone walls, and other mouse habitats) has been shown to dramatically reduce the number of ticks on the mice, prevalence of infection with *B. burgdorferi* in the mice, and host-seeking tick populations in the treated residences (M. Dolan et al., unpublished data). At the time of this writing, a commercial version of the fipronil-based bait box (Maxforce Tick Management System, Bayer Environmental Science, Montvale, N.J.) has been registered with the EPA and has been commercially available since late 2004.

Pheromone-Mediated Control Methods

Pheromones are messenger chemicals used by animals to modify behavior in members of the same species. Tick pheromones, broadly classified as assembly, aggregation-attachment, or sex-attractant phero-

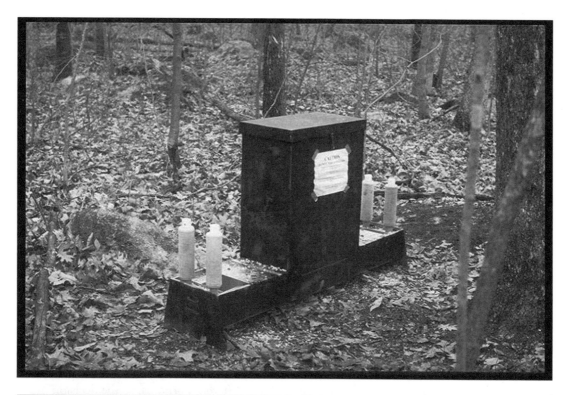

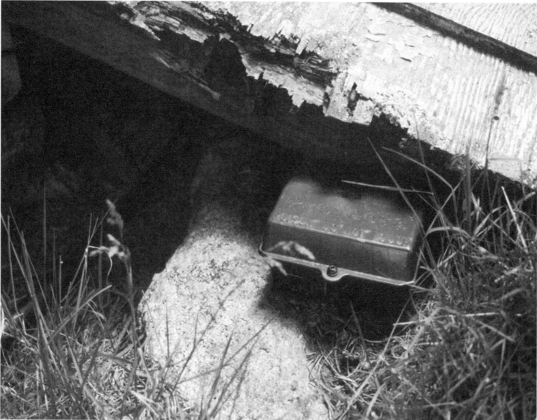

Figure 2. Host-targeted acaricide control. (Top) The 4-poster passive topical treatment device for controlling ticks on white-tailed deer consists of a central bin and two feeding and acaricide application stations on either side of the bin. Deer contact the vertical rollers treated with an acaricide as they place their heads into the bait port to feed. (Bottom) Fipronil-based rodent bait box used in initial trials for control of *I. scapularis* on white-footed mice in Connecticut that contained a nontoxic attractant bait and a yarn-like wick. Photographs by K. C. Stafford.

mones, are used by various tick species to control and modulate tick movement and mating behavior. Readers are referred to Sonenshine (183) for a more detailed review of pheromone types and methods for the identification of tick pheromones.

Tick pheromones and related chemicals are potential tools that could be applied to managing ticks by disrupting tick behavior and reproduction. Little is known about the regulation of behavior and mating in *Ixodes* ticks. Tick mating behavior is governed in a discrete series of phases by several sex pheromones, especially in non-*Ixodes* ticks, in which sperm development proceeds only after attachment and commencement of feeding (184). Sex pheromones may involve an attractant pheromone (for long-range attraction of males to feeding females), a mounting pheromone (for crawling upon and recognition of the female), and a genital sex pheromone (for location of the gonopore and copulation). The chemical 2,6-dichlorophenol is the sex attractant secreted by at least 14 species of ticks (72), but it is not the sex attractant for *Ixodes* ticks, which still needs to be characterized. In *Ixodes* ticks, mating may occur on the host or off the host in the vegetation, as male gamete development is not dependent upon tick feeding. The existence of sex and assembly pheromones has been reported for *I. ricinus* (66, 71).

Assembly pheromones are present in many, although not all, tick species and induce clustering of free-living ticks in the environment. Assembly pheromones in *Ixodes* could potentially be used against free-living ticks prior to feeding on people and transmission of disease. The presence of assembly pheromones, which appear to be purines or purine-like substances attractive to nymphal and adult *I. scapularis*, has recently been documented by using bioassays of cast skins and exudates from molted ticks (3, 8). Identified components of assembly pheromones in soft ticks (Argasidae) also elicit assembly responses.

Assembly pheromones or other attractants could be used to enhance the efficacy of a toxicant delivery system. Research has focused on use of pheromones as a lure to attract ticks to a toxicant or in a baited decoy system to attract and kill male ticks (184). For example, aggregation-attachment pheromones, produced by male ticks of several *Amblyomma* species, strongly attract unfed adults and sometimes nymphal ticks and induce attachment in areas where male ticks are feeding. This allows identification of tick-infested hosts, clustering of ticks on the host, and facilitation of mating (131). The combination of 2,6-dichlorophenol with an acaricide kills mate-seeking male *D. variabilis* and disrupts the mating process (186, 187). Pheromone-acaricide formulations on cattle have been shown to kill ticks more effectively than an acaricide alone (5, 6, 132). The use of a pheromone-cyfluthrin impregnated tail-tag provided 94.9 to 99.3% control of the bont tick, *Amblyomma hebraeum*, and other tick species on cattle (132). Development of controlled-release formulations containing assembly pheromone and acaricide could potentially improve area control of ticks with better efficacy and less toxicant. Other attractant chemicals could potentially be utilized in a similar manner. For example, Carroll (23, 24) reported that *I. scapularis* is attracted to host-derived chemicals secreted by white-tailed deer, which would serve to concentrate ticks in areas with increased likelihood of finding a host. The potential to use host-associated chemicals in tick baits remains to be explored.

IPM FOR TICKS

Tick control has several different purposes: (i) to lower direct damage to animals from ticks (e.g., loss of vigor), (ii) to prevent transmission of tick-borne diseases to animals, (iii) to lower nuisance to humans from ticks, and (iv) to prevent tick-borne diseases of humans. The reasons for tick management differ for these different purposes, so the decision-making process can differ as well. The concept of IPM was developed for agriculture and depends on a cost/benefit ratio to make management decisions. The economic injury level (EIL) is the pest population size at which the cost of intervention is equal to the value of the crop protected by the intervention. Control is applied to prevent the pest population from reaching the EIL. This type of reasoning clearly applies to tick control on farm animals (where the dollar value of lowering tick numbers can be calculated) and can sometimes be applied to tick control to prevent nuisance problems (e.g., to prevent loss of revenue from reduced tourism). However, this approach does not apply well to prevention of human disease or even to disease prevention for pets, because the dollar value of the benefit is not easily estimable and is not equivalent to the cost of a control measure. A cost-efficiency analysis provides a more appropriate model of IPM for disease management (57, 112, 113, 138), where the purpose is to allocate resources as efficiently as possible to minimize the number of cases of human disease with the funds available. Thus, there are two fundamentally different approaches to tick management: IPM for commodity protection (similar to traditional IPM for agricultural pests) and IPM for disease prevention (Table 1). We discuss these approaches separately below.

IPM for Commodity Protection

IPM involves the selection, integration, and implementation of several pest control actions based on

Table 1. IPM for ticks and tick-borne diseases

Purpose of management	Example	Analysis	Decision making
Protect commodity	Ticks on cattle, nuisance ticks in tourist area	Cost/benefit	Lower tick numbers in effective, cost-efficient manner
Manage tick-borne disease of humans	Ticks carrying Lyme borreliosis, TBE, rickettsioses	Cost-efficiency	Allocate available resources to maximally lower the number of human cases of disease

expected ecological, economic, and sociological consequences with the goal of managing, not eradicating, the pest population. The cost/benefit analysis for pest management decisions is most straightforward in the agricultural setting. In some cases, the costs of tick control are not justified in terms of the value of increased product that results (137). Recent IPM programs for *B. microplus* on cattle have shown that integration of Bm86-based vaccine (Gavac) with traditional methods provides cost effective management by lowering the number of acaricide treatments required (38, 150). Decisions on how to integrate methods for management of tick-borne diseases of farm animals can use methods similar to those described below for management of tick-borne human disease.

For the management of tick nuisance to humans, IPM analysis requires some threshold tick density before action is taken. Acceptable thresholds would be tied to the perception of nuisance and would be different for residential areas, recreational areas, and less-visited parts of woodland parks. Economic injury levels could theoretically be calculated based on expected economic losses resulting from decreased tourism or decreased value of property compared to the cost of tick control, but these are complex calculations with numerous variables that are difficult to estimate. In terms of human nuisance, an economic threshold of 0.65 tick per h in a carbon dioxide sample was proposed for the lone star tick based on an attack rate of <1 tick per human visitor per day (119). The increased effectiveness of control resulting from integration of various tick control measures has been estimated. In a project to manage lone star tick populations in a recreation area, combinations of three tick control methods (acaricides, vegetation management, and exclusion of white-tailed deer by a fence) provided greater tick reductions than each method alone (14). All three methods together produced the greatest reduction with 92 to 99% control of lone star larvae, nymphs, and adults.

IPM for Disease Prevention

Human tick-borne illnesses, such as Lyme borreliosis, tick-borne encephalitis, babesiosis, and ehrlichiosis, require an ecologically based integrated management approach to reduce the risk of disease. Tick control still often focuses on short-term suppression over small geographic areas, primarily through the use of broadcast applications of pesticides. Large-scale pesticide applications are generally no longer acceptable, particularly in residential settings, and environmentally acceptable approaches are needed to manage tick populations and reduce the risk of acquiring disease. No single methodology can address the cycle of tick vector, vertebrate reservoirs, pathogens, and exposure by the susceptible human population. Many novel methods are still experimental or speculative and not yet available for use in an integrated tick management program. Integrated studies on managing ticks and focused efforts to actually impact the incidence of tick-borne disease are few.

Theory of IPM for tick-borne diseases

The risk of tick-borne disease depends on the probability of being bitten by a tick and on the proportion of ticks that are infective to humans (102). The probability of being bitten depends on tick density, proximity of tick populations to human populated areas, and human behavior as it influences exposure to questing ticks (175). The proportion of ticks infected depends on numerous ecological factors that affect transmission dynamics (e.g., tick abundance, host abundance and diversity, and reservoir competence of the various host species present) (97, 101). Therefore, tick management methods can be divided into those that influence the number of tick bites and those that influence the proportion of ticks infected. The goal of an IPM program to prevent human cases of tick-borne disease is to lower the number of human cases as much as possible, with the funding and resources available. Therefore, the decision-making process for IPM for tick-borne diseases is a cost-efficiency analysis that determines how the available money and resources should be allocated so as to have the greatest possible effect on the number of human cases. This is not merely an economic analysis, because the more efficiently control techniques are applied (and the more efficiently money is spent), the fewer people will get sick. To determine how to integrate control measures to have the greatest effect on the number of human cases, it is necessary to estimate the effect on transmission to humans from the various control methods available, alone and in combination. This can be accomplished by extensive field trials and/or by modeling the expected effects of the various possible interventions.

Since the probability of exposure to a pathogen depends on both exposure to ticks and infection prevalence in ticks, the probability of human exposure is nonlinear, similar to the probability of exposure to infected individuals in the Reed-Frost epidemic model (46, 50). For example, a reduction in the number of tick bites does not always result in a similar reduction in the number of people exposed to the pathogen. If tick density and pathogen prevalence in ticks are both high, for example, the probability of exposure to the pathogen is only slightly diminished by a moderate reduction in tick numbers. When tick density and/or pathogen prevalence is low, the effect of tick reduction on the probability of human infection is more linear (55). Therefore, the efficacy of a control method depends on initial tick densities and pathogen prevalence in ticks.

The efficacy of integrating management methods that lower the number of tick bites (e.g., personal protection, habitat modification, and acaricide applications) with methods that lower pathogen prevalence in ticks (e.g., host-targeted acaricides or vaccines) was studied using a simple model of the probability of being bitten by a single infected tick (57). Lowering the number of tick bites to zero, or lowering pathogen prevalence in ticks to zero, eliminates any disease risk. However, dividing the same level of resources between methods that lower tick bites and methods that lower pathogen prevalence does not eliminate disease risk because some number of infected ticks remains. The closer control gets to zero tick bites, or to zero ticks infected, the fewer human cases of disease. Therefore, all else being equal, more human cases will be prevented by integrating methods that have the same effect (methods that lower tick bites, or methods that lower pathogen prevalence in ticks) than by integrating a method that lowers tick bites with one that lowers pathogen prevalence. Of course, differences in the costs or in the marginal efficiencies of the various techniques can change the outcome of this analysis.

To apply IPM to tick-borne disease in the real world, estimates of the cost and effectiveness of each available control method are needed. Expected effects on disease incidence of various combinations of techniques can be estimated and used to make pest management decisions. This approach allows environmental concerns to be taken explicitly into the decision-making process (56), because the costs of an environmentally benign combination of techniques can be compared directly to the costs of environmentally more destructive techniques that provide the same level of public

health protection. Since local factors influence the effectiveness of any control technique, it is essential to collect data on the effectiveness of a management program during its application. Information on the effects of management on the number of tick bites and on pathogen prevalence can be used to improve management in subsequent years. This approach is a form of adaptive management (78), in which analysis of current management outcomes is used to improve future effectiveness.

Current IPM practices for tick-borne diseases

Individuals make economic and risk decisions when they elect to implement prevention measures, obtain tick control services, alter their landscape, or use pesticides. The use of personal protection and tick control measures is influenced by perception of disease risk, degree of inconvenience in engaging in a protective activity, and concerns over the safety and environmental impacts of vector control options. The risk of infection with *B. burgdorferi* from a known tick bite is low (28, 125, 177) and transmission of spirochetes from an infected tick is low during the first 24 to 28 h of attachment by *I. scapularis* (40, 133, 140, 141). Thus, prompt removal of ticks can prevent infection and frequent detection of ticks appears to be a major incentive for engaging in prevention behaviors (i.e., tick checks or use of a repellent) (176). While it is difficult to put a value on a human disease, the consequences of misdiagnosis and mismanagement can be high (178). However, even when the disease is considered a serious problem, usage of some tick control measures, such as spraying pesticides, remains low.

On a practical basis, reducing the risk of tick bite and, consequently, human cases of disease has been limited to personal protection measures, the use of acaricides, and habitat modifications around the home. In the case of Lyme borreliosis in North America, the program LYMESIM has been used to examine a number of tick management and Lyme disease prevention strategies (75, 120, 121). The acaricidal treatment of deer was the most cost-effective, long-term strategy for larger areas, but the model also suggested deer density reductions to be an important element. However, area-wide acaricide application, vegetation reduction, or a combination of the two was most effective in small recreational or residential sites. Simulated 50 and 100% reductions in vegetation reduced infected nymphal abundance (by 89 and >99% by year 3, respectively). Simulations of area-wide acaricides applied annually to each stage reduced larvae, nymphs, and adults by 82, 91, and 93%, respectively. The combination of acaricides and vegetation reduction in the LYMESIM simulation produced a 96% reduction in the seasonal abundance of infected nymphal *I. scapularis*. Hayes et al. (75) used LYMESIM to assess the effectiveness of eight interventions in a hypothetical community of 10,000 people over 4 years with an annual incidence rate of Lyme disease of 0.01 case per person per year. The interventions simulated were area-wide acaricide, acaricide to nesting mice, acaricide to white-tailed deer, removal of white-tailed deer, fencing out deer, reduction of habitat vegetation, repellent and tick checks, and the Lyme vaccine. Various estimates of intervention use were based, in part, on published surveys of people on Lyme borreliosis-related behaviors and experimental efficacy of the intervention. The number of Lyme disease cases prevented was determined under varying assumptions for baseline, worst-case, and best-case scenarios for each intervention. The impact of the interventions was dependent upon the level of engagement. Reduction in tick habitat vegetation by 40% of residents with 90% habitat reduction on lawns, 80% habitat reduction in ecotone, and 10% reduction in forested areas resulted in the prevention of only 94 cases. The acaricidal treatment of deer prevented the most cases (113 to 306) of Lyme borreliosis under all scenarios except the best-case use of the Lyme vaccine. Removal or exclusion of deer also decreased disease incidence, although risk increased for the first 2 years, reflecting an increase in the proportion of infected nymphs. Use of the vaccine protects only vaccinated individuals and is dependent upon a high level of engagement, while some other interventions may prevent cases of Lyme borreliosis in neighbors who do not engage in these interventions. If these hypothetical results were applied to an actual endemic area, it would be important to collect the appropriate data to assess the accuracy of the predictions and to improve the model so that its effectiveness could be enhanced for future applications.

Management programs for tick-borne diseases require careful planning. Effectiveness of various control methods and of integrated programs involving multiple methods can be assessed by using theoretical analyses, simulation models, and data from field trials of the various techniques. Management programs can be designed that satisfy local requirements for disease management, environmental protection, and other considerations that are deemed important. However, ecological conditions, composition of host communities, transmission dynamics, and nature of human exposure to ticks vary considerably from site to site. Therefore, prediction of the efficacy of a management program at any given site must be considered tentative. Sampling programs to assess the effectiveness of management programs and to determine ways to improve the programs in future applications should be routine features of IPM programs for tick-borne diseases.

CONCLUSION

The mainstays of tick management and protection from tick-borne diseases have traditionally been personal precautions and the application of acaricides. These techniques maintain their value, and current innovations hold considerable promise for future improvement in effective targeting of materials for tick control. Furthermore, an explosion of research in the past few decades has resulted in the development and expansion of several novel and potentially valuable approaches to tick control, including vaccination against tick-borne pathogen transmission and against tick attachment, host management, use of natural enemies (especially entomopathogenic fungi), and pheromone-based techniques. The situations that require tick management are diverse and occur under varied ecological conditions. Therefore, the likelihood of finding a single "magic bullet" for tick management is low. In practical terms, the approach to tick management or to management of tick-borne disease must be tailored to the specific conditions at hand. One area that needs increased attention is the decision-making process in applying IPM to tick control. Further development of novel tick control measures and increased efficiency in their integration and application to achieve desired goals hold great promise for effective future management of ticks and tick-borne diseases.

REFERENCES

1. **Akhurst, R. J.** 1982. Antibiotic activity of *Xenorhabdus* spp. bacteria symbiotically associated with the insect pathogenic nematodes of the families Heterorhabditidae and Steinernematidae. *J. Gen. Microbiol.* **128:**3061–3065.

2. **Alexander, G. I.** 1984. The development of the Australian Friesian Sahiwal: a tick-resistant dairy breed. *World Anim. Rev.* **51:**27–34.

3. **Allan, S. A.** 1999. Pheromonal attraction in ticks, p. 18. National Conference on the Prevention and Control of Tick-borne Diseases. American Lyme Disease Foundation, New York, N.Y.

4. **Allan, S. A., and M. J. Appel.** 1993. Acquired resistance to *Ixodes dammini:* comparison of hosts, p. 255–262. *In* D. Borovsky and A. Spielman (ed.), *Host Regulated Developmental Mechanisms in Vector Arthropods.* University of Florida, Vero Beach, Fla.

5. **Allan, S. A., N. Barre, D. E. Sonenshine, and M. J. Burridge.** 1998. Efficacy of tags impregnated with pheromone and acaricide for the control of *Amblyomma variegatum. Med. Vet. Entomol.* **12:**141–150.

6. **Allan, S. A., R. A. I. Norval, D. E. Sonenshine, and M. J. Burridge.** 1996. Control of the bont tick, *Amblyomma hebraeum,* on cattle using tail-tag decoys. *Ann. N. Y. Acad. Sci.* **791:**85–94.

7. **Allan, S. A., and L. A. Patrican.** 1995. Reduction of immature *Ixodes scapularis* (Acari: Ixodidae) in woods by application of desiccant and insecticidal soap formulations. *J. Med. Entomol.* **32:**16–20.

8. **Allan, S. A., and D. E. Sonenshine.** 2002. Evidence of an assembly pheromone in the black-legged deer tick, *Ixodes scapularis. J. Chem. Ecol.* **28:**15–27.

9. **Allen, J. R.** 1992. An overview of progress in characterizing host immunity to ticks, p. 206–211. *In* U. G. Munderloh and T. J. Kurtti (ed.), First International Conference on Tick-borne Pathogens at the Host-Vector Interface: An Agenda for Research. University of Minnesota, St. Paul.

10. **Aventis.** 2000. *Fipronil Worldwide Technical Bulletin*, p. 27. *Aventis CropScience*, Lyon, France.

11. **Barnard, D. R.** 1986. Density perturbation in populations of *Amblyomma americanum* (Acari: Ixodidae) in beef cattle forage areas in response to two regimens of vegetation management. *J. Econ. Entomol.* **79:**122–127.

12. **Barrett, P. N., S. Schober-Bendixen, and H. J. Ehrlich.** 2003. History of TBE vaccines. *Vaccine* **21**(Suppl. 1):S41–S49.

13. **Benjamin, M. A., E. Zhioua, and R. S. Ostfeld.** 2002. Laboratory and field evaluation of the entomopathogenic fungus *Metarhizium anisopliae* (Deuteromycetes) for controlling questing adult *Ixodes scapularis* (Acari: Ixodidae). *J. Med. Entomol.* **39:**723–728.

14. **Bloemer, S. R., G. A. Mount, T. A. Morris, R. H. Zimmerman, D. R. Barnard, and E. L. Snoddy.** 1990. Management of lone star ticks (Acari: Ixodidae) in recreational areas with acaricide applications, vegetative management, and exclusion of white-tailed deer. *J. Med. Entomol.* **27:**543–550.

15. **Bloemer, S. R., E. L. Snoddy, J. C. Cooney, and K. Fairbanks.** 1986. Influence of deer exclusion on populations of lone star ticks and American dog ticks (Acari: Ixodidae). *J. Econ. Entomol.* **79:**679–683.

16. **Bonsma, J. C.** 1981. Breeding tick-repellent cattle, p. 67–77. *In* G. B. Whitehead and J. D. Gibson (ed.), *Tick Biology and Control: Proceedings of an International Conference*. Rhodes University, Grahamstown, South Africa.

17. **Boucias, D. G., and J. C. Pendland.** 1998. *Principles of Insect Pathology*. Kluwer, Boston, Mass.

18. **Bowman, A. S., L. B. Coons, G. R. Needham, and J. R. Sauer.** 1997. Tick saliva: recent advances and implications for vector competence. *Med. Vet. Entomol.* **11:**277–285.

19. **Brossard, M., and S. K. Wikel.** 1997. Immunology of interactions between ticks and hosts. *Med. Vet. Entomol.* **11:**270–276.

20. **Brown, R. S., C. F. Reichelderfer, and W. R. Anderson.** 1970. An endemic disease among laboratory populations of *Dermacentor andersoni* (*D. venustus*) (Acarina: Ixodidae). *J. Invert. Pathol.* **16:**142–143.

21. **Brum, J. G. W., and M. O. Teixeira.** 1992. Acaricidal activity of *Cedecea lapagei* on engorged females of *Boophilus microplus* exposed to the environment. *Arq. Bras. Med. Vet. Zool.* **44:**543–544.

22. **Camicas, J.-L., J.-P. Hervy, F. Adam, and P.-C. Morel.** 1998. Les tiques du monde. *Orstom editions*, Paris, France.

23. **Carroll, J. F.** 1998. Kairomonal activity of white-tailed deer metatarsal gland substances: a more sensitive behavioral bioassay using *Ixodes scapularis* (Acari: Ixodidae). *J. Med. Entomol.* **35:**90–93.

24. **Carroll, J. F.** 2001. Interdigital gland substances of white-tailed deer and the response of host-seeking ticks (Acari: Ixodidae). *J. Med. Entomol.* **38:**114–117.

25. **Carroll, M. C., H. S. Ginsberg, K. E. Hyland, and R. Hu.** 1992. Distribution of *Ixodes dammini* (Acari: Ixodidae) in residential lawns on Prudence Island, Rhode Island. *J. Med. Entomol.* **29:**1052–1055.

26. **Clymer, B. C., D. E. Howell, and J. A. Hair.** 1970. Environmental alteration in recreational areas by mechanical and chemical treatment as a means of lone star tick control. *J. Econ. Entomol.* **63:**504–509.

27. **Cochet, P., P. Birckel, M. Bromet-Petit, N. Bromet, and A. Weil.** 1997. Skin distribution of fipronil by microautoradiography following topical administration to the beagle dog. *Eur. J. Drug Metab. Pharmacokinet.* **22:**211–216.

28. **Costello, C. M., A. C. Steere, R. E. Pinkerton, and J. H. M. Feder.** 1989. A prospective study of tick bites in an endemic area for Lyme disease. *J. Infect. Dis.* **159:**136–139.

29. **Curran, K. L., D. Fish, and J. Piesman.** 1993. Reduction of nymphal *Ixodes dammini* (Acari: Ixodidae) in a residential suburban landscape by area application of insecticides. *J. Med. Entomol.* **30:**107–113.

30. **Curran, K. L., and G. R. Needham.** 1996. The effects of temperature and humidity on laboratory survival and development of nymphal *Ixodes scapularis* Say (Ixodidae), p. 501–504. *In* R. Mitchell, D. J. Horn, G. R. Needham, and W. C. Welborne (ed.), *Acarology IX*, vol. 1. Proceedings. Ohio Biological Survey, Columbus, Ohio.

31. **Daniel, M., J. Kolar, P. Zeman, K. Pavelka, and J. Sadlo.** 1998. Predictive map of *Ixodes ricinus* high-incidence habitats and a tick-borne encephalitis risk assessment using satellite data. *Exp. Appl. Acarol.* **22:**417–433.

32. **Daniels, T. J., and D. Fish.** 1995. Effect of deer exclusion on the abundance of immature *Ixodes scapularis* (Acari: Ixodidae) parasitizing small and medium-sized mammals. *J. Med. Entomol.* **32:**5–11.

33. **Daniels, T. J., D. Fish, and R. C. Falco.** 1991. Evaluation of host-targeted acaricide for reducing risk of Lyme disease in southern New York state. *J. Med. Entomol.* **28:**537–543.

34. **Daniels, T. J., D. Fish, and I. Schwartz.** 1993. Reduced abundance of *Ixodes scapularis* (Acari: Ixodidae) and Lyme disease risk by deer exclusion. *J. Med. Entomol.* **30:**1043–1049.

35. **Deblinger, R. D., and D. W. Rimmer.** 1991. Efficacy of permethrin-based acaricide to reduce the abundance of *Ixodes dammini* (Acari: Ixodidae). *J. Med. Entomol.* **28:**708–711.

36. **Deblinger, R. D., M. L. Wilson, D. W. Rimmer, and A. Spielman.** 1993. Reduced abundance of immature *Ixodes dammini* (Acari: Ixodidae) following incremental removal of deer. *J. Med. Entomol.* **30:**144–150.

37. **de la Fuente, J., M. Rodriguez, and J. C. Garcia-Garcia.** 2000. Immunological control of ticks through vaccination with *Boophilus microplus* gut antigens. *Ann. N. Y. Acad. Sci.* **916:**617–621.

38. **de la Fuente, J., M. Rodriguez, M. Redondo, C. Montero, J. C. Garcia-Garcia, L. Mendez, E. Serrano, M. Valdes, A. Enriquez, M. Canales, E. Ramos, O. Boue, H. Machado, R. Lleonart, C. A. de Armas, S. Rey, J. L. Rodriguez, M. Artiles, and L. Garcia.** 1998. Field studies and cost-effectiveness analysis of vaccination with Gavac against the cattle tick *Boophilus microplus*. *Vaccine* **16:**366–373.

39. **Dennis, D. T., T. S. Nekomoto, J. C. Victor, W. S. Paul, and J. Piesman.** 1998. Reported distribution of *Ixodes scapularis* and *Ixodes pacificus* (Acari: Ixodidae) in the United States. *J. Med. Entomol.* **35:**629–638.

40. **des Vignes, F., J. Piesman, R. Heffernan, T. L. Schulze, K. C. Stafford III, and D. Fish.** 2001. Effect of tick removal on transmission of *Borrelia burgdorferi* and *Ehrlichia phagocytophila* by *Ixodes scapularis* nymphs. *J. Infect. Dis.* **183:**773–778.

41. **Dizij, A., S. Arndt, H. M. Seitz, and K. Kurtenbach.** 1994. *Clethrionomys glareolus* acquires resistance to *Ixodes ricinus*: a mechanism to prevent spirochete inoculation? p. 228–231. *In* R. Cevenini, V. Sambri, and M. LaPlaca (ed.), *Advances in Lyme Borreliosis Research. Proceedings of the VI Interna-*

tional Conference on Lyme Borreliosis. Esculapio, Bologna, Italy.

42. Dowling, D. F. 1980. Adaptability of low cost tick-resistant cattle for growth. *Aust. Vet. J.* 56:552–554.

43. Drummond, R. O., J. E. George, and S. E. Kunz. 1988. *Control of Arthropod Pests of Livestock: A Review of Technology.* CRC Press, Inc., Boca Raton, Fla.

44. Duffy, D. C., R. Downer, and C. Brinkley. 1992. The effectiveness of Helmeted Guineafowl in the control of the deer tick, the vector of Lyme disease. *Wilson Bull.* 104:342–345.

45. Falco, R. C., D. McKenna, T. J. Daniels, R. B. Nadelman, J. Nowakowski, D. Fish, and G. P. Wormser. 1999. Temporal relation between *Ixodes scapularis* abundance and risk for Lyme disease associated with erythema migrans. *Am. J. Epidemiol.* 149:771–776.

46. Fine, P. E. M. 1981. Epidemiological principles of vector-mediated transmission, p. 77–91. *In* J. J. McKelvey, B. F. Eldridge, and K. Maramorosch (ed.), *Vectors of Disease Agents: Interactions with Plants, Animals, and Man.* Praeger, New York, N.Y.

47. Fish, D., and T. J. Daniels. 1990. The role of medium sized mammals as reservoirs of *Borrelia burgdorferi* in southern New York. *J. Wildl. Dis.* 26:339–345.

48. Flexner, J. L., B. Lighthart, and B. A. Croft. 1986. The effects of microbial pesticides on non-target, beneficial arthropods. *Agric. Ecosyst. Environ.* 16:203–254.

49. Fragoso, H., P. H. Rad, M. Ortiz, M. Rodriguez, M. Redondo, L. Herrera, and J. de la Fuente. 1998. Protection against *Boophilus annulatus* infestations in cattle vaccinated with the *B. microplus* Bm86-containing vaccine Gavac. *Vaccine* 16:1990–1992.

50. Frost, W. H. 1976. Some conceptions of epidemics in general. *Am. J. Epidemiol.* 103:141–151.

51. Garcia-Garcia, J. C., C. Montero, M. Redondo, M. Vargas, M. Canales, O. Boue, M. Rodriguez, M. Joglar, H. Machado, I. L. Gonzalez, M. Valdes, L. Mendez, and J. de la Fuente. 2000. Control of ticks resistant to immunization with Bm86 in cattle vaccinated with the recombinant antigen Bm95 isolated from the cattle tick, *Boophilus microplus. Vaccine* 18:2275–2287.

52. Gebbia, J. A., E. M. Bosler, R. D. Evans, and E. M. Schneider. 1995. Acquired resistance in dogs to repeated infestation with *Ixodes scapularis* (Acari: Ixodidae) reduces tick viability and reproductive success. *Exp. Appl. Acarol.* 19:593–605.

53. George, J. E. 1992. Naturally acquired immunity as an element in strategies for the control of ticks on livestock. *Insect Sci. Appl.* 13:515–524.

54. Ginsberg, H. S. 1992. *Ecology and Management of Ticks and Lyme Disease at Fire Island National Seashore and Selected National Parks.* Scientific monograph NPS/NRSUNJ/NRSM-92/20. U.S. Department of the Interior National Park Service, Washington, D.C.

55. Ginsberg, H. S. 1993. Transmission risk of Lyme disease and implications for tick management. *Am. J. Epidemiol.* 138:65–73.

56. Ginsberg, H. S. 1994. Lyme disease and conservation. *Conserv. Biol.* 8:343–353.

57. Ginsberg, H. S. 2001. Integrated pest management and allocation of control efforts for vector-borne diseases. *J. Vector Ecol.* 26:32–38.

58. Ginsberg, H. S., M. Butler, and E. Zhioua. 2002. Effect of deer exclusion by fencing on abundance of *Amblyomma americanum* (Acari: Ixodidae) on Fire Island, New York, USA. *J. Vector Ecol.* 27:215–221.

59. Ginsberg, H. S., and C. P. Ewing. 1989. Habitat distribution of *Ixodes dammini* (Acari: Ixodidae) and Lyme disease spirochetes on Fire Island, NY. *J. Med. Entomol.* 26:183–189.

60. Ginsberg, H. S., C. P. Ewing, A. F. O'Connell, Jr., E. M. Bosler, and M. W. Sayre. 1991. Increased population densities of *Amblyomma americanum* (Acari: Ixodidae) on Long Island, New York. *J. Parasitol.* 77:493–495.

61. Ginsberg, H. S., K. E. Hyland, R. Hu, T. J. Daniels, and R. C. Falco. 1998. Tick population trends and forest type. *Science* 281:349–350.

62. Ginsberg, H. S., R. A. LeBrun, K. Heyer, and E. Zhioua. 2002. Potential nontarget effects of *Metarhizium anisopliae* (Deuteromycetes) used for biological control of ticks (Acari: Ixodidae). *Environ. Entomol.* 31:1191–1196.

63. Ginsberg, H. S., and E. Zhioua. 1996. Nymphal survival and habitat distribution of *Ixodes scapularis* and *Amblyomma americanum* ticks (Acari: Ixodidae) on Fire Island, New York, USA. *Exper. Appl. Acarol.* 20:533–544.

64. Ginsberg, H. S., and E. Zhioua. 1999. Influence of deer abundance on the abundance of questing adult *Ixodes scapularis* (Acari: Ixodidae). *J. Med. Entomol.* 36:379–381.

65. Glass, G. E., B. S. Schwartz, J. M. Morgan III, D. T. Johnson, P. M. Noy, and E. Israel. 1995. Environmental risk factors for Lyme disease identified with geographic information systems. *Amer. J. Public Health* 85:944–948.

66. Graf, J. F. 1975. Ecologie and ethologie d'*Ixodes ricinus* L. en Suisse (Ixodoidea: Ixodidae). Cinquieme note: Mise un evidence d'une pheromone sexuelle chez *Ixodes ricinus. Acarologia* 17:436–441.

67. Gray, J. S., O. Kahl, C. Janetzki, and J. Stein. 1992. Studies on the ecology of Lyme disease in a deer forest in County Galway, Ireland. *J. Med. Entomol.* 29:915–920.

68. Grobler, J. H. 1979. The re-introduction of oxpeckers *Buphagus africanus* and *B. erythrorhynchus* to Rhodes Matopos National Park, Rhodesia. *Biol. Conserv.* 15:151–158.

69. Guerra, M., E. Walker, C. Jones, S. Paskewitz, M. R. Cortinas, A. Stancil, L. Beck, M. Bobo, and U. Kitron. 2002. Predicting the risk of Lyme disease: habitat suitability for *Ixodes scapularis* in the north central United States. *Emerg. Infect Dis.* 8:289–297.

70. Hajek, A. E., S. R. A. Butler, J. C. Walsh, F. P. Silver, F. P. Hain, F. L. Hastings, T. M. O'Dell, and D. R. Smitley. 1996. Host range of the gypsy moth (Lepidoptera: Lymantridae) pathogen *Entomophaga maimaiga* (Zygomycetes: Entomophthorales) in the field versus laboratory. *Environ. Entomol.* 25:709–721.

71. Hajkova, Z., and M. G. Leahy. 1982. Pheromone-regulated aggregation in larvae, nymphs, and adults of *Ixodes ricinus* (L.)(Acarina: Ixodidae). *Folia Parasitol.* 29:61–67.

72. Hamilton, J. G. C. 1992. The role of pheromones in tick biology. *Parasitol. Today* 8:130–133.

73. Hassan, S. M., O. O. Dipeolu, and D. M. Munyinyi. 1992. Influence of exposure period and management methods on the effectiveness of chickens as predators of ticks infesting cattle. *Vet. Parasitol.* 43:301–309.

74. Hassanain, M. A., M. F. El Garhy, F. A. Abdel-Ghaffar, A. El Sharaby, and N. Abdel-Mageed-Kadria. 1997. Biological control studies of soft and hard ticks in Egypt: I. The effect of *Bacillus thuringiensis* varieties on soft and hard ticks (Ixodidae). *Parasitol. Res.* 83:209–213.

75. Hayes, E. B., G. O. Maupin, G. A. Mount, and J. Piesman. 1999. Assessing the prevention effectiveness of local Lyme disease control. *J. Public Health Manag. Pract.* 5:84–92.

76. Hill, D. E. 1998. Entomopathogenic nematodes as control agents of developmental stages of the black-legged tick, *Ixodes scapularis. J. Parasitol.* 84:1124–1127.

77. Hoch, A. L., R. W. Barker, and J. A. Hair. 1971. Further observations on the control of lone star ticks (Acarina: Ixodidae) through integrated control procedures. *J. Med. Entomol.* 8:731–734.

78. Holling, C. S. (ed.). 1978. *Adaptive Environmental Assessment and Management.* John Wiley, New York, N.Y.

79. Hu, R., K. E. Hyland, and T. N. Mather. 1993. Occurrence and distribution in Rhode Island of *Hunterellus hookeri* (Hymenoptera: Encyrtidae), a wasp parasitoid of *Ixodes dammini.* *J. Med. Entomol.* 30:277–280.

80. Jenkins, D. W. 1964. Pathogens, parasites and predators of medically important arthropods. *Bull. W. H. O.* 30(Suppl.): 1–150.

81. Johnston, T. H., and M. J. Bancroft. 1918. A tick-resistant condition in cattle. *Proc. R. Soc. Queensland* 30:219–317.

82. Jones, C. G., R. S. Ostfeld, M. P. Richard, E. M. Schauber, and J. O. Wolff. 1998. Chain reactions linking acorns to gypsy moth outbreaks and Lyme disease risk. *Science* 279: 1023–1026.

83. Kaaya, G. P., and S. Hassan. 2000. Entomogenous fungi as promising biopesticides for tick control. *Exp. Appl. Acarol.* 24:913–926.

84. Kaaya, G. P., E. N. Mwangi, and E. A. Ouna. 1996. Prospects for biological control of livestock ticks, *Rhipicephalus appendiculatus* and *Amblyomma variegatum*, using the entomogenous fungi *Beauveria bassiana* and *Metarhizium anisopliae.* *J. Invertebr. Pathol.* 67:15–20.

85. Kalsbeek, V., F. Frandsen, and T. Steenberg. 1995. Entomopathogenic fungi associated with *Ixodes ricinus* ticks. *Exp. Appl. Acarol.* 19:45–51.

86. Kamrin, M. A. (ed.). 1997. *Pesticide profiles: toxicity, environmental impact, and fate.* Lewis Publications, CRC Press, Boca Raton, Fla.

87. Kartman, L. 1958. An insecticide bait-box method for the control of sylvatic plague vectors. *J. Hyg.* 56:455–465.

88. Kilpatrick, H. J., S. M. Spohr, and G. G. Chasko. 1997. A controlled deer hunt on a state-owned coastal reserve in Connecticut: controversies, strategies, and results. *Wildl. Soc. Bull.* 25:451–456.

89. Kitron, U., and J. Kazmierczak. 1997. Spatial analysis of the distribution of Lyme disease in Wisconsin. *Am. J. Epidemiol.* 145:558–566.

90. Knipling, E. F., and C. D. Steelman. 2000. Feasibility of controlling *Ixodes scapularis* ticks (Acari: Ixodidae), the vector of Lyme disease, by parasitoid augmentation. *J. Med. Entomol.* 37:645–652.

91. Kocan, K. M., T. Halbur, E. F. Blouin, V. Onet, J. de la Fuente, J. C. Garcia-Garcia, and J. T. Saliki. 2001. Immunization of cattle with *Anaplasma marginale* derived from tick cell culture. *Vet. Parasitol.* 102:151–161.

92. Kocan, K. M., M. S. Pidherney, E. F. Blouin, P. L. Claypool, M. Samish, et al. 1998. Interaction of entomopathogenic nematodes (Steiniernematidae) with selected species of ixodid ticks (Acari: Ixodidae). *J. Med. Entomol.* 35:514–520.

93. Kurtenbach, K., A. Dizij, H. M. Seitz, G. Margos, S. E. Moter, M. D. Kramer, R. Wallich, U. E. Schaible, and M. M. Simon. 1994. Differential immune responses to *Borrelia burgdorferi* in European wild rodent species influence spirochete transmission to *Ixodes ricinus* L. (Acari: Ixodidae). *Infect. Immun.* 62:5344–5352.

94. Kurtenbach, K., A. Dizij, P. Voet, P. Hauser, and M. M. Simon. 1997. Vaccination of natural reservoir hosts with recombinant lipidated OspA induces a transmission-blocking immunity against Lyme disease spirochetes associated with high levels of LA-2 equivalent antibodies. *Vaccine* 15:1670–1674.

95. Kurtenbach, K., H. Kampen, A. Dizij, S. Arndt, H. M. Seitz, U. E. Schaible, and M. M. Simon. 1995. Infestation of rodents with larval *Ixodes ricinus* (Acari: Ixodidae) is an important factor in the transmission cycle of *Borrelia burgdorferi* s.l. in German woodlands. *J. Med. Entomol.* 32:807–817.

96. Larousse, F., A. G. King, and S. B. Wolbach. 1928. The overwintering in Massachusetts of Ixodiphagus caucertei. *Science* 67:351–353.

97. LoGiudice, K., R. S. Ostfeld, K. A. Schmidt, and F. Keesing. 2003. The ecology of infectious disease: effects of host diversity and community composition on Lyme disease risk. *Proc. Nat. Acad. Sci. USA* 100:567–571.

98. Luke, C. J., R. C. Heubner, V. Kasmiersky, and A. G. Barbour. 1997. Oral delivery of purified lipoprotein OspA protects mice from systemic infection with *Borrelia burgdorferi.* *Vaccine* 15:739–746.

99. Martin, P. A. W., and E. T. Schmidtmann. 1998. Isolation of aerobic microbes from *Ixodes scapularis* (Acari: Ixodidae), the vector of Lyme disease in the eastern United States. *J. Econ. Entomol.* 91:864–868.

100. Mather, T. N., D. C. Duffy, and S. R. Campbell. 1993. An unexpected result from burning vegetation to reduce Lyme disease transmission risks. *J. Med. Entomol.* 30:642–645.

101. Mather, T. N., and H. S. Ginsberg. 1994. Vector-host-pathogen relationships: transmission dynamics of tick-borne infections, p. 68–90. *In* D. E. Sonenshine and T. N. Mather (ed.), *Ecological Dynamics of Tick-Borne Zoonoses.* Oxford University Press, Oxford, United Kingdom.

102. Mather T. N., M. C. Nicholson, E. F. Donnelly, and B. T. Matyas. 1996. Entomologic index for human risk of Lyme disease. *Am. J. Epidemiol.* 144:1066–1069.

103. Mather, T. N., J. Piesman, and A. Spielman. 1987. Absence of spirochaetes (*Borrelia burgdorferi*) and piroplasms (*Babesia microti*) in deer ticks (*Ixodes dammini*) parasitized by chalcid wasps (*Hunterellus hookeri*). *Med. Vet. Entomol.* 1: 3–8.

104. Mather, T. N., J. M. C. Ribeiro, and A. Spielman. 1987. Lyme disease and babesiosis: acaricide focused on potentially infected ticks. *Am. J. Trop. Med. Hyg.* 36:609–614.

105. Mauléon, H., N. Barré, and S. Panoma. 1993. Pathogenicity of 17 isolates of entomophagous nematodes (Steinernematidae and Heterorhabditidae) for the ticks *Amblyomma variegatum* (Fabricius), *Boophilus microplus* (Canestrini) and *Boophilus annulatus* (Say). *Exp. Appl. Entomol.* 17:831–838.

106. Maupin, G. O. 1999. Innovations in acaricides and delivery methods against ticks, p. 16. National Conference on the Prevention and Control of Tick-borne Diseases. American Lyme Disease Foundation, New York, N.Y.

107. Maupin, G. O., D. Fish, J. Zultowsky, E. G. Campos, and J. Piesman. 1991. Landscape ecology of Lyme disease in a residential area of Westchester County, New York. *Am. J. Epidemiol.* 133:1105–1113.

108. McGraw, L., and J. McBride. 2001. Out of the Lyme-light, p. 4–7. Agricultural Research.

109. Mejlon, H. A., T. G. T. Jaenson, and T. N. Mather. 1995. Evaluation of host-targeted applications of permethrin for control of *Borrelia*-infected *Ixodes ricinus* (Acari: Ixodidae). *Med. Vet. Entomol.* 9:207–210.

110. Meyer, J. A., J. J. L. Lancaster, and J. S. Simco. 1982. Comparison of habitat modification, animal control, and standard spraying for control of the lone star tick. *J. Econ. Entomol.* 75:524–529.

111. Miller, J. A., G. I. Garris, J. E. George, and D. D. Oehler. 1989. Control of lone star ticks (Acari: Ixodidae) on Spanish goats and white-tailed deer with orally administered ivermectin. *J. Econ. Entomol.* 82:1650–1656.

112. Mills, A. 1994. The economics of vector control strategies for controlling tropical diseases. *Am. J. Trop. Med. Hyg.* 50(Suppl.):151–159.

113. Mills, A., and M. Drummond. 1987. Value for money in the health sector: the contribution of primary health care. *Health Policy Plan.* 2:107–128.

114. Milne, A. 1948. Pasture improvement and the control of sheep tick (*Ixodes ricinus* L.). *Ann. Appl. Biol.* 35:369–378.

115. Milne, A. 1949. The ecology of the sheep tick, *Ixodes ricinus* L.: host relationships of the tick. 2. Observations on hill and moorland grazings in northern Ireland. *Parasitology* 39: 173–197.

116. Milner, R. J., J. A. Staples, and G. G. Lutton. 1997. The effect of humidity on germination and infection of termites by the Hyphomycete, *Metarhizium anisopliae. J. Invertebr. Pathol.* 69:64–69.

117. Monsen, S. E., L. R. Bronson, J. R. Tucker, and C. R. Smith. 1999. Experimental and field evaluations of two acaracides for control of *I. pacificus* (Acari: Ixodidae) in northern California. *J. Med. Entomol.* 36:660–665.

118. Mount, G. A. 1981. Control of the lone star tick in Oklahoma parks through vegetative management. *J. Econ. Entomol.* 74:173–175.

119. Mount, G. A., and J. E. Dunn. 1983. Economic thresholds for lone star ticks (Acari: Ixodidae) in recreational areas based on a relationship between CO_2 human subject sampling. *J. Econ. Entomol.* 76:327–329.

120. Mount, G. A., D. G. Haile, and E. Daniels. 1997. Simulation of blacklegged tick (Acari: Ixodidae) population dynamics and transmission of *Borrelia burgdorferi. J. Med. Entomol.* 34:461–484.

121. Mount, G. A., D. G. Haile, and E. Daniels. 1997. Simulation of management strategies for the blacklegged tick (Acari: Ixodidae) and the Lyme disease spirochete, *Borrelia burgdorferi. J. Med. Entomol.* 34:672–683.

122. Mwangi, E. N., O. O. Dipeolu, R. M. Newson, G. P. Kaaya, and S. M. Hassan. 1991. Predators, parasitoids and pathogens of ticks: a review. *Biocontrol Sci. Tech.* 1:147–156.

123. Mwangi, E. N., S. M. Hassan, G. P. Kaaya, and S. Essuman. 1997. The impact of *Ixodiphagus hookeri*, a tick parasitoid, on *Amblyomma variegatum* (Acari: Ixodidae) in a field trial in Kenya. *Exp. Appl. Acarol.* 21:117–126.

124. Mwangi, E. N., and G. P. Kaaya. 1997. Prospects of using tick parasitoids (Insecta) for tick management in Africa. *Int. J. Acarol.* 23:215–219.

125. Nadelman, R. B., J. Nowakowski, D. Fish, R. C. Falco, K. Freeman, D. McKenna, P. Welch, R. Marcus, M. E. Aguero-Rosenfeld, D. T. Dennis, and G. P. Wormser. 2001. Prophylaxis with single-dose doxycycline for the prevention of Lyme disease after an *Ixodes scapularis* tick bite. *N. Engl. J. Med.* 345:79–84.

126. Needham, G. R. 1985. Evaluation of five popular methods for tick removal. *Pediatrics* 75:997–1002.

127. Needham, G. R., and P. D. Teel. 1986. Water balance by ticks between bloodmeals, p. 100–164. *In* J. R. Saur and J. A. Hair (ed.), *Morphology, Physiology, and Behavioral Ecology of Ticks.* Ellis Horwood, Chichester, United Kingdom.

128. Needham, G. R., and P. D. Teel. 1991. Off-host physiological ecology of ixodid ticks. *Annu. Rev. Entomol.* 36:659–681.

129. Nicholson, M. C., and T. N. Mather. 1996. Methods for evaluating Lyme disease risks using geographic information systems and geospatial analysis. *J. Med. Entomol.* 33:711–720.

130. Noda, H., U. G. Munderloh, and T. J. Kurtti. 1997. Endosymbionts of ticks and their relationship to *Wolbachia* spp.

and tick-borne pathogens of humans and animals. *Appl. Environ. Microbiol.* 63:3926–3932.

131. Norval, R. A. I., J. H. R. Andrew, and C. E. Yunker. 1989. Pheromone-mediation of host selection in bont ticks (hebraeum). *Science* 243:364–365.

132. Norval, R. A. I., D. E. Sonsenshine, S. A. Allan, and M. J. Burridge. 1996. Efficacy of pheromone-acaricide-impregnated tail-tag decoys for controlling the bont tick, *Amblyomma hebraeum* (Acari: Ixodidae), on cattle in Zimbabwe. *Exp. Appl. Acarol.* 20:31–46.

133. Ohnishi, J., J. Piesman, and A. M. de Silva. 2001. Antigenic and genetic heterogeneity of *Borrelia burgdorferi* populations transmitted by ticks. *Proc. Natl. Acad. Sci USA* 98: 670–675.

134. Ostfeld, R. S., E. M. Schauber, C. D. Canham, F. Keesing, C. G. Jones, and J. Wolff. 2001. Effects of acorn production and mouse abundance on abundance and *Borrelia burgdorferi* infection prevalence of nymphal *Ixodes scapularis* ticks. *Vector Borne Zoonotic Dis.* 1:55–63.

135. Patrican, L. A., and S. A. Allan. 1995. Laboratory evaluation of desiccants and insecticidal soap applied to various substrates to control the deer tick *Ixodes scapularis. Med. Vet. Entomol.* 9:293–299.

136. Patrican, L. A., and S. A. Allan. 1995. Application of desiccant and insecticidal soap treatments to control *Ixodes scapularis* (Acari: Ixodidae) nymphs and adults in a hyperendemic woodland site. *J. Med. Entomol.* 32:859–863.

137. Pegram, G. R. 1991. The economic impact of cattle tick control in central Africa. *Insect Sci. Appl.* 12:139–146.

138. Phillips, M., A. Mills, and C. Dye. 1993. *Guidelines for Cost-Effectiveness Analysis of Vector Control.* WHO/CWS/93.4. World Health Organization, Geneva, Switzerland.

139. Piesman, J., and M. C. Dolan. 2002. Protection against Lyme disease spirochete transmission provided by prompt removal of nymphal *Ixodes scapularis* (Acari: Ixodidae). *J. Med. Entomol.* 39:509–512.

140. Piesman, J., T. N. Mather, R. J. Sinsky, and A. Spielman. 1987. Duration of tick attachment and *Borrelia burgdorferi* transmission. *J. Clin. Microbiol.* 25:557–558.

141. Piesman, J., B. S. Schneider, and N. S. Zeidner. 2001. Use of quantitative PCR to measure density of *Borrelia burgdorferi* in the midgut and salivary glands of feeding tick vectors. *J. Clin. Microbiol.* 39:4145–4148.

142. Poland, G. A. 2001. Prevention of Lyme disease: a review of the evidence. *Mayo Clin. Proc.* 76:713–724.

143. Pound, J. M., J. A. Miller, and C. A. LeMeilleur. 1994. Device and method for use as an aid in control of ticks and other ectoparasites on wildlife. U.S. Patent 5,367,983.

144. Pound, J. M., J. A. Miller, and J. E. George. 2000. Efficacy of amitraz applied to white-tailed deer by the '4-poster' topical treatment device in controlling free-living lone star ticks (Acari: Ixodidae). *J. Med. Entomol.* 37:878–884.

145. Pound, J. M., J. A. Miller, J. E. George, and C. A. Lemeilleur. 2000. The '4-poster' passive tropical treatment device to apply acaricide for controlling ticks (Acari: Ixodidae) feeding on white-tailed deer. *J. Med. Entomol.* 37:588–594.

146. Pound, J. M., J. A. Miller, J. E. George, D. D. Oehler, and D. E. Harmel. 1996. Systemic treatment of white-tailed deer with ivermectin-medicated bait to control free-living populations of lone star ticks (Acari: Ixodidae). *J. Med. Entomol.* 33:385–394.

147. Ramoska, W. A. 1984. The influence of relative humidity on *Beauveria bassiana* infectivity and replication in the chinch bug, *Blissus leucopterus. J. Invertebr. Pathol.* 43:389–394.

148. Rand, P. W., E. H. Lacombe, M. S. Holman, C. Lubelczyk, and R. P. Smith, Jr. 2000. Attempt to control ticks (Acari:

Ixodidae) on deer on an isolated island using ivermectin-treated corn. *J. Med. Entomol.* **37**:126–133.

149. **Randolph, S. E., and G. M. Steele.** 1985. An experimental evaluation of conventional control measures against the sheep tick, *Ixodes ricinus* (L.) (Acari: Ixodidae). II. The dynamics of the tick-host interaction. *Bull. Entomol. Res.* **75**:501–518.

150. **Redondo, M., H. Fragoso, M. Ortiz, C. Montero, J. Lona, J. A. Medellin, R. Fria, V. Hernandez, R. Franco, H. Machado, M. Rodriguez, and J. de la Fuente.** 1999. Integrated control of acaricide-resistant *Boophilus microplus* populations on grazing cattle in Mexico using vaccination with Gavac and amidine treatments. *Exp. Appl. Acarol.* **23**:841–849.

151. **Ribeiro, J. M. C.** 1987. *Ixodes dammini*: salivary anticomplement activity. *Exp. Parasitol.* **149**:3648–3653.

152. **Ribeiro, J. M. C.** 1989. Role of saliva in tick/host interactions (review). *Exp. Appl. Acarol.* **7**:15–20.

153. **Ribeiro, J. M. C., G. T. Makoul, J. Levine, D. R. Robinson, and A. Spielman.** 1985. Antihemostatic, antiinflammatory and immunosuppressive properties of the saliva of a tick, *Ixodes dammini. J. Exp. Med.* **161**:332–344.

154. **Ribeiro, J. M. C., G. T. Makoul, and D. R. Robinson.** 1988. *Ixodes dammini*: evidence for salivary prostacyclin secretion. *J. Parasitol.* **74**:1068–1069.

155. **Ribeiro, J. M. C., and A. Spielman.** 1986. *Ixodes dammini*: salivary anaphylatoxin inactivating activity. *Exp. Parasitol.* **62**:292–297.

156. **Ribeiro, J. M., J. J. Weis, and S. R. Telford III.** 1990. Saliva of the tick *Ixodes dammini* inhibits neutrophil function. *Exp. Parasitol.* **70**:382–388.

157. **Rogers, A. J.** 1953. *A Study of the Ixodid Ticks of Northern Florida, including the Biology and Life History of Ixodes scapularis.* Ph.D. Dissertation, University of Maryland, College Park.

158. **Samish, M., and E. Alekseev.** 2001. Arthropods as predators of ticks (Ixodoidea). *J. Med. Entomol.* **38**:1–11.

159. **Samish, M., E. A. Alekseev, and I. Glazer.** 1998. The effect of soil composition on anti-tick activity of entomopathogenic nematodes. *Ann. N. Y. Acad. Sci.* **849**:398–399.

160. **Samish, M., G. Gindin, E. Alekseev, and I. Glazer.** 2001. Pathogenicity of entomopathogenic fungi to different developmental stages of *Rhipicephalus sanguineus* (Acari: Ixodidae). *J. Parasitol.* **87**:1355–1359.

161. **Samish, M., and I. Glazer.** 1992. Infectivity of entomopathogenic nematodes (Steinernematidae and Heterorhabditidae) to female ticks of *Boophilus annulatus* (Arachnida: Ixodidae). *J. Med. Entomol.* **29**:614–618.

162. **Samish, M., and I. Glazer.** 2001. Entomopathogenic nematodes for the biocontrol of ticks. *Trends Parasitol.* **368**:371.

163. **Samish, M., and J. Rehacek.** 1999. Pathogens and predators of ticks and their potential in biological control. *Annu. Rev. Entomol.* **44**:159–182.

164. **Samsinakova, A., S. Kalalova, M. Daniel, F. Dusbábek, E. Honzakova, and V. Cerny.** 1974. Entomopathogenic fungi associated with the tick *Ixodes ricinus* L. *Folia Parasitol.* **21**:39–48.

165. **Schmidtmann, E. T.** 1994. Ecologically based strategies for controlling ticks, p. 240–280. *In* D. E. Sonenshine and T. N. Mather (ed.), *Ecological Dynamics of Tick-Borne Zoonoses.* Oxford University Press, New York, N.Y.

166. **Schoeler, G. B., and S. K. Wikel.** 2001. Modulation of host immunity by haematophagus arthropods. *Ann. Trop. Med. Parasitol.* **95**:755–771.

167. **Schulze, T. L., and R. L. Harrison.** 1995. Potential influence of leaf litter depth on effectiveness of granular carbaryl against subadult *Ixodes scapularis* (Acari: Ixodidae). *J. Med. Entomol.* **32**:205–208.

168. **Schulze, T. L., R. A. Jordan, and R. W. Hung.** 1995. Suppression of subadult *Ixodes scapularis* (Acari: Ixodidae) following removal of leaf litter. *J. Med. Entomol.* **32**:730–733.

169. **Schulze, T. L., R. Jordan, and R. Hung.** 2000. Effects of granular carbaryl application on sympatric populations of *Ixodes scapularis* and *Amblyomma americanum* (Acari: Ixodidae) nymphs. *J. Med. Entomol.* **37**:121–125.

170. **Schulze, T. L., R. A. Jordan, R. W. Hung, R. C. Taylor, D. Markowski, and M. S. Chomsky.** 2001. Efficacy of granular deltamethrin against *Ixodes scapularis* and *Amblyomma americanum* (Acari: Ixodidae) nymphs. *J. Med. Entomol.* **38**:344–346.

171. **Schulze, T. L., R. A. Jordan, L. M. Vasvary, M. S. Chomsky, D. C. Shaw, M. A. Meddis, R. C. Taylor, and J. Piesman.** 1994. Suppression of *Ixodes scapularis* (Acari: Ixodidae) nymphs in a large residential community. *J. Med. Entomol.* **31**:206–211.

172. **Schulze, T. L., W. M. McDevitt, W. E. Parkin, and J. K. Shisler.** 1987. Effectiveness of two insecticides in controlling *Ixodes dammini* (Acari: Ixodidae) following an outbreak of Lyme disease in New Jersey. *J. Med. Entomol.* **24**:420–424.

173. **Schulze, T. L., G. C. Taylor, R. A. Jordan, E. M. Bosler, and J. K. Shisler.** 1991. Effectiveness of selected granular acaricide formulations in suppressing populations of *Ixodes dammini* (Acari: Ixodidae): short-term control of nymphs and larvae. *J. Med. Entomol.* **28**:624–629.

174. **Schulze, T. L., R. C. Taylor, G. C. Taylor, and E. M. Bosler.** 1991. Lyme disease: a proposed ecological index to assess areas of risk in the northeastern United States. *Am. J. Public Health* **81**:714–718.

175. **Schwartz, B. S., and M. D. Goldstein.** 1991. Lyme disease in outdoor workers: risk factors, preventive measures, and tick removal methods. *Am. J. Epidemiol.* **133**:754–755.

176. **Shadick, N. A., L. H. Daltroy, C. B. Phillips, U. S. Lang, and M. H. Lang.** 1997. Determinants of tick-avoidance behaviors in an endemic area for Lyme disease. *Am. J. Prev. Med.* **13**:265–270.

177. **Shapiro, E. D., M. A. Gerber, N. B. Holabird, A. T. Berg, H. M. Feder, G. L. Bell, P. N. Rys, and D. H. Persing.** 1992. A controlled trial of antimicrobial prophylaxis for Lyme disease after deer-tick bites. *N. Engl. J. Med.* **327**:1769–1773.

178. **Sigal, L. H.** 1996. The Lyme disease controversy—social and financial costs of misdiagnosis and mismanagement. *Arch. Intern. Med.* **156**:1493–1500.

179. **Sigal, L. H., J. M. Zahradnik, P. Lavin, S. J. Patella, G. Bryant, R. Haselby, E. Hilton, M. Kunkel, D. Adler-Klein, T. Doherty, J. Evans, P. J. Molloy, A. L. Seidner, J. R. Sabetta, H. J. Simon, M. S. Klempner, J. Mays, D. Marks, S. E. Malawista, et al.** 1998. A vaccine consisting of recombinant Borrelia burgdorferi outer-surface protein A to prevent Lyme disease. *N. Engl. J. Med.* **339**:216–222.

180. **Smith, C. N., and M. M. Cole.** 1943. Studies of parasites of the American dog tick. *J. Econ. Entomol.* **36**:569–572.

181. **Solberg, V. B., J. A. Miller, T. Hadfield, R. Burge, J. M. Schech, and J. M. Pound.** 2003. Control of *Ixodes scapularis* (Acari: Ixodidae) with topical self-application of permethrin by white-tailed deer inhabiting NASA, Beltsville, Maryland. *J. Vector Ecol.* **28**:117–134.

182. **Solberg, V. B., K. Neidhardt, M. R. Sardelis, F. J. Hoffman, R. Stevenson, L. R. Boobar, and H. J. Harlan.** 1992. Field evaluation of two formulations of cyfluthrin for control of Ixodes dammini and Amblyomma americanum (Acari: Ixodidae). *J. Med. Entomol.* **29**:634–638.

183. **Sonenshine, D. E.** 1991. *Biology of Ticks*, vol. 1. Tick pheromones, p. 331–369. Oxford University Press, New York, N.Y.

184. Sonenshine, D. E. 1993. *Biology of Ticks*, vol. 2. Oxford University Press, New York, N.Y.

185. Sonenshine, D. E., S. A. Allan, R. A. Norval, and M. J. Burridge. 1996. A self-medicating applicator for control of ticks on deer. *Med. Vet. Entomol.* **10**:149–154.

186. Sonenshine, D. E., and G. Haines. 1985. A convenient method for controlling populations of the American dog tick, *Dermacentor variabilis* (Acari: Ixodidae) in the natural environment. *J. Med. Entomol.* **22**:577–583.

187. Sonenshine, D. E., J. G. C. Hamilton, J. S. Philips, K. P. Ellis, and R. A. I. Norval. 1992. Innovative techniques for control of tick disease vectors using pheromones, p. 308–313. *In* U. G. Munderloh and T. J. Kurtti (ed.), *First International Conference on Tick-Borne Pathogens at the Host-Vector Interface: An Agenda for Research*. University of Minnesota, St. Paul.

188. Stafford, K. C., III. 1991. Effectiveness of carbaryl applications for the control of *Ixodes dammini* (Acari: Ixodidae) nymphs in an endemic residential area. *J. Med. Entomol.* **28**:32–36.

189. Stafford, K. C., III. 1991. Effectiveness of host-targeted permethrin in the control of *Ixodes dammini* (Acari: Ixodidae). *J. Med. Entomol.* **28**:611–617.

190. Stafford, K. C., III. 1992. Third-year evaluation of host-targeted permethrin for the control of *Ixodes dammini* (Acari: Ixodidae) in southeastern Connecticut. *J. Med. Entomol.* **29**:717–720.

191. Stafford, K. C., III. 1993. Reduced abundance of *Ixodes scapularis* (Acari: Ixodidae) with exclusion of deer by electric fencing. *J. Med. Entomol.* **30**:986–996.

192. Stafford, K. C., III. 1994. Survival of immature *Ixodes scapularis* (Acari: Ixodidae) at different relative humidities. *J. Med. Entomol.* **31**:310–314.

193. Stafford, K. C., III. 1997. Pesticide use by licensed applicators for the control of *Ixodes scapularis* (Acari: Ixodidae) in Connecticut. *J. Med. Entomol.* **34**:552–558.

194. Stafford, K. C., III. 1998. Impact of controlled burns on the abundance of *Ixodes scapularis* (Acari: Ixodidae). *J. Med. Entomol.* **35**:510–513.

195. Stafford, K. C., III, M. L. Cartter, L. A. Magnarelli, S. Ertel, and P. A. Mshar. 1998. Temporal correlations between tick abundance and prevalence of ticks infested with *Borrelia burgdorferi* and increasing incidence of Lyme disease. *J. Clin. Microbiol.* **36**:1240–1244.

196. Stafford, K. C., III, A. J. DeNicola, and H. J. Kilpatrick. 2003. Reduced abundance of *Ixodes scapularis* (Acari: Ixodidae) and the tick parasitoid *Ixodiphagus hookeri* (Hymenoptera: Encyrtidae) with reduction of white-tailed deer. *J. Med. Entomol.* **40**:642–652.

197. Stafford, K. C., III, A. J. DeNicola, and L. Magnarelli. 1996. Presence of *Ixodiphagus hookeri* (Hymenoptera: Encyrtidae) in two Connecticut populations of *Ixodes scapularis* (Acari: Ixodidae). *J. Med. Entomol.* **33**:183–188.

198. Stafford, K. C., III, and U. Kitron. 2002. Environmental management for Lyme borreliosis control, p. 301–334. *In* J. S. Gray, O. Kahl, R. S. Lane, and G. Stanek (ed.), *Lyme Borreliosis*. CAB International, Wallingford, United Kingdom.

199. Stafford, K. C., III, and L. A. Magnarelli. 1993. Spatial and temporal patterns of *Ixodes scapularis* (Acari: Ixodidae) in southcentral Connecticut. *J. Med. Entomol.* **30**:762–771.

200. Steere A. C., V. K. Sikand, F. Meurice, D. L. Parenti, E. Fikrig, R. T. Schoen, J. Nowakowski, C. H. Schmid, S. Laukamp, C. Buscarino, D. S. Krause, et al. 1998. Vaccination against Lyme disease with recombinant *Borrelia burgdorferi* outer-surface lipoprotein A with adjuvant. *N. Engl. J. Med.* **339**:209–215.

201. Telford, S. T., III. 1993. Forum: management of Lyme disease, p. 164–167. *In* H. S. Ginsberg (ed.), *Ecology and Environmental Management of Lyme Disease*. Rutgers University Press, New Brunswick, N.J.

202. Trager, W. 1939. Acquired immunity to ticks. *J. Parasitol.* **25**:57–81.

203. Tsao, J., A. G. Barbour, C. J. Luke, E. Fikrig, and D. Fish. 2001. OspA immunization decreases transmission of *Borrelia burgdorferi* spirochetes from infected *Peromyscus leucopus* mice to larval *Ixodes scapularis* ticks. *Vector Borne Zoonotic Dis.* **1**:65–74.

204. Wanjohi, J. M., J. N. Ngeranwa, R. M. Rumberia, G. R. Muraguri, and S. K. Mbogo. 2001. Immunization of cattle against East Coast fever using *Theileria parva* (Marikebuni) and relaxation of tick control in North Rift, Kenya. *Onderspoort J. Vet. Res.* **68**:217–233.

205. White, D. J., H. G. Chang, J. L. Benach, E. M. Bosler, S. C. Meldrum, R. G. Means, J. G. Debbie, G. S. Birkhead, and D. L. Morse. 1991. The geographic spread and temporal increase of the Lyme disease epidemic. *JAMA* **266**:1269–1270.

206. Wikel, S. K. 1996. Host immunity to ticks. *Annu. Rev. Entomol.* **41**:1–22.

207. Wikel, S. K. 1999. Tick modulation of host immunity: an important factor in pathogen transmission. *Int. J. Parasitol.* **29**:851–859.

208. Wikel, S. K., and F. J. Alarcon-Chaidez. 2001. Progress toward molecular characterization of ectoparasite modulation of host immunity. *Vet. Parasitol.* **101**:275–287.

209. Wikel, S. K., D. K. Bergman, and R. N. Ramachandra. 1996. Immunological-based control of blood-feeding arthropods, p. 290–315. *In* S. K. Wikel (ed.), *The Immunology of Host-Ectoparasitic Arthropod Relationships*. CAB International, Wallingford, United Kingdom.

210. Wikel, S. K., R. N. Ramachandra, and D. K. Bergman. 1992. Immunological strategies for suppression of vector arthropods. *Bull. Soc. Vector Ecol.* **17**:10–19.

211. Wikel, S. K., R. N. Ramachandra, D. K. Bergman, T. R. Burkot, and J. Piesman. 1997. Infestation with pathogen-free nymphs of the tick *Ixodes scapularis* induces host resistance to transmission of *Borrelia burgdorferi* by ticks. *Infect. Immun.* **65**:335–338.

212. Wilkinson, P. R. 1957. The spelling of pasture in cattle tick control. *Aust. J. Agric. Res.* **8**:414–423.

213. Willadsen, P., and F. Jongejan. 1999. Immunology of the tick-host interaction and the control of ticks and tick-borne diseases. *Parasitol. Today* **15**:258–262.

214. Wilson, M. L. 1986. Reduced abundance of adult *Ixodes dammini* (Acari: Ixodidae) following destruction of vegetation. *J. Econ. Entomol.* **79**:693–696.

215. Wilson, M. L., and R. D. Deblinger. 1993. Vector management to reduce the risk of Lyme disease, p. 126–156. *In* H. S. Ginsberg (ed.), *Ecology and Environmental Management of Lyme Disease*. Rutgers University Press, New Brunswick, N.J.

216. Wilson, M. L., A. M. Ducey, T. S. Litwin, T. A. Gavin, and A. Spielman. 1990. Microgeographic distribution of immature *Ixodes dammini* ticks correlated with that of deer. *Med. Vet. Entomol.* **4**:151–159.

217. Wilson, M. L., S. R. Telford III, J. Piesman, and A. Spielman. 1988. Reduced abundance of immature *Ixodes dammini* (Acari: Ixodidae) following elimination of deer. *J. Med. Entomol.* **25**:224–228.

218. Yeh, M.-T. 1994. Vector competence in Lyme disease: studies on *Ixodes scapularis*, *Dermacentor variabilis*, and *Amblyomma americanum*. Ph.D. thesis. University of Rhode Island, Kingston.

219. **Yoder, J. A., and A. Spielman.** 1992. Differential capacity of larval deer ticks (*Ixodes dammini*) to imbibe water from sub-saturated air. *J. Insect Physiol.* **38:**863–869.

220. **Zeidner, N., M. Dreitz, D. Belasco, and D. Fish.** 1996. Suppression of acute *Ixodes scapularis*-induced *Borrelia burgdorferi* infection using tumor necrosis factor-alpha, interleukin-2, and interferon-gamma. *J. Infect. Dis.* **173:**187–195.

221. **Zhioua, E., M. Browning, P. W. Johnson, H. S. Ginsberg, and R. A. LeBrun.** 1997. Pathogenicity of the entomopathogenic fungus *Metarhizium anisopliae* (Deuteromycetes) to *Ixodes scapularis* (Acari: Ixodidae). *J. Parasitol.* **83:**815–818.

222. **Zhioua, E., H. S. Ginsberg, R. A. Humber, and R. A. LeBrun.** 1999. Preliminary survey for entomopathogenic fungi associated with *Ixodes scapularis* (Acari: Ixodidae) in southern New York and New England, USA. *J. Med. Entomol.* **96:**635–637.

223. **Zhioua, E., K. Heyer, M. Browning, H. S. Ginsberg, and R. A. LeBrun.** 1999. Pathogenicity of *Bacillus thuringiensis* variety *kurstaki* to *Ixodes scapularis* (Acari: Ixodidae). *J. Med. Entomol.* **36:**900–902.

224. **Zhioua, E., R. A. LeBrun, H. S. Ginsberg, and A. Aeschlimann.** 1995. Pathogenicity of *Steinernema carpocapsae* and *S. glaseri* (Nematoda: Steinernematidae) to *Ixodes scapularis* (Acari: Ixodidae). *J. Med. Entomol.* **32:**900–905.

225. **Zimmerman, G.** 1993. The entomopathogenic fungus *Metarhizium anisopliae* and its potential as a biocontrol agent. *Pestic. Sci.* **37:**375–379.

Chapter 5

Clinical Approach to the Patient
with a Possible Tick-Borne Illness

JESSE L. GOODMAN

OVERVIEW

There are many challenges in the clinical recognition, management, and treatment of patients with tick-borne diseases. The first and most important step for clinicians is to simply consider the possibility of a tick-borne infection in patients who, through their place of residence, occupational or recreational activities, or travels, may have been exposed to ticks that are vectors of human disease. In such a setting, considering the possibility of a tick-transmitted disease is critical because the disease manifestations are often both nonspecific and multisystemic, there are seldom definitive clinical or laboratory diagnostic findings present at the time of presentation, and the consequences of failure to treat can be fatal. As a result, prompt presumptive therapy is often appropriate and may, in fact, be lifesaving. The objective of this chapter is to provide an overview of differential diagnosis and points to consider related to certain clinical and laboratory manifestations of disease as well as empiric treatment. More detailed information about exposure factors, clinical manifestations, diagnosis, and treatment of each disease is available in the disease-specific chapters of this book. The geographic distributions of tick-borne diseases and their vectors are comprehensively addressed in Chapter 21 and the Color Map section.

WHEN TO CONSIDER A TICK-BORNE ILLNESS

It is often the clinical presentation that first raises the question of whether a tick-borne illness may be responsible. Suggestive findings include otherwise-unexplained acute fevers (especially without typical symptoms of viral respiratory infection or gastroenteritis); unexplained skin rashes (either localized or general), particularly in febrile patients; and fever accompanied by neurological findings. Fever with non-specific alterations in hepatic function, depressed platelet counts, or normal or depressed neutrophil counts also should suggest the possibility of a tick-borne infection. The failure of antibiotic therapies directed at common bacterial infections (e.g., cephalosporins, penicillins, and macrolides) to elicit a clinical response is also a circumstance where tick-borne diseases, particularly rickettsial and ehrlichial infections, must be considered. While most tick-borne infections are "equal opportunity employers," infecting primarily healthy, active individuals who tend to have more outdoor exposure, severe babesial infection should be considered as a cause of febrile illness in patients who have been transfused and/or are immunosuppressed (including due to human immunodeficiency virus [HIV]) or are asplenic. Similarly, clinical infection with *Ehrlichia ewingii* has most often been reported in immunosuppressed individuals, perhaps reflecting a low inherent pathogenicity for human hosts. In all of these settings, careful questioning regarding known and potential opportunities for tick exposure is critical. In some instances, patients themselves or relatives may raise the issue of whether outdoor exposures, travels, or recalled tick bites may be related to the symptoms being experienced.

RESIDENCE, TRAVEL, OCCUPATION, SEASON, AND TICK EXPOSURE

Almost anyone has some risk for tick exposure, although tick-borne disease would rarely be an important consideration in an individual who has exclusively been in densely populated, unwooded urban areas. However, even within such areas tick-borne disease transmission may occur in sites with vegetation, particularly large parks, brushy areas, and sometimes backyards. Exposures of city dwellers are most likely to occur during vacations and other trips away from the city. Exposure to ticks is much more common in

Jesse L. Goodman • Center for Biologics Evaluation and Research, U.S. Food and Drug Administration, 1401 Rockville Pike, Suite 200N, HFM-1, Rockville, MD 20852. Dr. Goodman's affiliation is provided for identification purposes. The views expressed in this book are those of the author and do not necessarily reflect those of the Food and Drug Administration or of the U.S. Department of Health and Human Services.

suburban and rural environments and, as human populations and residences spread out from cities, has become an increasing problem in many regions, especially the northeastern corridor of the United States from Maine to Maryland, where Lyme borreliosis, ehrlichiosis, and babesiosis are rapidly emerging tick-borne diseases.

Any patient, child or adult, with an unexplained febrile illness should have a careful exposure and travel history taken by a skilled clinician. If a patient is unable to provide this information, other informants such as friends or relatives must be contacted. Patients often do not spontaneously mention travel or exposure that they consider unremarkable or low risk. Therefore, all patients with acute onset febrile illness should be asked where they live and where they have traveled in the preceding 30 days; this period should be extended when considering potential later disease manifestations, for example, of Lyme disease or babesiosis, which may occur years following exposure. In some instances, tick-borne infections occur less commonly in children (e.g., babesiosis and ehrlichiosis), likely reflecting decreased susceptibility. In other cases (e.g., Rocky Mountain spotted fever [RMSF]), it has been suggested that children may more commonly be infected, for reasons that are unclear. Certain occupations (e.g., forestry, park service, farming, landscaping, and construction) and hobbies (e.g., gardening, hiking, fishing, hunting, and boating) may make tick exposure more likely and be associated with increased seroprevalence of certain tick-borne diseases. In certain instances, potential contact not only with ticks but also with competent zoonotic reservoir hosts may provide an important diagnostic clue to tick-borne or other routes of infection (e.g., ruminants for Q fever and rabbits for tularemia).

Patients may not mention seeing or being exposed to ticks unless specifically asked and therefore should be prompted with questions such as the following. Have you been in an area where you could have been exposed to ticks? Have you noticed ticks on yourself, your pets, or others? Finally, for diseases transmitted by smaller ticks, such as Lyme disease, babesiosis, and human granulocytic anaplasmosis (also known as human granulocytic ehrlichiosis or HGE) (all transmitted predominantly in the United States by the nymphal stage of *Ixodes scapularis*), a tick bite or even tick exposure is frequently not noted. (Throughout this chapter, the disease previously referred to as HGE is termed human granulocytic anaplasmosis [HGA] based on recent genetic findings. [See Chapter 13 for further discussion.]) Therefore, even in the absence of recalled tick exposure, the potential for exposure to ticks through residence, activities, or travel should always raise the question of a tick-borne illness

when symptoms, signs, or laboratory findings are consistent with such a process.

Most tick-borne diseases have a distinct seasonality based on feeding activity of the infective tick stages. In temperate or cool areas, transmission of tick-borne disease is uncommon in winter and is most common during late spring and summer. However, in areas where winters are mild or in the tropics, disease transmission may take place year-round. Activity of most ticks falls during periods of dryness.

GEOGRAPHIC CONSIDERATIONS

The distribution of tick-borne infections generally follows that of their vector and zoonotic hosts and is discussed in detail in individual disease-specific chapters and reviewed and mapped in Chapter 21 and the Color Map section, respectively. Here (see also Table 1), we review broad considerations that may be helpful if a patient has recently traveled to or resided in an area that the clinician is not directly familiar with as well as points to consider in differential diagnosis in patients exposed in nontemperate climates. For many diseases, the lack of evidence of their occurrence in areas of the world without active surveillance does not necessarily mean that the disease is not present. The range of tick-borne infectious diseases (and, indeed, the number of species identified as tick transmitted) is being constantly expanded as new knowledge becomes available. Some tick-borne infections have a global distribution, including Q fever (found on every continent) and tularemia (found throughout the temperate northern hemisphere); toxin-mediated tick paralysis is a possibility wherever ticks are present.

In North America, Lyme disease and HGA cases are concentrated in areas where *I. scapularis* and *Ixodes pacificus* ticks are most prevalent, particularly the northeast and mid-Atlantic regions, the upper Midwest, and northern California, although cases have been reported from many other states and from Canada. Babesiosis cases have been clustered in coastal New England and Long Island and nearby islands such as Nantucket, but cases have also occurred in other areas including the Midwest, California, and Washington State. Human monocytotropic ehrlichiosis (HME) has been most common in the southeast and south-central regions, but cases have also occurred in California. RMSF has been reported from nearly all continental states, but the disease has its highest incidence not in the Rockies but in the mid-Atlantic, southeast, and south-central regions. Tick-borne relapsing fever occurs almost exclusively west of the Mississippi basin, primarily in mountainous western states. Col-

Table 1. Major clinical and laboratory characteristics of tick-borne diseases[a]

Disease	Geographic region	Fever	Recurrences, chronicity, sequelae	Skin rash	CNS finding(s)	Other clinical findings	Nonspecific laboratory findings	Agent-specific laboratory findings useful in acute disease diagnosis
Viral								
Tick-borne encephalitis	Eurasia (endemic), North America	Yes	Typically biphasic; early nonspecific febrile illness, followed in 7–8 days by manifestations of meningoencephalitis	None	Ataxia, meningitis, encephalitis	Early nonspecific symptoms of URI, myalgias, and arthralgias	Leukopenia, thrombocytopenia, transaminase elevations	Specific IgM in acute-phase serum, isolation in mice or cell culture, PCR of blood or tissues, acute and convalescent serologies
CCHF and other HF viral infections	Africa, Middle East, Eurasia	Yes	Acute illness with fatality ratio about 30%; in survivors, improvement begins about day 9, and full convalescence may take weeks; peripheral neuritis, amnesia, confusion may persist for months	Petechial, purpuric rash typical	May have intracranial bleeding; stupor, coma from hepatic failure	Severe headache, neck pain and stiffness, mental status changes, back pain, myalgia, conjunctivitis, hepatomegaly, petechiae, purpura, GI bleeding; suspected CCHF cases should be isolated	Leukopenia, thrombocytopenia, coagulopathy, elevated transaminase	As above
Tick paralysis	Worldwide	No	Rapid recovery usual after tick removal but long-term sequelae may occur in severe cases	None	Ascending flaccid paralysis, bulbar findings; may progress to respiratory paralysis	Myocarditis (rare)	None (CSF normal)	No specific tests available
CTF	North America (western US, Canada)	Yes	Biphasic fever pattern typical; may have prolonged convalescence with persistent fatigue and lethargy	Transient macular rash (5–10%)	Meningitis, encephalitis in severe cases	Myopericarditis, pneumonitis, hepatitis, epididymo-orchitis, conjunctivitis, reported as unusual complications	Leukopenia characteristic	Virus may be seen after 5 days by antibody staining of RBCs

Continued on following page

89

Table 1. *Continued*

Disease	Geographic region	Fever	Recurrences, chronicity, sequelae	Skin rash	CNS finding(s)	Other clinical findings	Nonspecific laboratory findings	Agent-specific laboratory findings useful in acute disease diagnosis
Spirochetal Lyme borreliosis (*B. burgdorferi*)	North America, Eurasia	Yes[a]	If early disease not treated, recurrent illness and late sequelae (arthritic, neurologic, cardiac, cutaneous) may occur	Characteristic EM rash (~80%)	Meningitis, encephalitis, cranial and peripheral neuropathy (late) may occur	Early localized: solitary EM, cranial neuropathy, often accompanied by fever, malaise, myalgias. Early disseminated: multiple EM, aseptic meningitis, peripheral neuritis, carditis. Late systemic: arthritis, peripheral neuropathy, encephalopathy, acrodermatitis atrophica	Usually unremarkable in early localized infection, may have mild leukocytosis, anemia, elevated ESR, transaminases, total IgM in early disseminated; lymphocytic pleocytosis in aseptic meningitis; atrioventricular conduction disturbance in carditis; inflammatory joint fluid in arthritis	EIA combined with Western blot (serology positive in only ~50% presenting with early disease); culture on modified BSK medium; PCR of affected tissues (both specialized)
Tick-borne relapsing fever	Americas, Africa, Middle East, Eurasia	Yes	Relapsing episodes of high fever lasting 2–7 days alternating with periods of relative well-being lasting days to weeks; untreated, up to 10 relapses may occur	Macular, petechial (up to 50%)	Meningoencephalitis in ~10%, sometimes with focal findings; cranial nerve palsies; in severe disease, myocarditis, bleeding, hepatic failure	Fever, chills (rigors), sweats, myalgia, arthralgia, headache, cough, conjunctivitis, uveitis-iritis (uncommon), pleuritis, epistaxis, tender hepatomegaly, splenomegaly	Moderate thrombocytopenia, mild hyperbilirubinemia-transaminase elevations	Spirochetes seen in stained blood smears during fever (~70%); culture in modified BSK, antigen detection assays; mouse inoculation (latter three all specialized)

90

Organism	Geographic distribution		Long-term sequelae	CNS involvement	Rash	Other clinical features	Laboratory findings	Diagnosis
Rickettsia								
RMSF (*R. rickettsii*)	Americas	Yes	No relapses; rare neurological sequelae	Meningoencephalitis in severe cases	>80%; ranges from maculopapular to petechial to purpuric	Myalgia, arthralgia, headache, nausea, vomiting, abdominal pain; in complicated cases, renal and respiratory failure, vasculitis, DIC	Mild-moderate illness: normal or slightly lowered leukocyte count, thrombocytopenia. More severe infection: elevated immature neutrophils (bands) hyponatremia, transaminase and bilirubin elevations, prerenal azotemia, DIC, CSF lymphocytic pleocytosis	Immunostaining or PCR of skin biopsies (~70–90%); serology usually negative at presentation
Other spotted fevers and tick-borne typhus syndromes (e.g., caused by *R. conorii*, *R. africae*, *R. siberica*, *R. japonica*, *R. australis*, *R. honei*, *R. slovaka*)	Eurasia, Middle East, Africa, Australia		No relapses or permanent sequelae	Meningoencephalitis in severe cases	Maculopapular rash common, majority with eschar (tache noir) at bite site	Myalgia, arthralgia, headache, nausea, vomiting, abdominal pain; in complicated cases, renal and respiratory failure, vasculitis, DIC		
Q fever (*Coxiella burnetii*)	Worldwide	Yes	In untreated cases, chronic infection may occur, including endocarditis and other endovascular infections, osteomyelitis, arthritis, hepatitis, and pneumonitis	Meningitis, meningoencephalitis	None	Acute illness usually presents as undifferentiated fever, hepatitis, atypical pneumonitis, or both; endocarditis most common chronic manifestation	WBC normal or increased, elevated transaminases common, other findings depending on organ involvement	Specific IgG and/or IgM antibodies usually positive at clinical presentation; isolation from blood (dangerous to laboratory personnel); immunohistochemical staining, PCR of tissues; PCR of blood
Ehrlichiosis								
Human granulocytic ehrlichiosis (anaplasmosis) (*A. phagocytophilum*)	North America US, especially northeast and northern Midwest; Europe	Yes	None known	Rare (aseptic meningitis)	Uncommon (maculopapular)	Myalgia, arthralgia, headache	Leukopenia, thrombocytopenia, transaminase elevations	Stained peripheral blood, buffy coat (~40–80%, with organisms seen in PMN); PCR blood 70–90%, cultivation (70–>90%, specialized), serology usually negative at presentation

Continued on following page

Table 1. *Continued*

Disease	Geographic region	Fever	Recurrences, chronicity, sequelae	Skin rash	CNS finding(s)	Other clinical findings	Nonspecific laboratory findings	Agent-specific laboratory findings useful in acute disease diagnosis
HME (*E. chaffeensis*)	North America (south central, southeastern US)	Yes	None known	Maculopapular rash 30%	Aseptic meningitis (~20%)	Myalgia, arthralgia, headache	Leukopenia, thrombocytopenia, transaminase elevations	Stained peripheral blood, buffy coat (~10–40%, with organisms seen in monocytes; PCR, blood 70–90%; serology usually negative at presentation
E. ewingii ehrlichiosis	North America (south central, southeastern US)	Yes	None known	Uncommon (maculo-papular)	Uncommon (aseptic meningitis)	Myalgia, arthralgia, headache	Leukopenia, thrombo-cytopenia, transaminase elevations	Stained peripheral blood, buffy coat (~20–80% with organisms seen in PMN) PCR blood (? sensitivity); serology usually negative at presentation (may cross-react with *E. chaffeensis*)
Other infections Tularemia (*Francisella tularensis*)	North America, Eurasia	Yes	Untreated illness may result in protracted course, prolonged convalescence; rare chronic sequelae include endocarditis, infection of prosthetic devices, joint infection	Ulcerative (70%), often with eschar; Erythema marginatum; Erythema nodosum common in Scandinavia	Meningitis in "typhoidal" or septicemic tularemia	Fever, chills, myalgia, arthralgia, headache, nausea, vomiting, abdominal pain, lymphadenopathy common in early infection; other syndromes include ulceroglandular, glandular, pneu-monic, typhoidal, ocular, pharyngeal, meningeal	Sterile pyuria, hyponatremia, elevated CPK common in severe infection	Culture blood, tissues, exudates antigen capture, serology; PCR, immunohistochemical staining of tissues, exudates
Babesiosis (*Babesia microti*, *B. divergens*, *B. bovis*, WA-1)	North America (US, especially Northeast, Midwest, CA and WA), Europe	Yes	Chronic fever, anemia, fatigue common if untreated	Rare	None	Fever, anorexia, fatigue, hepatosple-nomegaly	Thrombocytopenia, hemolytic anemia with reticulocytosis, increased LDH, bilirubin	Blood smears positive for intraerythrocytic organ-isms in most acute infections; smears fre-quently negative but serologies positive in chronic disease; PCR of blood

[a] Abbreviations: BSK, Barbour-Stoenner-Kelly; CA, California; CNS, central nervous system; CPK, creatine phosphokinase; DIC, disseminated intravascular coagulation; EIA, enzyme immunoassay; ESR, erythrocyte sedimenta-tion rate; GI, gastrointestinal; LDH, lactate dehydrogenase; PMN, polymorphonuclear leukocytes; RBCs, red blood cells; URI, upper respiratory infection; US, United States; WA, Washington; WBC, white blood cells.

orado tick fever (CTF) despite its name, occurs not only in Colorado but throughout mountainous areas of the West at elevations above 1,000 m. Tick paralysis has been associated with multiple tick species and, while most common in the northwest and Rocky Mountain regions, has been reported in most areas of the country. Powassan virus is a rare cause of encephalitis in the northern United States and adjacent Canada. Tularemia occurs predominantly in the western and south-central regions, although cases have occurred throughout the continental United States. Cases most commonly arise from contact exposures to contaminated animal carcasses but can occur through bites by ticks and deer flies and from inhalation of infective aerosols, including during lawn mowing.

In Europe, ixodid ticks are widely distributed, and cases of Lyme disease, HGA, and babesiosis, while most common in central and eastern Europe, Russia, and Scandinavia, have been documented widely. Tick-borne encephalitis (TBE) also occurs widely throughout Europe and Russia. Cases of HME have only rarely been reported, and transmission has not been well documented in Europe. A variety of acute rickettsial infections other than RMSF occur in Europe, including several species causing spotted fever and/or "tick typhus" syndromes (characterized by an eschar at the bite site). Q fever is widespread, and outbreaks are common in sheep-raising areas. Relapsing fever due to *Borrelia hispanica* has been reported in Spain and Portugal. Crimean-Congo hemorrhagic fever (CCHF) virus has a wide range that includes much of Europe and the former Soviet Union.

RMSF has been documented in a number of Central and South American countries. Tick-borne relapsing fever occurs in Mexico and Central and South America.

In Asia, Lyme borreliosis is endemic in forested areas of northeastern China and Japan. Multiple species of spotted fever rickettsia are present in mainland Asia, and *Rickettsia australis* occurs in eastern Australia. Tick-borne relapsing fever occurs in scattered foci throughout the Middle East, central Asia, the Indian subcontinent, and China. CCHF is widespread throughout the area, and Kyasanur Forest disease causes hemorrhagic fever in southwestern India. TBE and Omsk hemorrhagic fever virus infections occur in eastern Russia.

In Africa, tick-borne relapsing fever is widespread, occurring in North Africa and the Near and Middle Eastern regions. CCHF and Q fever occur throughout the African region. Rickettsial infections causing spotted fever and tick typhus syndromes are common in both Mediterranean and sub-Saharan Africa. There is no conclusive evidence for transmission of Lyme disease or ehrlichiosis in Africa.

In assessing the possibility of a tick-borne illness in a patient who has recently resided in or traveled to tropical regions, a number of acute infectious diseases less common or seldom considered in North America or Europe should be kept in mind as part of the differential diagnosis. These include malaria; visceral leishmaniasis; typhoid fever; leptospirosis; tuberculosis; brucellosis; bartonellosis; louse-borne relapsing fever; flea- and louse-borne typhus; scrub typhus; mosquito-borne viral fevers such as dengue, chikungunya, o'nyong-nyong, Ross River, and Rift Valley fevers; arenaviral hemorrhagic fevers; Lassa fever; viral hemorrhagic fevers with neurological syndromes, such as Ebola-Marburg disease and yellow fever; and neurotropic viral diseases such as Venezuelan equine encephalitis, rabies, and polio.

Given that specific treatment is effective and may be urgently needed, it is particularly important to carefully evaluate blood smears in all cases of unexplained febrile illness from South and Central America, Africa, Oceania, and Asia to exclude the possibility of malaria.

CLINICAL SYNDROMES AND FINDINGS SUGGESTIVE OF TICK-BORNE DISEASES AND THEIR DIFFERENTIAL DIAGNOSES

Acute or Recurrent Unexplained Febrile Illness

Most tick-borne infectious diseases (see Table 1 for summary information) present as nonspecific acute febrile illnesses occurring days to weeks after potential tick exposure. Rickettsial and ehrlichial infections typically are abrupt in onset, and fever may be high and debilitating. Common accompanying symptoms include headache, myalgias, and arthralgias. A localized lesion or rash at the site of the infecting tick bite may be present (see below) but usually is not. Nonspecific acute febrile presentations often suggest community-acquired viral infection, although the typical localizing symptoms or signs suggestive of a primary respiratory or gastrointestinal viral illness are usually lacking. In those diseases in which the pathogens replicate intracellularly (for example, tularemia or ehrlichiosis), the pulse may be relatively low for the degree of fever, as is classically observed in typhoid fever. Patients with rickettsial or ehrlichial or HGA infections may have received treatment with antibiotics such as penicillins, macrolides, or cephalosporins with no response. Some patients may have what appears to be a biphasic illness (e.g., with an initial illness followed by improvement and then additional manifestations); this pattern is typical of CTF, TBE, and CCHF and sometimes occurs in patients with Lyme borreliosis.

Table 2. Tick-borne and other causes of recurrent fevers

Fever pattern	Infectious disease	Noninfectious process
May be periodic	Tick-borne relapsing fever Malaria (often every 2 to 3 days)[a] Rat bite fever	Deep venous thrombosis, pulmonary emboli, systemic emboli Neoplasms (especially lymphoma and Hodgkin's disease) Factitious or self-induced fever
Usually continuous but may be remitting or irregular	Bacterial endocarditis Brucellosis Bacterial abscesses (e.g., hepatic) Biliary disease Amebic liver abscess Granulomatous infections (e.g., TB, fungi) Visceral leishmaniasis	Nonbacterial (marantic) endocarditis Vasculitis Autoimmune and inflammatory diseases (SLE, rheumatoid arthritis) Inflammatory bowel disease, temporal arteritis, polymyalgia rheumatica Atrial myxoma Drug-related fever

[a] Malarial fevers may be continuous or irregular, particularly in nonimmune individuals (e.g., travelers) and early in infection. TB, tuberculosis; SLE, systemic lupus erythematosus.

Recurrent fevers (Table 2) should always raise the question of whether a patient may have been exposed to relapsing fever or malaria, either of which can be fatal without prompt specific treatment. As opposed to most patients with acute bacterial infections of similar severity (e.g., bacterial pneumonia or sepsis), leukocyte counts in tick-borne diseases are most often normal or low.

Fever with Skin Lesions

Unexplained fevers with skin rash should always raise the suspicion of an acute infectious disease, including many potential tick-borne infections. In particular, a hemorrhagic or petechial rash in a febrile patient may signal a life-threatening illness needing urgent intervention (Table 3). Tick-borne infections that may manifest such a rash include viral hemorrhagic fevers, rickettsial infections including RMSF, and relapsing fever borrelial infections. These rickettsial and borrelial infections require urgent treatment. Several non-tick-borne bacterial infections that must be considered when purpura is present and require urgent diagnosis and intervention include bacterial septicemias, most importantly meningococcemia. Noninfectious diseases that can mimic these infections include leukemia, thrombotic thrombocytopenic purpura (TTP), Henoch-Schönlein purpura, dysproteinemias, snake bite, vasculitides, and drug-induced purpura. In most instances, these disorders should be suspected based on history, other clinical findings, or basic laboratory evaluation.

Other types of skin rashes commonly accompany tick-borne diseases and provoke other considerations in their differential diagnoses (Table 4). A distinct localized erythematous rash, erythema migrans (EM) (see Color Plate 6A), often accompanied by regional lymphadenopathy, is typical of early Lyme disease, occurring in at least two-thirds of infections. It is a painless, usually circular or ovoid lesion that slowly expands over days from the site of a tick bite (which may not be recognized), typically reaching several inches in size and often clearing centrally with a resulting target-like or bull's-eye appearance. When untreated, dissemination and multiple lesions, which may be in one or multiple areas of the body, may develop. The EM lesion may be mimicked by an allergic reaction to a tick; by fly, spider, or other arthropod bites; or by localized infections, such as streptococcal cellulitis, which may occur at the site of any kind of bite or other cutaneous compromise.

Generalized erythematous macular or maculopapular rashes are common manifestations of many infectious diseases, including most cases of rickettsia and CTF. A maculopapular rash occurs in approximately one-third of cases of HME but is very uncommon in HGA. A multitude of viral infections, many of which are self limited and benign, can cause such rashes. A pruritic rash with arthralgia can occur during acute hepatitis B infection, and rash and headache are common in primary HIV infection. The classic rash of RMSF usually starts after 1 to 6 days of fever and spreads from the distal extremities to the trunk and face (see Color Plate 11A). Like secondary syphilis, the RMSF rash commonly involves the palms and soles. Unlike secondary syphilis, the lesions in RMSF are erythematous and typically evolve over days into a more purpuric rash that may then ulcerate. As they become purpuric, the lesions in RMSF may be difficult to distinguish from the rash often seen in meningococcemia, although lesions in meningococcemia tend to be fewer. Furthermore, virtually any maculopapular

Table 3. Diffuse petechial or hemorrhagic rash: tick-borne, other infectious, and noninfectious etiologies[a]

Etiology	Tick-borne infectious disease	Other infectious disease	Noninfectious condition
Viral	CCHF Omsk HF Kyasanur Forest disease CTF (rare)	Viral HFs Arenavirus, filovirus infections Echovirus Coxsackievirus Adenovirus Severe measles	
Rickettsial	RMSF Other spotted fever and tick typhus syndromes (rarely and in severe illness)	Louse-borne typhus	
Bacterial	Relapsing fever borreliosis	*Staphylococcus aureus* *Neisseria menigitidis* Disseminated *Neisseria gonorrhoeae* infection *P. aeruginosa* and other gram negatives Salmonellosis *Yersinia pestis*	
Other			Thrombocytopenic and coagulation disorders, including leukemia, TTP, ITP Venomous snake bite Vasculitis, due to SLE, Henoch-Schönlein purpura Drug reactions

[a] ITP, idiopathic thrombocytopenic purpura; SLE, systemic lupus erythematosus; TTP, thrombotic thrombocytopenic purpura.

eruption may become hemorrhagic in patients with thrombocytopenia and/or other coagulopathy. The rash of measles typically begins on the face and rapidly becomes confluent. Typhoid fever may be accompanied by a difficult-to-detect transient eruption, so-called rose spots, a salmon-colored maculopapular rash that is usually truncal.

An ulcerative lesion with accompanying localized lymphadenopathy occurs early in most patients with tick or fly bite transmission of tularemia (see Color Plate 7A and B) and may be confused with a variety of other infectious diseases, including fungal and mycobacterial infections, cutaneous leishmaniasis, and (in the genital area) lymphogranuloma venereum or chancroid, all of which are typically of more gradual onset than tularemia. An eschar sometimes covers the tularemia ulcer. In a patient with a relevant geographic exposure history, a cutaneous eschar should raise the possibilities of Mediterranean spotted fever due to *Rickettsia conorii* (Color Plate 13A) or African tick bite fever due to *Rickettsia africae* (Color Plate 14A). A similar eschar may be seen with mite-borne scrub typhus, tularemia, and (occasionally) plague. Some EM lesions may vesicate, but the underlying nature of the lesion should remain apparent. Vesicular skin lesions may be seen in *R. africae* infection, as well as with *R. australis* (so-called Queensland tick typhus) infection. Generalized vesicular rashes are most commonly manifestations of herpesvirus and poxvirus infections but are also characteristic of rickettsialpox (*Rickettsia akari*, transmitted to humans by mouse mites).

Fever with Neurologic Manifestations: Major Considerations in Evaluation

Neurologic manifestations accompanying an acute febrile illness raise a number of specific possibilities, including several tick-borne infectious diseases (Table 1). Diffuse central nervous system dysfunction ranging from subtle mental status changes to frank meningoencephalitis is characteristic of the tick-borne encephalitides (in which ataxia is also common) and also occurs in ~5 to 25% of relapsing fever patients, as well as in severe cases of CTF and in many rickettsial infections, including RMSF. Septicemic tularemia may cause lymphocytic predominant meningitis, which may also be seen in a minority of cases of HME. While neurologic manifestations of Lyme disease typically occur

Table 4. Nonhemorrhagic skin manifestations and their differential diagnoses[a]

Diagnosis	Erythematous		Ulcer(s)	Eschar(s)	Vesicle(s)
	Localized	Generalized maculopapular			
Tick-borne	*B. burgdorferi* EM Allergic reaction to tick bite	CTF, RMSF, other spotted fevers and tick typhus syndromes Other rickettsial infections Ehrlichiosis (less common)	Tularemia, at site of inoculation (usually with lymphadenopathy); affected nodes may suppurate and form draining sinus tracts to skin	African tick bite fever (*R. africae*) Mediterranean spotted fever (*R. conorii*), tick typhus and African tick-bite fever syndromes	EM African tick-bite fever (*R. africae*), Queensland tick typhus (*R. australis*), tick typhus due to *R. conorii*
Other infections	Cellulitis (e.g., streptococcal, staphylococcal); usually painful	Most common viruses (e.g., measles, rubella, adenovirus, EBV, hepatitis B, parvovirus B19, HIV) Mycoplasma Leptospirosis Salmonellosis, especially typhoid Secondary syphilis	Lymphogranuloma venereum or chancroid (typically inguinal) Fungi: sporotrichosis, cryptococcus Parasitic: leishmaniasis Anthrax: painless, asymptomatic Atypical mycobacteria Dracunculiasis	Scrub typhus Rickettsialpox (*R. akari*) Gram-negative septicemia[b] Aspergillus (compromised host)[b] Tularemia Plague	Rickettsialpox (*R. akari*) Poxviruses (smallpox, cowpox, monkeypox) Herpesviruses (HSV, VZV) Enterovirus infections
Noninfectious	Allergic or toxic reactions to bites by arthropods other than ticks	Drug reactions Autoimmune and inflammatory diseases	Neoplasm Vasculitis	Vascular insufficiency, embolism[b]	Drug reactions

[a] EBV, Epstein-Barr virus; HSV, herpes simplex virus; VZV, varicella-zoster virus.
[b] These lesions are primarily necrotic and embolic in origin but may be similar in appearance to an eschar at a local site of infection.

weeks after the initial infection, facial nerve palsy (at times bilateral, which would be highly unusual in idiopathic Bell's palsy) and/or lymphocytic meningitis occurs in 10 to 15% of untreated patients; both may be seen as the initial presentation of illness because a skin rash either did not occur, was not noted, or resolved spontaneously. Other neurologic manifestations of Lyme disease include encephalopathy and peripheral neuropathy, but these almost always occur months to years after initial infection and are typically not accompanied by fever.

A febrile illness with neurologic abnormalities can occur in a wide variety of infectious and noninfectious diseases, and prompt consideration of a number of treatable but potentially severe disease entities is critical. Bacterial meningitis, sepsis, endocarditis, and treatable viral encephalitis (e.g., due to herpes simplex) must always be considered. In travelers, particular considerations for treatable infections include cerebral malaria, typhoid fever, tuberculous meningitis, trypanosomiasis, and, if travel to Latin America has occurred, neurocysticercosis.

If localizing findings are present, brain imaging (e.g., magnetic resonance imaging [MRI] or computed tomography with contrast) should be obtained to evaluate the possibility of a mass lesion such as a bacterial brain abscess or tuberculoma. An MRI may show signs of viral encephalitis and, in particular, characteristic frontotemporal changes suggestive of a treatable herpes simplex virus infection. Blood cultures are usually indicated to rule out bacterial sepsis and endocarditis, which is not always accompanied by a cardiac murmur. In all but mild illnesses, lumbar puncture with cell counts, chemistry, Gram stain, and cultures are indicated to rule out acute bacterial meningitis. Specific testing may confirm another diagnosis (e.g., PCR for herpes simplex virus or cerebrospinal fluid [CSF] antibodies for *Borrelia burgdorferi* in a patient whose blood has not yet seroconverted). In contrast to bacterial meningitis, the tick-borne infectious diseases generally cause either minimal abnormalities of the CSF or a lymphocytic pleocytosis.

Unexplained Neurologic, Cardiac, or Joint Findings in Patients from Areas Where Lyme Disease Is Known To Be Endemic

As described above and in Chapter 11, later manifestations of Lyme disease may occur without a recognized initial EM rash. For this reason, individuals who have resided in or traveled in areas of known Lyme disease transmission who have otherwise unexplained neurological, joint, or cardiac findings should be evaluated for *B. burgdorferi* infection. The neurological findings that should particularly raise this concern include lymphocytic meningitis, facial nerve palsy (usually occurring within weeks to months of exposure), and peripheral neuropathy (often only years later). Acute myopericarditis and especially unexplained and usually transient atrioventricular cardiac conduction disturbances typically occur within weeks to months of initial infection. Finally, unexplained recurrent monoarticular, migratory, or pauciarticular arthritis, usually involving large joints and often with culture-negative effusions containing large numbers of granulocytes, should always raise the question of *B. burgdorferi* infection, typically months to years earlier. In all of these settings, with the exception of earlier neurologic manifestations, the overwhelming majority of patients (>90%) will have positive blood *B. burgdorferi* antibody titers and confirmatory Western blot findings.

ROLE OF THE LABORATORY

Suggestive Laboratory Findings

In the setting of an otherwise unexplained acute febrile illness in potentially exposed individuals, certain laboratory findings should prompt the consideration of tick-borne pathogens. In particular, a high fever with normal or reduced leukocyte counts, while often seen in viral infections and in overwhelming sepsis, should always raise the question of a rickettsial, spirochetal, or ehrlichial infection. Ehrlichiosis should be particularly suspected when both leukopenia and thrombocytopenia are present; such cytopenias typically become apparent or more severe with increased duration of untreated infection. Mild to moderate increases in serum hepatic transaminase levels are common in a variety of rickettsial and ehrlichial infections, sometimes causing confusion with viral hepatitis. Finally, diagnostic abnormalities on a blood smear may be present in certain tick-borne infections (Table 1; see also "Initial Laboratory Evaluation," below) but may not be recognized by observers as specific intraleukocytic, intraerythrocytic, or free infectious organisms. Unexplained findings on blood smears should always prompt further investigation, observation, and, where needed, consultation with experienced observers.

Initial Laboratory Evaluation and Potentially Diagnostic Findings Early in Infection

General findings and studies

Patients with a significant but unexplained acute febrile illness should almost always have a basic laboratory evaluation that includes a complete blood count with a manual (not just automated) examination of the blood smear to allow detection of organisms, basic chemistry profiling including hepatic and renal functions, and a chest radiograph. If the patient is severely ill, if a diagnosis is not readily apparent, or if there are findings suggestive of bacterial infection, appropriate cultures (e.g., of blood, sputum, and urine) should usually be obtained. As described above, when neurologic findings are present, CSF examination and cultures are almost always indicated; neuroimaging should be obtained (usually prior to lumbar puncture) whenever focal findings are present.

Direct detection of organisms: blood smears

In patients with potential exposure in areas where disease is endemic, an examination of Wright- or Giemsa-stained peripheral blood should be performed for organisms within granulocytes (seen in 40 to 80% of patients with *Anaplasma phagocytophilum* infection [Color Plate 8A] and in a smaller proportion of patients with *E. ewingii* [Color Plate 9F]). Ehrlichial organisms may also be seen in monocytes but in only 10 to 40% of patients with *Ehrlichia chaffeensis* infection (Color Plate 9A). Because these organisms are often scarce early in infection (typically present in <1% of the relevant cell type) and difficult to find when leukocyte counts are depressed, examination of large numbers of fields, buffy coat preparations, and serial examinations over time may be very useful if the diagnosis is suspected. Toxic granulations and staining artifacts are frequently mistaken for ehrlichia and vice versa. Similarly, careful examination of blood smears may reveal the presence of typical ring-like, irregular, or cross-like (tetrad) intraerythrocytic inclusions in cases of babesiosis (see Color Plate 17). These organisms may be mistaken for malarial parasites and vice versa, for Howell-Jolly bodies seen in the very asplenic patients most prone to babesiosis, and for other inclusions. The percentage of infected red blood cells may range from <1%, typical in otherwise healthy individuals, to >50%, frequently seen in the asplenic or severely immunosuppressed.

In relapsing fever, spirochetemia is detectable in the majority of patients by examining Giemsa-stained blood smears (see Color Plate 10) obtained during febrile periods. Levels of organisms in the blood decline rapidly as the patient defervesces and are usually not noted during intervening afebrile periods. Examination of acridine orange-stained blood smears by fluorescence microscopy may enhance the sensitivity of detection.

In CTF, while the needed reagents are not commonly available, orbivirus inclusions may be noted by specific direct antibody staining of blood clots and/or cellular elements within days of infection.

Direct detection of organisms: other studies

In RMSF patients with typical acute petechial or purpuric rashes, immunostaining by direct fluorescent antibody shows *Rickettsia rickettsii* antigens in 70 to 90% of biopsies. However, given the urgency of initiating treatment for RMSF and the occurrence of false-negative results, treatment should be initiated based on clinical and epidemiological findings and should be neither delayed by obtaining such studies nor dependent on a positive result (see below).

In early Lyme disease, skin biopsy of typical EM lesions, examined by silver staining (Color Plate 6D), immunofluorescent staining with *B. burgdorferi* antibodies, or PCR amplification of DNA, will reveal evidence of spirochetes in 50 to 90% of lesions. However, the need for a biopsy, the delays involved in obtaining results, and the generally diagnostic nature of the EM rash itself make such studies of limited usefulness.

Nucleic acid amplification, including PCR

Nucleic acid amplification technologies and PCR in particular allow detection of pathogen-specific DNA or RNA sequences from extremely small numbers of organisms in patient blood, other body fluid, and tissue samples. Therefore, nucleic acid amplification tests have been widely explored as tools in the early diagnosis of a broad variety of infectious diseases, including most tick-borne infections. For example, PCR testing is more sensitive than microscopy in the diagnosis of acute ehrlichiosis and anaplasmosis and in the detection of recurrent babesiosis. While nucleic acid amplification tests are becoming more widely available and may in some cases be reliable and useful for early diagnosis, a number of concerns must be kept in mind when considering ordering such tests and interpreting the results. First, for most infections where very small numbers of organisms may be present in the material being sampled (e.g., ehrlichiosis, HGA, or babesiosis) or where the presence of the organism may be transient, a negative result may not be sufficient to exclude the diagnosis and obviate the need for empiric treatment (below). Second, not only do such false negatives occur, but due to the extreme sensitivity of the tests, laboratory cross-contamination is common. False-positive test results may be found, particularly in inexperienced laboratories, and may not be recognized as such unless sufficient numbers of control samples are included. Given these caveats and the fact that assays with well-characterized clinical sensitivity and specificity are not widely available for most pathogens, PCR tests for tick-borne pathogens should be ordered and interpreted in a carefully considered manner. Negative results should generally not mitigate against presumptive treatment of seriously ill patients.

Early antibody response

Most patients with acute tick-borne infectious diseases do not have diagnostic levels of specific antibodies detectable at the time of clinical presentation, although the majority of immunocompetent patients will ultimately develop such antibodies, usually within 2 to 4 weeks of disease onset. This is true even where sensitive immunoglobulin M (IgM) assays are available. For example, less than half of patients with early Lyme disease, acute babesiosis, or any of the ehrlichioses (including HGA) will have a positive antibody test at the time of presentation. In addition, while a variety of newer antibody testing methods, such as those measuring antibodies against pathogen-specific recombinant proteins or peptides, appear to have enhanced specificity, frequent cross-reactions are noted among members of related species causing tick-borne infections, for example, between *B. burgdorferi* and relapsing fever spirochetes, between *E. chaffeensis* and *E. ewingii*, and among multiple rickettsial species. For these reasons, antibody testing for acute tick-borne infectious diseases, including rickettsioses, ehrlichioses, HGA, and Lyme disease, is primarily useful for confirmatory purposes. Noteworthy exceptions include the tick-borne encephalitides, where positive IgM antibody levels in the blood are usually noted at the time of clinical presentation, likely because meningoencephalitis typically does not become evident until at least 10 days after initial infection. In addition, serodiagnosis is highly useful in chronic infections such as chronic babesiosis and later Lyme disease, which are accompanied by positive IgG antibody titers in >90% of infected patients.

INITIAL THERAPY: WHEN TO CONSIDER EMPIRIC TREATMENT

If not promptly suspected or recognized and appropriately treated, several of the acute tick-borne infections can result in progressive and severe illness, often with nervous system involvement or organ failure. While poor outcomes are more common among elderly individuals and those with underlying medical conditions, fatalities occur even among healthy young adults. Most notable are RMSF and some other spotted fever and tick-borne typhus syndromes, which can be rapidly fatal. In addition, the morbidity and mortality of untreated tick-borne relapsing fever, while lower than that of louse-borne disease, may be significant with death rates as high as 5 to 10%. Q fever, if clinically evident and not appropriately treated, can be a progressive disease with an overall mortality rate of ~5% and result in a broad range of clinical mani-festations, the most serious of which is endocarditis. Even ehrlichial and anaplasma infections, which tend to resolve spontaneously without treatment, can have a severe or fatal course in ~5% of patients not receiving prompt and appropriate treatment, particularly the elderly, and respiratory and renal failure can occur. Prior to the availability of effective antimicrobials, up to one-third of patients with tularemia developed complications such as disseminated intravascular coagulation, meningitis, encephalitis, or renal failure and died. Finally, the failure to recognize and treat early Lyme disease results in dissemination of the spirochete and development of cardiac or neurologic disease in ~10% of patients and development of arthritis in approximately one-half. Thus, early and effective treatment is important in reducing morbidity, including disability.

As discussed above, commonly available serodiagnostic tests are seldom sensitive early in acute infection with organisms such as rickettsia, ehrlichia, anaplasma, and spirochetes; most patients are seronegative at the time they present clinically. A careful search of blood smears can be extremely helpful and establish a diagnosis of babesiosis or relapsing fever in the majority of cases and less often may be diagnostic in ehrlichial infections. However, blood smears are insufficiently sensitive to exclude these diagnoses and should not be relied upon for such a purpose in seriously ill individuals with possible exposure and clinically consistent illnesses.

For all of these reasons, while each case must be evaluated carefully, it is highly appropriate after obtaining needed tests and while awaiting confirmation to treat most individuals with potential tick exposure and unexplained clinical findings consistent with relevant rickettsial, ehrlichial, anaplasmal, or tick-borne spirochetal infections with empiric antimicrobial therapy aimed at the suspected pathogen(s). Common scenarios where such treatment should be strongly considered include the following:

- fever with maculopapular, petechial, or hemorrhagic rash, and/or severe headache or neurological findings, where RMSF or related rickettsial infection, possible ehrlichiosis, anaplasmosis, or a possible first episode of tick-borne relapsing fever should be suspected;
- fever with eschar, where tick-borne typhus syndrome or tularemia should be suspected;
- recurrent acute febrile paroxysms, where malaria should be ruled out and relapsing fever suspected;
- fever with leukopenia and thrombocytopenia, where ehrlichiosis or anaplasmosis should be suspected;

- fever with thrombocytopenia, anemia, and/or evidence of hemolysis, where babesiosis should be suspected;
- an EM-like skin lesion(s), with or without fever, where early Lyme disease should be suspected; note that pain or purulent drainage is more suggestive of pyogenic infection (e.g., with staphylococci or streptococci);
- ulcerative skin lesion with fever, where tularemia should be suspected.

Despite the extensive range of diagnoses in most of these situations, an extremely helpful fact is that nearly all of the most serious tick-borne infections that may benefit from urgent treatment are susceptible to doxycycline. This includes rickettsial infections, all pathogens causing ehrlichiosis and anaplasmosis, and the bacterial organisms causing relapsing fever, tularemia, and Lyme borreliosis. Doxycycline treatment of suspected early Lyme borrreliosis also has the advantage of treating possible coinfection with *A. phagocytophilum* (and vice versa). An exception is babesiosis, which is not susceptible to doxycycline or most antimicrobials; it is usually treated with quinine and clindamycin.

Therefore, after obtaining appropriate samples, usually including bacterial blood cultures, and in the absence of clinical evidence for another acute bacterial infection requiring urgent treatment (e.g., meningococcemia, sepsis, or endocarditis) or a protozoal infection (e.g., malaria or babesiosis), therapy with doxycycline should be initiated promptly with an individual presenting with these syndromes, provided they have had an opportunity for exposure to the relevant tick vector and do not have mild or improving symptoms. In cases of mild illness and particularly when there is evidence to support another etiology, careful clinical observation or other antimicrobial treatment may be appropriate. However, in such circumstances and particularly when fever persists on typical broad-spectrum antimicrobial regimens (such as the cephalosporins or penicillins) or in the face of worsening clinical or laboratory findings, presumptive therapy with doxycycline should be reconsidered and administered in most cases. Doxycycline can be safely administered to most individuals 9 years of age or older. With younger children, pregnant women, or those rare individuals with a history of severe allergic reactions, alternative therapies may need to be considered. Penicillins, ceftriaxone, and macrolides, although inactive against rickettsial infections, ehrlichiosis, and HGA, are active in spirochetal infections including Lyme disease and relapsing fever, though failures and recurrences appear more commonly following macrolide treatment. Rifampin, the newer fluoroquinolones, and chloramphenicol may be alternatives in other situations, including some rickettsial, ehrlichial, and anaplasma infections, although doxycycline is generally the treatment with the clearest efficacy and may be indicated in severe disease, even when relative contraindications (such as age of <9 years) are present. Aminoglycocides or fluoroquinolones are the agents of choice in treating tularemia. Antimicrobial therapy is discussed in more depth in the disease-specific chapters, and a knowledgeable specialist should be consulted in difficult cases including treatment decisions for young children and pregnant women.

Empiric treatment with doxycycline usually results in a rapid and dramatic clinical response in patients with rickettsial spotted fever, tick-borne typhus syndromes, ehrlichiosis, HGA, tularemia, and relapsing fever. Patients usually become afebrile within 24 h and, except for patients treated late in the course of infection, improve significantly in overall clinical status within 24 to 72 h. Where organisms were present in the blood, the numbers of those organisms are diminished. Failure to observe a dramatic response in both fever and overall clinical status should prompt doubt as to the diagnosis and lead to further consideration of other possibilities, such as those discussed above, as well as complicating factors such as secondary nosocomial infections or drug allergies.

CONCLUSIONS

In patients with unexplained febrile illnesses, a careful travel and exposure history is critical. In individuals with outdoor exposures where infection is endemic, tick-borne infections should always be part of the differential diagnosis of acute, severe, persistent, or recurrent fevers, particularly when typical clinical and laboratory findings of common community-acquired viral and bacterial infections are absent. In addition to known tick exposure or bites in areas of endemicity, clinical findings particularly suggestive of a possible tick-borne infection may include leukopenia and/or thrombocytopenia and persistent fevers despite use of broad-spectrum antimicrobials, as well as negative routine cultures and the presence of otherwise unexplained skin rashes or lesions (particularly if petechial, hemorrhagic, or eschar) or central nervous system abnormalities. However, numerous other possibilities, including a broad variety of infectious and noninfectious processes, must usually be considered. Among the most urgent to always consider are meningococcemia, bacterial infections of the central nervous system, and, with an appropriate exposure history, malaria.

While the organisms causing ehrlichiosis, babesiosis, and relapsing fever may be seen on appropriately examined blood smears in a varying proportion of patients and more often with severe untreated infection, false negatives do occur. In these and the other treatable tick-borne infectious diseases, including rickettsial infections, antibodies are usually not present at the time of acute illness. There are at present no other readily available and reliable rapid diagnostics sufficiently sensitive and specific to promptly or definitively diagnose or rule out infection. An exception is viral TBE, for which no effective antiviral treatment is currently available. Thus, empiric antimicrobial therapy, most often with doxycycline, is appropriate in most cases of significant clinical illness where rickettsiosis, ehrlichiosis, anaplasmosis, tularemia, or borrelial infections are epidemiologically suspected and may be lifesaving. The lack of a clear-cut clinical response to empiric treatment should result in timely and comprehensive reconsideration of the preliminary diagnosis. Conversely, most patients with currently treatable tick-borne infectious diseases where the diagnosis is suspected and treated early respond dramatically to appropriate antimicrobial treatment and recover completely.

Acknowledgments.   I thank Colin Jordan and David Dennis for their helpful comments.

REFERENCES

1. Aguero-Rosenfeld, M. E. 2003. Laboratory aspects of tick-borne diseases: lyme, human granulocytic ehrlichiosis and babesiosis. *Mt. Sinai J. Med.* **70:**197–206.
2. Cunha, B. A. (ed.). 2000. *Tickborne Infectious Diseases: Diagnosis and Management.* Marcel Dekker, New York, N.Y.
3. Donovan, B. J., D. J. Weber, J. C. Rublein, and R. H. Raasch. 2002. Treatment of tick-borne diseases. *Ann. Pharmacother.* **36:**1590–1597.
4. Faul, J. L., R. L. Doyle, P. N. Kao, and S. J. Ruoss. 1999. Tick-borne pulmonary disease: update on diagnosis and management. *Chest* **116:**222–230.
5. Gantz, N. M., R. B. Brown, S. L. Berk, A. L. Esposito, and R. A. Gleckman (ed.). 1999. *Manual of Clinical Problems in Infectious Diseases,* 4th ed., p. 245–303. Lippincott, Williams and Wilkins, Philadelphia, Pa.
6. Goodman, J. L. 1999. Ehrlichiosis—ticks, dogs, and doxycycline. *N. Engl. J. Med.* **341:**195–197.
7. Masters, E. J., G. S. Olson, S. J. Weiner, and C. D. Paddock. 2003. Rocky Mountain spotted fever: a clinician's dilemma. *Arch. Intern. Med.* **163:**769–774.
8. McGinley-Smith, D. E., and S. S. Tsao. 2003. Dermatoses from ticks. *J. Am. Acad. Dermatol.* **49:**363–392.
9. Parola, P. 2004. Tick-borne rickettsial diseases: emerging risks in Europe. *Comp. Immunol. Microbiol. Infect. Dis.* **27:**297–304.
10. Ryan, E. T., M. E. Wilson, and K. C. Kain. 2002. Current concepts: illness after international travel. *N. Engl. J. Med.* **347:**505–516.
11. Smego, R. A., Jr., M. Castiglia, and M. O. Asperilla. 1999. Lymphocutaneous syndrome. A review of non-sporothrix causes. *Medicine (Baltimore)* **78:**38–63.

Tick-Borne Diseases of Humans
Jesse L. Goodman et al.
© 2005 ASM Press, Washington, D.C.

Chapter 6

The Human Reaction to Ticks

UWE U. MÜLLER-DOBLIES AND STEPHEN K. WIKEL

INTRODUCTION

Ticks evolved from free-living mites as hematophagous parasites of reptiles, birds, and mammals more than 94 million years ago, based on the oldest argasid record (96). More than 50 species of ticks will feed on humans (49, 67). They belong to two families, the soft ticks (Argasidae) and the hard ticks (Ixodidae). Humans are not the principal, but rather the serendipitous, host for most tick species and play no or an insignificant role in the endemic cycles of tick-borne diseases. Diseases transmitted by ticks are the primary concern when dealing with human infestation. Only over the past 2 decades has it become widely accepted that ticks play a pivotal role in pathogen transmission beyond mechanical inoculation (87, 149, 168, 183). This role may turn out to be the Achilles heel of maintaining pathogen cycles, because successful immune responses to specific tick saliva antigens may allow us to impair this role of the tick and thus block pathogen transmission (104, 150, 215). Our knowledge of human reactions is largely based on case reports and retrospective studies, whereas most of our understanding of the tick-host interface is derived from experimental work with domestic and laboratory animals.

To accomplish a successful blood meal, a tick has to (i) attach to the host, (ii) impair local itching and pain responses to stay undetected, (iii) prepare the tissue for blood extraction, (iv) prevent the blood-clotting cascade, and (v) suppress the local immune and inflammatory responses (204). The resulting local milieu is advantageous for colonization by pathogens, which enter the skin with tick saliva. Molecules secreted in saliva have to satisfy all these needs for the entire duration of feeding, sometimes for more than 12 days. Given the complexity of host responses, it is intriguing and not understood how some tick species successfully feed on a large spectrum of hosts; i.e., the same developmental stage and species of tick may feed successfully on several species of reptiles, birds, and mammals. Several hypotheses must be considered. (i) The importance of overcoming or avoiding host responses may be largely overestimated. (ii) Ticks may have developed a universal skeleton key to overcome host responses. (iii) Most likely, ticks are equipped with an array of molecules tailored to the natural host range, with sufficiently overlapping and redundant activities to warrant the cross-reactivity required for feeding on novel or serendipitous host species, like humans. The last hypothesis is supported by recent findings that the tick's pharmacological arsenal is under intense selection pressure and is probably finely tuned for a set of local host species (109, 110). Saliva composition varies significantly between ticks from the same laboratory population, suggesting that molecular variation at the individual level may be part of the strategy for avoiding the development of host resistance (205).

The diversity of molecules in tick saliva is considerable and far from fully characterized. Whether or not a tick can specifically adjust its saliva composition appropriately to the response it elicits is unclear. Much work remains to be done to define these relationships. In the past few years, dozens of molecules and biochemical activities in tick saliva and tick salivary glands have been described. However, all these activities explain only a tiny proportion of the genes expressed in tick salivary glands. A large proportion of RNA messages identified so far encode proteins without sequence homology to any current database entries (19, 40, 77, 112, 145, 201).

In the following synopsis, the common features of tick biology and pharmacology will be discussed in the context of the physiology of tick feeding. Immunological reactions will then be treated before separately reviewing the pathological conditions caused by ticks in their own right, i.e., local skin reactions and systemic toxicoses. Finally, current research directions will be explored briefly, as they are rapidly changing our perception of the tick-host interface and have led to the use of ticks as innovative pharmacological repositories.

Uwe U. Müller-Doblies and Stephen K. Wikel • Center for Microbial Pathogenesis, School of Medicine, University of Connecticut Health Center, 263 Farmington Ave., Farmington, CT 06030.

THE PHYSIOLOGY OF TICK FEEDING

Biology and Morphology

The Argasidae and Ixodidae differ fundamentally in their life histories and feeding habits (186). Members of the Argasidae (Color Plate 2A to E) predominantly parasitize nidicolous hosts, such as nesting birds, roosting bats, or mammals with nests or burrows. Apart from a few species that also live in human dwellings, like *Ornithodoros moubata*, human exposures are usually associated with animal nesting sites or caves, while most hard ticks quest for suitable hosts on vegetation (12). The argasid life cycle is characterized by two to eight nymphal instars, while the ixodid life cycle is characterized by only one nymphal instar. Argasid larvae may feed either slowly or rapidly. However, argasid nymphs and adults are rapid feeders, engorging in a matter of minutes to a few hours. Argasid females feed repeatedly and oviposit several hundred eggs after each blood meal (186). Ixodid larvae, nymphs, and females feed once; the female dies after ovipositing thousands of eggs (186). Ixodid feeding occurs over a period of days, with the shortest duration of feeding for larvae and the longest for females, which feed slowly for several days and then rapidly at the end of engorgement (95, 186). A female argasid consumes a blood volume that can be several times her unfed size, while the blood meal of a female ixodid might exceed 100 times her prefed weight (186). Differences in cuticle structure accommodate the different patterns of feeding observed in the two families (95).

Mouthpart structure, host attachment, and feeding of selected argasid (soft) and ixodid (hard) tick species have been topics of both thorough studies and reviews (14, 17, 69, 95, 136, 186). Basic mouthpart structures are similar for soft and hard ticks (14, 186) (Color Plate 2F to H). The capitulum consists of the hypostome, chelicerae, and cheliceral sheaths, which merge proximally to form the basis capituli (14). The ixodid tick capitulum is anterior and clearly visible, while the argasid capitulum is located in a subterminal, ventral position (186). The ventral aspect of the capitulum consists of the hypostome, which is covered on its ventral surface by rows of retrograde denticles with smaller teeth at the tip (14). The dorsal aspect of the hypostome is concave and covered above by the two cheliceral sheaths, forming the canal for delivery of saliva and uptake of food (186). The chelicerae are covered by cheliceral sheaths. The apex of the cheliceral shaft bears the cheliceral digits, with sharp denticles for cutting host skin (186). Cheliceral digits contain mechano- and chemosensory structures, which appear to have a key function in feeding behavior (204).

Attachment

Upon finding a suitable host, the tick raises its body at an angle to the skin surface and the chelicerae begin to cut the epidermis with an outward movement (95, 186). The hypostome is inserted with a rocking motion and serves the function of a holdfast organ (186). The tick may detach after a few minutes and begin the attachment process at another site (186). Mouthpart lengths differ significantly, with lengths in *Dermacentor*, *Haemaphysalis*, and *Rhipicephalus* extending to the dermis-epidermis interface, while the mouthparts of *Amblyomma* and *Ixodes* species extend well into the dermis (Fig. 1 and Color Plate 2H and I) (95, 136). When the mouthparts are fully inserted, the palps are splayed laterally on the skin surface (14).

Cement

Salivary glands of ixodid ticks generally secrete an attachment cement (95), which is believed to serve as an adhesive and to seal the bite lesion by bridging the cleft between mouthparts and host tissue (136). Attachment cement secretion begins within minutes after skin penetration and hardens into a tube surrounding the mouthparts and in some species forms an elevated cone on the epidermal surface (14, 95). Additional cement layers are secreted over the next 3 days of feeding (186). Hard tick species differ widely in the size and shape of the cement cones they form at the feeding site, and some *Ixodes* species apparently do not produce any cement at all (95). Figure 1 illustrates the spectrum of mouthpart and cement configurations encountered in different hard ticks (136). However, the association with a particular genus is not as clear as indicated. Argasid nymphs and adults do not utilize cement for attachment, likely due to their brief feeding periods (186).

Mechanics

Cutting action and mouthpart insertion produce an expanding hemorrhagic pool within the tissues (186), which is aided by anticoagulants, vasodilators, and platelet aggregation inhibitors in tick saliva (175). Mouthpart mechanical actions alone are not sufficient to account for the lesion (Color Plate 2J) (14). The lesion is characterized by a large blood-filled cavity, which led to the term pool feeding or telmophagy. This is a strategy used by many hematophagous arthropod species (108, 186). Ixodid tick blood uptake and saliva secretion are not continuous (186). The first few days of hard tick feeding are referred to as the slow-feeding phase, which coincides with cuticle growth to accommodate the blood meal. Next, the rapid-feeding

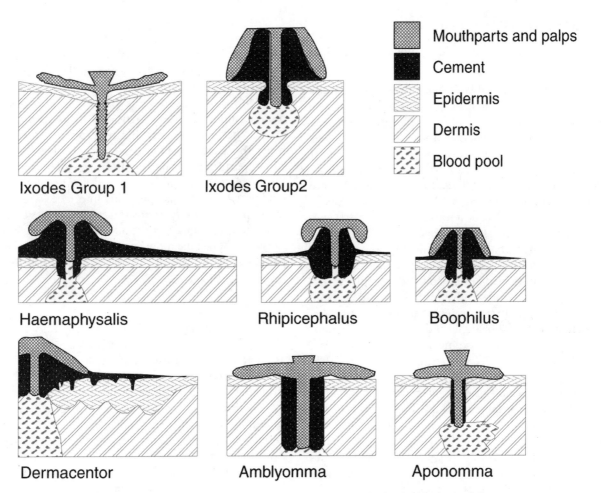

Figure 1. Schematic representation of tick attachment variants in hard ticks. The depth of feeding and the cement cone structure show a high degree of variability between different genera and species of hard ticks. This has important implications for the physiological and immunological structure of the tick-host interface. Adapted from Moorhouse (136) with the permission of the publisher.

phase is characterized by the uptake of very large quantities of blood. The onset of the rapid-feeding phase requires successful mating; thus, rapid feeding may be delayed for up to a week (204). The increase in size during the 7- to 10-day slow-feeding phase can be 10-fold, with an additional 10-fold increase during the rapid-feeding phase (93). This increase actually underestimates the amount of blood consumed, since fluid from the blood meal is reintroduced into the host during salivation (93). The amount of blood taken up is also affected by the host species and host hematocrit (93).

MOLECULAR AND BIOCHEMICAL ASPECTS OF TICK FEEDING

Ticks evolved strategies to overcome host hemostasis, pain and itch responses, inflammation, and immune defenses by secreting saliva, which contains a complex array of pharmacologically active molecules.

Tick salivary gland pharmacology has been reviewed elsewhere (30, 167, 175). Indicative of their importance, redundant mechanisms exist within individual ticks to counteract host defenses (175), and different tick species utilize different strategies for modulating or counteracting the same host defensive pathway (168). Our current knowledge is based on the small proportion of salivary molecules that have been functionally characterized. Thus, the data are far from complete; when discussing the functions of these bioactive compounds, we present a collage of many species. Although the overall picture is fragmentary, it can provide an understanding of the varying roles and common features inherent in this complex mixture.

Proteases and Protease Inhibitors

As mentioned earlier, the mechanical activity of the chelicerae will most certainly not entirely explain the relatively large blood-filled tissue cavity that is characteristic of feeding ticks. It may thus be safe to assume that enzymatic activities contribute greatly to the formation of these lesions. A number of proteolytic activities and proteases have been characterized from various tick species, e.g., two papain-like cysteine proteases and two serine proteases were found in *Haemaphysalis longicornis* (138). At the same time, many putative serine protease inhibitors have been identified, based on sequence homology data from *Boophilus microplus* (GenBank accession no. AJ304447) (191), *Ixodes ricinus* (112), *Ixodes scapularis* (201), *H. longicornis* (139), and *Rhipicephalus appendiculatus* (140). This coexpression of proteases and protease inhibitors may appear contradictory at first glance. But it is likely to be explained by diverging substrate specificities, which are still largely unknown, and pH changes between alkaline saliva and near-neutral host tissue. Most of the tick-derived proteases and protease inhibitors characterized to date inhibit components of the complement and coagulation cascades as well as the kinin system, all to be discussed below. In vivo data on how and where proteases and protease inhibitors act will aid our understanding of how the hematoma-like cavity is created and maintained throughout the feeding period without noticeable repair mechanisms blocking it.

Pain and Itch

Pain and/or itching are important host responses that alert an individual to the presence of a tick, resulting in grooming behavior that removes the tick. Bradykinin is a peripheral mediator of the sensations of itching (4) and pain (37). A serine protease inhibitor from *B. microplus* is effective for inhibiting the protease kallikrein, which transforms inactive plasma kininogens into vasodilatory bradykinin and kallidin (191). *I. scapularis* saliva contains a metallodipeptidyl carboxypeptidase capable of degrading active bradykinin (172). Bradykinin also has roles in inflammation and increases vascular permeability (159). Histamine is one of several mediators that transmit the sensation of itching through peripheral sensory nerve endings (4), but it is also an important mediator of innate and acquired immune responses (discussed below). Furthermore, a combination of histamine and serotonin, a further mediator of itching, inhibited tick feeding (153). Histamine-binding proteins are produced by the salivary glands of many tick species. Histamine-blocking activity was initially observed in the salivary gland homogenates of partially fed adult *Rhipicephalus sanguineus* (33). *R. appendiculatus* has three closely related histamine-binding proteins, two of which occur in females and one of which occurs in males (151). These proteins are unique lipocalins in that they possess one high-affinity site and a second binding site with low affinity for histamine (152). That second binding site of a *Dermacentor reticulatus* histamine-binding lipocalin is now known to bind serotonin, while the first binding site binds histamine (179). This lipocalin has higher affinity for serotonin than membrane receptors on target cells (179). A dual-binding lipocalin likely reflects the need to modulate combinations of mediators produced by diverse host species (179).

Additional histamine-binding proteins were identified by characterization of cDNAs prepared from mRNAs of salivary glands of *I. scapularis* (201) and *Amblyomma americanum* (19). As genomic and proteomic studies of tick salivary glands progress, additional molecules that modulate these important mediators will almost certainly be described.

Blood Coagulation and Tick Anticoagulants

Blood coagulation is a critical mechanism to prevent blood loss from the vasculature; it poses a major obstacle for blood-feeding parasites, including ticks. Blood coagulation results from activation of the extrinsic tissue factor and intrinsic pathways, which converge to form activated factor X (Xa), which initiates the common pathway of coagulation (116). Factor Xa and activated factor V (Va) convert prothrombin to thrombin, which in turn converts fibrinogen into fibrin, the basis of all blood clots (116, 161). The intrinsic pathway is approximately 50 times more efficient at activating factor X than the extrinsic pathway (116). Pharmacologists are focusing considerable attention on factor X as a key target for development of novel drugs to control coagulation (161).

Blood-feeding arthropods are expert pharmacologists, and ticks in particular have developed numerous redundant and complementary ways to inhibit coagulation, as shown in Fig. 2. Ticks block host blood coagulation predominantly by targeting factor Xa and thrombin (54). Inhibitors of factor Xa have been reported from the saliva or salivary glands of the following tick species: *O. moubata* (212), *R. appendiculatus* (114), *Hyalomma truncatum* (88), *Ornithodoros savignyi* (89), *Hyalomma dromedarii* (82), and *I. scapularis* (143). *I. scapularis* saliva contains a further inhibitor of extrinsic factor X activation, Ixolaris, which is believed to utilize both factors X and Xa as scaffolds for the inhibition of activated factor VII/tissue factor complex (54). Blocking the action of thrombin prevents conversion of fibrinogen to fibrin (116). Thrombin inhibitors are produced by the salivary glands of *Ixodes holocyclus* (11), *I. ricinus* (79), *A. americanum* (229), and *O. savignyi* (146). *Dermacentor andersoni* salivary glands contain inhibitors of factor V, an integral part of the complex with Xa that converts prothrombin to thrombin, and factor VII, a component of

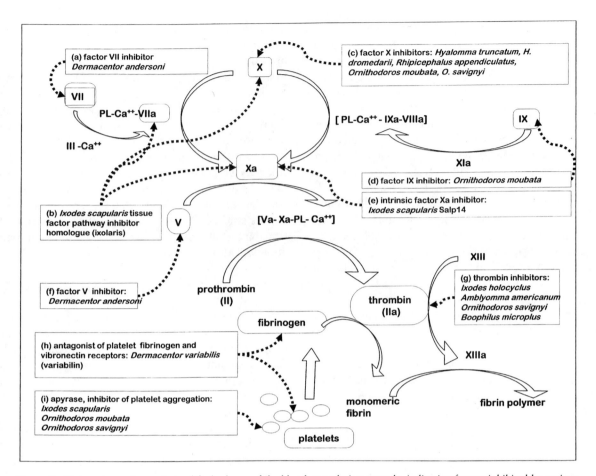

Figure 2. Tick anticoagulants. A simplified scheme of the blood coagulation cascade, indicating factors inhibited by various tick species. Green arrows indicate the conversion of a factor. Factors targeted by tick molecules are highlighted in pink. Phospholipids (PL) and Ca^{2+} (Ca^{++}) are cofactors in several steps. The analysis of all the inhibitors identified to date indicates evolutionary significant inhibition targets that may also be useful targets for the pharmacological control of blood clotting. (a) *D. andersoni* inhibitor of factor VII (65) and (b) the *I. scapularis* tissue factor pathway inhibitor homologue Ixolaris (54) both inhibit the extrinsic pathway. (c) Factor X inhibitors have been identified in numerous species, e.g., *H. truncatum* (88), *H. dromedarii* (82), *R. appendiculatus* (114), *O. moubata* (212), or *O. savignyi* (89). (d) A second activity in targeting the intrinsic pathway is *O. moubata* factor IX inhibitor, which was described more than 35 years ago (72). (e) Recently Salp14, a third intrinsic pathway inhibitor, was described from *I. scapularis* (143). The common pathway of coagulation is targeted by *D. andersoni* factor V inhibitor (65). (g) Thrombin, the activated factor II, is inhibited by *I. holocyclus* (11), americanin from *A. americanum* (229), and savignin from *O. savignyi* (146). The inhibition of thrombin prevents the conversion of fibrinogen into fibrin as well as the activation of factor XIII, which contributes to the polymerization of fibrin monomers. (h) *D. variabilis* produces variabilin, an antagonist of platelet fibrinogen and vibronectin receptors. (i) Platelet aggregation is also inhibited by the apyrase activity detected in *I. scapularis* (168, 171), *O. moubata* (169), and *O. savignyi* (117, 118).

the extrinsic pathway (65). *O. moubata* produces an inhibitor of the intrinsic pathway component, factor IX (72).

Inhibition of Platelet Aggregation

Platelet aggregation can be inhibited by apyrase, which hydrolyzes both ATP and ADP to AMP and inorganic phosphate (168). Salivary apyrases are present in *O. moubata* (169), *O. savignyi* (117), *I. scapularis* (171), and many other blood-feeding arthropods (168). *O. moubata* can inhibit platelet aggregation with a disintegrin-like molecule (91) and an inhibitor

of collagen-mediated platelet aggregation (211). *Dermacentor variabilis* salivary glands inhibit platelet aggregation with an antagonist of fibrinogen and vibronectin receptors (210). Metalloproteases degrade extracellular matrix (165). Snake venom metalloproteases prevent platelet aggregation by altering platelet binding to fibrin (189). Genes encoding putative metalloproteases are present in the salivary glands of *I. scapularis* (201). Tick saliva metalloproteases could provide another means of preventing platelet aggregation. In addition, the disruption of the extracellular matrix likely contributes to maintaining the feeding lesion around tick mouthparts.

Lipid Metabolites

In addition to inhibiting platelet aggregation, prostaglandin E_2 (PGE_2) is also a vasodilator. PGE_2 occurs in the salivary glands of *B. microplus* (46, 76), *I. scapularis* (171), and *A. americanum* (170). Vasodilation increases blood flow to the bite site, which is beneficial to engorging ticks. It should be noted that PGE_2 is also involved in signaling within the salivary glands (160); other properties of PGE_2 will be addressed in the context of immune interaction. A more quantitative analysis of the very divergent potential roles of PGE_2 would greatly enhance our current understanding. Saliva of *A. americanum* contains phospholipase A2, which possesses hemolytic activity (230), likely valuable in maintaining the feeding site and uptake of blood.

Calreticulin

Rapid advances are being made in identification of tick salivary gland molecules that modify inflammation, as well as innate and specific acquired immune responses. Many of those molecules likely possess additional activities. *A. americanum* calreticulin was the first tick salivary gland gene cloned and expressed (85). Calreticulin is a highly conserved molecule with a wide range of biological functions: it acts as a molecular chaperone, regulates integrin-mediated adhesion, and interferes with the action of complement component C1q (39, 98). Antibodies to *A. americanum* calreticulin revealed that it is secreted in saliva of both *A. americanum* and *D. variabilis* females (85). *B. microplus* calreticulin is expressed during each developmental phase in all tissues (53). Repeatedly infested cattle do not develop antibodies to *B. microplus* calreticulin (53). However, some humans bitten by *I. scapularis* develop cross-reactive serum antibodies to *A. americanum* calreticulin (177). It will be interesting to see which activities, if any, tick calreticulin exhibits in mammalian skin.

TICK INTERACTIONS WITH THE HOST IMMUNE SYSTEM

The outcome of tick feeding and pathogen inoculation is governed by the interplay of the tick's salivary pharmacologic repertoire and the host's innate and adaptive immune responses. From many in vitro and in vivo studies, it is apparent that ticks manipulate host immune responses. Interest in these interactions was stimulated by two lines of observations. (i) Hosts can acquire immune-mediated resistance to hard ticks (6, 196) and soft ticks (144). (ii) Tick saliva facilitates the transmission of pathogens, also referred to as saliva-activated transmission or SAT (87, 149). Based on current understanding, the pharmacological effects of tick saliva profoundly modify the feeding site to facilitate feeding and to avoid adverse immune reactions; thus, the threshold for infectious inocula is lowered. This turns out to be a rather complex host-parasite interaction, which surprisingly functions across a variety of host and tick species (109). However, the tick's pharmacological arsenal is constantly being shaped by the predominant host species in a region, resulting in matching pairs of tick and "natural" host species (110). This point needs to be considered when investigating vector competency in the laboratory and extends further to correctly matching pathogen and tick biotype (228). The feeding success of ticks on unnatural hosts may be explained by the homology of target molecules across different mammalian hosts and redundant as well as complementary activities in tick saliva (64, 201).

Resistance Models

Before dealing with the individual components that define the immunological tick-host interface, a brief account will highlight key features of host resistance. Host resistance results in reduced engorgement, decreased reproductive success, and increased mortality in affected ticks, but in all of the animal models a percentage of ticks will feed sufficiently to lay eggs or molt to the next life cycle stage. At a mechanistic level, the effects on ticks have not been characterized conclusively. This being said, immunological resistance is being successfully used to control *B. microplus* (222). Tick resistance has been examined with numerous tick-host systems (6, 29, 126). Resistance to *D. andersoni*, the Rocky Mountain wood tick, has been studied extensively. The resistance in several host species is clearly multifactorial: transfer experiments identified lymph node cells (218), high-titer antibodies (213), and complement factor C3 (219) as contributing to resistance. In particular, guinea pig resistance to ticks is associated with a dominant basophil influx (cutaneous basophil hypersensitivity) (6), and their pivotal role in the expression of resistance has been demonstrated by the effects of the depletion of basophils with specific hyperimmune serum (28).

Mast cells have a crucial role in another model, which consists of repeated infestations of mice with larval *H. longicornis*, resulting in >80% resistance (125, 126). It was concluded that mast cells (125) and immunoglobulin E (IgE) (126) are essential in this resistance. It is unclear whether mast cells and IgE alone are sufficient or rather pivotal in the subsequent recruitment of eosinophils and T cells from the blood

(199). In the same model, the role of gamma interferon (IFN-γ) was assessed using IFN-γ-deficient mice. Although initial larval feeding was more successful in the IFN-$\gamma^{-/-}$ mice, the mice too developed resistance after repeated infestations, indicating that IFN-γ contributed to innate resistance. The increased levels of interleukin-4 (IL-4) in these mice were not sufficient to prevent resistance (15).

Until now, success in counteracting tick strategies of manipulating the immune system has been limited. A better understanding of the immune factors governing the outcome of infestation and pathogen inoculation would be valuable to induce immune responses to ticks that are beneficial for the control of ticks and tick-borne zoonoses. When considering potential vaccine applications, a clear line must be drawn between veterinary objectives and clinical (human) medical objectives. The ideal vaccine for human use would deter the tick from feeding by providing sufficient negative feedback signals during the attachment process or by restoring itch and pain responses, which would lead to the detection and removal of the tick before pathogens are being transmitted. A less ambitious and likely more feasible vaccine would aim at preventing pathogen transmission by blocking the tick interference with the immune system. The only vaccine accomplished to date is for veterinary use and interferes with successful tick feeding by targeting concealed antigens of the tick gut and salivary glands (162, 222, 223). This leads to diminished viability and population control of the cattle tick B. microplus.

Components of the Innate and Adaptive Immune System at the Tick-Host Interface

The mechanisms by which ticks undermine host immune defenses are the subject of numerous reviews (24, 150, 217, 220, 221). The molecules and cells defining the innate and adaptive tick-host interactions are intimately intertwined. Teasing these components apart will be very instructive in understanding the mechanisms that prevent and underlie acquired resistance to ticks and facilitate or block transmission of tick-borne pathogens. Ticks target common proinflammatory pathways of cell activation and recruitment, such as bioactive amines, chemokines, and the complement system. In this process, adaptive immune responses are affected. Hence, the effects of tick infestation on adaptive immune responses are not easily separated from the inhibition of innate responses. Numerous studies have identified changes in the cytokine expression pattern of T cells upon tick infestation in animal models (24) and humans (99). How these observations relate to histopathologic and clinical findings is, as yet, unclear. The changes described in cyto-kine expression profiles were not associated with success in tick feeding or pathogen transmission. The following is an attempt to make this field more accessible, but it is certainly not intended to be comprehensive.

Complement Inhibition

The complement system is involved in pathogen opsonization, processing of immune complexes, and proinflammatory signaling, among other functions (123). Three distinct pathways lead to the cleavage of the central factor C3 into C3a and C3b, which in turn constitutes the central component of the multiprotein C5 convertase. The activation of C5 leads to the formation of the membrane attack complex, which perforates foreign cell membranes. In regards to tick-host interaction, anaphylatoxins (C4a, C3a, and C5a) are likely important for cell recruitment and activation. The classical pathway is triggered by antigen-antibody complexes and thus relies on the acquired immune system. Innate pattern recognition is responsible for activating the two other pathways, i.e., the alternative pathway, which relies on the direct binding and activation of C3 to hydroxyl or amine groups on cell-surface molecules, and the recently discovered lectin pathways (also referred to as mannose-binding pathways), which respond to sugar groups (in particular, mannose). C4 is required in the classical pathway and subsets of the lectin pathway but is apparently not required for the expression of resistance to D. andersoni (214), while its substrate, C3, is required for expression of this acquired resistance (219). This suggests that the alternative pathway and/or the lectin pathway plays an important role in this resistance, which these pathways apparently do not play during primary infestation with D. andersoni larvae. This area merits revisiting with current tools. I. scapularis saliva contains inhibitors of both the alternative pathway and anaphylatoxins (166, 173). Tick-host range has been linked to the ability to impair host alternative pathway function (110). An I. scapularis anti-complement protein (ISAC) was purified from saliva, cloned, and expressed (200). This inhibitor accelerates the uncoupling of factor Bb from the alternative pathway C3 convertase and inhibits C3b binding (200). At concentrations inhibitory to the alternative pathway, the classical pathway was not affected. These tick molecules are thereby blocking the innate recognition of foreign molecules through the two antibody-independent complement pathways. This prevents anaphylatoxin C5a from eliciting a proinflammatory signal amplification through C5a receptors on a range of cells, including endothelial cells and mast cells, which recruit inflammatory cells from the blood through upregulation of adhesion molecules and release of other proinflammatory mediators.

Antibodies

Logically, antibodies are probably the most effective host response to inactivate soluble bioactive saliva constituents. Indeed, resistance or partial resistance to tick feeding was transferred with high-titer serum from animals that acquired resistance through repeated infestations (22, 26, 196, 213). However, soluble protein antigens, like saliva antigens, often are not very amenable to antibody induction, which may play to the tick's advantage in other tick-host systems. The specificity of resistance conferring antibodies is not defined. However, as mentioned previously, early work on the role of complement in tick resistance suggests that antibodies are neutralizing inhibitors of C3 activation in one or both of the two C4 independent complement activation pathways (127), i.e., the alternative pathway or the mannose-binding lectin-associated serine protease 1 (MASP-1)-dependent C3 activation. Another mechanism of antibody-mediated resistance is Fc receptor dependent (225).

Salivary gland extracts of *Amblyomma variegatum*, *Ixodes hexagonus*, and *R. appendiculatus* each contain IgG-binding proteins (IGBPs), which have different molecular weights for each tick species (208). Two additional IGBPs were observed in the salivary glands of male, but not female, *R. appendiculatus* ticks after 6 days of feeding (207). Host Igs in the blood meal pass from the digestive tract into the hemolymph (181). IGBPs may form part of a tick Ig excretion system (TIES) as transporters that translocate Igs from the tick gut via the hemolymph into the salivary glands for excretion (209). Such a specific transport is indirectly supported by observations that IgG and IgM are translocated more efficiently into the hemolymph than are other smaller proteins (83). IgG as well as IgG-binding proteins occur in the hemolymph and salivary glands (206). However, only one of the three male tick-specific IGBPs appears to be secreted into the saliva (209). The biologic role of a TIES is uncertain: it has been proposed that excreted antibodies would be harmless and would compete with potentially harmful antibodies for Fc receptors (209). However, there is no evidence that the secretion mechanism is selective for certain antibodies. Another hypothesis proposed that TIES is the disposal mechanism for the large amounts of Igs taken up with the blood meal (83), but this is not supported by the quantity of antibodies transported by this mechanism (83). A third explanation is that tick mouthparts break the skin integrity, thereby allowing skin flora to enter the bite site. The tick would almost inevitably be infected with these germs. But as these microorganisms are part of the host flora, the host antibodies can be exploited as an antibody-mediated immune system for the tick. This hypothesis is indirectly supported by the observation that host antibodies retain their antigen-binding capacity during passage through the tick (2, 55). More direct support comes from observations related to the *Borrelia burgdorferi* vaccine, which targets the spirochetal lipoprotein OspA. OspA-specific antibodies prevent spirochete transmission by clearing the infection within the tick (164). In the case of *Borrelia*, this vaccine-induced antibody response is "unnatural," but for natural skin-colonizing microorganisms, host antibodies may serve as a form of passive immunization.

Macrophages and Reactive Oxygen and Nitrogen Metabolites

A combination of pathogen-associated molecular patterns (PAMPs) (130) and instructive cytokine signals activate recruited macrophages to acquire several distinct effector phenotypes (66), three of which will be mentioned here.

First, IFN-γ is the prototype inducer of classical macrophage activation. It involves production of proinflammatory cytokines (IL-6, tumor necrosis factor alpha [TNF-α], and IL-1) and upregulation of radical-forming enzymes, ultimately leading to respiratory burst. The formed reactive oxygen species (ROS) and nitrogen species kill a wide range of microorganisms at the expense of concomitant local tissue damage. Whether ROS are effective at harming ticks is yet unclear, but two distinct groups of antioxidants are produced in ticks and tick salivary glands: peroxiredoxin in *H. longicornis* (198) and a glutathione peroxidase in *I. scapularis* (42). Sera from tick-sensitized rabbits react with tick glutathione peroxidase; thus, it is believed to be secreted with saliva despite lacking a secretory signal peptide. Another peroxidase activity is located within the salivary gland vesicles of *A. americanum* (D. Müller-Doblies, unpublished observations).

Second, innate macrophage activation through pattern recognition receptors for PAMPs leads to the increased expression of costimulatory molecules and the production of NO-ROS and alpha and beta interferons (IFN-α and -β) (type I interferons) (66), which in turn invoke an antiviral state in surrounding tissue that will be discussed later.

Third, IL-4 and/or IL-13 stimulation of macrophages leads to the alternative macrophage activation, which is characterized by high production of lysozyme, upregulation of arginase, and expression of mannose-binding receptors (66). This phenotype is more likely associated with tissue repair and parasitic infections (66). Along these lines, macrophages treated with *I. ricinus* salivary gland extracts are less capable of killing tick-transmitted *Borrelia afzelii* spirochetes (103), possibly due to alternative activation. The increase in expression of IL-10 in some tick models (51, 97) and of PGE$_2$ at the bite site (170, 180) may contribute to this phenotype, but on the other hand IL-10 could also induce macrophage deactivation, which leads to the secretion of anti-inflammatory cytokines, e.g., transforming growth factor β (66). Macrophages are clearly recruited to the tick feeding sites, and it remains to be shown whether one of the macrophage phenotypes is associated with resistance for pathogen transmission or tick feeding. The initiation of this response requires IL-4, derived from a cell of the innate immune response and/or from T cells (48).

IFN-α/β

IFN-α and IFN-β are important proinflammatory cytokines, which induce a plethora of antiviral molecules in immune and nonimmune cells (176). MX proteins are among the better-characterized IFN response proteins (71). They are potent inhibitors of orthomyxoviruses and several arthropod-borne viruses (178). Mx-mediated IFN-α/β activity is compromised in Thogoto virus infection if the virus is transmitted by ticks (45). This may be one of the key factors underlying SAT of viruses. Interestingly, the IFN-α/β are produced by innately stimulated macrophages but not by alternatively stimulated macrophages (66).

Natural Killer Cells

Adult *D. reticulatus*, *A. variegatum*, and *Haemaphysalis inermis* salivary gland extracts inhibited human natural killer cells (NK), while *I. ricinus* and *R. appendiculatus* had no effect (101, 102). IL-2, an important growth factor for NK cells and T cells, is blocked through a putative IL-2-binding protein in the saliva of *I. scapularis* (63).

Chemokines

Chemokines recruit immune cells, such as neutrophils, basophils, lymphocytes, and monocytes to the site of a tissue insult. IL-8, which attracts and activates neutrophils and basophils, is inhibited by activities in the saliva of several hard ticks (*R. appendiculatus*, *D. reticulatus*, *A. variegatum*, *I. ricinus*, and *H. inermis*) (70). Other chemokines with similar activities, like the complement-derived anaphylatoxins C3a and C5a, are inhibited by *I. scapularis* (173). These and probably other mechanisms inhibit the immediate influx and activation of neutrophils (174).

Macrophage Migration Inhibitory Factor (MIF)

An intriguing finding is the expression of a homologue of the proinflammatory cytokine, macrophage MIF in the salivary glands and midgut of *A. americanum* (84). This pleotropic lymphocyte/macrophage cytokine is reported to possess oxidoreductase activity, inhibit lysis by NK cells, act as a neurohumoral mediator, prevent random migration of macrophages, inhibit delayed type hypersensitivity, generate antigen-specific B- and T-lymphocyte responses in vivo (115, 158), and play an essential role in neovascularization (31). Specific roles of this molecule in tick saliva and midgut are undefined.

IL-4

IL-4 upregulation in response to ticks appears to be a consistent finding (15, 24, 36, 57, 131). The effects of IL-4 on macrophages have already been discussed, and IL-4's effect on other cells will be addressed. The source of IL-4 in most of these studies is likely to be T cells. T cells only express significant amounts of IL-4, about 4 to 5 days after their initial priming. Innate sources of IL-4 (e.g., mast cells, basophils, eosinophils, and NK-T-cells) may be important for the differentiation of the acquired immune response. In some mouse models, IL-4 increases were interpreted as a tick-beneficial cytokine response which does maintain tick susceptibility (24, 52, 100). Similarly, IL-10 is up-regulated in several systems and may contribute to reduced IFN-γ responsiveness (24, 51, 97, 99). However, at this point we lack conclusive evidence for the role of IL-4 or other cytokines in tick susceptibility, tick resistance, and the transmission of tick-borne pathogens. It has been proposed that ticks purposely promote IL-4-polarized T-helper cells to avoid immune-mediated host resistance, but to date evidence in support of that hypothesis is inconclusive.

T Cells and T-Cell Cytokines

CD4$^+$ T-helper cells play an important role in orchestrating adaptive immune responses. Numerous tick species have developed different strategies to affect T cells. *I. scapularis* saliva contains an IL-2-binding protein that complexes with IL-2 in the fluid phase rather than by acting directly upon the cytokine-producing cell (63). This IL-2-binding protein can potentially influence any IL-2-responsive cell population, and it has similar affinities for both human and mouse IL-2 (63). *D. andersoni* inhibits proliferation and priming of T cells through p36 (18), a mannose-glycosylated protein (3), by blocking antigen-specific T-cell priming (Müller-Doblies, unpublished) and mitogen concanavalin A (ConA)-induced proliferation directly. Antibodies to native p36 cross-reacted with polypeptides of 33 and 101 kDa in *D. variabilis* salivary gland extract (18). Salp15 from *I. scapularis* inhibits activation of CD4 T cells by repressing T-cell receptor engagement-initiated calcium signals (13). An *I. ricinus* salivary gland protein (Iris) inhibits ConA-driven in vitro proliferation of mouse splenocytes (111). With human peripheral blood mononuclear cells stimulated with the T-cell mitogen phytohemagglutinin (PHA), Iris reduced the number of cells producing IFN-γ but did not alter the number of cells producing IL-10. Similarly, cells stimulated with multiple activators produced reduced amounts of IFN-γ, IL-6, IL-8, and TNF-α in the presence of Iris (111). In general, Iris inhibits proinflammatory cytokines. *D. andersoni* p36 antiproliferative properties affect CD8 T cells (Müller-Doblies, unpublished), but the biological function of p36 is still unclear.

The effects of tick saliva and tick feeding on T-cell cytokines have been studied extensively using in vitro mitogen stimulation. The common denominator of these observations for several species is a reduced IFN-γ response and an upregulation of IL-4 (34, 35, 51, 52, 99, 100, 182). Upregulation of IL-10 is not as consistently observed (51, 52, 97, 100), but upregulation of IL-4 and IL-10, individually or combined, may account for the reduced IFN-γ induction (97, 134, 142).

Mast Cells, Basophils and Their Mediators

Mast cells and basophils are well known as primary effector cells in allergic inflammation, and they represent a major source of inflammatory mediators (83). Among the major secretions of mast cells are histamine, serotonin, heparin, and several cytokines including IL-4 and the two proteases tryptase and chymase (113). Through the release of histamine, mast cells mediate local itch responses and facilitate leukocyte infiltration. Interestingly, mast cells degranulate at the site of a tick bite even in the absence of homocytotropic antibodies, and they do not increase in number at bite sites after presensitization of the host (7). This is consistent with the idea that mast cells differentiate in situ from bone marrow-derived precursor cells (197) and are not acutely recruited. Histamine is reported to alter immune regulation by changing the Th1-Th2-polarizing capacity of immature dendritic cells, modifying cytokine production by monocytes, and stimulating IL-10 production (90).

Shortly after a histamine-neutralizing activity in the salivary gland extracts of *R. sanguineus* was described (33), Willadsen et al. (224) showed that mepyramin, an H1 receptor antagonist, inhibited skin hypersensitivity in resistant cattle. In a later study involving guinea pigs, a combination of H1 and H2 receptor antagonists was not able to inhibit the antibody-mediated resistance of guinea pigs to *A. americanum* (27). In a mouse model, mast cells were shown to convey resistance to the larvae of the Japanese tick *H. longicornis*

in an IgE-dependent fashion (124–126) and contributed to the resistance against larvae of *D. andersoni* (44). It was later shown that the mast cell function possibly provided chemotactic signals to eosinophils (199) rather than being the immediate effector cell. This would also explain why the pharmacological blockade of histamine receptors did not reverse resistance in other models (216).

Whether histamine is directly toxic to ticks in vivo needs to be conclusively established. A large proportion of *B. microplus* larvae detached from artificial feeding membranes upon histamine encounter and from skin after histamine injection (94). In an artificial feeding model, *D. andersoni* females stopped blood intake and salivation 1.5 to 7.5 min after a combination of histamine and serotonin was added to the blood meal (153). At the same time, individual components (i.e., histamine, serotonin, PGE$_1$, PGF$_{2\alpha}$, and dopamine) had no effect on the feeding process. The discovery of histamine-neutralizing activity (33) eventually led to the identification of histamine-binding proteins (HBPs) in the saliva of *R. appendiculatus* (151). HBPs have most recently been identified in numerous other hard tick species, based on analyses of sequence homologies, suggesting that HBPs are a common strategy (19, 179, 201). HBPs bind histamine with a higher affinity than histamine receptors and thereby prevent inflammation and potentially toxic effects on the tick. Low levels of histamine may, however, increase the local blood flow and temperature, with the cosecreted heparin contributing as an anticoagulant. Thus, the tick may have to carefully balance the availability of histamine to keep the tissue levels below the level of an inflammatory or itch response, yet high enough to increase local blood supply. In this regard, lipocalins may regulate the bioavailability of histamine at the bite site, while preventing to some extent histamine dissemination, which leads to chemotaxis and other proinflammatory events. The differential expression of three different lipocalin genes in larvae and adult males and females is unexplained, but it may reflect different requirements of larvae and males and females to maintain certain histamine levels throughout their blood meal. It would be of further interest whether the heparin released from the mast cells is advantageous to the feeding process by preventing blood clotting. Mechanisms of histamine inactivation, e.g., salivary histamine-inactivating enzymes or the induction of such enzymes in the host, have not yet been described.

In conclusion, mast cells play an important role in anti-tick resistance, although it remains to be shown whether this is by creating a local environment that is hostile for the tick (e.g., by recruiting T cells and eosinophils to the site of infestation) or by directly affecting the tick through toxic mast cell products.

Basophils are bone marrow-derived granulocytes that comprise up to 2% of blood leukocytes. The most pertinent properties shared between them and mast cells are the production of histamine and the surface Fc$_\varepsilon$ receptor I. Histological examination of tick feeding sites implicated basophils as mediators of resistance (6, 7). In resistant guinea pigs and cattle, basophil infiltrates build up within 24 h after attachment. This phenomenon was further investigated experimentally and referred to as cutaneous basophil hypersensitivity, because of the unusually strong contribution of basophils to the cellular infiltrate. The particular recruitment requirements for this tick-resistant state are not understood.

Other Cell Types at the Tick-Host Interface

Many cell types have been implicated in the immunological responses to ticks, but they have not been studied in detail. Langerhans cells and other dendritic cells mop up tick antigens and prime T cells in the skin draining lymph nodes (8, 9, 147, 148). Neutrophils appear early in tick bite lesions, but their contribution to resistance is uncertain (1, 23, 43). On the other hand, neutrophils may contribute to the formation of the feeding lesion (192). Eosinophils appear in the lesions of sensitized hosts, but their role in resistance remains unclear (43, 128, 190, 199).

HUMAN PATHOLOGY ASSOCIATED WITH TICK FEEDING

Clinical Findings

Medical attention to tick bites is largely directed at transmitted pathogens, which are covered in other chapters. Before the identification and isolation of these tick-borne pathogens, tick bite sequelae were often regarded as toxic or autoimmune tick-associated phenomena, including the B. burgdorferi sensu lato-associated lesions termed erythema migrans and acrodermatitis chronica atrophicans (68). In the light of the variety of pathogens described as being tick transmitted during the past 25 years (154), the clinical findings related to tick bites need to be reassessed. The typical local tick bite reaction begins as a somewhat indurated lesion with an erythematous halo, which develops over a period of 2 to 4 days and may either resolve as the tick falls off or progress to a persistent, pruritic papule or nodule (155). Ticks are mostly able to prevent itching and pain responses by inactivating bradykinin (172, 173), by binding histamine (33, 151), and probably by other means yet to be characterized. Tick-induced local anesthesia during the feeding process explains why the lesions are often discovered only after the tick has detached.

The response patterns change dramatically with host species and the degree of sensitization. To understand the diversity of clinical presentations, a number of points should be considered (106): (i) the species and stage involved, (ii) prior sensitization to tick antigens, (iii) persistence of antigenic material in the skin, (iv) pathogen transmission, and (v) secondary infections of the bite lesion. For instance, guinea pigs are prone to a dominant basophil infiltration (20 to 60%) only upon sensitization, which is associated with a high degree of resistance, while basophils in humans usually contribute less than 5% of infiltrating cells and, rarely, as many as 15% (48, 56). The clinical conditions that result from tick bites either are directly caused by the tick and tick antigen in the skin or result from the mechanical lesion that provides immediate access for microorganisms to the deeper strata of the dermis. The local immune-compromised environment created by the tick may particularly promote secondary infections, e.g., Staphylococcus dermatitis (68). At the same time, saliva-derived deposits (8, 9), as well as mouthpart fragments, may persist in the skin and cause chronic reactive inflammatory and/or lymphoproliferative disorders (194, 227).

Alopecia Areata

A transient alopecia areata, which is probably widely underreported, may appear within a 3- to 4-cm radius around bite sites within a week after the removal of a hard tick (5, 74, 120, 121, 163). Regrowth of hair usually occurs within 3 months, but permanent hair loss has also been reported after D. variabilis bites (reviewed in reference 121). Although this finding was already cited by Plinius in the year 77 AD (74), the mechanism is not well understood, and the tick species responsible have been recorded in only a few instances, e.g., Dermacentor marginatus in Europe (163). In dogs, similar hair loss has been caused by Hyalomma and Amblyomma species in South Africa (121). Inappropriate mechanical removal of a tick may result in a bolus of saliva and/or gut content being inoculated into the bite (154). As mechanical tick removal from the scalp precedes the local hair loss, it is possibly a sequela to the involuntary inoculation of a saliva bolus and/or regurgitated blood during removal.

Allergic Reactions

Ticks account for only a minority of the allergic reactions induced by arthropods; in a study from Queensland, Australia, ticks accounted for only 0.7% of all allergic responses to arthropods (185). The reactions to tick bites are as diverse as can be expected when dealing with such a large number of species with multiple blood-feeding developmental stages. The nature of the allergenic antigens has not been systematically examined; thus, it is not known to which extent different life stages and species share allergenic determinants.

Immediate Hypersensitivity

Type I hypersensitivity reactions to tick bites range from local painful pruritic erythematous and papular lesions at the bite site to rare life-threatening systemic anaphylaxis (25, 58, 62, 107, 135). The local reactions arise over minutes to hours and last for more than a week. The bite site may remain itchy for several weeks (58). The role of IgE in mediating the response has been established for *I. holocyclus* (58–61), *I. ricinus* (16), and the soft tick, *Argas reflexus* (132, 184, 202, 203), which commonly infests pigeons. With *I. holocyclus*, an IgE immunoblot analysis identified several distinct allergens (59, 61). The majority of patients with positive skin test reactions reacted specifically with two dominant allergens of approximately 28 and 35 kDa and several minor allergens (61). Intense type I hypersensitivity reactions to *I. ricinus* were decribed in a study of forest workers in France with elevated levels of total IgE and tick extract-specific IgE. Intradermal skin testing with whole-tick extracts produced immediate skin reactions of 55-mm-diameter lesions with surrounding erythema, as well as a delayed reaction at 48 h (16).

Delayed-Type Hypersensitivity

Ornithodoros capensis is a soft tick predominantly feeding on seabirds. Human skin reactions to tick extracts from *O. capensis* peaked in severity at 35 to 40 h and were interpreted as delayed type IV hypersensitivity, characterized by pruritus, blistering (a major feature), erythema, weeping lesions, lymphangitis, dull ache, rheumatic pain, general lassitude, and intense discomfort (80). A pruritic delayed-type skin reaction following *I. ricinus* exposure revealed inflammation in the dermis with some protein-rich, leukocyte-poor vesicles at the epidermis-dermis junction and perivascular mononuclear cell infiltrates dominated by CD8$^+$ T cells and CD1$^+$ Langerhans cells. No deposits of IgG, IgA, IgM, C1q, or C3 were detected in the same biopsy (16).

Lesions Caused by Tick Larvae

Tick larvae of most hard tick species preferentially feed on smaller hosts, but occasionally larvae of certain species will feed on humans. Unlike nymphs and adults, larvae have six rather than eight legs. Due to their small size (<0.6 mm long), they are difficult to recognize as arthropods while attached to the skin. This complicates the attempts at a correct diagnosis (41). They are often referred to as seed ticks in North America (e.g., *A. americanum*) (21, 47, 86), pepper ticks in Africa (*R. appendiculatus* and others), or scrub-itch in Autralia (*I. holocyclus*) (137, 188). Intraepithelial blisters may develop towards the end of feeding at the larval bite site (137). The bite sites in humans may be characterized by local erythema and intense pruritus, both of which can persist for days to weeks after detachment (137). Hundreds of larvae originating from one clutch of eggs can simultaneously attack a suitable host. Thus, the lesions can be rather numerous and can mimic eczemata. They have to be differentiated from chigger mite infestations (Trombiculidae) (75, 78). It is not well established whether these reactions to larval feeding are allergies in the strict sense or whether they are directly caused by larval saliva.

Chronic Lesions

Chronic lesions caused by tick bites have been described as tick bite granuloma (194), dermal eosinophilic granuloma (5), pseudoepitheliomatous hyperplasia (5), or as a cutaneous lymphoid hyperplasia (CLH) (32). They appear as plaques, papules, nodules, or (rarely) miliary lesions. A solitary nodule of up to 4 cm in diameter with doughy to firm consistency is the most common presentation. It may be associated with ulceration and pruritus. Such lesions frequently persist for months or even years (81). In some cases, the cellular infiltrate has been noted to contain Sternberg-Reed cells like those seen in Hodgkins lymphoma (5).

Recently, several studies have linked adolescent hypersensitivity to mosquito bites to a syndrome of chronic active Epstein-Barr virus (EBV) infection and NK cell leukemia-lymphoma (195). Due to the generally high prevalence of EBV in human populations and the low prevalence of this syndrome, more studies will be needed to corroborate this association. In the case of ticks, similar lymphoproliferative lesions have been reported as chronic sequelae of tick bites. They were observed with Lyme patients, but the epidemiological link to Lyme disease could not be substantiated (141). Similar lesions may be neoplastic or associated with other forms of foreign antigens and various drugs, as reviewed by Chesney (32). The pathogenesis of chronic lesions is not understood, but a viral cofactor like EBV is an alternative hypothesis to local antigen persistence.

Histology

Depending on the tick species and local skin thickness, the lesions may reach from the superficial dermis in the case of metastriate species to the deep dermis and subcutis in the case of prostriate adult females (10, 136). The mouthparts frequently break off during detachment and remain in the skin, where they induce a foreign body granuloma (194). The serrated edges of the hypostome may facilitate the drift of hypostome fragments deeper into the skin, where they cause a foreign-body reaction. Cement residues and saliva components may also contribute to the antigenic stimulus locally elicited by the tick. Histologically, the lesions range from mixed cellular dermal infiltrate in subacute lesions to a granulomatous and fibrotic picture in chronic lesions (155), which may be mixed in cellular composition and contain lymphocytes, eosinophiles, polymorphonuclear leukocytes, plasma cells, histiocytes, and mast cells. Giant cells may be present in some cases. Older lesions may progress to a nodular-to-diffuse dermatitis dominated by mononuclear cells, which resemble or reflect neoplastic changes (5, 227).

TICK TOXICOSES

Tick toxicoses are a less-common tick bite complication, which left untreated is often fatal. The symptoms are attributed to toxins inoculated with the saliva. To date, 69 of the approximately 870 recognized tick species have been associated with intoxication syndromes (67). The toxic etiology is proven for only a very few species, while for most of the species evidence is only circumstantial (67). The implication of toxicosis is based on (i) the lack of evidence for any causative pathogen and (ii) the often-rapid clinical recovery after the removal of a feeding tick from the patient. Unless stated otherwise, the following is based on the comprehensive monograph on tick toxicosis by Gothe (67). Gothe lists 11 separate forms of toxicosis, most of which are only known from animals. Toxins have been characterized in *I. holocyclus* (60, 122), *Rhipicephalus evertsi* (67), and *O. savignyi* (119). The identification of toxins has been complicated by variable patterns of toxin production. Toxin production varies within a given species, between and within populations, by sex, by developmental stage, and by feeding phase. Human cases of tick toxicosis fall almost exclusively into the category of tick paralysis (67). The predominantly systemic manifestation of tick paralysis may distract from the thorough examination of the patient's skin for undetected ticks; fatal cases have occurred when ticks were not removed in time. Because tick toxicoses are rarely encountered, the primary danger is a lack of awareness of the potential for a direct link between the syndrome and an undetected feeding tick. The tick species implicated in human toxicosis syndromes are listed in Table 1. Children are much more frequently affected than adults (67). The

geographical distribution indicates that toxicosis-competent ticks exist in all continents, with the exception of Antarctica. Three species of hard ticks account for the vast majority of reported human tick paralysis cases: *I. holocyclus* in Australia, and *D. andersoni* and *D. variabilis* in North America. Australian tick paralysis is the most common and best-studied human tick toxicosis and will be described in more detail.

Australian Tick Paralysis

Clinical presentation

I. holocyclus, the Australian paralysis tick, is a natural parasite of bandicoots (Peramelidae) in the eastern coastal region of Australia. Adult females and, rarely, nymphs cause paralysis while feeding on humans, livestock, and companion animals. The toxin is secreted beginning on the third day of attachment. Paralysis symptoms occur on the fourth or fifth day of infestation, which coincides with the onset of the rapid engorgement phase and is accompanied by an increase in the size of the tick salivary glands (187).

The initial symptoms of tick paralysis are loss of appetite and voice, followed by ascending flaccid paralysis, ocular irritation, excessive salivation, asymmetric pupillary dilation, and vomiting. Bell's palsy has occurred repeatedly following tick attachment to the head (133). Untreated, the condition progresses into full-limb paralysis and death due to respiratory failure (187). After removal of the tick, clinical recovery is often preceded by a worsening of symptoms (156). This is a peculiar feature of *I. holocyclus* paralysis and has not been established for other paralysis ticks (187).

Pathogenesis

Experimental data suggest that the toxin inhibits the release of acetylcholine at the neuromuscular synapse, an effect which is partially reversed by the lowering of temperature (38). The time between onset of symptoms and death ranges between 18 and 30 h. The toxic saliva fraction of *I. holocyclus* is resistant to digestion with pepsin, trypsin, and papain; heating to 75°C for 15 min; and moderate pH changes (187). In older studies, paralytic activity was associated with molecules of 40 to 80 kDa (reviewed in reference 122). Three toxin fractions of similar size were designated holocyclotoxin 1 (HT1, HT2, and HT3). HT1 has been cloned and sequenced (193). The calculated molecular mass of the polypeptide is 5.8 kDa, a size which corresponds to that of other arachnid toxins. HT2 and HT3 have not been characterized. However, several toxins may be responsible for the clinical picture. The discrepancy of the molecular weight described earlier and the

Table 1. Tick species implicated in human toxicosis and paralysis syndromes[a]

Species	Geographic range	Syndrome[b]	Status[c]
Prostriate hard ticks (Ixodidae)			
Ixodes cornuatus	Australia (Tasmania, Victoria)	P	+
Ixodes gibbosus	Eastern Mediterranean	P	+
I. holocyclus	Australia, New Guinea	P	+++
I. muris	Northeastern North America	T	+
I. redikorzevi	Israel	T	++
I. scapularis	Eastern North America	P	+
I. ricinus	Europe	P/T	?
Ixodes tancitarius	Mexico	P	?
Metastriate hard ticks (Ixodidae)			
A. americanum	North America, South America	P	++
Amblyomma hebraeum	Africa, Caribbean	P	?
Amblyomma maculatum	Southern North America	P	?
Amblyomma ovale	Central and South America	P	?
D. andersoni	Northwestern North America	P	+++
D. variabilis	Eastern North America	P	+++
H. truncatum	Africa, Asia	P/T	+
Rhipicephalus praetextatus	Uganda	P	++
R. sanguineus	Worldwide	P	?
Rhipicephalus simus	Africa	P	?
Soft ticks (Argasidae)			
Ornithodoros gurneyi	Australia	T	+
O. coriaceus	Western North America	T	+

[a] The species implicated in human tick paralysis and other toxicosis syndromes were compiled from Gothe (67). The geographic region indicates where the clinical syndromes were described and does not necessarily match the species' full distribution.

[b] Most species are implicated as causing paralysis (P). In several species, the clinical presentation lacked signs of paralysis and is therefore referred as a toxicosis syndrome (T).

[c] The status of a species was defined as follows: ?, inconclusive reports on cases with humans; +, well-established veterinary cases but only inconclusive reports of humans; ++, less than five conclusive case reports of humans; +++, well-established human clinical relevance.

molecular mass described for HT1 may be a result of heavy glycosylation or may indicate that the toxin is secreted in a high-molecular-mass complex.

Treatment

Treatment relies on the removal of all attached ticks and supportive critical care. This is basically the same for all forms of tick toxicoses. Tick removal should be attempted without exerting pressure on the distending tick body (as this might force more saliva or gut contents into the skin lesion) by grasping the capitulum and mouthparts with a fine forceps and applying gentle traction until the tick dislodges. Dogs infested with increasing numbers of *I. holocyclus* females develop toxin-neutralizing antibodies. Canine serum preparations have successfully been used to treat symptomatic humans and animals and are commercially available in Australia.

North American Tick Paralysis

In the northwestern United States and Canada, particularly in Washington State and British Columbia,

D. andersoni regionally causes paralysis in humans and livestock. All documented cases occurred during the months of February to August and coincide with the peak activity of adult *D. andersoni* ticks. In the southern and eastern United States, *D. variabilis* is responsible for the majority of human tick paralysis cases, but a number of other tick species also have to be considered (Table 1).

Other Forms of Human Tick Toxicosis

Two forms of human tick toxicosis without evidence of paralysis will be mentioned briefly. First, *Ixodes redikorzevi* toxicosis is known from several case reports in Israel, which clearly implicate adult females of *I. redikorzevi*, a species occurring in the Near and Middle East. The clinical findings include local pain in the area of the bite site, fever, vomiting, and torticollis. The symptoms improved rapidly after the removal of the ticks (92, 226). Second, *Ixodes muris* bites may cause extreme pain and swelling at the bite site; as the tick feeds toward engorgement, symptoms of lethargy, anorexia, and high fever may be observed (105) in the patient. The toxin has not been identified for either species. *Ornithodoros coriaceus*, the pajaroello tick, occurs in the coastal mountains of California and adjoining Mexico, where it is referred to as talaja. It readily feeds on humans (73). The bite causes a painful local swelling that may extend over large areas of the body. The affected area may feel irritable and subsequently become numb. Exudate forms at the bite site over several weeks from under a small scab (73). This syndrome has been regarded as a toxicosis; however, the reaction is likely to have an allergic component (50). *H. truncatum* is implicated in human cases of tick paralysis. In addition, it is responsible for four other toxicosis syndromes found in domestic animals across southern and central Africa: sweating sickness, mhlosinga, magudu, and possibly also a necrotic stomatitis nephrosis syndrome (67). Sweating sickness is the best characterized. It is accompanied by systemic hyperemia and heavy exudation from skin and mucous membranes. Clinical symptoms develop beginning on the fourth day of infestation (pyrexia, skin hyperemia and hyperesthesia, anorexia, lacrimation, rhinitis, muscle tremor, and dysphagy) and may lead to death within 3 days, even with low tick burdens (<20 ticks). Histologically, the tentative toxin specifically affects epithelia leading to skin necrosis and fibrinous to pseudomembranous necrotic inflammation of gastrointestinal mucous membranes. Surviving cattle develop antitoxic immunity, which does protect from sweating sickness and from mhlosinga, but not from magudu (reviewed in reference 67). This indicates that different toxins occur independently of each other within the same species. Tick toxins may be pharmacologically active across a broad range of host species and through an array of toxic mechanisms, which are yet to be identified. *Ixodes rubicundus*, the Karroo paralysis tick of South Africa, causes tick paralysis in domestic and wild ungulates as well as dogs and jackals. One case in a child was also mentioned (67).

CONCLUSIONS AND FUTURE DIRECTIONS

The idea of immunological control of ticks dates back to 1939 (196). An anti-tick vaccine for the cattle tick *B. microplus* has been quite successful in controlling tick numbers but falls short of eliminating the tick from cattle herds. Although these field results were satisfactory in controlling tick numbers, they did not fulfill the heightened expectations founded on the overwhelming effects of acaricides in similar settings. However, environmental advantages of anti-tick vaccines may outweigh the benefits of acaricides in many settings. The concept of saliva-activated pathogen transmission has led to the idea of novel transmission-blocking vaccines. These would also be of interest for

human use and are currently being explored in several laboratories. In this case, the aim of the vaccine is not to impede the tick feeding but rather to impede pathogen transmission. Although proof of principle has been provided, the mechanisms and target antigens remain to be identified. Recent advances in the characterization of salivary gland proteins and messages are rapidly expanding our understanding of molecular events that facilitate feeding. However, quantitative data on the in vivo activities of salivary proteins are much needed to assess the contributions of individual components. Even in the most robust models of natural tick resistance, there is a significant percentage of successful feeders. It is not understood how they overcome the host response. A recent paradigm of the molecular individuality of ticks (205) might explain this phenomenon, but full understanding will require the development of a whole new research area on tick population genetics and the regulation of gene expression in salivary glands.

REFERENCES

1. Abdul-Amir, I. M., and J. S. Gray. 1987. Resistance of sheep to laboratory infestations of the tick, *Ixodes ricinus*. *Res. Vet. Sci.* 43:266–267.
2. Ackerman, S., F. B. Clare, T. W. McGill, and D. E. Sonenshine. 1981. Passage of host serum components, including antibody, across the digestive tract of *Dermacentor variabilis* (Say). *J. Parasitol.* 67:737–740.
3. Alarcon-Chaidez, F. J., U. U. Müller-Doblies, and S. K. Wikel. 2003. Characterization of a recombinant immunomodulatory protein from the salivary glands of *Dermacentor andersoni*. *Parasite Immunol.* 25:69–77.
4. Alexander, J. 1986. The physiology of itch. *Parasitol. Today* 2:345–351.
5. Allen, A. C. 1948. Persistent "insect bites" (dermal eosinophilic granulomas) simulating lymphoblastoma, histiocytoses and squamous cell carcinoma. *Amer. J. Pathol.* 24:367–373.
6. Allen, J. R. 1973. Tick resistance: basophils in skin reactions of resistant guinea pigs. *Int. J. Parasitol.* 3:195–200.
7. Allen, J. R., B. M. Doube, and D. H. Kemp. 1977. Histology of bovine skin reactions to *Ixodes holocyclus* Neumann. *Can. J. Comp. Med.* 41:27–35.
8. Allen, J. R., H. M. Khalil, and J. E. Graham. 1979. The location of tick salivary antigens, complement and immunoglobulin in the skin of guinea-pigs infested with *Dermacentor andersoni* larvae. *Immunology* 38:467–472.
9. Allen, J. R., H. M. Khalil, and S. K. Wikel. 1979. Langerhans cells trap tick salivary gland antigens in tick-resistant guinea pigs. *J. Immunol.* 122:563–565.
10. Amosova, L. I. 1997. Ultrastructural features of histopathologic changes at the site of attachment of the larva of the Ixodid tick Haemaphysalis longicornis to the body of the host. *Parazitologiia* 31:514–520.
11. Anastopoulos, P., M. J. Thurn, and K. W. Broady. 1991. Anticoagulant in the tick *Ixodes holocyclus*. *Aust. Vet. J.* 68:366–367.
12. Anderson, J. F. 2002. The natural history of ticks. *Med. Clin. North Am.* 86:205–218.

13. Anguita, J., N. Ramamoorthi, J. W. Hovius, S. Das, V. Thomas, R. Persinski, D. Conze, P. W. Askenase, M. Rincon, F. S. Kantor, and E. Fikrig. 2002. Salp15, an *Ixodes scapularis* salivary protein, inhibits CD4(+) T cell activation. *Immunity* 16:849–859.

14. Balashov, Y. S. 1972. Bloodsucking ticks (Ixodoidea)—vectors of disease of man and animals. *Entomol. Soc. Amer. Misc. Publ.* 8:163–376.

15. Battsetseg, B., K. Mamiro, N. Inoue, L. Makala, H. Nagasanw, Y. Iwakura, Y. Toyoda, T. Mikami, and K. Fujisaki. 2002. Immune responses of interferon gamma (IFN-gamma) knock out mice to repeated *Haemaphysalis longicornis* (Acari: Ixodidae) nymph infestations. *J. Med. Entomol.* 39:173–176.

16. Beaudouin, E., G. Kanny, B. Guerin, L. Guerin, F. Plenat, and D. A. Moneret-Vautrin. 1997. Unusual manifestations of hypersensitivity after a tick bite: report of two cases. *Ann. Allergy Asthma. Immunol.* 79:43–46.

17. Bergman, D. 1996. Mouthparts and feeding mechanisms of haematopgagous arthropods, p. 30–61. *In* S. Wikel (ed.), *The Immunology of Host-Ectoparasitic Arthropod Relationships.* CAB International, Wallingford, United Kingdom.

18. Bergman, D. K., M. J. Palmer, M. J. Caimano, J. D. Radolf, and S. K. Wikel. 2000. Isolation and molecular cloning of a secreted immunosuppressant protein from *Dermacentor andersoni* salivary gland. *J. Parasitol.* 86:516–525.

19. Bior, A. D., R. C. Essenberg, and J. R. Sauer. 2002. Comparison of differentially expressed genes in the salivary glands of male ticks, *Amblyomma americanum* and *Dermacentor andersoni. Insect Biochem. Mol. Biol.* 32:645–655.

20. Bird, J. J., D. R. Brown, A. C. Mullen, N. H. Moskowitz, M. A. Mahowald, J. R. Sider, T. F. Gajewski, C. R. Wang, and S. L. Reiner. 1998. Helper T cell differentiation is controlled by the cell cycle. *Immunity* 9:229–237.

21. Bode, D., P. Speicher, and H. Harlan. 1987. A seed tick infestation of the conjunctiva: *Amblyomma americanum* larva. *Ann. Ophthalmol.* 19:63–64.

22. Brossard, M. 1977. Rabbits infested with the adults of Ixodes ricinus L.: passive transfer of resistance with immune serum. *Bull. Soc. Pathol. Exot. Filiales* 70:289–294.

23. Brossard, M., and V. Fivaz. 1982. *Ixodes ricinus* L.: mast cells, basophils and eosinophils in the sequence of cellular events in the skin of infested or re-infested rabbits. *Parasitology* 85:583–592.

24. Brossard, M., and S. K. Wikel. 1997. Immunology of interactions between ticks and hosts. *Med. Vet. Entomol.* 11:270–276.

25. Brown, A. F., and D. L. Hamilton. 1998. Tick bite anaphylaxis in Australia. *J. Accid. Emerg. Med.* 15:111–113.

26. Brown, S. J., and P. W. Askenase. 1981. Cutaneous basophil responses and immune resistance of guinea pigs to ticks: passive transfer with peritoneal exudate cells or serum. *J. Immunol.* 127:2163–2167.

27. Brown, S. J., and P. W. Askenase. 1985. Rejection of ticks from guinea pigs by anti-hapten-antibody-mediated degranulation of basophils at cutaneous basophil hypersensitivity sites: role of mediators other than histamine. *J. Immunol.* 134:1160–1165.

28. Brown, S. J., S. J. Galli, G. J. Gleich, and P. W. Askenase. 1982. Ablation of immunity to *Amblyomma americanum* by anti-basophil serum: cooperation between basophils and eosinophils in expression of immunity to ectoparasites (ticks) in guinea pigs. *J. Immunol.* 129:790–796.

29. Brown, S. J., and F. W. Knapp. 1981. Response of hypersensitized guinea pigs to the feeding of *Amblyomma americanum* ticks. *Parasitology* 83:213–223.

30. Champagne, D. E., and J. G. Valenzuela. 1996. Pharmacology of haemathopgagous arthropod saliva, p. 85–106. *In* S. Wikel (ed.), *The Immunology of Host-Ectoparasitic Arthropod Relationships.* CAB International, Wallingford, United Kingdom.

31. Chesney, J., C. Metz, M. Bacher, T. Peng, A. Meinhardt, and R. Bucala. 1999. An essential role for macrophage migration inhibitory factor (MIF) in angiogenesis and the growth of a murine lymphoma. *Mol. Med.* 5:181–191.

32. Chesney, T. M. 2000. Non-infectious predominantly deep inflammatory diseases, p. 635–641. *In* A. F. Hood (ed.), *Pathology of the Skin.* McGraw-Hill, New York, N.Y.

33. Chinery, W. A., and E. Ayitey-Smith. 1977. Histamine blocking agent in the salivary gland homogenate of the tick *Rhipicephalus sanguineus sanguineus. Nature* 265:366–367.

34. Christe, M., B. Rutti, and M. Brossard. 1998. Susceptibility of BALB/c mice to nymphs and larvae of *Ixodes ricinus* after modulation of IgE production with anti-interleukin-4 or anti-interferon-gamma monoclonal antibodies. *Parasitol. Res.* 84:388–393.

35. Christe, M., B. Rutti, and M. Brossard. 1999. Influence of the genetic background and parasite load of mice on the immune response developed against nymphs of *Ixodes ricinus. Parasitol. Res.* 85:557–561.

36. Christe, M., B. Rutti, and M. Brossard. 2000. Cytokines (IL-4 and IFN-gamma) and antibodies (IgE and IgG2a) produced in mice infected with *Borrelia burgdorferi* sensu stricto via nymphs of *Ixodes ricinus* ticks or syringe inoculations. *Parasitol. Res.* 86:491–496.

37. Clark, W. G. 1979. *Handbook of Experimental Pharmacology*, vol. 25, p. 311–356. Springer-Verlag, Berlin, Germany.

38. Cooper, B. J., and I. Spence. 1976. Temperature-dependent inhibition of evoked acetylcholine release in tick paralysis. *Nature* 263:693–695.

39. Coppolino, M. G., and S. Dedhar. 1998. Calreticulin. *Int. J. Biochem. Cell Biol.* 30:553-558.

40. Crampton, A. L., C. Miller, G. D. Baxter, and S. C. Barker. 1998. Expressed sequenced tags and new genes from the cattle tick, *Boophilus microplus. Exp. Appl. Acarol.* 22:177–186.

41. Culp, J. S. 1987. Seed ticks. *Am. Fam. Physician* 36:121–123.

42. Das, S., G. Banerjee, K. DePonte, N. Marcantonio, F. S. Kantor, and E. Fikrig. 2001. Salp25D, an *Ixodes scapularis* antioxidant, is 1 of 14 immunodominant antigens in engorged tick salivary glands. *J. Infect. Dis.* 184:1056–1064.

43. denHollander, N., and J. R. Allen. 1985. *Dermacentor variabilis*: acquired resistance to ticks in BALB/c mice. *Exp. Parasitol.* 59:118–129.

44. denHollander, N., and J. R. Allen. 1985. *Dermacentor variabilis*: resistance to ticks acquired by mast cell-deficient and other strains of mice. *Exp. Parasitol.* 59:169–179.

45. Dessens, J. T., and P. A. Nuttall. 1998. Mx1-based resistance to thogoto virus in A2G mice is bypassed in tick-mediated virus delivery. *J. Virol.* 72:8362–8364.

46. Dickinson, R. G., J. E. O'Hagan, M. Schotz, K. C. Binnington, and M. P. Hegarty. 1976. Prostaglandin in the saliva of the cattle tick *Boophilus microplus. Aust. J. Exp. Biol. Med. Sci.* 54:475–486.

47. Duckworth, P. F., Jr., G. F. Hayden, and C. N. Reed. 1985. Human infestation by *Amblyomma americanum* larvae ("seed ticks"). *South. Med. J.* 78:751–753.

48. Dvorak, H. F., M. C. Mihm, Jr., A. M. Dvorak, R. A. Johnson, E. J. Manseau, E. Morgan, and R. B. Colvin. 1974. Morphology of delayed type hypersensitivity reactions in man. I. Quantitative description of the inflammatory response. *Lab. Investig.* 31:111–130.

49. Estrada-Pena, A., and F. Jongejan. 1999. Ticks feeding on humans: a review of records on human-biting Ixodoidea with special reference to pathogen transmission. *Exp. Appl. Acarol.* **23:**685–715.

50. Failing, R. M., C. B. Lyon, and J. E. McKittrick. 1972. The pajaroello tick bite. The frightening folklore and the mild disease. *Calif. Med.* **116:**16–19.

51. Ferreira, B. R., and J. S. Silva. 1998. Saliva of *Rhipicephalus sanguineus* tick impairs T cell proliferation and IFN-γ-induced macrophage microbicidal activity. *Vet. Immunol. Immunopathol.* **64:**279–293.

52. Ferreira, B. R., and J. S. Silva. 1999. Successive tick infestations selectively promote a T-helper 2 cytokine profile in mice. *Immunology* **96:**434–439.

53. Ferreira, C. A., I. Da Silva Vaz, S. S. da Silva, K. L. Haag, J. G. Valenzuela, and A. Masuda. 2002. Cloning and partial characterization of a *Boophilus microplus* (Acari: Ixodidae) calreticulin. *Exp. Parasitol.* **101:**25–34.

54. Francischetti, I. M., J. G. Valenzuela, J. F. Andersen, T. N. Mather, and J. M. Ribeiro. 2002. Ixolaris, a novel recombinant tissue factor pathway inhibitor (TFPI) from the salivary gland of the tick, *Ixodes scapularis:* identification of factor X and factor Xa as scaffolds for the inhibition of factor VIIa/ tissue factor complex. *Blood* **99:**3602–3612.

55. Fujisaki, K., T. Kamio, and S. Kitaoka. 1984. Passage of host serum components, including antibodies specific for *Theileria sergenti*, across the digestive tract of argasid and ixodid ticks. *Ann. Trop. Med. Parasitol.* **78:**449–450.

56. Galli, S. J., and H. E. Dvorak. 1979. Basophils and mast cells: structure, function and role in hypersensitivity, p. 1–53. *In* S. Gupta and R. A. Good (ed.), *Comprehensive Immunology*, vol. 6. Plenum Medical Book Company, New York, N.Y.

57. Ganapamo, F., B. Rutti, and M. Brossard. 1995. In vitro production of interleukin-4 and interferon-gamma by lymph node cells from BALB/c mice infested with nymphal *Ixodes ricinus* ticks. *Immunology* **85:**120–124.

58. Gauci, M., R. K. Loh, B. F. Stone, and Y. H. Thong. 1989. Allergic reactions to the Australian paralysis tick, *Ixodes holocyclus:* diagnostic evaluation by skin test and radioimmunoassay. *Clin. Exp. Allergy* **19:**279–283.

59. Gauci, M., R. K. Loh, B. F. Stone, and Y. H. Thong. 1990. Evaluation of partially purified salivary gland allergens from the Australian paralysis tick *Ixodes holocyclus* in diagnosis of allergy by RIA and skin prick test. *Ann. Allergy* **64:**297–299.

60. Gauci, M., B. F. Stone, and Y. H. Thong. 1988. Detection in allergic individuals of IgE specific for the Australian paralysis tick, *Ixodes holocyclus. Int. Arch. Allergy Appl. Immunol.* **85:**190–193.

61. Gauci, M., B. F. Stone, and Y. H. Thong. 1988. Isolation and immunological characterisation of allergens from salivary glands of the Australian paralysis tick *Ixodes holocyclus. Int. Arch. Allergy Appl. Immunol.* **87:**208–212.

62. Gaunder, B. N. 1986. Insect bites and stings: managing allergic reactions. *Nurse Pract.* **11:**16, 19–22, 27–28.

63. Gillespie, R. D., M. C. Dolan, J. Piesman, and R. G. Titus. 2001. Identification of an IL-2 binding protein in the saliva of the Lyme disease vector tick, *Ixodes scapularis. J. Immunol.* **166:**4319–4326.

64. Gillespie, R. D., M. L. Mbow, and R. G. Titus. 2000. The immunomodulatory factors of bloodfeeding arthropod saliva. *Parasite Immunol.* **22:**319–331.

65. Gordon, J. R., and J. R. Allen. 1991. Factors V and VII anticoagulant activities in the salivary glands of feeding Dermacentor andersoni ticks. *J. Parasitol.* **77:**167–170.

66. Gordon, S. 2003. Alternative activation of macrophages. *Nat. Rev. Immunol.* **3:**23–35.

67. Gothe, R. 1999. *Zeckentoxikosen—Tick toxicoses.* Hieronymus Buchreproduktions GMBH, Munich, Germany.

68. Götz, H., and C. Patiri. 1975. Zeckenbißbedingte Dermatosen. *Med. Klin.* **70:**1332–1339.

69. Gregson, J. D. 1960. Morphology and functioning of the mouthparts of *Dermacentor andersoni. Acta Trop.* **17:**46–79.

70. Hajnicka, V., P. Kocakova, M. Slavikova, M. Slovak, J. Gasperik, N. Fuchsberger, and P. A. Nuttall. 2001. Antiinterleukin-8 activity of tick salivary gland extracts. *Parasite Immunol.* **23:**483–489.

71. Haller, O., and G. Kochs. 2002. Interferon-induced mx proteins: dynamin-like GTPases with antiviral activity. *Traffic* **3:** 710–717.

72. Hellmann, K., and R. I. Hawkins. 1967. The action of tick extracts on blood coagulation and fibrinolysis. *Thromb. Diath. Haemorrh.* **18:**617–625.

73. Herms, W. B., and M. T. James. 1961. *Medical Entomology*, 5th ed. The Macmillan Company, New York, N.Y.

74. Heyl, T. 1982. Tick bite alopecia. *Clin. Exp. Dermatol.* **7:** 537–542.

75. Heyne, H., E. A. Ueckermann, and L. Coetzee. 2001. First report of a parasitic mite, *Leptotrombidium (Hypotrombidium) subquadratum* (Lawerence) (Acari: Trombiculidae: Trombiculinae), from dogs and children in the Bloemfontein area, South Africa. *J. S. Afr. Vet. Assoc.* **72:**105–106.

76. Higgs, G. A., J. R. Vane, R. J. Hart, C. Potter, and R. G. Wilson. 1976. Prostaglandins in the saliva of the cattle tick, *Boophilus microplus* (Canestrini) (Acarina, Ixodidae). *Bull. Entomol. Res.* **66:**665–670.

77. Hill, C. A., and J. A. Gutierrez. 2000. Analysis of the expressed genome of the lone star tick, *Amblyomma americanum* (Acari: Ixodidae) using an expressed sequence tag approach. *Microb. Comp. Genomics* **5:**89–101.

78. Hoeppli, R., and H. H. Schumacher. 1962. Histological reactions to trombiculid mites with special reference to "natural" and "unnatural" hosts. *Z. Tropenmed. Parasitol.* **13:** 419–428.

79. Hoffmann, A., P. Walsmann, G. Riesener, M. Paintz, and F. Markwardt. 1991. Isolation and characterization of a thrombin inhibitor from the tick *Ixodes ricinus. Pharmazie* **46:**209–212.

80. Humphery-Smith, I., Y. H. Thong, D. Moorhouse, C. Creevey, M. Gauci, and B. Stone. 1991. Reactions to argasid tick bites by island residents on the Great Barrier Reef. *Med. J. Aust.* **155:**181–186.

81. Hwong, H., D. Jones, V. G. Prieto, C. Schulz, and M. Duvic. 2001. Persistent atypical lymphocytic hyperplasia following tick bite in a child: report of a case and review of the literature. *Pediatr. Dermatol.* **18:**481–484.

82. Ibrahim, M. A., A. H. Ghazy, T. M. Maharem, and M. I. Khalil. 2001. Factor Xa (FXa) inhibitor from the nymphs of the camel tick *Hyalomma dromedarii. Comp. Biochem. Physiol. B. Biochem. Mol. Biol.* **130:**501–512.

83. Jasinskas, A., D. C. Jaworski, and A. G. Barbour. 2000. *Amblyomma americanum:* specific uptake of immunoglobulins into tick hemolymph during feeding. *Exp. Parasitol.* **96:**213–221.

84. Jaworski, D. C., A. Jasinskas, C. N. Metz, R. Bucala, and A. G. Barbour. 2001. Identification and characterization of a homologue of the pro-inflammatory cytokine macrophage migration inhibitory factor in the tick, *Amblyomma americanum. Insect Mol. Biol.* **10:**323–331.

85. Jaworski, D. C., F. A. Simmen, W. Lamoreaux, L. B. Coons, M. T. Muller, and G. R. Needham. 1995. A secreted calreticulin protein in ixodid tick (*Amblyomma americanum*) saliva. *J. Insect Physiol.* **41:**369–375.

86. Jones, B. E. 1981. Human 'seed tick' infestation. *Amblyomma americanum* larvae. *Arch. Dermatol.* **117:**812–814.

87. Jones, L. D., E. Hodgson, T. Williams, S. Higgs, and P. A. Nuttall. 1992. Saliva activated transmission (SAT) of Thogoto virus: relationship with vector potential of different haematophagous arthropods. *Med. Vet. Entomol.* **6:**261–265.

88. Joubert, A. M., J. C. Crause, A. R. Gaspar, F. C. Clarke, A. M. Spickett, and A. W. Neitz. 1995. Isolation and characterization of an anticoagulant present in the salivary glands of the bont-legged tick, *Hyalomma truncatum. Exp. Appl. Acarol.* **19:**79–92.

89. Joubert, A. M., A. I. Louw, F. Joubert, and A. W. Neitz. 1998. Cloning, nucleotide sequence and expression of the gene encoding factor Xa inhibitor from the salivary glands of the tick, *Ornithodoros savignyi. Exp. Appl. Acarol.* **22:**603–619.

90. Jutel, M., T. Watanabe, M. Akdis, K. Blaser, and C. A. Akdis. 2002. Immune regulation by histamine. *Curr. Opin. Immunol.* **14:**735–740.

91. Karczewski, J., R. Endris, and T. M. Connolly. 1994. Disagregin is a fibrinogen receptor antagonist lacking the Arg-Gly-Asp sequence from the tick, *Ornithodoros moubata. J. Biol. Chem.* **269:**6702–6708.

92. Kassis, I., I. Ioffe-Uspensky, I. Uspensky, and K. Y. Mumcuoglu. 1997. Human toxicosis caused by the tick *Ixodes redikorzevi* in Israel. *Isr. J. Med. Sci.* **33:**760–761.

93. Kaufman, W. R. 1989. Tick-host interaction: a synthesis of current concepts. *Parasitol. Today* **5:**47–56.

94. Kemp, D. H., and A. Bourne. 1980. *Boophilus microplus:* the effect of histamine on the attachment of cattle-tick larvae—studies in vivo and in vitro. *Parasitology* **80:**487–496.

95. Kemp, D. H., B. F. Stone, and K. C. Binnington. 1982. Tick attachment and feeding: role of the mouthparts, feeding apparatus, salivary gland secretions and the host response, p. 119–168. *In* F. D. Obenchain and R. Galun (ed.), *Physiology of Ticks,* vol. 1. Pergamon Press, Oxford, United Kingdom.

96. Klompen, H., and D. Grimaldi. 2001. First mesozoic record of a parasitiform mite: a larval argasid tick in cretaceous amber (Acari: Ixodida: Argasidae). *Ann. Entomol. Soc. Am.* **94:**10–15.

97. Kopecky, J., M. Kuthejlova, and J. Pechova. 1999. Salivary gland extract from *Ixodes ricinus* ticks inhibits production of interferon-gamma by the upregulation of interleukin-10. *Parasite Immunol.* **21:**351–356.

98. Kovacs, H., I. D. Campbell, P. Strong, S. Johnson, F. J. Ward, K. B. Reid, and P. Eggleton. 1998. Evidence that C1q binds specifically to CH2-like immunoglobulin gamma motifs present in the autoantigen calreticulin and interferes with complement activation. *Biochemistry (Moscow)* **37:**17865–17874.

99. Kovar, L., J. Kopecky, and B. Rihova. 2001. Salivary gland extract from Ixodes ricinus tick polarizes the cytokine profile toward Th2 and suppresses proliferation of T lymphocytes in human PBMC culture. *J. Parasitol.* **87:**1342–1348.

100. Kovar, L., J. Kopecky, and B. Rihova. 2002. Salivary gland extract from Ixodes ricinus tick modulates the host immune response towards the Th2 cytokine profile. *Parasitol. Res.* **88:**1066–1072.

101. Kubes, M., N. Fuchsberger, M. Labuda, E. Zuffova, and P. A. Nuttall. 1994. Salivary gland extracts of partially fed *Dermacentor reticulatus* ticks decrease natural killer cell activity in vitro. *Immunology* **82:**113–116.

102. Kubes, M., P. Kocakova, M. Slovak, M. Slavikova, N. Fuchsberger, and P. A. Nuttall. 2002. Heterogeneity in the effect of different ixodid tick species on human natural killer cell activity. *Parasite Immunol.* **24:**23–28.

103. Kuthejlova, M., J. Kopecky, G. Stepanova, and A. Macela. 2001. Tick salivary gland extract inhibits killing of *Borrelia*

afzelii spirochetes by mouse macrophages. *Infect. Immun.* **69:**575–578.

104. Labuda, M., O. Kozuch, E. Zuffova, E. Eleckova, R. S. Hails, and P. A. Nuttall. 1997. Tick-borne encephalitis virus transmission between ticks cofeeding on specific immune natural rodent hosts. *Virology* **235:**138–143.

105. Lacombe, E. H., P. W. Rand, and R. P. Smith, Jr. 1999. Severe reaction in domestic animals following the bite of *Ixodes muris* (Acari: Ixodidae). *J. Med. Entomol.* **36:**227–232.

106. Latif, A. A., J. N. Maina, T. S. Dhadialla, and S. Nokoe. 1990. Histological reactions to bites of *Amblyomma variagatum* and *Rhipicephalus appendiculatus* (Acari: Ixodidae) fed simultaneously on naive or sensitized rabbits. *J. Med. Entomol.* **27:**316–323.

107. Lavaud, F., F. Bouchet, P. M. Mertes, and S. Kochman. 1999. Allergy to the bites of blood-sucking insects: clinical manifestations. *Allerg. Immunol. (Paris)* **31:**311–316.

108. Lavoipierre, M. M. 1965. Feeding mechanism of blood-sucking arthropods. *Nature* **208:**302–303.

109. Lawrie, C. H., and P. A. Nuttall. 2001. Antigenic profile of *Ixodes ricinus:* effect of developmental stage, feeding time and the response of different host species. *Parasite Immunol.* **23:**549–556.

110. Lawrie, C. H., S. E. Randolph, and P. A. Nuttall. 1999. *Ixodes* ticks: serum species sensitivity of anticomplement activity. *Exp. Parasitol.* **93:**207–214.

111. Leboulle, G., M. Crippa, Y. Decrem, N. Mejri, M. Brossard, A. Bollen, and E. Godfroid. 2002. Characterization of a novel salivary immunosuppressive protein from *Ixodes ricinus* ticks. *J. Biol. Chem.* **277:**10083–10089.

112. Leboulle, G., C. Rochez, J. Louahed, B. Ruti, M. Brossard, A. Bollen, and E. Godfroid. 2002. Isolation of Ixodes ricinus salivary gland mRNA encoding factors induced during blood feeding. *Am. J. Trop. Med. Hyg.* **66:**225–233.

113. Li, L., S. W. Reddel, and S. A. Krilis. 2000. Phenotypic similarities and differences between human basophils and mast cells, p. 97–130. *In* S. J. Galli (ed.), *Mast Cells and Basophils.* Academic Press, San Diego, Calif.

114. Limo, M. K., W. P. Voigt, A. G. Tumbo Oeri, R. M. Njogu, and O. K. Ole MoiYoi. 1991. Purification and characterization of an anticoagulant from the salivary glands of the ixodid tick *Rhipicephalus appendiculatus. Exp. Parasitol.* **72:**418–429.

115. Lue, H., R. Kleemann, T. Calandra, T. Roger, and J. Bernhagen. 2002. Macrophage migration inhibitory factor (MIF): mechanisms of action and role in disease. *Microbes Infect.* **4:**449–460.

116. Mann, K. G. 1999. Biochemistry and physiology of blood coagulation. *Thromb. Haemost.* **82:**165–174.

117. Mans, B. J., A. R. Gaspar, A. I. Louw, and A. W. Neitz. 1998. Apyrase activity and platelet aggregation inhibitors in the tick *Ornithodoros savignyi* (Acari: Argasidae). *Exp. Appl. Acarol.* **22:**353–366.

118. Mans, B. J., A. I. Louw, and A. W. Neitz. 2002. Savignygrin, a platelet aggregation inhibitor from the soft tick *Ornithodoros savignyi,* presents the RGD integrin recognition motif on the Kunitz-BPTI fold. *J. Biol. Chem.* **277:**21371–21378.

119. Mans, B. J., C. M. Steinmann, J. D. Venter, A. I. Louw, and A. W. Neitz. 2002. Pathogenic mechanisms of sand tampan toxicoses induced by the tick, *Ornithodoros savignyi. Toxicon* **40:**1007–1016.

120. Marshall, J. 1966. Alopecia after tick bite. *S. Afr. Med. J.* **40:**555–556.

121. Marshall, J. 1967. Ticks and the human skin. *Dermatologica* **135:**60–65.

122. Masina, S., and K. W. Broady. 1999. Tick paralysis: development of a vaccine. *Int. J. Parasitol.* **29:**535–541.

123. Mastellos, D., and J. D. Lambris. 2002. Complement: more than a 'guard' against invading pathogens? *Trends Immunol.* 23:485–491.

124. Matsuda, H., K. Fukui, Y. Kiso, and Y. Kitamura. 1985. Inability of genetically mast cell-deficient W/Wv mice to acquire resistance against larval *Haemaphysalis longicornis* ticks. *J. Parasitol.* 71:443–448.

125. Matsuda, H., T. Nakano, Y. Kiso, and Y. Kitamura. 1987. Normalization of anti-tick response of mast cell-deficient W/Wv mice by intracutaneous injection of cultured mast cells. *J. Parasitol.* 73:155–160.

126. Matsuda, H., N. Watanabe, Y. Kiso, S. Hirota, H. Ushio, Y. Kannan, M. Azuma, H. Koyama, and Y. Kitamura. 1990. Necessity of IgE antibodies and mast cells for manifestation of resistance against larval *Haemaphysalis longicornis* ticks in mice. *J. Immunol.* 144:259–262.

127. Matsushita, M., S. Thiel, J. C. Jensenius, I. Terai, and T. Fujita. 2000. Proteolytic activities of two types of mannose-binding lectin-associated serine protease. *J. Immunol.* 165:2637–2642.

128. Mbow, M. L., M. Christe, B. Rutti, and M. Brossard. 1994. Absence of acquired resistance to nymphal *Ixodes ricinus* ticks in BALB/c mice developing cutaneous reactions. *J. Parasitol.* 80:81–87.

129. Mbow, M. L., B. Rutti, and M. Brossard. 1994. IFN-γ IL-2, and IL-4 mRNA expression in the skin and draining lymph nodes of BALB/c mice repeatedly infested with nymphal *Ixodes ricinus* ticks. *Cell. Immunol.* 156:254–261.

130. Medzhitov, R., and C. A. Janeway, Jr. 1997. Innate immunity: impact on the adaptive immune response. *Curr. Opin. Immunol.* 9:4–9.

131. Mejri, N., N. Franscini, B. Rutti, and M. Brossard. 2001. Th2 polarization of the immune response of BALB/c mice to *Ixodes ricinus* instars, importance of several antigens in activation of specific Th2 subpopulations. *Parasite Immunol.* 23:61–69.

132. Miadonna, A., A. Tedeschi, E. Leggieri, P. Falagiani, M. Nazzari, M. Manzoni, and C. Zanussi. 1982. Anaphylactic shock caused by allergy to the venom of *Argas reflexus*. *Ann. Allergy* 49:293–294.

133. Miller, M. K. 2002. Massive tick (*Ixodes holocyclus*) infestation with delayed facial-nerve palsy. *Med. J. Aust.* 176:264–265.

134. Mocellin, S., M. C. Panelli, E. Wang, D. Nagorsen, and F. M. Marincola. 2003. The dual role of IL-10. *Trends Immunol.* 24:36–43.

135. Moneret-Vautrin, D. A., E. Beaudouin, G. Kanny, L. Guerin, and J. F. Roche. 1998. Anaphylactic shock caused by ticks (*Ixodes ricinus*). *J. Allergy Clin. Immunol.* 101:144–145.

136. Moorhouse, D. E. 1969. The attachment of some ixodid ticks to their natural hosts, p. 319–327. *In Proceedings of the Second International Congress of Acarology*. Hungarian Academy of Sciences, Budapest, Hungary.

137. Moorhouse, D. E. 1981. Ticks and their medical importance: a problem in human disease, p. 63–69. *In* J. Pearn (ed.), *Animal Toxins and Man: Human Poisoning by Toxic Australian Venomous Creatures*. Division of Health Education and Information, Brisbane, Australia.

138. Mulenga, A., C. Sugimoto, G. Ingram, K. Ohashi, and M. Onuma. 1999. Molecular cloning of two *Haemaphysalis longicornis* cathepsin L-like cysteine proteinase genes. *J. Vet. Med. Sci.* 61:497–502.

139. Mulenga, A., M. Sugino, M. Nakajima, C. Sugimoto, and M. Onuma. 2001. Tick-encoded serine proteinase inhibitors (serpins); potential target antigens for tick vaccine development. *J. Vet. Med. Sci.* 63:1063–1069.

140. Mulenga, A., A. Tsuda, M. Onuma, and C. Sugimoto. 2003. Four serine proteinase inhibitors (serpin) from the brown ear tick, Rhiphicephalus appendiculatus; cDNA cloning and preliminary characterization. *Insect Biochem. Mol. Biol.* 33:267–276.

141. Munksgaard, L., M. Frisch, M. Melbye, and H. Hjalgrim. 2000. Incidence patterns of Lyme disease and cutaneous B-cell non-Hodgkin's lymphoma in the United States. *Dermatology* 201:351–352.

142. Murphy, K. M., and S. L. Reiner. 2002. The lineage decisions of helper T cells. *Nat. Rev. Immunol.* 2:933–944.

143. Narasimhan, S., R. A. Koski, B. Beaulieu, J. F. Anderson, N. Ramamoorthi, F. Kantor, M. Cappello, and E. Fikrig. 2002. A novel family of anticoagulants from the saliva of *Ixodes scapularis*. *Insect Mol. Biol.* 11:641–650.

144. Need, J. T., and J. F. Butler. 1991. Sequential feedings by two species of argasid tick on laboratory mice: effects on tick survival, weight gain, and attachment time. *J. Med. Entomol.* 28:37–40.

145. Needham, G. R., D. C. Jaworski, F. A. Simmen, N. Sherif, and M. T. Muller. 1989. Characterization of ixodid tick salivary-gland gene products, using recombinant DNA technology. *Exp. Appl. Acarol.* 7:21–32.

146. Nienaber, J., A. R. Gaspar, and A. W. Neitz. 1999. Savignin, a potent thrombin inhibitor isolated from the salivary glands of the tick *Ornithodoros savignyi* (Acari: Argasidae). *Exp. Parasitol.* 93:82–91.

147. Nithiuthai, S., and J. R. Allen. 1984. Significant changes in epidermal Langerhans cells of guinea-pigs infested with ticks (*Dermacentor andersoni*). *Immunology* 51:133–141.

148. Nithiuthai, S., and J. R. Allen. 1985. Langerhans cells present tick antigens to lymph node cells from tick-sensitized guinea-pigs. *Immunology* 55:157–163.

149. Nuttall, P. A., L. D. Jones, M. Labuda, and W. R. Kaufman. 1994. Adaptations of arboviruses to ticks. *J. Med. Entomol.* 31:1–9.

150. Nuttall, P. A., G. C. Paesen, C. H. Lawrie, and H. Wang. 2000. Vector-host interactions in disease transmission. *J. Mol. Microbiol. Biotechnol.* 2:381–386.

151. Paesen, G. C., P. L. Adams, K. Harlos, P. A. Nuttall, and D. I. Stuart. 1999. Tick histamine-binding proteins: isolation, cloning, and three-dimensional structure. *Mol. Cell* 3:661–671.

152. Paesen, G. C., P. L. Adams, P. A. Nuttall, and D. L. Stuart. 2000. Tick histamine-binding proteins: lipocalins with a second binding cavity. *Biochim. Biophys. Acta* 1482:92–101.

153. Paine, S. H., D. H. Kemp, and J. R. Allen. 1983. In vitro feeding of *Dermacentor andersoni* (Stiles): effects of histamine and other mediators. *Parasitology* 86:419–428.

154. Parola, P., and D. Raoult. 2001. Ticks and tickborne bacterial diseases in humans: an emerging infectious threat. *Clin. Infect. Dis.* 32:897–928.

155. Patterson, J. W., J. E. Fitzwater, and J. Connell. 1979. Localized tick bite reaction. *Cutis* 24:168–169, 172.

156. Pearn, J. 1977. The clinical features of tick bite. *Med. J. Aust.* 2:313–318.

157. Reference deleted.

158. Petrovsky, N., and R. Bucala. 2000. Macrophage migration inhibitory factor (MIF). A critical neurohumoral mediator. *Ann. N. Y. Acad. Sci.* 917:665–671.

159. Proud, D., and A. P. Kaplan. 1988. Kinin formation: mechanisms and role in inflammatory disorders. *Annu. Rev. Immunol.* 6:49–83.

160. Qian, Y., R. C. Essenberg, J. W. Dillwith, A. S. Bowman, and J. R. Sauer. 1997. A specific prostaglandin E2 receptor and its role in modulating salivary secretion in the female tick, *Amblyomma americanum* (L.). *Insect Biochem. Mol. Biol.* 27:387–395.

161. Rai, R., P. A. Sprengeler, K. C. Elrod, and W. B. Young. 2001. Perspectives on factor Xa inhibition. *Curr. Med. Chem.* **8:**101–119.

162. Rand, K. N., T. Moore, A. Sriskantha, K. Spring, R. Tellam, P. Willadsen, and G. S. Cobon. 1989. Cloning and expression of a protective antigen from the cattle tick *Boophilus microplus. Proc. Natl. Acad. Sci. USA* **86:**9657–9661.

163. Raoult, D., A. Lakos, F. Fenollar, J. Beytout, P. Brouqui, and P. E. Fournier. 2002. Spotless rickettsiosis caused by *Rickettsia slovaca* and associated with *Dermacentor* ticks. *Clin. Infect. Dis.* **34:**1331–1336.

164. Rathinavelu, S., A. Broadwater, and A. M. de Silva. 2003. Does host complement kill *Borrelia burgdorferi* within ticks? *Infect. Immun.* **71:**822–829.

165. Ravanti, L., and V. M. Kahari. 2000. Matrix metalloproteinases in wound repair (review). *Int. J. Mol. Med.* **6:**391–407.

166. Ribeiro, J. M. 1987. *Ixodes dammini*: salivary anti-complement activity. *Exp. Parasitol.* **64:**347–353.

167. Ribeiro, J. M. 1989. Role of saliva in tick/host interactions. *Exp. Appl. Acarol.* **7:**15–20.

168. Ribeiro, J. M. 1995. Blood-feeding arthropods: live syringes or invertebrate pharmacologists? *Infect. Agents Dis.* **4:**143–152.

169. Ribeiro, J. M., T. M. Endris, and R. Endris. 1991. Saliva of the soft tick, *Ornithodoros moubata*, contains anti-platelet and apyrase activities. *Comp. Biochem. Physiol. A* **100:**109–112.

170. Ribeiro, J. M., P. M. Evans, J. L. MacSwain, and J. Sauer. 1992. *Amblyomma americanum*: characterization of salivary prostaglandins E2 and F2 alpha by RP-HPLC/bioassay and gas chromatography-mass spectrometry. *Exp. Parasitol.* **74:**112–116.

171. Ribeiro, J. M., G. T. Makoul, J. Levine, D. R. Robinson, and A. Spielman. 1985. Antihemostatic, antiinflammatory, and immunosuppressive properties of the saliva of a tick, *Ixodes dammini. J. Exp. Med.* **161:**332–344.

172. Ribeiro, J. M., and T. N. Mather. 1998. *Ixodes scapularis*: salivary kininase activity is a metallo dipeptidyl carboxypeptidase. *Exp. Parasitol.* **89:**213–221.

173. Ribeiro, J. M., and A. Spielman. 1986. *Ixodes dammini*: salivary anaphylatoxin inactivating activity. *Exp. Parasitol.* **62:**292–297.

174. Ribeiro, J. M., J. J. Weis, and S. R. Telford III. 1990. Saliva of the tick *Ixodes dammini* inhibits neutrophil function. *Exp. Parasitol.* **70:**382–388.

175. Ribeiro, J. M. C. 1995. How ticks make a living. *Parasitol. Today* **11:**91–93.

176. Samuel, C. E. 2001. Antiviral actions of interferons. *Clin. Microbiol. Rev.* **14:**778–809.

177. Sanders, M. L., G. E. Glass, R. B. Nadelman, G. P. Wormser, A. L. Scott, S. Raha, B. C. Ritchie, D. C. Jaworski, and B. S. Schwartz. 1999. Antibody levels to recombinant tick calreticulin increase in humans after exposure to *Ixodes scapularis* (Say) and are correlated with tick engorgement indices. *Am. J. Epidemiol.* **149:**777–784.

178. Sandrock, M., M. Frese, O. Haller, and G. Kochs. 2001. Interferon-induced rat Mx proteins confer resistance to Rift Valley fever virus and other arthropod-borne viruses. *J. Interferon Cytokine Res.* **21:**663–668.

179. Sangamnatdej, S., G. C. Paesen, M. Slovak, and P. A. Nuttall. 2002. A high affinity serotonin- and histamine-binding lipocalin from tick saliva. *Insect Mol. Biol.* **11:**79–86.

180. Sauer, J. R., R. C. Essenberg, and A. S. Bowman. 2000. Salivary glands in ixodid ticks: control and mechanism of secretion. *J. Insect Physiol.* **46:**1069–1078.

181. Sauer, J. R., J. L. McSwain, and R. C. Essenberg. 1994. Cell membrane receptors and regulations of cell function in ticks and blood-sucking insects. *Int. J. Parasitol.* **24:**33–52.

182. Schoeler, G. B., S. A. Manweiler, and S. K. Wikel. 1999. *Ixodes scapularis*: effects of repeated infestations with pathogen-free nymphs on macrophage and T lymphocyte cytokine responses of BALB/c and C3H/HeN mice. *Exp. Parasitol.* **92:**239–248.

183. Schoeler, G. B., and S. K. Wikel. 2001. Modulation of host immunity by haematophagous arthropods. *Ann. Trop. Med. Parasitol.* **95:**755–771.

184. Sirianni, M. C., G. Mattiacci, B. Barbone, A. Mari, F. Aiuti, and J. Kleine-Tebbe. 2000. Anaphylaxis after *Argas reflexus* bite. *Allergy* **55:**303.

185. Solley, G. O. 1990. Allergy to stinging and biting insects in Queensland. *Med. J. Aust.* **153:**650–654.

186. Sonenshine, D. E. 1991. *Biology of Ticks*, vol. 1. Oxford University Press, New York, N.Y.

187. Stone, B. F. 1988. Tick paralysis, particularly involving *Ixodes holocyclus* and other *Ixodes* species. *Adv. Dis. Vector Res.* **5:**61–85.

188. Sutherst, R. W., and D. E. Moorhouse. 1971. *Ixodes holocyclus* larvae and 'scrub-itch' in southeast Queensland. *Southeast Asian J. Trop. Med. Public Health* **2:**82–83.

189. Swenson, S., L. R. Bush, and F. S. Markland. 2000. Chimeric derivative of fibrolase, a fibrinolytic enzyme from southern copperhead venom, possesses inhibitory activity on platelet aggregation. *Arch. Biochem. Biophys.* **384:**227–237.

190. Szabo, M. P., and G. H. Bechara. 1999. Sequential histopathology at the *Rhipicephalus sanguineus* tick feeding site on dogs and guinea pigs. *Exp. Appl. Acarol.* **23:**915–928.

191. Tanaka, A. S., R. Andreotti, A. Gomes, R. J. Torquato, M. U. Sampaio, and C. A. Sampaio. 1999. A double headed serine proteinase inhibitor—human plasma kallikrein and elastase inhibitor—from *Boophilus microplus* larvae. *Immunopharmacology* **45:**171–177.

192. Tatchell, R. J., and D. E. Moorhouse. 1970. Neutrophils: their role in the formation of a tick feeding lesion. *Science* **167:**1002–1003.

193. Thurn, M., A. Gooley, and K. W. Broady. 1992. Identification of the neurotoxin from the Australian paralysis tick *Ixodes holocyclus. In* C. K. Tan (ed.), *Recent Advances in Toxicology Research*, vol. 2. Venom and Toxin Research Group, National University of Singapore, Singapore.

194. Tobias, N. 1949. Tickbite granuloma. *J. Invest. Dermatol.* **12:**255–259.

195. Tokura, Y., S. Ishihara, S. Tagawa, N. Seo, K. Ohshima, and M. Takigawa. 2001. Hypersensitivity to mosquito bites as the primary clinical manifestation of a juvenile type of Epstein-Barr virus-associated natural killer cell leukemia/lymphoma. *J. Am. Acad. Dermatol.* **45:**569–578.

196. Trager, W. 1939. Acquired immunity to ticks. *J. Parasitol.* **25:**57–81.

197. Tsai, M., C. S. Lantz, and S. J. Galli. 2000. Regulation of mast cell and basophil development by stem cell factor and interleukin 3, p. 3–20. *In* S. J. Galli (ed.), *Mast Cells and Basophils*. Academic Press, San Diego, Calif.

198. Tsuji, N., T. Kamio, T. Isobe, and K. Fujisaki. 2001. Molecular characterization of a peroxiredoxin from the hard tick *Haemaphysalis longicornis. Insect Mol. Biol.* **10:**121–129.

199. Ushio, H., S. Hirota, T. Jippo, S. Higuchi, Y. Kitamura, and H. Matsuda. 1995. Mechanisms of eosinophilia in mice infested with larval *Haemaphysalis longicornis* ticks. *Immunology* **84:**469–475.

200. Valenzuela, J. G., R. Charlab, T. N. Mather, and J. M. Ribeiro. 2000. Purification, cloning, and expression of a novel

salivary anticomplement protein from the tick, *Ixodes scapularis*. *J. Biol. Chem.* **275**:18717–18723.

201. Valenzuela, J. G., I. M. Francischetti, V. M. Pham, M. K. Garfield, T. N. Mather, and J. M. Ribeiro. 2002. Exploring the sialome of the tick *Ixodes scapularis*. *J. Exp. Biol.* **205**: 2843–2864.

202. Veraldi, S., M. Barbareschi, R. Zerboni, and G. Scarabelli. 1998. Skin manifestations caused by pigeon ticks (*Argas reflexus*). *Cutis* **61**:38–40.

203. Veraldi, S., G. Scarabelli, and R. Grimalt. 1996. Acute urticaria caused by pigeon ticks (*Argas reflexus*). *Int. J. Dermatol.* **35**:34–35.

204. Waladde, S. M., and M. J. Rice. 1982. The sensory basis of tick feeding behaviour, p. 71–118. *In* F. D. Obenchain and R. Galun (ed.), *Physiology of Ticks*, vol. 1. Pergamon Press, Oxford, United Kingdom.

205. Wang, H., W. R. Kaufman, W. W. Cui, and P. A. Nuttall. 2001. Molecular individuality and adaptation of the tick *Rhipicephalus appendiculatus* in changed feeding environments. *Med. Vet. Entomol.* **15**:403–412.

206. Wang, H., and P. A. Nuttall. 1994. Excretion of host immunoglobulin in tick saliva and detection of IgG-binding proteins in tick haemolymph and salivary glands. *Parasitology* **109**:525–530.

207. Wang, H., and P. A. Nuttall. 1995. Immunoglobulin G binding proteins in male *Rhipicephalus appendiculatus* ticks. *Parasite Immunol.* **17**:517–524.

208. Wang, H., and P. A. Nuttall. 1995. Immunoglobulin-G binding proteins in the ixodid ticks, *Rhipicephalus appendiculatus*, *Amblyomma variegatum* and *Ixodes hexagonus*. *Parasitology* **111**:161–165.

209. Wang, H., and P. A. Nuttall. 1999. Immunoglobulin-binding proteins in ticks: new target for vaccine development against a blood-feeding parasite. *Cell. Mol. Life Sci.* **56**:286–295.

210. Wang, X., L. B. Coons, D. B. Taylor, S. E. Stevens, Jr., and T. K. Gartner. 1996. Variabilin, a novel RGD-containing antagonist of glycoprotein IIb-IIIa and platelet aggregation inhibitor from the hard tick *Dermacentor variabilis*. *J. Biol. Chem.* **271**:17785–17790.

211. Waxman, L., and T. M. Connolly. 1993. Isolation of an inhibitor selective for collagen-stimulated platelet aggregation from the soft tick *Ornithodoros moubata*. *J. Biol. Chem.* **268**: 5445–5449.

212. Waxman, L., D. E. Smith, K. E. Arcuri, and G. P. Vlasuk. 1990. Tick anticoagulant peptide (TAP) is a novel inhibitor of blood coagulation factor Xa. *Science* **248**:593–596.

213. Whelen, A. C., and S. K. Wikel. 1993. Acquired resistance of guinea pigs to *Dermacentor andersoni* mediated by humoral factors. *J. Parasitol.* **79**:908–912.

214. Wikel, S. K. 1979. Acquired resistance to ticks: expression of resistance by C4-deficient guinea pigs. *Am. J. Trop. Med. Hyg.* **28**:586–590.

215. Wikel, S. K. 1980. Host resistance to tick-borne pathogens by virtue of resistance to tick infestation. *Ann. Trop. Med. Parasitol.* **74**:103–104.

216. Wikel, S. K. 1982. Histamine content of tick attachment sites and the effects of H1 and H2 histamine antagonists on the expression of resistance. *Ann. Trop. Med. Parasitol.* **76**:179–185.

217. Wikel, S. K. 1999. Tick modulation of host immunity: an important factor in pathogen transmission. *Int. J. Parasitol.* **29**: 851–859.

218. Wikel, S. K., and J. R. Allen. 1976. Acquired resistance to ticks. I. Passive transfer of resistance. *Immunology* **30**:311–316.

219. Wikel, S. K., and J. R. Allen. 1978. Acquired resistance to ticks. III. Cobra venom factor and the resistance response. *Immunology* **32**:457–465.

220. Wikel, S. K., and D. Bergman. 1997. Tick-host immunology: significant advances and challenging opportunities. *Parasitol. Today* **13**:383–389.

221. Willadsen, P., and F. Jongejan. 1999. Immunology of the tick-host interaction and the control of ticks and tick-borne diseases. *Parasitol. Today* **15**:258–262.

222. Willadsen, P., G. A. Riding, R. V. McKenna, D. H. Kemp, R. L. Tellam, J. N. Nielsen, J. Lahnstein, G. S. Cobon, and J. M. Gough. 1989. Immunologic control of a parasitic arthropod. Identification of a protective antigen from *Boophilus microplus*. *J. Immunol.* **143**:1346–1351.

223. Willadsen, P., D. Smith, G. Cobon, and R. V. McKenna. 1996. Comparative vaccination of cattle against *Boophilus microplus* with recombinant antigen Bm86 alone or in combination with recombinant Bm91. *Parasite Immunol.* **18**: 241–246.

224. Willadsen, P., G. M. Wood, and G. A. Riding. 1979. The relation between skin histamine concentration, histamine sensitivity, and the resistance of cattle to the tick, *Boophilus microplus*. *Z. Parasitenkd.* **59**:87–93.

225. Worms, M. J., P. W. Askenase, and S. J. Brown. 1988. Requirement for host Fc receptors and IgG antibodies in host immune responses against *Rhipicephalus appendiculatus*. *Vet. Parasitol.* **28**:153–161.

226. Yeruham, I., A. Hadani, I. Aroch, F. Galker, H. Gilor, and S. Rodrig. 2000. Cases of apparent tick toxicosis in humans and dogs, caused by *Ixodes redikorzevi* s.l. *Ann. Trop. Med. Parasitol.* **94**:413–415.

227. Yesudian, P., and A. S. Thambiah. 1973. Persistent papules after tick-bites. *Dermatologica* **147**:214–218.

228. Zeidner, N. S., B. S. Schneider, M. S. Nuncio, L. Gern, and J. Piesman. 2002. Coinoculation of *Borrelia* spp. with tick salivary gland lysate enhances spirochete load in mice and is tick species-specific. *J. Parasitol.* **88**:1276–1278.

229. Zhu, K., A. S. Bowman, D. L. Brigham, R. C. Essenberg, J. W. Dillwith, and J. R. Sauer. 1997. Isolation and characterization of americanin, a specific inhibitor of thrombin, from the salivary glands of the lone star tick *Amblyomma americanum* (L.). *Exp. Parasitol.* **87**:30–38.

230. Zhu, K., J. W. Dillwith, A. S. Bowman, and J. R. Sauer. 1997. Identification of hemolytic activity in saliva of the lone star tick (Acari: Ixodidae). *J. Med. Entomol.* **34**:160–166.

Tick-Borne Diseases of Humans
Jesse L. Goodman et al.
© 2005 ASM Press, Washington, D.C.

Chapter 7

Tick Systematics and Identification

JAMES E. KEIRANS AND LANCE A. DURDEN

INTRODUCTION

Ticks are obligate ectoparasites of terrestrial vertebrates (amphibians, reptiles, birds, and mammals). They belong to the class Arachnida, which as a group are distinguished from the class Insecta by having four pairs of legs as nymphs and adults, lacking both antennae and wings, and having two pairs of appendages associated with their mouthparts, i.e., chelicerae and pedipalps. All ticks and some mites are the only members of the Arachnida that are parasitic. In terms of size, ticks are the largest acarines and can be recognized by their dorsoventrally flattened appearance and by one component of the mouthparts, a hypostome with recurved teeth that acts as a holdfast organ, anchoring the tick to its host. They also possess a unique sensory apparatus, called Haller's organ on the tarsus of each foreleg. Ticks can be divided into three families, the Argasidae (soft ticks), Ixodidae (hard ticks), and Nuttalliellidae. The last-named family includes a single species from Africa that is infrequently collected, but the other two families are widespread and include many species, some of which may bite humans. The main morphological features of an adult male and female tick are shown in Fig. 1. Immature ticks are represented by larvae which have six legs, followed by nymphs which have eight legs but which lack the ventral genital apertures of adults. Nymphal argasids are very similar to adults except for this feature. A representative larval ixodid tick is shown in Fig. 2, a nymphal ixodid is shown in Fig. 3, and a larval argasid is shown in Fig. 4.

Ticks are found on all continents of the world, including Antarctica. There are relatively few species (~865), but their small numbers belie their importance as vectors of pathogens. They are second only to mosquitoes in their importance as vectors of disease agents to humans and are undoubtedly the prime vectors of pathogenic organisms to both wild and domestic animals.

While several species of ticks may occasionally attach to humans, relatively few species commonly bite humans, and some of these are vectors of disease-causing pathogens. In this chapter, we mostly consider ticks that are frequently recorded as biting humans. Table 1 lists identification guides for ticks that occur in the world's different zoogeographic regions.

KEY TO ADULT STAGES OF HUMAN-BITING TICK GENERA WORLDWIDE

1. Scutum absent; capitulum ventral (sometimes partially recessed); spiracular plates small; coxae unarmed (lacking spurs) (soft ticks: Argasidae) 2
Scutum present (entire in males, partial in females); capitulum anterior and terminal; spiracular plates large (posterior to coxa IV); coxae armed (with spurs) in most species (hard ticks: Ixodidae) 3
2. Margin of body narrow and acute with a distinct sutural line separating the dorsal and ventral surfaces (cosmopolitan) . . . . . *Argas*
Margin of body thick, rounded, and lacking a distinct sutural line between the dorsal and ventral surfaces (cosmopolitan) . . . . *Ornithodoros*
3. Eyes and festoons (rectangular areas separated by distinct grooves on posterior margin of dorsum) absent; anal groove extending anteriorly around anus (cosmopolitan) . . . . *Ixodes*
Eyes and festoons present; anal groove not extending anteriorly around anus . . . 4
4. Palps much longer than basis capituli; palpal article 2 much longer than broad 5
Palps about as long as basis capituli; palpal article 2 about as long as broad 6

(*key continues on page 128*)

James E. Keirans and Lance A. Durden • Institute of Arthropodology and Parasitology and Department of Biology, Georgia Southern University, Statesboro, GA 30460–8056.

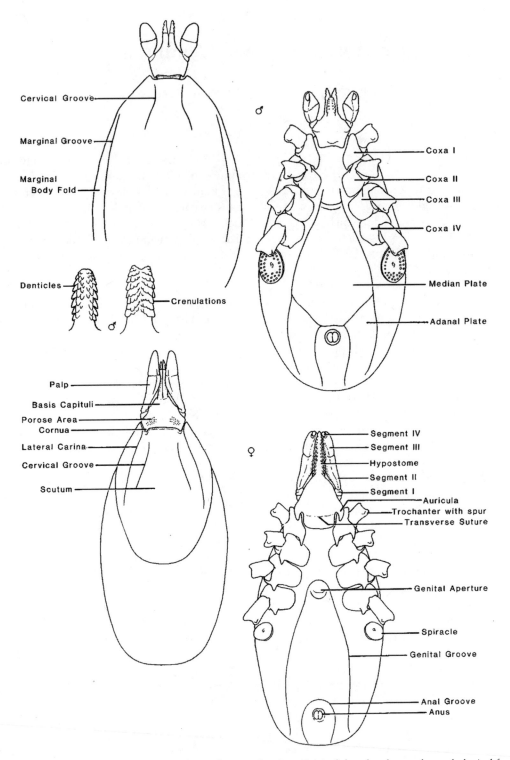

Figure 1. Line drawings of an ixodid (hard) tick (*Ixodes* sp.), showing prinicipal dorsal and ventral morphological features, including enlargements of two types of male hypostomes with denticles or crenulations (from reference 47 with permission).

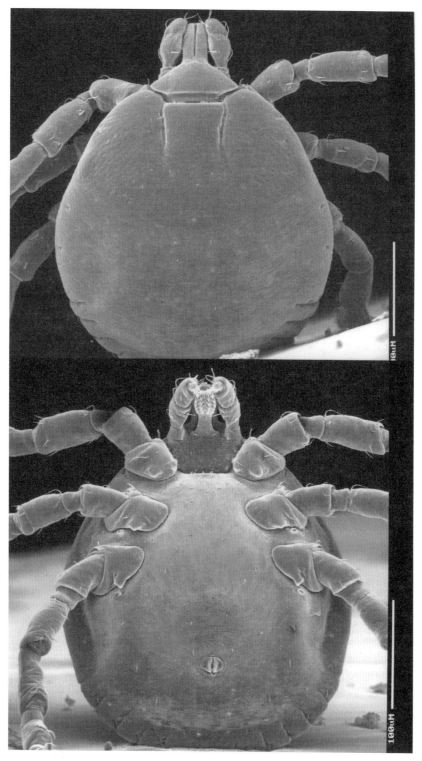

Figure 2. Scanning electron micrographs (SEMs) showing dorsal (top) and ventral (bottom) morphology of a larval ixodid (hard) tick. Scale bars, 100 μm. The specimen is *Amblyomma falsomarmoreum* from the Afrotropical region.

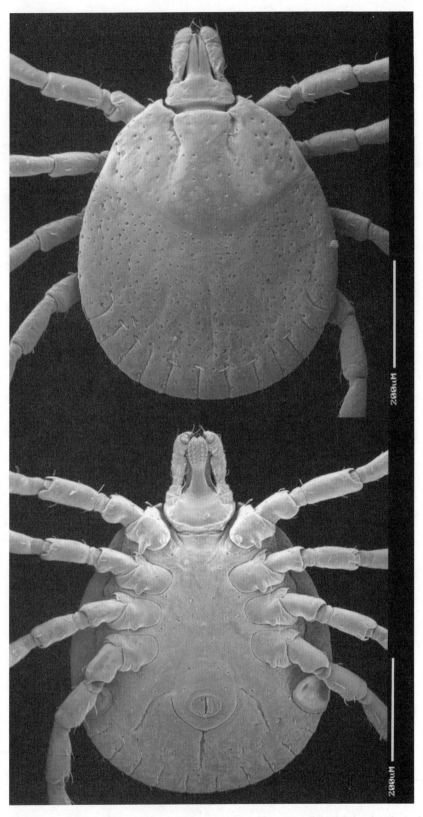

Figure 3. SEMs showing dorsal (top) and ventral (bottom) morphology of a nymphal ixodid (hard) tick. Scale bars, 200 μm. The specimen is *Amblyomma cajennense* from the Neotropical and southern Nearctic regions.

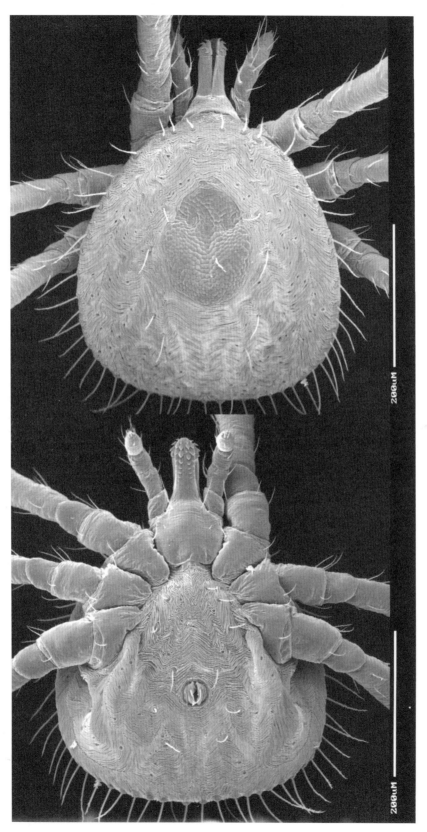

Figure 4. SEMs showing dorsal (top) and ventral (bottom) morphology of a larval argasid (soft) tick. Scale bars, 200 μm. The specimen is *Argas cucumerinus* from the Neotropical region.

Table 1. Tick identification references organized by zoogeographic region

Region	Country or area	Reference(s)
Afrotropical	General	6, 25, 62, 79, 86, 88
	Botswana	89
	Cameroon	61
	Central Africa	21–24, 83
	Ethiopia	60
	Kenya	87
	Madagascar	40, 82
	South Africa	44, 88
	Sudan	41
	Tanzania	91
	Uganda	56
	Zambia	33
Australian	General	25, 29, 67
Nearctic	United States, Canada, northern Mexico	9–12, 14–20, 25, 32, 35, 39, 47–49, 57, 66, 72, 92
Neotropical	General	25, 36, 37, 46, 92
	Argentina	3
	Belize	84
	Brazil	2, 4, 68
	Mexico	39
	Panama	27
	Venezuela	46
Oriental	General	25, 45, 85
	China	77, 78
	India	34, 59, 69, 81
	Indochina	80
	Indonesia	1, 52
	Japan, Korea, Ryuku Islands	90
	Malaysia	7, 52
	Micronesia	51
	Philippines	50
	Taiwan	74
	Thailand	75, 76
Palearctic	General	25, 30, 31, 54, 85
	Balkans	58, 63
	Belgium	26
	Central Europe	8
	Czech Republic, Slovakia	13
	Egypt	42
	Greece	64
	Italy	73
	Northwestern Europe	38
	Poland	70
	Romania	28
	Russia	30, 31, 65
	Saudi Arabia	43
	Turkey	53
	United Kingdom	5, 55, 71

(key continued from page 123)
5. Scutum inornate (lacking colored markings); festoons irregular, partially coalesced; males with additional ventral plates (adanal and subanal plates) (Africa, Asia, Europe) . . . . *Hyalomma*

Scutum usually ornate; festoons regular, not coalesced; males without additional ventral plates (worldwide in tropical, subtropical, and southern temperate regions) . . . . *Amblyomma*
6. Basis capituli hexagonal dorsally; usually inornate (cosmopolitan between latitudes of about 60° north and south, but most species occur in Africa) . . . . *Rhipicephalus*

Basis capituli rectangular dorsally; usually ornate (widespread) . . . . *Dermacentor*

ARGASIDAE CANESTRINI

Argas Latreille

This genus is characterized by a marginal suture encircling flattened dorsal and ventral body surfaces. Disks (small flattened projections) are present on both aspects of the body. Birds and cave-dwelling bats are hosts for many of the 60 or so species (Fig. 5).

Argas persicus (Oken) is established in most areas of the world and was introduced into the United States at some time in the past. It is believed to have originated in Central Asia and is a parasite of poultry. There have been numerous reports of this species attacking humans, but it appears that all reports are based on hearsay, although isolated instances of human tick bites may have occurred.

Ornithodoros Koch

These are thick, leathery, rounded ticks that are often difficult to find. There are about 115 species; unlike the genus *Argas*, whose members usually parasitize birds and bats, most members of the genus *Ornithodoros* parasitize mammals, including bats, but feed less often on birds (Fig. 6)

Known as the eyeless tampan, *Ornithodoros moubata* (Murray) (Color Plate 2A) is found in sub-Saharan Africa under arid conditions. Forty years ago, this species was broken up into four species representing "wild" and "domestic" populations, with wild populations tending to be larger and to be found in burrows of relatively large mammals such as warthogs. The typical *O. moubata* tick is the only known vector of *Borrelia duttoni* (Novy and Knapp), the organism responsible for human relapsing fever in eastern, central, and southern Africa. Humans are the only known reservoir host for this spirochete.

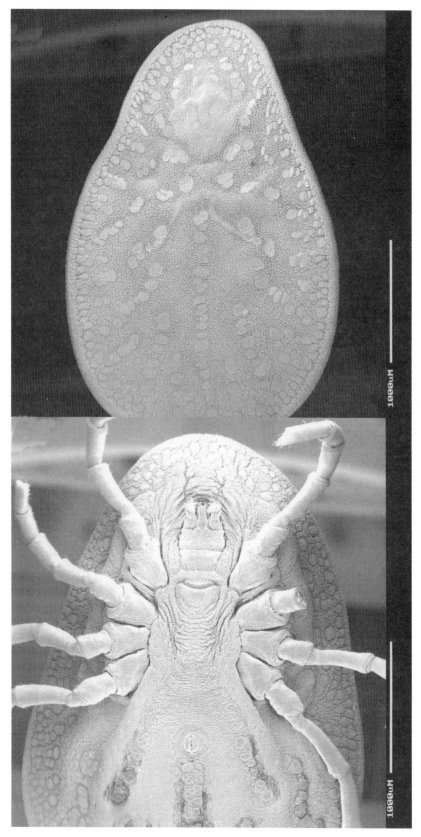

Figure 5. SEMs showing dorsal (top) and ventral (bottom) morphology of an adult *Argas* sp. soft tick. Scale bars, 1,000 μm. The upper specimen is a male *Argas reflexus* from the Palearctic region; the lower specimen is a female *A. cucumerinus* from the Neotropical region.

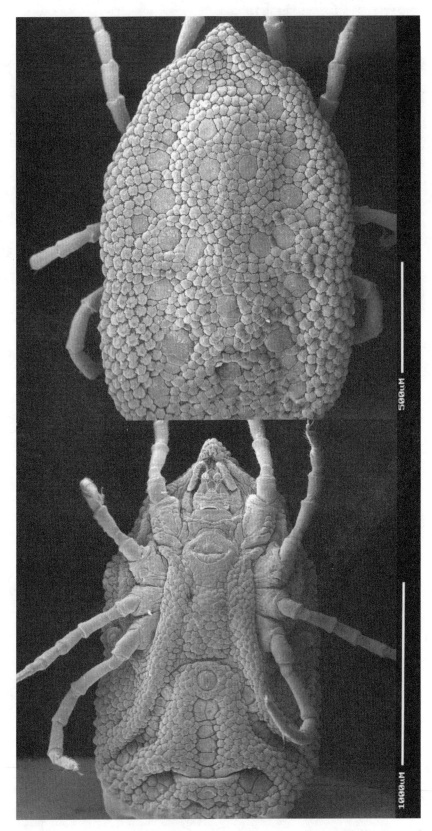

Figure 6. SEMs showing dorsal (top) and ventral (bottom) morphology of an adult *Ornithodoros* sp. soft tick. Scale bars, 500 μm (top) and 1,000 μm (bottom). The specimens are male *Ornithodoros capensis* ticks; this species occurs almost worldwide in tropical, subtropical, and warm temperate maritime regions.

Ornithodoros hermsi Wheeler, Herms, and Meyer is the vector of *Borrelia hermsii* (Davis), the organism that causes relapsing fever in humans in the western United States and southern British Columbia, Canada. In the United States, this tick species is found in Arizona, California, Colorado, Idaho, Montana, Nevada, New Mexico, Oregon, and Washington. It is probably also resident in Utah. This tick is primarily a parasite of ground squirrels and other rodents, but when their habitat (the nests of these rodents are often in old buildings) is eliminated, *O. hermsi* ticks will feed on humans.

IXODIDAE KOCH

Amblyomma Koch

There are approximately 120 species of *Amblyomma*, most of which are found in tropical and subtropical regions of the world. They can be found on all classes of terrestrial vertebrates, and all are three-host ticks (Fig. 7).

Amblyomma americanum (L.), the lone star tick (Color Plates 1A and 2F), is abundant in the Gulf Coast and the south-Atlantic and south-central United States; in recent decades, its range has extended north as far as Maine. This species can occur in vast numbers on a host, and all active stages (larva, nymph, and adult) will feed on humans. It is the vector of *Ehrlichia chaffeensis* Anderson, Dawson, Jones, and Wilson, the agent of human monocytic ehrlichiosis, and of *Borrelia lonestari* Barbour, Maupin, Teltow, Carter, and Piesman, an organism that has recently been cultivated and that is said to cause a Lyme-like illness.

Amblyomma variegatum (Fabricius) is an African tick species that was imported into islands in the Caribbean in the 19th century. It has become established on several islands; although an eradication program is underway, it is still a threat to the mainland United States. It occurs south of the Sahel transition zone of Africa across the continent from Senegal to Sudan and Ethiopia. From there, it extends southward to the Caprivi Strip and northern Zimbabwe. It is not found in the arid areas of the horn of Africa and northern Kenya. Hosts for adult ticks are domestic stock and many wild animals, especially larger antelopes. Immature ticks feed on the same host as adult ticks and on small mammals such as hares and on ground-dwelling birds.

Dermacentor Koch

This genus comprises about 30 species and is found primarily in the New World, but some species are also found in Asia, Africa, and Europe. With the exception of two species, all are three-host ticks (Fig. 8).

Dermacentor andersoni Stiles, the Rocky Mountain wood tick, is distributed in Canada from the coastal range of mountains in British Columbia eastward to eastern Saskatchewan. In the United States, it is found from the eastern-facing slopes of the Cascade Mountains to extreme western South Dakota and Nebraska and southward to northern Arizona and New Mexico. Although this tick does not feed on birds or reptiles, it is found on a wide variety of mammals. Immature ticks are found on rodents of all sizes but very rarely on large mammals. Adults will feed on almost any large mammal, including humans. In western North America, *D. andersoni* (Color Plates 2H and I) is the primary vector of *Rickettsia rickettsii* (Wolbach), which causes Rocky Mountain spotted fever, and of Colorado tick fever virus, among other pathogens. Females of this tick species can also cause tick paralysis.

Dermacentor variabilis (Say), the American dog tick (Color Plate 1B), is found in the states bordering the Atlantic westward to eastern Montana and Wyoming and southward through Nebraska, Kansas, and Oklahoma, to west-central Texas. There is also a large population of these ticks along coastal California and southern Oregon, and another in eastern Washington and the panhandle of Idaho. Like *D. andersoni*, immature *D. variabilis* ticks feed on rodents, with adults feeding on a large variety of mammals. It is the primary vector of the rickettsia of Rocky Mountain spotted fever in the eastern United States. Like the previous species, females of this species can also cause tick paralysis.

Dermacentor occidentalis Marx, the Pacific Coast tick, occurs along the Pacific Coast of North America from Oregon to Baja California, Mexico. Adults of this tick species sometimes bite humans, and it can transmit the agents of Rocky Mountain spotted fever, Colorado tick fever, tularemia [*Francisella tularensis* (McCoy and Chapin)] and Q fever [*Anaplasma burnetii* (Derrick)], formerly placed in the genus *Coxiella*. Females of this tick species can also cause tick paralysis, mainly in livestock.

Dermacentor reticulatus (Fabricius) is distributed in Eurasia from Britain in the west to central Asia in the east. The tick inhabits most ecotypes from grasslands to pastures and woodlands. Adults feed on large mammals, including domestic animals such as cattle, horses, sheep, and dogs, and wild mammals, such as deer, foxes, hares, and hedgehogs. Humans are also often bitten. Immature ticks feed on rodents, insectivores, and occasionally birds. It is a human vector of tick-borne encephalitis (TBE) virus, *Rickettsia conorii* Brumpt, the agent of Mediterranean spotted fever (boutonneuse fever), and of *F. tularensis*, the agent of tularemia.

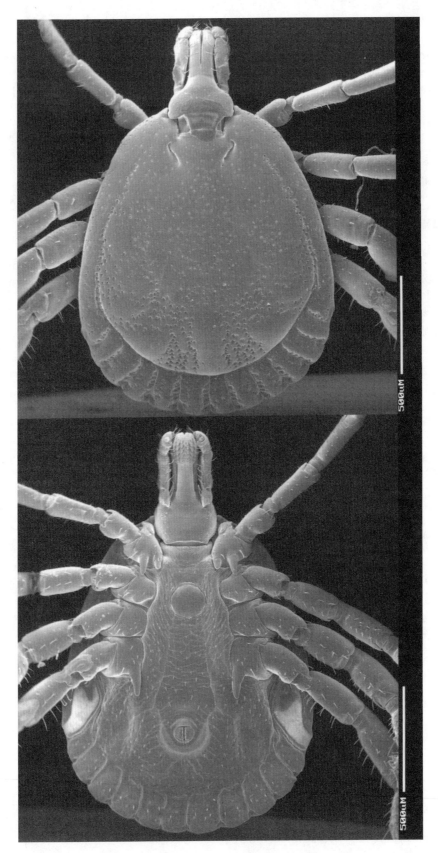

Figure 7. SEMs showing dorsal (top) and ventral (bottom) morphology of an adult *Amblyomma* sp. hard tick. Scale bars, 500 μm. The specimen (both figures) is a male *A. cajennense* tick; this species occurs in the Neotropical and southern Nearctic regions.

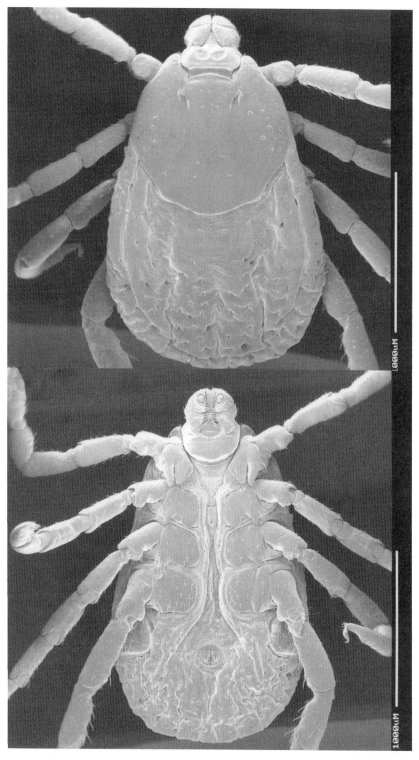

Figure 8. SEMs showing dorsal (top) and ventral (bottom) morphology of an adult *Dermacentor* sp. hard tick. Scale bars, 1,000 μm. The specimen is a female *D. andersoni* tick; this species occurs in the Nearctic region.

Dermacentor marginatus (Sulzer) is found in Germany, Switzerland, southern and central France, Italy, and Spain and eastwards into Central Asia. It also occurs in Morocco. Adults feed on large mammals such as humans, sheep, and cattle but also on dogs and hedgehogs. Immature ticks feed on rabbits, other small mammals, and ground-nesting birds such as quail. It is a vector of *A. burnetii,* the agent of Q fever, and of TBE virus.

Hyalomma Koch

The genus *Hyalomma* comprises about 30 species or subspecies. Members of this genus are found in southern Europe and Africa and eastward to the Indian subcontinent. These are large, inornate ticks of great morphological variability that are found in low-altitude areas of long, hot, dry conditions (Fig. 9).

Hyalomma marginatum rufipes Koch is primarily a tick of the drier areas of Africa, although it is also found in Yemen, Israel, Iraq, Turkey, and Russia. Immature *H. marginatum rufipes* ticks are carried northward on migrating birds, which may account for the scattered far-flung populations of this tick. It is an efficient vector of Crimean Congo hemorrhagic fever virus to humans. Some other members of this genus also sometimes bite humans.

Ixodes Latreille

The genus *Ixodes* is the largest tick genus with about 240 species and with representative species found on all of the world's continents. All, so far as is known, are three-host ticks, and all, except for one species that feeds on reptiles in all active stages, are found as adults on birds or mammals (Fig. 10).

Ixodes pacificus Cooley and Kohls, the western black-legged tick, is found from western British Columbia southward along the Pacific coast through the states of Washington, Oregon, and California and into northern Mexico. Populations have also been found in Arizona, Idaho, Nevada, New Mexico, and Utah. This species feeds on reptiles, birds, and mammals. Adults are often found on medium-sized or large mammals, including humans, and immature forms occur on lizards, birds, or small mammals. In the western United States, it is the primary vector of *Borrelia burgdorferi* Johnson, Schmid, Hyde, Steigerwalt, and Brenner, the agent of Lyme disease. This tick also transmits *Anaplasma* (formerly *Ehrlichia*) *phagocytophilum* (Foggie), the agent of human granulocytic ehrlichiosis (HGE).

Ixodes scapularis Say (synonym, *Ixodes dammini*), the black-legged tick (or the deer tick of some authors) is found in eastern North America from Prince Edward Island in the north and southward through New England, New York, and the mid-Atlantic states to central Florida. It is also found in the upper Midwest, in Oklahoma, Kansas, Missouri, Tennessee, Arkansas, the Gulf Coast states, and Texas. Adult ticks prefer large mammals, especially white-tailed deer. The white-footed mouse is the primary host for the larval stage in the north; but in the southern states, the cotton mouse and lizards are hosts for larvae. It is the primary Lyme disease agent vector in the north-central and eastern United States. It also transmits the agents of HGE and human babesiosis [*Babesia microti* (Franca)].

Ixodes ricinus (L.), the sheep tick (or castor bean tick), is found in Ireland in the west through Great Britain, all of Europe southward to the Caspian Sea, northern Iran, and western Russia. The adult stage typically feeds on domestic mammals, deer, other herbivores, and carnivores. Nymphs are found mainly on lizards, voles, and mice; larvae are found mainly on lizards, insectivores, rodents, and birds. It is a vector of the virus of TBE, the bacterium of Lyme disease, and the rickettsiae of boutonneuse fever and HGE.

Ixodes persulcatus Schulze, the taiga tick, is found from Poland in the west, and eastward through Russia to Siberia, the Primor (far eastern Russia), and Japan. It has also been recorded in the Korean peninsula. Like *I. ricinus*, *I. persulcatus* typically feeds on wild and domestic ungulates, dogs, and other mammals in its adult stage, with immature ticks feeding on small mammals such as the dormouse, the hedgehog, and occasionally birds. Throughout its range, it is the primary vector of the *Borrelia* of Lyme disease. It also transmits TBE-complex viruses.

Rhipicephalus Koch

The genus *Rhipicephalus* contains about 75 species; all but 3 or 4 species are three-host ticks. All but four species are unornamented. They are concentrated primarily in Africa, but a few are found in the Palearctic, and one species is found throughout the world (Fig. 11).

Rhipicephalus evertsi evertsi Neumann, the red-legged tick, feeds on cattle, horses, sheep, and goats but is rarely found on pigs or dogs. It is also an avid feeder on wild herbivores but not carnivores. This tick species is the most widespread of any rhipicephaline in the Afrotropical region. It ranges from the Sudan in the north to South Africa in the south and from Senegal in the west to Somalia in the east. It has also been introduced into Saudi Arabia and Yemen. *R. evertsi evertsi* was also introduced into the United States, and it took 2 years before eradication efforts were successful. This tick species is not known to be an important vector of any human disease agent, but it is a very important vector of *Borrelia theileri* (Laveran), the causative agent of spirochetosis in cattle.

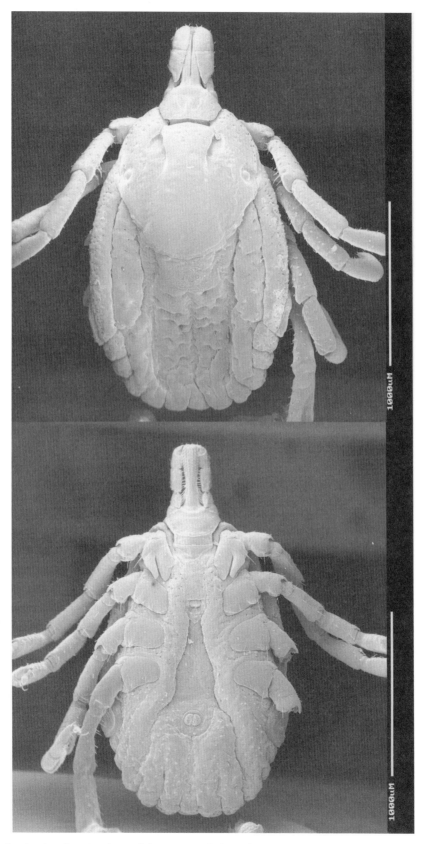

Figure 9. SEMs showing dorsal (top) and ventral (bottom) morphology of an adult *Hyalomma* sp. hard tick. Scale bars, 1,000 μm. The specimen is a female *H. truncatum* tick; this species occurs in the Afrotropical region, although a few have been collected from the southern Palearctic region. Note: some leg segments were removed from this specimen as part of another study.

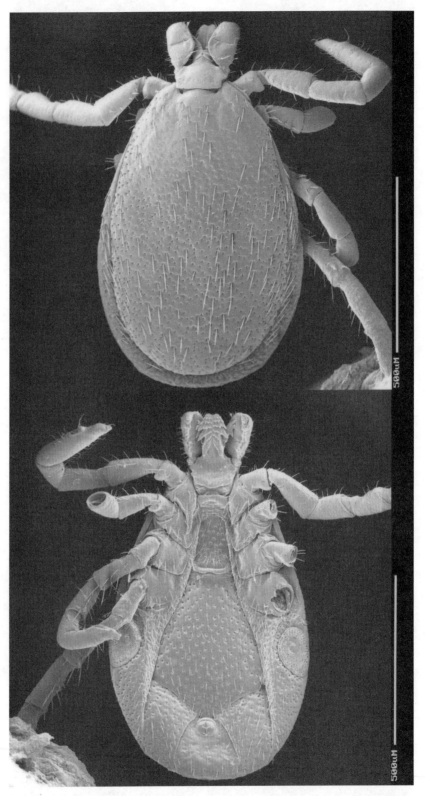

Figure 10. SEMs showing dorsal (top) and ventral (bottom) morphology of an adult *Ixodes* sp. hard tick. Scale bars, 500 μm. The specimen is a male *I. ricinus* tick; this species occurs in the Palearctic region. Note: some leg segments were removed from this specimen in connection with another study.

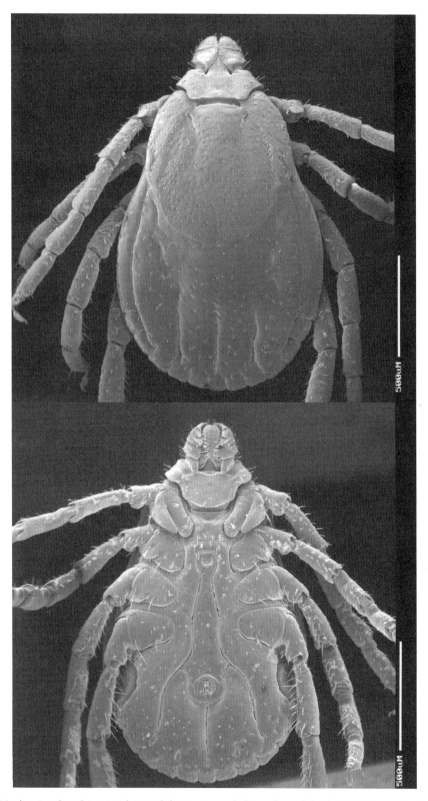

Figure 11. SEMs showing dorsal (top) and ventral (bottom) morphology of an adult *Rhipicephalus* sp. hard tick. Scale bars, 500 μm. The specimen is a female *Rhipicephalus appendiculatus* tick from the Afrotropical region.

Rhipicephalus sanguineus (Latreille), the brown dog tick (or kennel tick), is not, generally speaking, an ectoparasite of humans, although there have been several records of it feeding on humans in the United States. It is, however, the most widely distributed tick in the world and a true parasite of dogs. Originally from Africa, *R. sanguineus* is now found circumglobally on dogs, and it is one of the very few tick species that, in colder climates, completes its entire life cycle indoors. It is a vector of numerous pathogens to dogs and, where this tick species feeds on humans, a vector of the rickettsia of boutonneuse fever.

Acknowledgments.   Preparation of this chapter was supported, in part, by NIH grant 40729.

We are grateful to Jennifer Taylor for preparing the SEM figures.

REFERENCES

1. **Anastos, G.** 1950. The scutate ticks, or Ixodidae, of Indonesia. *Entomol. Am. New Ser.* 30:1–144.
2. **Aragão, H. De B.** 1911. Notas sobre ixódidas brazileiros. Notes sur les ixodidés du Brésil. *Mem. Inst. Oswaldo Cruz* 3:145–195.
3. **Aragão, H. De B.** 1935. Observações sobre os ixodideos da Republica Argentina. *Mem. Inst. Oswaldo Cruz* 30:519–533.
4. **Aragão, H. De B.** 1936. Ixodidas brasileiros e de alguns paizes limitrophes. *Mem. Inst. Oswaldo Cruz* 31:759–844.
5. **Arthur, D. R.** 1963. *British Ticks.* Butterworths, London, England.
6. **Arthur, D. R.** 1965. *Ticks of the Genus Ixodes in Africa.* The Athlone Press, University of London, England.
7. **Audy, J. R., M. Nadchatram, and B. L. Lim.** 1960. Malaysian parasites. XLIX. Host distribution of Malayan ticks (Ixodoidea). *Stud. Inst. Med. Res. Fed. Malaya* 29:225–246.
8. **Babos, S.** 1964. *Die Zeckenfauna Mittleuropas.* Akadémia Kiadó, Budapest, Hungary.
9. **Bequaert, J. C.** 1946. The ticks, or Ixodoidea of the northeastern United States and eastern Canada. *Entomol Am. New Ser.* 25:73–120, 121–184, 185–232.
10. **Brinton, E. P., and D. E. Beck.** 1963. Hard-bodied ticks of the western United States. Part I. Pictorial key for the separation of the genera. *Brigham Young Univ. Sci. Bull. Biol. Ser.* 2:1–28.
11. **Brinton, E. P., and D. E. Beck.** 1963. Hard-bodied ticks of the western United States. Part II and III. Pictorial keys for the separation of genera and nymphal and larval stages. *Brigh. Young Univ. Sci. Bull. Biol. Ser.* 3:1–21.
12. **Brinton, E. P., D. E. Beck, and D. M. Allred.** 1965. Identification of the adults, nymphs and larvae of ticks of the genus *Dermacentor* Koch (Ixodidae) in the western United States. *Brigham Young Univ. Sci. Bull. Biol. Ser.* 5:1–44.
13. **Černý, V.** 1972. The tick fauna of Czechoslovakia. *Folia Parasitol.* 19:87–92.
14. **Clifford, C. M., G. Anastos, and A. Elbl.** 1961. The larval ixodid ticks of the eastern United States (Acarina-Ixodidae). *Misc. Publ. Entomol. Soc. Am.* 2:213–237.
15. **Cooley, R. A.** 1938. The genera *Dermacentor* and *Otocentor* (Ixodidae) in the United States, with studies in variation. *Bull. Natl. Inst. Health* 171:1–89.
16. **Cooley, R. A.** 1946. The genera *Boophilus, Rhipicephalus,* and *Haemaphysalis* (Ixodidae) of the New World. *Bull. Natl. Inst. Health* 187:1–54.
17. **Cooley, R. A., and G. M. Kohls.** 1944. The genus *Amblyomma* (Ixodidae) in the United States. *J. Parasitol.* 30:77–111.
18. **Cooley, R. A., and G. M. Kohls.** 1944. The Argasidae of North America, Central America and Cuba. *Am. Midl. Nat. Monogr.* 1:1–152.
19. **Cooley, R. A., and G. M. Kohls.** 1945. The genus *Ixodes* in North America. *Bull. Natl. Inst. Health* 184:1–246.
20. **Durden, L. A., and J. E. Keirans.** 1996. *Nymphs of the Genus Ixodes (Acari: Ixodidae) of the United States: Taxonomy, Identification Key, Distribution, Hosts, and Medical/Veterinary Importance.* Thomas Say Publications in Entomology. Entomological Society of America, Lanham, Md.
21. **Elbl, A., and G. Anastos.** 1966. Ixodid ticks (Acarina, Ixodidae) of Central Africa. Vol. 1. Genus *Amblyomma* Koch, 1844. *Annales du Musée Royal de l'Afrique Centrale, Sciences Zoologiques* no. 145. Royal Museum for Central Africa, Tervuren, Belgium.
22. **Elbl, A., and G. Anastos.** 1966. Ixodid ticks (Acarina, Ixodidae) of Central Africa. Vol. 2. Genus *Ixodes* Latreille, 1795. *Annales du Musée Royal de l'Afrique Centrale, Sciences Zoologiques* no. 146. Royal Museum for Central Africa, Tervuren, Belgium.
23. **Elbl, A., and G. Anastos.** 1966. Ixodid ticks (Acarina, Ixodidae) of Central Africa. Vol. 3. Genus *Rhipicephalus* Koch, 1844. *Annales du Musée Royal de l'Afrique Centrale, Sciences Zoologiques,* no. 147. Royal Museum for Central Africa, Tervuren, Belgium.
24. **Elbl, A., and G. Anastos.** 1966. Ixodid ticks (Acarina, Ixodidae) of Central Africa. Vol. 4. Genera *Aponomma* Neumann, 1899, *Boophilus* Curtice, 1891, *Dermacentor* Koch, 1844, *Haemaphysalis* Koch, 1844, *Hyalomma* Koch, 1844 and *Rhipicentor* Nuttall and Warburton, 1908. *Annales du Musée Royal de l'Afrique Centrale, Sciences Zoologiques* no. 148. Royal Museum for Central Africa, Tervuren, Belgium.
25. **Estrada Peña, A., and F. Jongejan.** 1999. Ticks feeding on humans: a review of records on human-biting Ixodoidea with special reference to pathogen transmission. *Exp. Appl. Acarol.* 23:685–715.
26. **Fain, A.** 1990. Les tiques de Belgique (Acari: Ixodoidea). *Documents de Travail de l'Institut Royal des Sciences Naturelle de Belgique* 58:1–34.
27. **Fairchild, G. B., G. M. Kohls, and V. J. Tipton.** 1966. The ticks of Panama (Acarina: Ixidoidea), p. 167–219. *In* R. L. Wenzel and V. J. Tipton (ed.), *Ectoparasites of Panama.* Field Museum of Natural History, Chicago, Ill.
28. **Fieder, Z.** 1965. *Fauna Republicii Populare Române. Arachnida, vol. 5, fasc. 2. Acaromorpha, Suprafamilia Ixodoidea (Căpuşe).* Editura Academiei Republicii Populare Române, Bucharest, Romania. (In Romanian.)
29. **Fielding, J. W.** 1926. *Australian Ticks.* Service Publication no. 9. Division of Tropical Hygiene of the Commonwealth Department of Health, Melbourne, Australia.
30. **Fillippova, N. A.** 1966. *Argasid Ticks (Argasidae).* Fauna SSSR, Paukobraznye 4. Akademica Nauk, Moscow, Russia. (In Russian.)
31. **Fillippova, N. A.** 1977. *Ixodid Ticks of the Subfamily Ixodinae.* Fauna SSSR, Paukobraznye 4. Akademica Nauk, Moscow, Russia. (In Russian.)
32. **Furman, D. P., and E. C. Loonis.** 1984. The ticks of California (Acari: Ixodida). *Bull Cal. Insect Surv.* 25:1–239.
33. **Ganagarajah, M.** 1976. A preliminary check-list and host list of ticks of Zambia. Pest Research Report 1. National Council for Scientific Research, Lusaka, Zambia.
34. **Geevershese, G., and V. Dhanda.** 1987. *The Indian Hyalomma Ticks (Ixodoidea: Ixodidae).* Publications and Information Division, Indian Council of Agricultural Research, Krishi Anusandhan Bhavan, New Delhi, India.

35. **Gregson, J. D.** 1956. *The Ixodoidea of Canada.* Publication 930. Science Service, Entomology Division, Canada Department of Agriculture, Ottawa, Ontario, Canada.

36. **Guglielmone, A. A., A. Estrada-Peña, J. E. Keirans, and R. G. Robbins.** 2003. Ticks (Acari: Ixodida) of the neotropical region. International Consortium on Ticks and Tick-Borne Diseases (ICTTD-2), Utrecht, The Netherlands.

37. **Guimarães, J. H., E. C. Tucci, and D. M. Barros-Battesti.** 2001. *Ectoparasitos de Importância Veterinária.* Fundação de Amparo à Pesquisa do Estado de São Paulo, São Paulo, Brazil.

38. **Hillyard, P. D.** 1996. *Ticks of North-West Europe.* Synopses of the British fauna, new series, no. 52. Linnean Society of London and the Estuarine and Coastal Sciences Association. Field Studies Council Publications, Montford Bridge, United Kingdom.

39. **Hoffmann, A.** 1962. Monografia de los Ixodoidea de Mexico. *Rev. Soc. Mex. Hist. Nat.* 23:191–307.

40. **Hoogstraal, H.** 1953. Ticks (Ixodoidea) of the Malagasy Faunal Region (excepting the Seychelles). Their origins and host-relationships; with descriptions of five new *Haemaphysalis* species. *Bull. Mus. Comp. Zool. Harv. Coll.* 111:37–113.

41. **Hoogstraal, H.** 1956. African Ixodoidea. I. Ticks of the Sudan (*with Special Reference to Equatoria Province and with Preliminary Reviews of the Genera Boophilus, Margaropus, and Hyalomma*). Bureau of Medicine and Surgery, Department of the Navy, Washington, D.C.

42. **Hoogstraal, H., and M. N. Kaiser.** 1958. The ticks (Ixodoidea) of Egypt: a brief review and keys. *J. Egypt Public Health Assoc.* 33:51–85.

43. **Hoogstraal, H., H. Y. Wassef, and W. Büttiker.** 1981. Ticks (Acarina) of Saudi Arabia Fam. Argasidae, Ixodidae. *Fauna Saudi Arab.* 3:25–110.

44. **Horak, I. J., L. J. Fourie, H. Heyne, J. B. Walker, and G. R. Needham.** 2002. Ixodid ticks feeding on humans in South Africa: with notes on preferred hosts, geographic distribution, seasonal occurrence and transmission of pathogens. *Exp. Appl. Acarol.* 27:113–136.

45. **Itagaki, S., R. Noda, and T. Yamaguchi.** 1959. *Studies on the Ticks of the Domestic Animals in the Far East.* Japan Society for the Promotion of Science, Tokyo, Japan.

46. **Jones, E. K., C. M. Clifford, J. E. Keirans, and G. M. Kohls.** 1972. The ticks of Venezuela (Acarina: Ixodoidea) with a key to the species of *Amblyomma* in the Western Hemisphere. *Brigham Young Univ. Sci. Bull. Biol. Ser.* 17:1–40.

47. **Keirans, J. E., and C. M. Clifford.** 1978. The genus *Ixodes* in the United States: a scanning electron microscope study and key to the adults. *J. Med. Entomol. Suppl.* 2:1–149.

48. **Keirans, J. E., and L. A. Durden.** 1998. Illustrated key to nymphs of the tick genus *Amblyomma* (Acari: Ixodidae) found in the United States. *J. Med. Entomol.* 35:489–495.

49. **Keirans, J. E., and T. Litwak.** 1989. Pictorial key to the adults of hard ticks, family Ixodidae (Ixodida: Ixodidae), east of the Mississippi River. *J. Med. Entomol.* 26: 435–448.

50. **Kohls, G. M.** 1950. Ticks (Ixodoidea) of the Philippines. *Bull. Natl. Inst. Health* 192:1–28.

51. **Kohls, G. M.** 1957. Insects of Micronesia. Acarina: Ixodoidea. *Insects Micronesia* 3:85–104.

52. **Kohls, G. M.** 1957. Malaysian parasites. XVIII. Ticks (Ixodoidea) of Borneo and Malaya. *Stud. Inst. Med. Res. Fed. Malaya* 28:65–94.

53. **Kurtpinar, H.** 1954. *Turkish ticks (Ixodoidea). Morphology, biology, hosts, distribution and medical importance.* Guven Press, Ankara, Turkey. (In Turkish with English summary.)

54. **Marquez, F. J., P.-C. Morel, C. Guiguen, and J. Beaucournu.** 1992. Clef dichotomique des Ixodidae d'Europe. 1. Les larves du genre *Ixodes*. *Acarologia* 33:325–330.

55. **Martyn, K. P.** 1988. *Provisional Atlas of the Ticks (Ixodoidea) of the British Isles.* Biological Records Centre, Institute of Terrestrial Ecology, Monks Wood Experimental Station, Huntingdon, England.

56. **Matthysse, J. G., and M. H. Colbo.** 1987. *The Ixodid Ticks of Uganda Together with Species Pertinent to Uganda Because of Their Present Known Distribution.* Entomological Society of America, College Park, Md.

57. **Merten, H. A., and L. A. Durden.** 2000. A state-by-state survey of ticks recorded from humans in the United States. *J. Vector Ecol.* 25:102–113.

58. **Milutinović, M., Z. Miščević, and S. Katić-Radivojević.** 1995. Ticks (Acarina, Ixodoidea, Ixodidae) of Serbia: fauna and ecology. *Acta Vet. (Beograd)* 45:37–48.

59. **Miranpuri, G. S., and H. S. Gill.** 1983. *Ticks of India.* Lindsay & Macleod, Edinburgh, Scotland.

60. **Morel, P. C.** 1976. *Étude sur les tiques d'Éthiopie (acariens, ixodides).* Institut d'Élevage et de Médecine Vétérinaire des Pays Tropicaux, Maisons-Alfort, France.

61. **Morel, P. C., and J. Mouchet.** 1958. Les tiques du Cameroun (Ixodidae et Argasidae). *Ann. Parasitol. Hum. Comp.* 33:69–111.

62. **Okello-Onen, J., S. M. Hassan, and S. Essuman.** 1999. *Taxonomy of African ticks. An identification manual.* ICIPE Science Press, Nairobi, Kenya.

63. **Oswald, B.** 1939. On Yugoslavian (Balkan) ticks (Ixodoidea). *Parasitology* 31:271–280.

64. **Pantazi, G. P.** 1947. The ticks of Greece, p. 71–82. *Scientific Annual of the University of Athens.* Athens, Greece. (In Greek.)

65. **Pomerantzev, B. I.** 1950. *Ixodid ticks (Ixodidae)* Transl. A. Elbl, ed. G. Anastos. American Institute of Biological Sciences, Washington, D.C.

66. **Robbins, R. G., and J. E. Keirans.** 1992. *Systematics and ecology of the subgenus* Ixodiopsis *(Acari: Ixodidae: Ixodes)*, vol. 14. Thomas Say Foundation, Entomological Society of America, Lanham, Md.

67. **Roberts, F. H. S.** 1970. *Australian ticks.* Commonwealth Scientific and Industrial Research Orginization, Melbourne, Australia.

68. **Rohr, C. J.** 1909. *Estudos sobre ixódidas do Brasil.* Irmão & C. Gomes, Rio de Janeiro, Brazil.

69. **Sharif, M.** 1928. A revision of the Indian Ixodidae with special reference to the collection in the Indian Museum. *Rec. Ind. Mus.* 30:217–344.

70. **Siuda, K.** 1993. *Ticks of Poland (Acari: Ixodida). II. Taxonomy and distribution.* Polski Towarzystwo Parazytologiczne, Warsaw, Poland. (In Polish.)

71. **Snow, K. R.** 1978. Identification of larval ticks found on small mammals in Britain. *An Occasional Publication of the Mammalian Society*; Reading, Berkshire, England.

72. **Sonenshine, D. E.** 1979. Ticks of Virginia (Acari: Metastigmata). The insects of Virginia: No. 13. Research Division Bulletin 139, Agricultural Experiment Station, Virginia Polytechnic Institute and State University, Blacksburg.

73. **Starkoff, O.** 1958. *Ixodoidea d'Italia.* Studio monografico. Il Pensiero Scientifico, Rome, Italy.

74. **Sugimoto, M.** 1939. *Ticks of Taiwan.* Taihoku Imperial University, Taipei, Taiwan. (In Japanese.)

75. **Tanskul, P. L., H. E. Stark, and I. Inlao.** 1983. A checklist of ticks of Thailand (Acari: Metastigmata: Ixodoidea). *J. Med. Entomol.* 20:330–341.

76. **Tanskul, P. L., and I. Inlao.** 1989. Keys to adult ticks of *Haemaphysalis* Koch, 1844, in Thailand with notes on changes in taxonomy (Acari: Ixodoidea: Ixodidae). *J. Med. Entomol.* 26: 573–601.

77. Teng, K.-F. 1978. *Economic insect fauna of China*, fasc. 15. *Acari, Ixodoidea*. Science Press, Academica Sinica, Beijing, China. (In Chinese.)

78. Teng, K.-F., and Z. Jiang. 1991. *Economic insect fauna of China*, fasc. 39. *Acari, Ixodidae*. Science Press, Academica Sinica, Beijing, China. (In Chinese.)

79. Theiler, G. 1962. *The Ixodoidea Parasites of Vertebrates in Africa South of the Sahara (Ethiopian Region)*. Report of the Director of Veterinary Services, Onderstepoort. Project S.9958. Veterinary Institute, Onderstepoort, Republic of South Africa.

80. Toumanoff, C. 1944. *Les tiques (Ixodoidea) de l'Indochine*. Instituts Pasteur de l'Indochine, Saigon, Vietnam.

81. Trapido, H., M. G. R. Varma, P. K. Rajagopalan, K. R. P. Singh, and M. J. Rebello. 1964. A guide to the identification of all stages of the *Haemaphysalis* ticks of South India. *Bull. Entomol. Res.* 55:249–270.

82. Uilenberg, G., H. Hoogstraal, and J. M. Klein. 1980. Les tiques (Ixodoidea) de Madagascar et leur rôle vecteur. *Arch. Instit. Pasteur Madagascar* (special issue).

83. Van der Borght-Elbl, A. 1977. Ixodid ticks (Acarina, Ixodidae) of Central Africa. Vol. 5. The larval and nymphal stages of the genus *Amblyomma* Koch, 1844. *Annales du Musée Royal de l'Afrique Centrale, Sciences Zoologiques* no. 222. Royal Museum for Central Africa, Tervuren, Begium.

84. Varma, M. G. R. 1973. Ticks (Ixodidae) of British Honduras. *Trans R. Soc. Trop. Med. Hyg.* 67:92–102.

85. Volzit, O. V., and J. E. Keirans. 2002. A review of Asian *Amblyomma* species (Acari, Ixodida, Ixodidae). *Acarina* 10: 95–136.

86. Volzit, O. V., and J. E. Keirans. 2003. A review of African *Amblyomma* species (Acari, Ixodida, Ixodidae). *Acarina* 11: 135–214.

87. Walker, J. B. 1974. *The Ixodid Ticks of Kenya. A Review of Present Knowledge of Their Hosts and Distribution*. Commonwealth Institute of Entomology, London, England.

88. Walker, J. B. 1991. A review of the ixodid ticks (Acari, Ixodidae) occurring in southern Africa. *Onderstepoort J. Vet. Res.* 58:81–105.

89. Walker, J. B., D. Mehlitz, and G. E. Jones. 1978. Notes on the ticks of Botswana. *Deutsche Gesellschaft für Technische Zusammenarbeit (GTZ) GmbH*, no. 57. Eschborn, Germany.

90. Yamaguti, N., V. J. Tipton, H. L. Keegan, and S. Toshioka. 1971. Ticks of Japan, Korea, and the Ryukyu Islands. *Brigham Young Univ. Sci. Bull. Biol. Ser.* 15:1–226.

91. Yeoman, G. H., and J. B. Walker. 1967. *The Ixodid Ticks of Tanzania. A Study of the Zoogeography of the Ixodidae of an East African Country*. Commonwealth Institute of Entomology, London, England.

92. Yunker, C. E., J. E. Keirans, C. M. Clifford, and E. R. Easton. 1986. *Dermacentor* ticks (Acari: Ixodoidea: Ixodidae) of the New World: a scanning electron microscope atlas. *Proc. Entomol. Soc. Wash.* 88:609–627.

II. SPECIFIC DISEASES

Tick-Borne Diseases of Humans
Edited by Jesse L. Goodman et al.
© 2005 ASM Press, Washington, D.C.

Chapter 8

Colorado Tick Fever and Related *Coltivirus* Infections

ANTHONY A. MARFIN AND GRANT L. CAMPBELL

INTRODUCTION AND HISTORY

Accounts of "mountain fever" first appeared in the mid-19th century among Rocky Mountain settlers. Although this term likely included several infectious diseases, a relatively mild form of fever was endemic in the area, associated with headache, arthralgia, and myalgia that occurred in the spring and early summer and very likely represented Colorado tick fever (CTF) (7). In 1930, Becker suggested that mountain fever was associated with exposure to the Rocky Mountain wood tick (*Dermacentor andersoni*) and named it Colorado tick fever (5). In 1940, Topping and colleagues more fully described the illness (51). The viral cause of CTF was determined in a series of experiments by Florio and colleagues (26). Colorado tick fever virus (CTFV) is the prototypic member of the *Coltivirus* genus, a member of the family *Reoviridae*. A few other tick-borne coltiviruses have been associated with rare cases of human illness, including Salmon River virus isolated from a patient with CTF-like illness in Idaho and Eyach virus isolated in Europe.

ETIOLOGIC AGENT AND BIOLOGY

Classification

In addition to the coltiviruses, the *Reoviridae* family contains eight other virus genera. Members of three of these other genera, *Orthoreovirus*, *Rotavirus*, and *Orbivirus*, are known to infect humans; of these three, only *Orbivirus* contains arthropod-borne species (41, 53). Coltiviruses are distinguished from the closely related orbiviruses by containing 12 rather than 10 double-stranded RNA segments (35, 41, 52).

Historically, coltiviruses have been divided into subgroup A (North American and European species) and subgroup B (Asian species) based on genetic relatedness. More recently, researchers have suggested that these subgroups are only distantly related and that subgroup B should be separated into the *Seadornavirus* genus (3).

The four members of former subgroup A (CTFV; Salmon River virus; Eyach virus, isolated in Germany, France, and the Czech Republic; and a virus recovered from a hare and a ground squirrel in California) are antigenically related tick-borne viruses. Of these, CTFV and Salmon River virus are known to cause human disease; Eyach virus likely causes meningoencephalitis and polyradiculitis; and the virus recovered from a hare and a ground squirrel in California has yet to be associated with human disease (16, 17, 34, 36, 45).

Genetic Organization

Coltiviruses are double-capsid structures with icosahedral symmetry and an outer capsid diameter of approximately 80 nm (Color Plate 4). *Coltivirus* genomes comprise 12 double-stranded RNA segments with estimated sizes ranging from 0.24×10^6 Da (0.35 kbp) to 2.53×10^6 Da (3.7 kbp). The total size of the *Coltivirus* genome is approximately 18×10^6 Da (approximately 26 kbp).

Most *Coltivirus* proteins have yet to be characterized. If the genetic organization mirrors that of other members of the *Reoviridae*, it is likely that each segment encodes a monocistronic message and gene product. Although CTFV strains have similar polyacrylamide gel electrophoretic (PAGE) profiles, some genetic variability has also been shown by differential PAGE mobility of homologous RNA segments from different isolates obtained simultaneously from one location and by serum cross-neutralization studies (9, 34). By such analyses, RNA segments 4 and 6 appear to be more variable than other segments, with RNA segment 6 exhibiting the highest degree of variation. By analogy with other members of *Reoviridae*, RNA segments 4 and 6 probably encode the outer capsid proteins.

Anthony A. Marfin and Grant L. Campbell • Division of Vector-Borne Infectious Diseases, National Center for Infectious Diseases, Centers for Disease Control and Prevention, 3150 Rampart Road (Foothills Campus), Fort Collins, CO 80521.

In the laboratory, coltiviruses exhibit a high frequency of RNA segment reassortment, both in cell culture and in tick vectors. Reassortment in nature may permit the generation of potentially advantageous CTFV variants and allow the salvage of genes that have suffered deleterious mutations arising from the inherent infidelity of RNA genomic replication (47). RNA-RNA hybridization studies, however, have shown a relative conservation of gene sequences among CTFV isolates (6).

LIFE CYCLE AND ZOONOTIC HOSTS OF CTFV

Tick Vectors and Vertebrate Hosts

CTFV was first isolated from *D. andersoni* by Florio and colleagues, who demonstrated that these ticks can acquire infection by feeding on infected hamsters and subsequently transfer infection to naive animals (27). *Dermacentor occidentalis*, which occasionally feeds on humans, has also been found to be infected with CTFV but has not been established as a vector to humans (20, 21). In addition, CTFV has been isolated from several tick species that rarely feed on humans, including *Dermacentor albopictus*, *Dermacentor parumapertus*, *Otobius lagophilus*, *Ixodes sculptus*, *Ixodes spinipalpis*, and *Haemophysalis leporispalustris* (7). Although these may in some circumstances be important in maintaining natural cycles of the virus, epidemiological evidence indicates that *D. andersoni* is overwhelmingly the principal bridge vector between the enzootic transmission cycle and humans. All stages of *D. andersoni* can acquire the virus, and there is efficient vertical transmission of infection between life stages. However, transovarial transmission does not occur, and the virus must be horizontally transmitted to larval ticks from intermediate mammalian reservoirs to maintain the cycle. The CTFV titer in an infected adult tick is up to 10^5 times the mouse 50% lethal dose per milliliter of homogenized tissue, and infection can be maintained for up to 1 year (48).

CTFV is maintained in nature in a cycle involving *D. andersoni* ticks and a vertebrate reservoir in rodents and other small mammals (11, 19). In the usual cycle, larvae become infected when feeding on rodents, mainly in the summer. Infected larvae pass the infection transstadially as they molt to the nymphal stage. Infected nymphs usually overwinter before feeding on rodents in the following spring, transmitting CTFV as they feed. Engorged infected nymphs drop off the host and then pass CTFV to the adult stage as they molt. In the following year, adults seek medium-sized and large mammals (e.g., porcupines, canids, and deer) for blood meals prior to laying eggs. Adult ticks, the principal source of CTFV transmission to

humans, typically begin questing for hosts at the onset of snowmelt in February or March and maintain questing activity until June or early July, when surface water evaporates and they begin diapause. Nymphal ticks are most active in May and June, and larvae are most easily collected from animal hosts from June to September (7). The entire life cycle of *D. andersoni* takes 2 to 3 years.

Numerous mammalian genera have been found to be naturally infected with CTFV. Rodent hosts include *Peromyscus*, *Eutamias*, *Spermophilus*, *Sciurus*, *Tamiasciurus*, *Microtus*, *Perognathus*, *Dipodomys*, *Neotoma*, *Clethrionomys*, *Ochotona*, *Erethizon*, and *Marmota* spp. Evidence from field studies throughout the Rocky Mountain region indicates that the golden-mantled ground squirrel (*Spermophilus lateralis*), the least chipmunk (*Eutamias minimus*), the deer mouse (*Peromyscus maniculatus*), and the bushy-tailed woodrat (*Neotoma cinerea*) are among the most important reservoir hosts maintaining CTFV in nature (8, 11, 19). These virus-amplifying hosts develop apparently silent infections followed by persistent viremia that lasts for weeks to months. Hibernating animals may sustain viremia even longer, which has been proposed as one mechanism allowing CTFV to survive the winter and initiate a new transmission cycle when fed upon by immature stage ticks early the next year. Other mammalian hosts include *Lepus* and *Sylvilagus* spp. among lagomorphs, *Canis* spp. among carnivores, and *Cervus* and *Odocoileus* spp. among ungulates (7).

EPIDEMIOLOGY AND GEOGRAPHY OF CTF

Although most western states include CTF on their list of reportable diseases, CTF is not a nationally reportable disease. Surveillance for the disease is limited and nonstandardized, and surveillance data are almost certainly unreliable because of underdiagnosis and underreporting. From 1970 to 1984, there was a renewed scientific interest in CTF, and an annual average of 218 case reports was received by state health departments in the United States, with more than two-thirds of total cases reported in Colorado, followed by Utah and Montana (7). In the 15-year period spanning 1987 to 2001, a total of 777 CTF case reports was received by nine western state health departments, with Colorado (32 cases), Utah (8 cases), and Montana (7 cases) reporting the greatest annual averages (15) (Table 1). For unknown reasons, the number of reported cases has declined steadily during the past 2 decades. Nevertheless, CTF is almost certainly greatly underrecognized and underreported. One study in an area in Colorado in which CTF is hyperendemic revealed that only about 10% of cases occurring there were reported (7).

Table 1. CTF cases reported to state health departments, United States, 1987 to 2001

State	No. of CTF cases in:															Total no.
	1987	1988	1989	1990	1991	1992	1993	1994	1995	1996	1997	1998	1999	2000	2001	
Arizona	0	0	0	0	0	0	0	0	1	0	0	0	0	0	0	1
California	3	1	0	1	0	1	0	0	1	0	0	0	0	0	0	7
Colorado	74	43	60	59	54	39	32	25	33	27	9	10	7	2	2	476
Idaho	1	1	2	3	0	0	0	0	0	0	0	0	1	0	0	8
Montana	5	19	12	12	12	8	8	6	1	3	6	6	2	0	6	106
Nevada	0	0	0	0	0	0	0	1	1	0	0	0	0	0	0	2
New Mexico	0	0	0	0	0	0	0	0	0	0	0	0	0	0	0	0
Oregon	0	0	0	0	0	0	0	0	0	0	0	0	0	0	0	0
South Dakota	0	0	0	0	0	0	0	0	0	0	0	0	0	0	0	0
Utah	9	7	8	12	16	14	23	7	11	3	3	2	4	3	0	122
Washington	0	0	0	0	0	0	0	1	0	0	0	0	0	0	0	1
Wyoming	4	2	5	0	6	1	4	15	6	1	0	5	2	2	1	54
Total	96	73	87	87	88	63	67	55	54	34	18	23	16	7	9	777

CTFV is transmitted to humans throughout the geographic range of *D. andersoni* and only rarely outside this area. Risk factors for human transmission frequently cited include male sex, age from 10 to 49 years, and spring and early summer outdoor occupational and recreational activities at elevations from 1,200 to 3,000 meters in the Rocky Mountains from New Mexico to Canada, the Wasatch Range of Utah, the Black Hills of South Dakota, and the Sierra Nevada Range of Nevada and California (Fig. 1) (7, 10, 29). Conditions found on south-facing rock-covered slopes in the Colorado Rockies may be associated with greater risk of CTFV exposure among humans. These areas are characterized by open stands of ponderosa pine and juniper with underbrush that provides food and harborage for rodents and a moist microenvironment for ticks (39). Years in which higher than average precipitation or early snowmelt occurs may favor larger tick populations. At least one case of transfusion-associated CTF has been reported (14). The virus should be handled under biosafety level 3 conditions to minimize the risk to laboratory workers.

CLINICAL FEATURES OF CTF

Signs and Symptoms of Illness

More than 90% of CTF patients have a history of recent tick bite or exposure to an endemic site within 2 weeks of onset of illness, providing the basis for an estimated incubation period of 1 to 14 days (median, 4 days) (7, 14, 29). The onset of illness is usually sudden, with fever typically ranging from 38 to 40°C, chills, headache, generalized musculoskeletal aches, and malaise progressing to profound weakness and

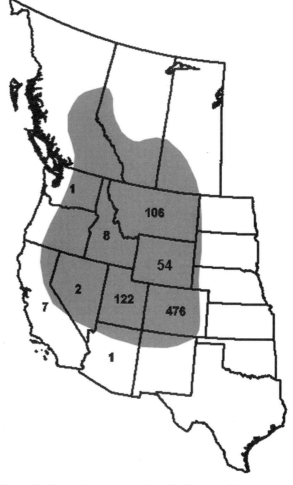

Figure 1. Approximate geographic distribution of *D. andersoni* (Rocky Mountain wood tick) and numbers of CTF cases reported to state health departments, United States, 1987 to 2001.

prostration (29, 49, 50). Nausea, vomiting, and other abdominal symptoms; photophobia; retroorbital pain; and sore throat are common but less prominent manifestations. Patients are usually bedridden during the acute illness, and in one case series as many as 14% of patients were hospitalized (29). On physical examination, patients appear weak and listless but show few specific signs of illness. Conjunctival injection, pharyngeal erythema, palatine enanthem, generalized lymphadenopathy, and mild hepatosplenomegaly may be found. A maculopapular or petechial rash involving the trunk and, less frequently, the extremities is seen in 5 to 12% of patients and may be confused with the rash of Rocky Mountain spotted fever (29, 50).

About half of all patients experience a biphasic illness in which, following several days of acute symptoms, there is a remission of fever and other symptoms, followed in a few days by a second short period of acute febrile illness that may be more severe than the first. Although a biphasic or saddleback fever curve is typical, some patients may experience no recrudescence, while a rare few have a third recrudescence. A prolonged convalescence characterized by weakness, lassitude, and fatigue is common and can continue for weeks. The duration of convalescence depends on patient age, typically continuing for 3 weeks or longer in patients at least 30 years of age and for 1 week or less in patients less than 20 years of age (29).

A small proportion of patients experience central nervous system (CNS) illness ranging from mild, self-limited aseptic meningitis to rare encephalitis with coma and death. CNS involvement may be manifested by severe headache, impaired sensorium, neck stiffness, and photophobia. Examination of the cerebrospinal fluid (CSF) in these patients typically demonstrates a lymphocytic pleocytosis (usually less than 500 cells/mm^3); the CSF may also show mild to moderately decreased glucose and elevated protein levels (50).

Clinical Pathology

Mild bleeding disorders associated with thrombocytopenia and petechiae occasionally occur in CTF patients aged less than 10 years. Life-threatening complications and deaths due to CTF are rare, and all such reported cases have been in children. Some have been associated with disseminated intravascular coagulation and bleeding, and some have involved severe damage to the CNS (28, 49, 50). The possibility of a concurrent *Rickettsia rickettsii* infection should be considered in such cases. In fatal cases of CTFV infection, pathological findings have included intravascular coagulation focal necrosis with mononuclear cell infiltrates in the brain, liver, spleen, heart, and intestinal tract; and acute renal tubular necrosis (13). In lab-

oratory studies, suckling mice and hamsters were similarly affected (30, 40).

Other reported complications have included hepatitis, epididymo-orchitis, pericarditis, myocarditis, and pneumonitis (13, 18, 25, 31, 37). Patients with hepatitis experience mild elevations of hepatic transaminase and creatine phosphokinase levels (29, 47, 50).

Pathogenesis

The tropism of CTFV for hematopoietic cells is demonstrated by the finding of viral antigen within erythrocytes and their precursors by immunofluorescence assay long after the acute phase of infection (1, 23, 24, 42, 44). Presumably, the intracellular location of CTFV shields it from immune clearance by neutralizing antibody throughout the natural life span of the red blood cell (24). In addition, CTFV can infect and replicate within human hematopoietic progenitor cell lines, which may explain the intraerythrocytic persistence as well as the frequently encountered leukopenia and thrombocytopenia. Low cell counts in these lines may be due to direct cytopathic effects of the virus on infected stem cells as they differentiate, host immune clearance of infected cells displaying viral antigen, decreased production of colony-stimulating factor by mononuclear cells, or circulating inhibitory factors such as lactoferrin or interferon. In early infection, high levels of alpha interferon can be detected in most CTF patients and are likely correlated with fever (2).

Leukopenia is the most characteristic laboratory finding in CTF. It is reported to be present in 70 to 100% of cases, variously described as falling to a mean of 3,900 total leukocytes/mm^3 5 to 6 days after the onset of illness (1) or to levels as low as 1,500 to 2,500 total leukocytes/mm^3 1 to 2 weeks after the onset of illness, with a rebound in the third week of illness (7, 43). Examination of peripheral blood smears reveals a left shift of polymorphonuclear leukocytes, a relative lymphocytosis, and the presence of atypical lymphocytes. Moderate thrombocytopenia, ranging from 20,000 to 60,000/mm^3, is common. Bone marrow examination reveals an arrest of granulocytic cell development and decreased megakaryocytes. Erythroblasts and primitive stem cells maintain infection throughout their development and carry CTFV with them into the circulation, but persistence of this virus in marrow cells has not been shown (44).

DIAGNOSIS OF CTF

Clinical Diagnosis

The provisional diagnosis of CTF depends heavily on clinical suspicion and a history of probable exposure to the Rocky Mountain wood tick. The differential diagnosis should include other vector-borne infectious diseases, including tularemia and Rocky Mountain spotted fever, also transmitted by hard ticks. Tick-borne relapsing fever, transmitted by soft ticks in the genus *Ornithodoros*, occurs in the range of CTFV and should also be considered. Because of their overlapping transmission seasons, CTF must also be distinguished from mosquito-borne arboviral fevers and a number of non-arthropod-borne viral diseases such as those caused by enteroviruses. Distinguishing CTF from Rocky Mountain spotted fever can be difficult early in the course of disease. However, the typical improvement after 2 to 3 days, the common appearance of a saddleback fever pattern, prominent leukopenia, and the absence (in adults) of a hemorrhagic rash that are seen in CTF weigh against a diagnosis of Rocky Mountain spotted fever. The geographic distributions of human anaplasmosis and ehrlichiosis do not overlap that of CTF.

Laboratory Diagnosis

Although a laboratory diagnosis of CTF can be made by virus isolation, detection of viral antigens or nucleic acids (e.g., by PCR), or serology, serologic tests remain the mainstay (4, 12, 22, 23, 33, 46). Available serologic tests include immunoglobulin M (IgM)-capture enzyme-linked immunosorbent assay (ELISA), immunofluorescent assay, plaque reduction neutralization, or (rarely) complement fixation tests. Tests of paired acute- and convalescent-phase serum specimens are often necessary. The "gold standard" for a laboratory diagnosis of CTF continues to be virus isolation from clinical material (especially blood), accompanied by demonstration of seroconversion in neutralization tests of acute- and convalescent-phase serum specimens. However, virus isolation and neutralization tests are available at only a few reference laboratories, including those of a few state health departments and the Centers for Disease Control and Prevention. In general, diagnostic tests for CTFV infection are unstandardized, and their accuracy has not been rigorously evaluated. The results of commercial laboratory tests for CTFV infection should be interpreted with particular caution and considered preliminary.

IgM detectable by IgM-capture ELISA usually appears at about the same time as neutralizing antibody (typically, 14 to 21 days after illness onset) or slightly before, but it often declines abruptly after 6 weeks, thus limiting the diagnostic usefulness of testing a single acute-phase serum sample by this method. Complement fixation antibodies may appear relatively late in the course of illness (22).

About one-third of CTF patients develop detectable neutralizing antibody titers within 10 days of illness onset; by 30 days, more than 90% have neutralizing antibody. Despite the presence of neutralizing antibody, nearly half of all patients continue to have detectable viremia by either immunofluorescent staining or virus culture, which is evidence of immunoprotective sequestration in erythrocytes (24, 32). Convalescence is accompanied by lasting immunity against reinfection. One case of a patient who experienced either relapse or reinfection a year after the initial infection (29) has been reported.

Isolation of CTFV by intracerebral or intraperitoneal inoculation of blood clot suspensions or red blood cells into suckling mice remains the most sensitive isolation technique, although virus isolation is also possible in Vero or BHK-21 cell cultures (in which cytopathic effects are observed). Mice sicken and die 4 to 8 days after inoculation. Specific virus isolation is confirmed by direct immunofluorescent staining of smears of mouse brain or blood or of cultured cells. Although less sensitive than isolation procedures, immunofluorescent staining is a rapid way to identify CTFV antigens in peripheral blood smears (23). The blood clot intended for virus isolation should be refrigerated but not frozen. When available, a source tick can be retained for speciation and virus isolation. Although diagnostic yield by either virus isolation or antigen detection is greatest during the acute phase of illness, viremia is at times detectable well into the period of convalescence. Nearly 50% of patients remain culture positive after 4 weeks, and 5 to 17% are culture positive up to 12 weeks after illness onset. Persistent CTFV antigens are detectable in red blood cells by direct fluorescence assay of samples from nearly 10% of patients up to 20 weeks after illness onset. There is no apparent relationship between the persistence of viremia and the duration of symptoms. PCR techniques are available to amplify and identify viral genomic products in clinical and experimental materials (33).

TREATMENT

No specific treatment for coltivirus infections is available. Management of CTF consists of supportive care with standard infection control precautions. Recovered patients wishing to donate blood should advise blood collection agencies of their prior illness and defer donation for a minimum of 6 months after illness recovery.

PREVENTION

Persons exposed to ticks during the spring and summer months in areas where CTF is endemic should take standard personal preventive measures against tick bites, such as wearing protective clothing, applying repellents as directed by the manufacturer, staying on trails and avoiding brushy areas, conducting periodic tick checks, and promptly removing any ticks found on clothing or skin. Repellents containing dimethylmetatoluamide (DEET) may be applied to skin and clothing, while those containing permethrin (which has a particularly long and durable residual effect) may be applied to clothing.

OTHER RELATED TICK-BORNE COLTIVIRUSES

A few scattered serologically diagnosed CTF-like cases have been reported in California from areas outside the known range of *D. andersoni* (36). A coltivirus that is antigenically distinct from CTFV has been isolated from a ground squirrel and a hare in these areas and has been suggested as the causative agent; *D. occidentalis* has been suggested as a possible vector. Salmon River virus, another coltivirus that is antigenically distinct from CTFV, was recovered from the blood of a person who developed a CTF-like illness following outdoor exposure in Idaho. This virus may be responsible for most CTF-like cases in Montana and Idaho (52). Eyach virus, a coltivirus that has been associated with cases of meningoencephalitis and polyradiculitis in the former Czechoslovakia, has been isolated from *Ixodes ricinus* and *Ixodes ventalloi* ticks in Germany and France (38, 45).

REFERENCES

1. **Andersen, R. D., M. A. Entringer, and W. A. Robinson.** 1985. Virus-induced leukopenia: Colorado tick fever as a human model. *J. Infect. Dis.* **151:**449–453.
2. **Ater, J. L., J. C. Overall, Jr., T. J. Yeh, R. T. O'Brien, and A. Bailey.** 1985. Circulating interferon and clinical symptoms in Colorado tick fever. *J. Infect. Dis.* **151:**966–968.
3. **Attoui, H., F. Billoir, P. Biagini, P. de Micco, and X. de Lamballerie.** 2000. Complete sequence determination and genetic analysis of Banna virus and Kadipiro virus: proposal for assignment to a new genus (*Seadornavirus*) within the family Reoviridae. *J. Gen. Virol.* **81:**1507–1515.
4. **Attoui, H., F. Billoir, J. M. Bruey, P. de Micco, and X. de Lamballerie.** 1998. Serologic and molecular diagnosis of Colorado tick fever viral infections. *Am. J. Trop. Med. Hyg.* **59:**763–768.
5. **Becker, F. E.** 1930. Tick-borne infections in Colorado. II. A survey of occurrence of infections transmitted by the wood tick. *Colorado Med.* **27:**87–95.
6. **Bodkin, D. K., and D. L. Knudson.** 1987. Genetic relatedness of Colorado tick fever virus isolates by RNA-RNA blot hybridization. *J. Gen. Virol.* **68:**1199–1204.
7. **Bowen, G. S.** 1988. Colorado tick fever, p. 159–166. *In* T. P. Monath (ed.), *The Arboviruses: Epidemiology and Ecology*, vol. 2. CRC Press, Boca Raton, Fla.
8. **Bowen, G. S., R. G. McLean, R. B. Shriner, D. B. Francy, K. S. Pokorny, J. M. Trimble, R. A. Bolin, A. M. Barnes, C. H. Calisher, and D. J. Muth.** 1981. The ecology of Colorado tick fever in Rocky Mountain National Park in 1974. II. Infection in small mammals. *Am. J. Trop. Med. Hyg.* **30:**490–496.
9. **Brown, S. E., B. R. Miller, R. G. McLean, and D. L. Knudson.** 1989. Co-circulation of multiple Colorado tick fever virus genotypes. *Am. J. Trop. Med. Hyg.* **40:**94–101.
10. **Burgdorfer, W.** 1977. Tick-borne diseases in the United States: Rocky Mountain spotted fever and Colorado tick fever. A review. *Acta Trop.* **34:**103–126.
11. **Burgdorfer, W., and C. M. Eklund.** 1959. Studies on the ecology of Colorado tick fever virus in western Montana. *Am. J. Hyg.* **69:**127–137.
12. **Calisher, C. H., J. D. Poland, S. B. Calisher, and L. A. Warmoth.** 1985. Diagnosis of Colorado tick fever virus infection by enzyme immunoassays for immunoglobulin M and G antibodies. *J. Clin. Microbiol.* **22:**84–88.
13. **Centers for Disease Control.** 1972. Colorado tick fever—Colorado. *Morb. Mortal. Wkly. Rep.* **21:**374.
14. **Centers for Disease Control.** 1975. Transmission of Colorado tick fever virus by blood transfusion—Montana. *Morb. Mortal. Wkly. Rep.* **24:**422, 427.
15. **Centers for Disease Control and Prevention.** Unpublished data.
16. **Chastel, C.** 1998. Erve and Eyach: two viruses isolated in France, neuropathogenic for man and widely distributed in Western Europe. *Bull. Acad. Natl. Med.* **182:**801–809. (In French.)
17. **Chastel, C., A. J. Main, A. Couatarmanac'h, G. Le Lay, D. L. Knudson, M. C. Quillien, and J. C. Beaucournu.** 1984. Isolation of Eyach virus (Reoviridae, Colorado tick fever group) from *Ixodes ricinus* and *I. ventalloi* ticks in France. *Arch. Virol.* **82:**161–171.
18. **Draughn, D. E., O. F. Sieber, Jr., and J. H. Umlauf, Jr.** 1965. Colorado tick fever encephalitis. *Clin. Pediatr. (Philadelphia)* **4:**626–628.
19. **Eklund, C. M.** 1962. Natural history of Colorado tick fever virus. *Lancet* **82:**172–174.
20. **Eklund, C. M., G. M. Kohls, and J. M. Brennan.** 1955. Distribution of Colorado tick fever and virus-carrying ticks. *JAMA* **157:**335–337.
21. **Eklund, C. M., G. M. Kohls, W. L. Jellison, W. Burgdorfer, R. C. Kennedy, and L. Thomas.** 1959. The clinical and ecological aspects of Colorado tick fever. *Proc. 6th Int. Congr. Trop. Med. Malariol.* **5:**197–203.
22. **Emmons, R. W., D. V. Dondero, V. Devlin, and E. H. Lennette.** 1969. Serologic diagnosis of Colorado tick fever. A comparison of complement-fixation, immunofluorescence, and plaque-reduction methods. *Am. J. Trop. Med. Hyg.* **18:**796–802.
23. **Emmons, R. W., and E. H. Lennette.** 1966. Immunofluorescent staining in the laboratory diagnosis of Colorado tick fever. *J. Lab. Clin. Med.* **68:**923–929.
24. **Emmons, R. W., L. S. Oshiro, H. N. Johnson, and E. H. Lennette.** 1972. Intra-erythrocytic location of Colorado tick fever virus. *J. Gen. Virol.* **17:**185–195.
25. **Emmons, R. W., and H. I. Schade.** 1972. Colorado tick fever simulating acute myocardial infarction. *JAMA* **222:**87–88.
26. **Florio, L., M. D. Stewart, and E. R. Mugrage.** 1946. The etiology of Colorado tick fever. *J. Exp. Med.* **83:**1–10.
27. **Florio, L., M. D. Stewart, and E. R. Mugrage.** 1944. The experimental transmission of Colorado tick fever. *J. Exp. Med.* **80:**165–188.
28. **Fraser, C. H., and D. W. Schiff.** 1962. Colorado tick fever encephalitis. Report of a case. *Pediatrics* **29:**187–190.
29. **Goodpasture, H. C., J. D. Poland, D. B. Francy, G. S. Bowen, and K. A. Horn.** 1978. Colorado tick fever: clinical, epidemiologic, and laboratory aspects of 228 cases in Colorado in 1973–1974. *Ann. Intern. Med.* **88:**303–310.

30. Hadlow, W. J. 1957. Histopathologic changes in suckling mice infected with the virus of Colorado tick fever. *J. Infect. Dis.* **101:**158–167.

31. Hierholzer, W. J., and D. W. Barry. 1971. Colorado tick fever pericarditis. *JAMA* **217:**825.

32. Hughes, L. E., E. A. Casper, and C. M. Clifford. 1974. Persistence of Colorado tick fever virus in red blood cells. *Am. J. Trop. Med. Hyg.* **23:**530–532.

33. Johnson, A. J., N. Karabatsos, and R. S. Lanciotti. 1997. Detection of Colorado tick fever virus by using reverse transcriptase PCR and application of the technique in laboratory diagnosis. *J. Clin. Microbiol.* **35:**1203–1208.

34. Karabatsos, N., J. D. Poland, R. W. Emmons, J. H. Mathews, C. H. Calisher, and K. L. Wolff. 1987. Antigenic variants of Colorado tick fever virus. *J. Gen. Virol.* **68:**1463–1469.

35. Knudson, D. L. 1981. Genome of Colorado tick fever virus. *Virology* **112:**361–364.

36. Lane, R. S., R. W. Emmons, V. Devlin, D. V. Dondero, and B. C. Nelson. 1982. Survey for evidence of Colorado tick fever virus outside of the known endemic area in California. *Am. J. Trop. Med. Hyg.* **31:**837–843.

37. Loge, R. V. 1985. Acute hepatitis associated with Colorado tick fever. *West. J. Med.* **142:**91–92.

38. Malkova, D., J. Holubova, J. M. Kolman, Z. Marhoul, F. Hanzal, H. Kulkova, K. Markvart, and L. Simkova. 1980. Antibodies against some arboviruses in persons with various neuropathies. *Acta Virol.* **24:**298.

39. McLean, R. G., R. B. Shriner, K. S. Pokorny, and G. S. Bowen. 1989. The ecology of Colorado tick fever in Rocky Mountain National Park in 1974. III. Habitats supporting the virus. *Am. J. Trop. Med. Hyg.* **40:**86–93.

40. Miller, J. K., V. N. Tompkins, and J. C. Sieracki. 1961. Pathology of Colorado tick fever in experimental animals. *Arch. Pathol.* **72:**149–157.

41. Nibert, M. L., and L. A. Schiff. 2001. Reoviruses and their replication, p. 1679–1728. *In* D. M. Knipe, P. M. Howley, D. E. Griffin, S. R. A. Lamb, M. A. Martin, B. Roizman, and S. E. Straus (ed.), *Fields Virology*, 4th ed. Lippincott Williams & Wilkins, Philadelphia, Pa.

42. Oshiro, L. S., D. V. Dondero, R. W. Emmons, and E. H. Lennette. 1978. The development of Colorado tick fever virus within cells of the haemopoietic system. *J. Gen. Virol.* **39:**73–79.

43. Philip, R. N., E. A. Casper, J. Cory, and J. Whitlock. 1975. The potential for transmission of arboviruses by blood transfusion with particular reference to Colorado tick fever, p. 175–195. *In* T. J. Greenwalt and G. A. Jamieson (ed.), *Transmissible Disease and Blood Transfusion.* Grune & Stratton, New York, N.Y.

44. Philipp, C. S., C. Callaway, M. C. Chu, G. H. Huang, T. P. Monath, D. Trent, and B. L. Evatt. 1993. Replication of Colorado tick fever virus within human hematopoietic progenitor cells. *J. Virol.* **67:**2389–2395.

45. Rehse-Kupper, B., J. Casals, E. Rehse, and R. Ackermann. 1976. Eyach—an arthropod-borne virus related to Colorado tick fever virus in the Federal Republic of Germany. *Acta Virol.* **20:**339–342.

46. Roehrig, J. 2002. Arboviruses, p. 727–734. *In* N. R. Rose, R. G. Hamilton, and B. Detrick (ed.), *Manual of Clinical Laboratory Immunology*, 6th ed. ASM Press, Washington, D.C.

47. Roy, P. 2001. Orbiviruses, p. 1835–1869. *In* D. M. Knipe, P. M. Howley, D. E. Griffin, S. R. A. Lamb, M. A. Martin, B. Roizman, and S. E. Straus (ed.), *Fields Virology*, 4th ed. Lippincott Williams & Wilkins, Philadelphia, Pa.

48. Rozeboom, L. E., and W. Burgdorfer. 1959. Development of Colorado tick fever virus in the Rocky Mountain wood tick, *Dermacentor andersoni. Am. J. Hyg.* **59:**138–145.

49. Silver, H. K., G. Meiklejohn, and C. H. Kempe. 1961. Colorado tick fever. *Am. J. Dis. Child* **101:**56–62.

50. Spruance, S. L., and A. Bailey. 1973. Colorado tick fever. A review of 115 laboratory confirmed cases. *Arch. Intern. Med.* **131:**288–293.

51. Topping, N. H., J. S. Cullyford, and G. E. Davis. 1940. Colorado tick fever. *Publ. Health Rep.* **55:**2224–2237.

52. Tsai, T. F. 2000. Coltiviruses (Colorado tick fever), p. 1694–1696. *In* G. L. Mandell, J. E. Bennett, and R. Dolin (ed.), *Principles and Practice of Infectious Diseases.* Churchill Livingstone, Philadelphia, Pa.

53. Tsai, T. F. 2000. Orthoreoviruses and orbiviruses, p. 1693–1694. *In* G. L. Mandell, J. E. Bennett, and R. Dolin (ed.), *Principles and Practice of Infectious Diseases.* Churchill Livingstone, Philadelphia, Pa.

Tick-Borne Diseases of Humans
Jesse L. Goodman et al.
© 2005 ASM Press, Washington, D.C.

Chapter 9

Tick-Borne Encephalitis

PATRICIA A. NUTTALL AND MILAN LABUDA

HISTORY

The many synonyms for tick-borne encephalitis (TBE) chart the history of this important tick-borne viral disease (Table 1). As early as the 18th century, descriptions suggestive of TBE were noted in church registers on the Åland islands, Finland. During the summer of 1927, Schneider, working in a hospital in Lower Austria, recognized several patients with encephalitis who had similar clinical findings. He discovered that this condition occurred regularly, although the numbers of cases varied, with peak incidence during the summer months. On the basis of clinical and epidemiological observations, the condition was called meningitis serosa epidemica and later Schneider's disease.

TBE was recognized clinically in Siberia and the Far East of Russia in the early 1930s. Severe cases of encephalitis were observed in humans residing in formerly uninhabited areas. A special expedition was organized in 1937 by Lev Zilber to determine the cause of the disease. Virus isolates were obtained from the blood of patients and from *Ixodes persulcatus* ticks. The disease was known by several names, including Russian spring-summer encephalitis (RSSE), Far Eastern encephalitis, and forest spring encephalitis.

A less-severe form of encephalitis, affecting humans residing in central Bohemia, now in the Czech Republic, was recorded in 1948. The virus recovered from the blood of a patient and from *Ixodes ricinus* ticks was related to isolates from RSSE cases. In the following year, similar or milder forms of the disease, called biphasic meningoencephalitis, were observed in other central and eastern European countries. In 1951, an outbreak of TBE was recorded in southern Slovakia associated with consumption of unpasteurized goats' milk.

Kumlinge disease was first described in the 1940s affecting inhabitants of, and visitors to, islands in the Baltic Sea. The causative agent, Kumlinge virus, was isolated in 1959 and later found to be related to a virus isolate from central Europe. In Sweden, the first case of

TBE was described in 1954; the virus was isolated in 1958 from a patient and from *I. ricinus* ticks. The disease was named Früh-Sommer-Meningo-Enzephalitis (FSME) to reflect its seasonal occurrence.

Many viruses isolated from ticks collected across Europe, Asia, and North America have been shown to be antigenically related to the virus species, *Tick-borne encephalitis virus* (TBEV). They have been grouped together into the TBEV serocomplex and subsequently recognized as members of the family *Flaviviridae* (7, 46). The name of the family is derived from the Latin *flavus* for yellow, referring to the type species, *Yellow fever virus*.

In addition to TBEV itself, two other TBEV serocomplex members cause encephalitis in humans: *Louping ill virus* (LIV) and *Powassan virus* (POWV) (Table 2). LIV derives its name from the Scots dialect word for leaping, referring to the gait of sheep suffering from the encephalomyelitic disease that has been recognized for at least 2 centuries in southern Scotland. POWV is named after the town in northern Ontario, Canada, where the first fatal human case of the disease was recognized. A virus was isolated from the patient, a 5-year-old boy who developed encephalitis and died in 1958. However, the virus had been isolated previously from a pool of ticks collected in 1952 in Colorado, although specific identification of the virus was not made at the time. The first isolation of POWV from the Asian continent was from a pool of ticks collected in southern Russia in 1972.

Deer tick virus (DTV), a close relative of POWV, was first isolated from *Ixodes scapularis* ticks collected in the northeastern United States (55). The virus was considered to warrant a distinct name based on apparent differences from POWV in vertebrate host, tick vector species, the lack of recognized cases of encephalitis among human residents in places where the virus was found, and molecular genetic data indicating that DTV strains form a distinct clade within the TBEV complex (9, 10, 30).

Patricia A. Nuttall • Centre for Ecology and Hydrology, Mansfield Rd., Oxford OX1 3SR, United Kingdom. **Milan Labuda** • Institute of Zoology, Slovak Academy of Sciences, Dubravska cesta 9, 845 06 Bratislava, Slovakia.

Table 1. Synonyms for TBE

Synonyms
Biundulant meningoencephalitis
Biphasic meningoencephalitis
Central European encephalitis (CEE)
Biphasic milk fever
Far Eastern encephalitis
Forest spring encephalitis
Früh-Sommer-Meningo-Enzephalitis (FSME)
Kumlinge disease
Russian spring-summer encephalitis (RSSE)
Schneider's disease

ETIOLOGIC AGENT AND BIOLOGY

TBEV is classified within the tick-borne viruses of the family *Flaviviridae* in the genus *Flavivirus* (25). Most of the viruses in this genus are arboviruses (arthropod-borne viruses). Many of them are transmitted by mosquitoes: these include such medically important pathogens as *Yellow fever virus*, *Japanese encephalitis virus*, *West Nile virus*, and the four serotypes of *Dengue virus*. Compared with tick-borne flaviviruses, mosquito-borne members of the genus cause larger and more widespread epidemics, attributed to the greater mobility and frequency of feeding of mosquitoes than ticks. Mosquito-borne flaviviruses also show a more rapid rate of evolution than their tick-borne relatives, perhaps reflecting the faster transmission cycle of mosquito-borne than tick-borne flaviviruses. Phylogenetic analyses indicate that tick- and

mosquito-borne flaviviruses diverged as two distinct and major genetic lineages 5,000 to 10,000 years ago (15).

Tick-borne flaviviruses currently comprise 12 species (25). They are classified into two groups: mammalian and seabird. In addition to the three mammalian species listed in Table 2, two species cause severe hemorrhagic disease in humans: *Kyasanur forest disease virus* (and its close relative, Alkhurma virus) and *Omsk hemorrhagic fever virus*. The remainder in the mammalian group are *Kadam virus*, *Langat virus*, and *Royal Farm virus* (and the related Karshi virus); they are not associated with human disease. None of the tick-borne flaviviruses of seabirds (*Gadgets Gully virus*, *Meaban virus*, *Saumarez Reef virus*, and *Tyuleniy virus*) have any disease associations. Three subtypes of TBEV are recognized: European virus (previously Central European encephalitis virus [CEE virus]), Far Eastern virus (previously RSSE virus), and Siberian virus (previously west Siberian virus).

Like all viruses, TBEV needs to infect a living cell to perpetuate itself and survive. As an arbovirus, the life cycle of TBEV depends on infection of both vertebrate and invertebrate (tick) cells. Mature TBE virions (individual virus particles) are roughly spherical, with a diameter of approximately 50 nm, and comprise a nucleocapsid core surrounded by a lipid envelope into which are anchored two surface proteins, E (envelope) and M (membrane) (Fig. 1).

Immature (intracellular) virions contain a precursor M protein (prM); cleavage of prM to M by a furin-like protease occurs during the exit of virions from

Table 2. TBEV and related viruses causing encephalitis in humans

Virus[a]	First isolated in:	Geographical distribution	Major vertebrate host species	Principal tick vector species
TBEV				
Far Eastern subtype	1937	Far East Russia	Rodents (e.g., *Clethrionomys rufocanus, Microtus arvalis*)	*I. persulcatus*
Siberian subtype	1963	Siberia	Rodents (e.g., *Apodemus agrarius, Apodemus peninsulae*)	*I. persulcatus*
European subtype	1940	Northern Europe	Rodents (e.g., *Apodemus flavicollis, Apodemus sylvaticus, Clethrionomys glareolus*)	*I. ricinus*
LIV	1930	Europe (United Kingdom, Ireland, Norway, Spain, Greece, Turkey)	Mountain hare (*Lepus timidus*), sheep, goat, red grouse (*Lagopus scoticus*)	*I. ricinus*
POWV	1952	Canada, United States, Russia	Rodents (e.g., *M. monax, A. peninsulae, C. rufocanus, Microtus* spp.)	*I. cookei, I. persulcatus, H. concinna, D. silvarum*
Deer tick[b]	1996[c]	Northeastern United States; Ontario, Canada	White-footed mouse (*P. leucopus*)	*I. scapularis*

[a] Species names of viruses and virus families cited in the text are given in italics, following the convention of the International Committee on Taxonomy of Viruses (25).
[b] A subtype of POWV.
[c] Some POWV strains isolated before this date are probably deer tick virus.

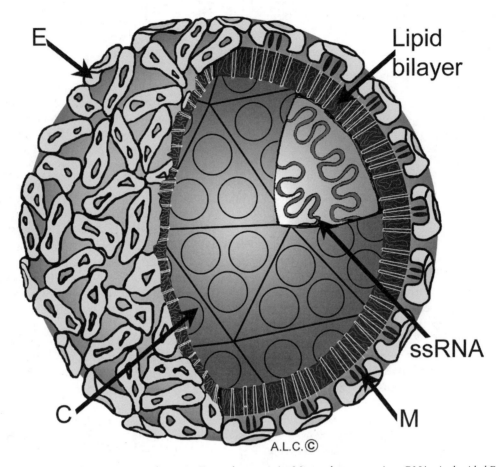

Figure 1. Structure of TBEV. C, capsid protein; E, envelope protein; M, membrane protein; ssRNA, single-sided RNA.

cells. The capsid protein (C) protects the viral genome, a single molecule of single-stranded RNA of approximately 11 kb, which is infectious. Infectivity of the virion RNA has facilitated mutational studies linking genes to function. The open reading frame of the virion RNA is flanked by 5′ and 3′ untranslated regions. These regions form secondary stem-loop structures that may have roles in amplification, translation, and packaging.

Flaviviral proteins are synthesized within the infected cell cytoplasm as a polyprotein of some 3,400 amino acids that is subsequently cleaved by viral and cellular proteases into the three structural proteins (C, M, and E) and seven nonstructural proteins (NS1, NS2A, NS2B, NS3, NS4A, NS4B, and NS5) (41). During the infectious cycle, the NS3 (helicase) and NS5 (RNA-dependent RNA polymerase) proteins form polymerase complexes that associate with cellular membranes through NS1 and NS2A. The NS1 protein was originally known as the soluble antigen and induces a protective immune response. Association of NS3 with NS2B provides virus-specific serine protease activity for the cleavage of newly synthesized viral polyprotein. The NS4A and NS4B proteins appear to help orientate the polyprotein within the intracellular mem-

branes to ensure correct cleavage and functioning of the viral polymerase complex.

The E glycoprotein is the major structural protein and plays an important role in membrane binding during cell infection and in inducing a protective immune response. It carries antigenic determinants, detected by neutralization (NT) and hemagglutination-inhibition (HI) tests, which are used to identify different flaviviral subgroups and species. Determination of the crystallographic structure of the E protein of TBEV revealed that, unlike the spikes seen on many viruses, the flavivirus E protein is situated parallel to the virion surface in the form of head-to-tail homodimeric rods (52). Based on studies of recombinant subviral particles formed by coexpression of E and pre-M, a model of the virion has been constructed that has icosahedral symmetry, with each face of the virion comprising three subunits (triangulation number [T] = 3) (12).

The E protein comprises three structural domains. The central domain I carries the N-glycosylation site thought to play a role in infectivity. Dimerization domain II makes contact with itself in the homodimer and is directly involved in the release of the viral genome into the cytoplasm. Domain III is believed to be the primary site of contact with the cellular receptor; many point mutations that change the virulence or cell tropism of the virus cluster within the protruding part of this domain. Although laminin receptors and binding to glycosaminoglycans appear to be utilized by TBEV for infecting mammalian cells, there is still little understanding of the nature of TBEV receptors, including receptors used to infect tick cells (24).

Organic solvents and detergents readily inactivate TBEV by attacking the lipid bilayer or envelope. Nonionic detergents, such as Triton X, solubilize the entire envelope, releasing M and E proteins; sodium deoxycholate appears to remove only E, leaving M associated with the nucleocapsid. Infectivity and viral hemagglutination are optimally stable at pH 8.4 to 8.8, although residual infectivity is detectable over a broad range (pH 1.4 to 9.2). At an acidic pH, the E protein undergoes conformational changes that reduce viral infectivity. Nevertheless, virions still remain infectious in curdled milk and gastric juice. This explains infections by TBEV through the alimentary route. Flaviviruses are rapidly inactivated at 50°C. Total inactivation of virus in blood occurs within 30 min at 56°C. By contrast, temperatures of −70°C preserve infectivity almost indefinitely. Aerosols (as water droplets or powder) present an infectious hazard in the laboratory and should be avoided by appropriate containment and handling. Flaviviruses are stable for at least 6 h in liquid aerosol suspension at room temperature and 23 to 80% humidity. In freeze-dried form, they survive almost indefinitely at room temperature. Flaviviruses are inactivated by light, gamma irradiation, and disinfectants (e.g., 3 to 8% formaldehyde, 2% glutaraldehyde, 2 to 3% hydrogen peroxide, or 500 to 5,000 ppm of available chlorine, 1% iodine, and phenol iodophors). Tick-borne flaviviruses appear to be relatively more resistant to these forms of treatment than mosquito-borne flaviviruses (6).

The relationships between TBEV and the other tick-borne flaviviruses causing encephalitis (LIV, POWV, and DTV) have been defined by genome sequencing and phylogenetic analyses (15). The phylogenetic tree shows divergence of the tick-borne flaviviruses into two major clades, one comprising Tyuleniy virus and Saumarez Reef virus (the seabird group) and the second clade comprising a monophyletic sister group of the TBE complex viruses (the mammalian group). In the latter group, POWV is at the deepest node, indicating that it emerged as the most ancestral lineage of the mammalian tick-borne flaviviruses; LIV is the most recent lineage.

On the basis of nucleotide sequence and phylogenetic analysis, DTV is considered to be sufficiently different from POWV to be a distinct subtype (11). Phylogenetic analysis of 15 strains of POW-related viruses

and the first recognized isolate of DTV (CT95) revealed two lineages, one including the prototype POWV (ON58) and the other DTV (30). The oldest isolate in the DTV lineage was obtained in 1952 from ticks collected in Colorado. An isolate from a fox obtained in 1977 was also found in the DTV lineage (11). Thus it appears that DTV has been circulating in North America for some years.

LIFE CYCLE—ZOONOTIC HOSTS, TRANSMISSION, AND SEASONAL ACTIVITY

The life cycle of TBEV can be represented by a triangle of parasitic interactions (Fig. 2). The interactions are between (i) virus-tick, (ii) virus-host, and (iii) tick-host. In virus-tick interactions (i), TBEV interacts with its tick vector, infecting and replicating within tick cells including those of the gut, hemocoel, and salivary glands. The goal of the virus is to infect the tick's salivary glands so that it can be transmitted in saliva when the infected tick feeds. The ability of a particular tick species to act as a vector depends on whether TBEV can survive and overcome several barriers within the tick, e.g., the environment within the midgut where the virus is initially taken up in the blood meal, the gut infection barrier, and the salivary gland infection barrier (45).

TBEV can be transmitted transovarially from the adult tick through the eggs to the larvae (49). The incidence of transovarial transmission may be too low to make a significant contribution to the TBEV life cycle. However, transovarial infections may be amplified to significant levels as a result of the aggregated questing and feeding behavior of TBEV tick vector larvae (32). Transovarial transmission and the ability of each parasitic stage of the tick vector to survive for relatively long periods (weeks to months and even years) without a blood meal greatly enhance the role of ticks as reservoirs of TBEV, helping the virus to persist in nature.

Experimental studies indicate that TBEV can replicate and be transmitted by a wide variety of ixodid tick species. This helps in studying virus transmission in the laboratory, but field studies reveal a different picture. Since the expedition of Zilber and colleagues (see "History" above), repeated field collections have identified *I. persulcatus* as the principal vector of Far Eastern and Siberian subtypes of TBEV. Similarly, following the first isolation of TBEV from *I. ricinus* ticks in the Czech Republic, large numbers of isolates have been obtained from *I. ricinus* in various geographic regions of Europe, reflecting the primary role of *I. ricinus* as a vector of the European TBE viral subtype. In some areas of Siberia and Far Eastern Russia, where *I. persulcatus* is not the predominant species, *Dermacentor*

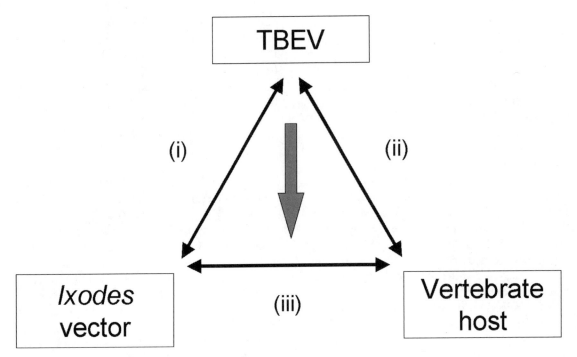

Figure 2. Schematic life cycle of TBEV.

reticulatus, Dermacentor silvarum, and *Haemaphysalis concinna* have been associated with local TBE outbreaks (19). In China, the virus has been isolated from *H. concinna* in the Hunchun area, Jilin province, and from *Ixodes ovatus* in the subtropical region of western Yunnan, 2,700 m above sea level near the Burmese border (54).

The virus-host interaction of the parasitic triangle involves virus infection of the vertebrate host (Fig. 2, ii). The outcome of infection depends on the viral tropism for specific host cell or tissue types or locations (e.g., central nervous tissue) and its pathogenic phenotype, and on the age and immune status of the host and genetic susceptibility to infection. Vertebrate host species that maintain the transmission cycle of TBEV in nature are partly determined by the host preferences of their tick vectors. The principal vectors of TBEV, *I. ricinus* and *I. persulcatus,* are three-host ticks: each parasitic stage feeds on a different individual host. Immature stages often feed on rodents and birds while adults feed on goats, deer, and other ungulates (see reference 43 and Fig. 1 therein). Several rodent species are highly competent in supporting tick-borne transmission of TBEV, whereas avian species are not (the reasons for this difference are unknown). Typically, an uninfected larva feeds on an infected rodent and becomes infected. The engorged larva drops off its host, moults in the undergrowth to an infected nymph, and then seeks out a new host. If the new host is susceptible to TBEV, it will become infected as the infected nymph feeds. The infected nymph also retains the infection

through to the adult stage. However, hosts of adult *I. ricinus* and *I. persulcatus* ticks are not usually susceptible to TBEV. Thus, the most important vertebrate species in the life cycle of TBEV are the hosts on which larvae and nymphs feed (Table 2). Humans are incidental hosts and do not contribute to the virus life cycle.

The third component of the triangle (Fig. 2, iii) is the interaction between the tick and its host. Blood feeding by the ixodid tick vectors of TBEV is a comparatively long and highly ordered process (see Chapter 2, "The Biology of Tick Vectors of Human Disease"). Feeding success relies on the actions of numerous pharmacologically active molecules produced in the tick salivary glands and secreted in the saliva. These overcome the host's hemostatic (vasoconstriction, blood coagulation, and platelet aggregation), inflammatory, and immune responses provoked by the physical and chemical processes involved in tick blood feeding. For example, adult *I. ricinus* ticks show numerous immunomodulatory activities (Table 3). In addition, they may produce inhibitors of the antiviral action of interferon alpha/beta. The evidence is based on increased vesicular stomatitis virus yields in mouse LX cells in the presence of salivary gland extracts from adult female *I. ricinus* ticks (reference 20 and unpublished data).

The pharmacopeia of *I. persulcatus* has not been explored, and little is known about the immature stages of *I. ricinus.* Nevertheless, increasing evidence indicates that the survival of TBEV depends on its ability to exploit the pharmacological activities of tick

Table 3. Pharmacopeia of adult *I. ricinus*

Activity	Target	Reference(s)
Antihemostatic	Thrombin	26
Anti-inflammatory	Alternative complement system (C3a anaphylatoxin)	38, 39
Anti-immune	B lymphocytes	23
	T lymphocytes	40
	Interleukin-2	22
	Interleukin-4	22
	Interleukin-8	21
	Eotaxin	22
	Macrophage inflammatory protein 1α	22
	Monocyte chemotactic protein 1	22
	RANTES	22
	IgG	56

saliva components. The phenomenon has been named saliva-activated transmission (SAT) and has been demonstrated for a number of tick-borne and insect-borne pathogens (44). It is represented in Fig. 2 by the large vertical arrow.

Evidence that SAT plays a critical role in the life cycle of TBEV is based on five key observations. (i) Successful transmission of TBEV between infected and uninfected ticks cofeeding on the same individual host does not depend on the presence of detectable levels of infectious virus circulating in the host's blood (so-called nonviremic transmission) (1, 33). (ii) Nonviremic transmission can be reproduced by syringe inoculation of susceptible vertebrate hosts with a mixture of TBEV and tick saliva or salivary gland extract (2, 34). (iii) Nonviremic transmission occurs with natural wild rodent hosts of TBEV (35). (iv) Nonviremic transmission can occur in hosts immune to TBEV (37). (v) Estimates of the basic reproductive number (R_0) of TBEV indicate that survival of the virus in nature relies on nonviremic transmission (47).

Nonviremic transmission is facilitated by the feeding behavior of the tick vectors of TBEV (48). Like most parasites, ticks show a typical negative binomial distribution on their hosts. Thus, at any one time point, a small number of individual animals are heavily infested with ticks, whereas the majority of the host population are uninfested or support low numbers of ticks. These multiinfested hosts appear to be ideally suited for nonviremic transmission. In addition, ticks are gregarious feeders. For example, >90% of immature *I. ricinus* ticks feed together on the ears of rodents or around the bills of birds. Feeding aggregation reduces the distance between cofeeding infected and uninfected ticks, thereby facilitating nonviremic transmission (36).

As described above, there is now compelling evidence that the interactions between tick vector and vertebrate host at the skin feeding site play a key part in the life cycle of TBEV. The virus depends on nonviremic transmission for its survival, and the mechanism underpinning nonviremic transmission is the exploitation by TBEV of the pharmacological activities of tick saliva at the skin feeding site (the basis of SAT).

The interactions between tick vector and vertebrate host (Fig. 2, iii) also determine the seasonality of TBEV infections. Development of the tick vectors of TBEV is synchronized through diapause with seasonal climatic changes (5). For engorged larvae and nymphs of *I. ricinus* and *I. persulcatus*, diapause appears as delayed metamorphosis. Whereas morphogenic diapause is accepted, there is some controversy about behavioral diapause (16). Thus, for example, it is disputed whether the inactivity of unfed *I. ricinus* ticks is merely a form of quiescence.

Although the developmental biology of *I. persulcatus* and *I. ricinus* is similar, the seasonal activity of *I. persulcatus* may be shorter, lasting only from the end of April to the beginning of June in colder biotopes. In Karelia, in the European part of Russia, the seasonal activity of *I. persulcatus* commences with adults attacking cattle from late April to July; larvae and nymphs parasitize small mammals throughout June and July (4). In most parts of its range, *I. ricinus* becomes active and feeds on hosts in spring and early summer, ticks occurring on vegetation and animals from late March onwards. Depending on environmental conditions, *I. ricinus* shows a bimodal activity pattern with spring and autumn peaks or a unimodal pattern (16).

Cofeeding studies have also demonstrated nonviremic transmission of LIV. This virus is mostly confined to upland regions of the United Kingdom and Ireland, where it is transmitted by *I. ricinus* to a range of mammalian and avian species, although sheep were once thought to be the key hosts in virus survival (50). Mountain hares (*Lepus timidus*) develop subthreshold levels of viremia following syringe inoculation with LIV and consequently were originally discounted from playing a significant epidemiological role. However, when LIV-infected and uninfected ticks were allowed to cofeed on trapped wild hares, 47% of uninfected nymphs became infected, although feeding on apparently nonviremic animals (28). Further studies have established the important role of mountain hares in the life cycle of LIV (42).

POWV is transmitted in enzootic cycles involving ixodid ticks, rodents, and carnivores. Lagomorphs and (in Russia) birds may also be involved (3). Studies of cofeeding nonviremic transmission of POWV have not been reported. In Canada, the most important enzootic vector, *Ixodes cookei*, feeds mainly on groundhogs

(*Marmota monax*), attacking other hosts (including humans) only rarely. POWV has also been isolated from *Ixodes angustus*, which often bites humans and cats, and *I. scapularis* and *Dermacentor variabilis*, which frequently bite humans and dogs. In Russia, POWV has been isolated from *I. persulcatus*, *Haemaphysalis longicornis*, *H. concinna*, and *D. silvarum*; the latter species is the most common source of virus isolations. Although the virus has been isolated from mosquitoes in the Far East, no insect vectors of POW virus have been identified in North America, and the role of mosquitoes in the enzootic cycle is unclear. However, it is intriguing that POWV has an extra amino acid in the E protein sequence, D_{336}, that is shared with mosquito-borne flaviviruses but not tick-borne flaviviruses (17).

The two phylogenetic lineages, POW-related viruses and DT-related viruses, appear to coexist independently in overlapping geographic distributions, at least in Ontario, Canada, and the northeastern United States. Whether this reflects different life cycles (tick vector species and/or vertebrate hosts) is as yet unknown. What little is known of DTV suggests its enzootic transmission cycle primarily involves the deer tick (*I. scapularis*) and white-footed mice (*Peromyscus leucopus*) (10).

SUMMARY OF EPIDEMIOLOGY AND MAP OF DISTRIBUTION

TBE is endemic over a wide geographic area, covering Europe, northern Asia, China, and Japan. The occurrence of TBE is largely determined by the distribution and activity of the principal tick vectors, *I. persulcatus* and the closely related *I. ricinus*, which re-

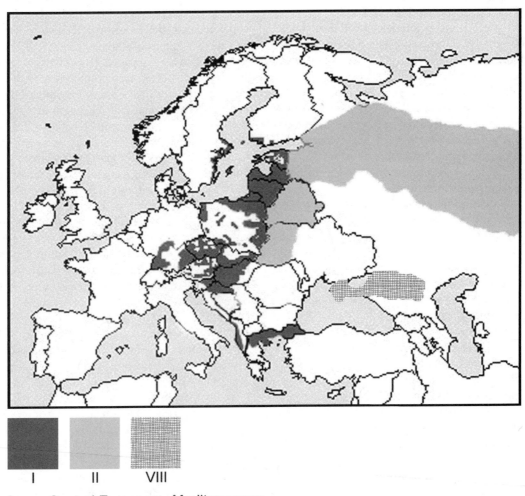

I   Central European - Mediterranean
II   Eastern European
VIII   Crimean - Caucasian

Figure 3. Distribution map of TBEV. (Left) European, Crimean, and Caucasian region; (right) Asian region.

places *I. ricinus* in northeast Europe, from the Baltic Sea and extending across northern Asia to Japan. The northern border for *I. persulcatus* extends across the forests of the central taiga. At least 30,000 natural foci of TBEV are considered to exist across the northern hemisphere from Europe to Japan. These have been divided into eight groups of focal regions (29), namely: I, Central-European–Mediterranean; II, Eastern European; III, Western Siberian; IV, Kazakh-Central Asian; V, Central Siberian–Transbaikalian; VI, Khingan–Amur; VII, Pacific; and VIII, Crimean–Caucasian (Fig. 3). They cover at least 25 European and 7 Asian countries.

In general, the peak incidence of human infections coincides with seasonal peaks of tick feeding activity: May and June and also September and October for *I. ricinus* and May and June for *I. persulcatus*. Although risk maps are available for Europe, they do not provide the complete picture. Thus, seasonal or annual variations in the incidence of TBE cases may vary according to changes in TBEV prevalence or merely reflect changes in human exposure (e.g., bad weather reducing outdoor activities). Seroprevalence cannot be used to generate risk maps because of the high level of immunization in some regions (e.g., >94% of children in Austria are vaccinated against TBEV) (54).

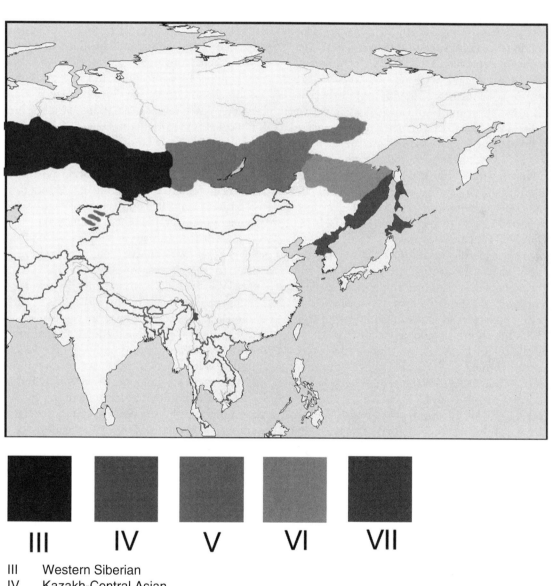

III	Western Siberian
IV	Kazakh-Central Asian
V	Central Siberian–Transbaikalian
VI	Khingan–Amur
VII	Pacific

Figure 3. *Continued.*

Worldwide, 10,000 to 12,000 cases of TBE in humans are recorded annually, with considerable variation from year to year and from one region to another (29, 54). The highest numbers of hospitalized cases are recorded for the pre-Ural and Ural regions and Siberia. During the 1950s and 1960s, the highest TBE occurrence was in forest workers, reaching 700 to 1,200 cases annually. However, following perestroika in the 1990s, the incidence of TBE increased, with up to 11,000 recorded cases per year among urban dwellers who became infected when they visited local forests or even when they worked in their gardens. The increase resulted from fewer people being immunized against TBEV and cessation of the use of pesticides to control ticks. In Western European countries, the total number of annual cases has averaged 3,000 for the last 5 years; most infections are contracted during leisure activities. The number of reported cases of TBE from various European countries and Russia for 1990 to 2001 is reported by Süss (see reference 54 and Table 1 therein). Little is known of the disease incidence in China; natural foci of TBEV have been reported in the Hunchun area of Jilin province, where the seroprevalence in humans was 11%, and in the subtropical region of western Yunnan near the Burmese border. On Hokkaido, the northern island of Japan, a severe case of TBE was diagnosed and several isolates related to the Far Eastern subtype of TBEV were identified.

Although TBE can affect people of all ages, the highest incidence usually occurs among 17- to 40-year-olds. The highest risk groups are agricultural and forestry workers; hikers, ramblers, and people engaged in outdoor sports that bring them into contact with tick habitats; and collectors of mushrooms and wild fruit. Most TBEV infections of humans result from an infected tick bite. The risk of infection and resulting morbidity rate are difficult to determine as tick bites often go unnoticed. References to tick bite in the case history of patients range from 10 to 85%. In Western Europe, the estimated risk of infection varies from 1:200 to 1:900 per tick bite. Serological surveys suggest that more than 70 to 95% of TBEV human infections in regions of Russia where TBEV is endemic are subclinical and indicate frequent exposure to infected ticks.

The incidence of clinically expressed forms of disease is dependent on several factors (for a review, see reference 19):

1. the number of exposures to infected ticks. In some endemic areas, up to 45% of the local population receives at least one tick bite per epidemic season.
2. infection prevalence in ticks. Infection prevalence varies in different years and in different regions, ranging from 0.1 to 5% in Europe and 4 to 39% in Asia.

3. concentration of infectious virus in ticks. Most people receive bites from ticks carrying low doses of virus, and only about 15% are bitten by highly infected ticks (29). Thus, an estimated one clinical case occurs for every 100 people bitten by ticks in regions of endemicity. These calculations correlate well with the 1.4% of people who develop TBE after knowingly being bitten by a tick.
4. virulence of the infecting TBEV strain, which affects severity of the disease (see "Clinical Manifestations," below).

In addition to tick-borne infections, sporadic cases and family outbreaks of alimentary TBEV infections are observed in Slovakia almost annually and in other countries in Central Europe and Russia where unpasteurized milk and milk products of goats, sheep, and cattle are consumed.

Unlike TBEV infections, LIV infections of humans are largely an occupational health hazard confined to laboratory workers, veterinarians, farmers, and abattoir workers (51, 53). In total, 26 of 39 human cases reported resulted from laboratory exposure. Serosurveys of patients with aseptic meningitis or encephalitis of unknown etiology identified 5 of 35 positive sera of patients in Ireland; examination of 775 sera from Scottish patients identified one case of LIV encephalitis in a farmer and one fatal case in a slaughterman. However, 8% of sera from abbatoir workers were positive despite the fact that only two clinical cases have been reported for this occupational health group.

LIV is the only flavivirus identified in the United Kingdom. There, it is mainly restricted to the rough, upland grazings and unimproved pastures of the western seaboard of the United Kingdom that are largely devoted to sheep farming, although the virus is also found in some areas of northeast Scotland, northern and southwest England, northern Wales, and Ireland. In the most common habitats, there is a thick mat of vegetation and the soil remains damp throughout the summer. The increase of LIV infections of grouse (*Lagopus scoticus*) in northern England has been associated with the spread of bracken, which provides a thick vegetation mat.

An encephalomyelitic disease in sheep, reported in Norway, is caused by LIV-infected sheep ticks (*I. ricinus*) introduced from mainland Britain (13). Sheep and goat encephalomyelitis has also been reported in Spain, Greece, and Turkey, and sequence analysis confirms an etiological association with LIV although the viruses that cause these infections are genetically distinct from LIV (15). They are thought to have emerged on the hillsides of Greece, Turkey, and Spain when sheep were introduced near wooded areas where TBEV was present.

POWV circulates in South Dakota, the eastern and western United States, Canada, and Far Eastern Russia. There appear to be differences in the epidemiology of POWV between North America and Asia, with a higher incidence but milder infections in Far Eastern Russia than in North America. At present, there is no explanation for these differences. Encephalitis due to POWV is seen only sporadically in Canada, with 27 reported cases in North America since 1958 (http://www.phac-aspc.ga.ca/msds-ftss/msds121e.html). A low incidence of encephalitis associated with POWV has been recorded in Russia. However, in Russia POWV cocirculates with TBEV; hence, the real incidence of encephalitis associated with POWV may be masked by the encephalitis produced by TBEV or even by mixed TBEV-POWV infections, which have been shown to occur (19).

Although DTV has not been associated with disease (11), one isolate (ON97) originally identified as POWV but phylogenetically more closely related to DTV was obtained from the brain of a 64-year-old man diagnosed as having "Powassan encephalitis" (14, 30). The patient had been bitten by an "unidentified insect" while camping in Ontario.

The geographic distribution of tick-borne flaviviruses is reflected in their phylogenetic tree (15). When genetic distance from the most recently emerged LIV in Scotland is plotted, increasing geographic distance between viruses correlates directly with genetic distance between the viruses. Thus, the TBE complex viruses appear to have evolved as a cline across the forests and sheep-rearing hillsides of the northern hemisphere (57). Examination of this clinal evolution and geographic distribution in relation to global satellite data has revealed another correlation. In Central Europe and southern Scandinavia, climatic conditions that favor coincident cofeeding transmission between *I. ricinus* larvae and nymphs appear to be predictors of geographic locations where TBEV is capable of causing significant epidemiological problems (48).

CLINICAL MANIFESTATIONS

Although not directly proven, the severity of clinical manifestations broadly correlates with the TBEV subtype. In general, Far Eastern subtypes cause severe disease in humans, with a mortality that can reach 50% in some outbreaks; disease associated with European subtypes is less severe, and mortality is usually under 5%. Based on genome analysis, a Siberian subtype has been established which characteristically induces a less-severe form of disease. Case fatality rates rarely exceed 8%, but patients may develop chronic forms of TBE.

About 70 to 95% of all TBEV infections are asymptomatic. When disease occurs, a variety of manifestations have been described, summarized as follows: (i) mild or moderate fever with complete recovery, (ii) subacute encephalitis with nearly complete recovery or residual symptoms that may or may not disappear over a long period of time, (iii) severe encephalitis associated with irreversible damage to the central nervous system (CNS), resulting in disability or death, and (iv) chronic infections. A variety of clinical symptoms are recognized by Russian medical authorities (for a review, see reference 18).

Regardless of disease severity, the incubation period of TBE is usually 7 to 14 days. Early symptoms include fatigue lasting 1 to 2 days, with pain in the neck, shoulders, and lower back. Headache may also occur. The classical symptoms appear suddenly, and patients can often recall the exact hour of onset. There is a sudden temperature elevation and nausea. Muscular pains become severe, and a sense of numbness can occur in the limbs. Some patients develop meningeal symptoms, such as neck stiffness, during this period. There may also be shortness of breath and flushing of the face, neck, and upper body.

In the febrile form of TBE, there are no neurological symptoms. Temperatures can reach 39°C, and fever may last for a few hours to 5 days. Approximately one-third of all diagnosed TBEV infections take this course. The most common severe form of TBE shows an onset similar to that of the febrile form, but with severe headaches and nausea. Vomiting occurs frequently, and the patient becomes photophobic and experiences eye pain. The fever lasts 7 to 14 days, and recovery is gradual. More severe but less common is the meningoencephalitic form of TBE in which there is damage to the CNS. Patients are weak and drowsy, hallucinate frequently, and may become unconscious. Symptoms include fibrillations, bradycardia, bradykinesis, stomach bleeding, hyperkinesia, hemiparesis, and hemiplegia. Some patients subsequently experience epileptic seizures. Up to 30% of cases are fatal. In survivors (particularly the elderly), hemiplegia is irreversible. Convalescence is slow, with signs of nervous exhaustion, malaise, and frequent mood changes.

The poliomyelitic form of TBE is characterized by a prodromal period of fatigue, periodic muscle contractions, and weakness or numbness in one of the limbs that develops into paralysis. Paresis of the neck, shoulder, and upper limbs intensifies during the first or second febrile period and lasts up to 2 weeks or even several months. Wrist drop is typical, and when the patient is standing, his or her head hangs down (the "hanged head" sign). Muscles begin to atrophy by the end of the second or third week. Paresis or paralysis of the lower limbs is rare. Recovery is slow, and only about half the patients recover partially from the neurological damage. Slow progressive deterioration is common. Damage to peripheral nerves occurs in the polyradiculoneuritic form of TBE; however, recovery is usually complete.

The slow, progressive form of TBE accounts for 2 to 5% of all cases in Russia, up to 8 to 13% in some regions. This chronic disease has been described in patients from Siberia and Far Eastern Russia but has not been reported in Europe. It is characterized by a long incubation period, sometimes with a latent period of years after the infective tick bite before encephalitis appears. The condition then slowly worsens over a period of months or years, eventually resulting in severe disability or death. The infectious etiology of such chronic forms of TBE, in both seropositive and seronegative patients, is confirmed by virus isolation following the onset of symptoms.

The incidence of different forms of TBE varies in different regions. For example, in Siberia about 80% of clinical infections present as a mild or moderate fever without neurological sequelae, although hospitalization and special medical care are frequently required. Paralytic forms comprise about 7 to 8%, and Kozshevnikov's epilepsy (a form of chronic TBE) comprises about 4 to 5% (58). Approximately 7% of patients die following acute encephalitis, but the proportion of fatalities varies in different regions, depending on TBEV subtype. Although the incidence of TBE in Far Eastern Russia is lower than in Siberia, fatality and disability rates are higher, reaching 60% in some regions. In European countries such as Austria, the case fatality rate was 1% prior to extensive vaccination.

Biphasic milk fever was the name given to the form of disease first associated with the consumption of goat's milk, which was drunk as a substitute for cow's milk in Russia and Central Europe following World War II. The course of the disease is biphasic, whereas in classical TBE, a biphasic course is observed in only 20 to 30% of cases. Meningoencephalitis, with slightly developed meningeal and parenchymal symptoms, is also characteristic. Differences in clinical manifestations between TBE contracted by tick bite or through the alimentary tract are explained by differences in the host immune response that depend on the route of virus penetration and the initial concentration of virus.

There have been few reported cases of encephalitis in humans resulting from LIV infections, and most cases have occurred in laboratory workers (8). The clinical picture is similar to that produced by European subtypes of TBEV, following a biphasic course. The first phase is characterized by fever lasting 2 to 11 days, followed by a remission of 5 to 6 days and then the reappearance of fever and meningoencephalitis, lasting 4 to 10 days. Leukopenia occurs during the first phase and leukocytosis occurs during the encephalitic phase. No deaths have been reported. In one laboratory-acquired case, a hemorrhagic diathesis developed, and the disease closely resembled Kyasanur Forest disease.

POWV infections in humans are characterized by a variable period of fever and nonspecific symptoms, followed by neurological signs, which are often severe. In North America, POWV causes severe encephalitis with a high incidence of neurological sequelae and a case fatality rate of up to 60%. In Far Eastern Russia, infections were described as milder than those produced by TBEV, and some differences were noted between the lesions in the CNS caused by POWV and TBEV.

A case reported as Powassan encephalitis included neuropathological changes similar to those seen in the first reported case of the disease (14, 30). However, the isolated virus (ON97) was subsequently shown to be related to DTV. This case suggests that DTV is capable of causing encephalitis in humans.

DIAGNOSIS

Clinical manifestations of TBE are often nonspecific; hence, diagnosis must rely on laboratory findings. However, laboratory results mainly serve for differential diagnosis, rather than determining therapy, as similar symptoms are observed in other infections.

Diagnosis can be made by reverse transcription-PCR, direct virus isolation from blood (serum or heparinized plasma) collected during the first phase of illness or from cerebrospinal fluid during the early encephalitic phase, or by serological methods. In the viremic phase of the early stages, virus can be identified in blood by electron microscopy. Infectious virus can be cultivated in suitable cell cultures (e.g., Vero cells) or by intracerebral inoculation of newborn mice. As signs of CNS infection are not usually observed until 2 to 4 weeks after the infecting tick bite, serum antibody tests are usually positive at the time of admission to hospital.

A recent infection with TBEV can sometimes be confirmed by a twofold or higher increase in antibody titer within a 2- to 4-week period. Serological techniques include complement fixation, NT, and HI, but enzyme-linked immunosorbent assay (ELISA) is most commonly used (27). Antibodies are produced locally in cerebrospinal fluid, and the serum:cerebrospinal fluid antibody ratio has also been employed for diagnosing infections.

Detection of immunoglobulin M (IgM) antibodies in serum using a μ-capture ELISA has proved a reliable method in most cases for diagnosing TBE in patients with CNS symptoms. Specific IgG antibodies and rheumatoid factor do not interfere with the test. IgM antibodies may persist and be detected in serum up to 9 months after infection.

Tests used to evaluate the antibody response following immunization against TBE virus include the NT and HI tests. IgG-specific ELISA methods have been associated with false-positive reactions.

Laboratory techniques for diagnosing TBEV infections are also applicable to diagnosis of infections caused by other tick-borne flaviviruses causing encephalitis. Obviously, specific antibodies and antigens and reference virus strains are needed for specific identification.

TREATMENT

Curative treatment for TBE is not available. Care given to patients is therefore supportive. Sera obtained from human convalescent patients or from hyperimmunized horses have produced favorable results in a number of human cases when cerebrospinal fluid injections of 10 to 15 ml were supplemented with intramuscular injections of 30 to 50 ml of serum. Immediate intramuscular injections of 40 to 50 ml of serum have been given to humans bitten by ticks in areas where TBE is endemic or following laboratory infection. To be successful, immunotherapy has to be administered on the first or second day of the disease and followed by two or three additional injections. Patients thus treated with repeated injections of convalescent serum have shown a drop in temperature and improvement in their general condition. IgG preparations for treatment of TBEV infections were previously available commercially but have since been withdrawn in Europe. The ability to engineer humanized antibodies offers a potentially useful means of preparing immunotherapies for the future.

There is currently no treatment available for POWV or LIV infections, although TBEV immunotherapy may provide some cross-protection. One patient infected with a virus related to DTV and diagnosed as having viral encephalitis was treated with acyclovir. The patient appeared to recover, but while awaiting physiotherapy suffered a cardiac arrest and died. Autopsy revealed a massive pulmonary embolism as the cause of death (14).

PREVENTION (PUBLIC HEALTH AND MEDICAL)

The most effective preventive measure is to avoid tick bites. Protective clothing is effective, particularly if light-colored, for easier detection of ticks. This may be undesirable during hot weather, and reliance should

then be placed on a thorough search of the body, at least daily, after exposure to a tick-infested habitat. Ticks that have become attached to the skin should be removed carefully with tweezers or forceps to grasp the mouthparts that are buried in the skin. The tick mouthparts have backward-pointing barbs so the action of removal should first be to push down and gently twist before pulling. Several tick repellents are available, but their efficacy in preventing infection with TBEV has not been fully elucidated. Large-scale tick control has been employed in Russia and Central Europe, including aerial application of DDT, and was effective in reducing tick numbers. However, large-scale control is no longer employed.

In areas where TBE is endemic, routine measures to raise public awareness of the risk of TBEV infection include (i) publicizing relevant information concerning potential sources of TBEV infection, methods of avoiding tick bites, and measures to take if a tick bite occurs (reporting to medical authorities); (ii) reminding owners of animals to treat the animals with acaricides; (iii) employing local people to cut the grass around houses prior to spraying the area with acaricides; and (iv) spraying nearby forested areas used by local residents for recreation.

Preventive measures directed at ticks are not foolproof, and vaccination is recommended for at-risk groups in areas where TBE is highly endemic. Vaccination of laboratory personnel is strongly recommended and in some countries is mandatory for anyone working with TBEV. The most common vaccine used in Europe is FSME-Immun, originally prepared by Immuno AG, Vienna, Austria, which is now owned by Baxter. This vaccine is a suspension of purified viral antigen derived from TBEV grown in chick embryo cells and inactivated with formaldehyde. Three doses given intramuscularly provide protection for at least 3 years. A booster dose is recommended every third year to maintain protective immunity. A protective rate of 96 to 98% is achieved after the third dose, and cases of TBE among fully immunized persons are rare. Adverse reactions are usually mild. In Austria, the vaccine is used extensively; although no controlled clinical trials have been reported, it is considered to have performed effectively because of the high levels of seroconversion and the progressive reduction observed in numbers of cases of TBE (31). A pediatric variant of the vaccine containing a smaller dose of antigen has been developed and is recommended for young children older than 6 months who live in high-risk regions. A new formulation of the Austrian vaccine without preservatives, the use of continuous-flow ultracentrifugation, and development of a patented syringe to improve handling have all helped to improve the vaccine.

In Russia, a similar vaccine has been produced, and up to 7 million doses have been administered. Owing to the high cost, use of the concentrated purified Russian vaccine has been limited mainly to laboratory personnel, whereas a nonconcentrated tissue culture vaccine based on another TBE strain, strain 205, is in use in many Russian regions and outperforms the earlier vaccine based on TBEV strain Pan.

Although the vaccine in Austria has been shown to be highly effective, there is concern that the same vaccine may not be as effective in Russia (19). This concern stems from the failure of Russian vaccines to afford high levels of protection, the comparatively high risk of exposure to infected ticks in many areas, and the diversity of strains, particularly of the Siberian and Far Eastern subtypes, which are more virulent than strains of the European subtype endemic in Western Europe. Several attempts have been made in Russia to produce a live attenuated vaccine based on either naturally attenuated (serial subculture) or mutated TBEV or Langat virus (a close relative of TBEV that does not appear to cause disease in humans), but these have been unsuccessful.

Recent developments in molecular virology have begun to explain many aspects of virus attenuation. They have also opened up new approaches for producing safe and effective live virus vaccines, including the use of recombinant subviral particles, naked DNA, and synthetic infectious RNA (24).

A vaccine to protect sheep against LIV was developed soon after the isolation of the etiological agent. The vaccine was grown in sheep kidney cell cultures, formalin inactivated, and concentrated by methanol precipitation. However, control of the disease in sheep relies primarily on acaricide treatment (by dipping or application of pour-on agents) to control tick infestations. There is no vaccine available for POWV or DTV.

REFERENCES

1. **Alekseev, A. N., and S. P. Chunikhin.** 1990. Exchange of tick-borne encephalitis virus between *Ixodidae* simultaneously feeding on animals with subthreshold levels of viremia. *Med. Parazitol. Parazit. Bolezni* 2:48–50.
2. **Alekseev, A. N., S. P. Chunikhin, M. Y. Rukhkyan, and L. F. Stefutkina.** 1991. Possible role of Ixodidae salivary gland substrate as an adjuvant enhancing arbovirus transmission. *Med. Parazitol. Parazit. Bolezni* 1:28–31.
3. **Artsob, H.** 1988. Powassan encephalitis, p. 29–49. *In* T. P. Monath (ed.), *The Arboviruses: Epidemiology and Ecology*, Vol. 4. CRC Press, Inc., Boca Raton, Fla.
4. **Balashov, Y. S.** 1972. Bloodsucking ticks (Ixodoidea)—vectors of diseases of man and animals. *Misc. Publ. Entomol. Soc. Am.* 8:161–376.
5. **Belozerov, V. N.** 1982. Diapause and biological rhythms in ticks, p. 469–500. *In* F. D. Obenchain and R. Galun (ed.), *Physiology of Ticks.* Current Themes in Tropical Science, vol. 1. Pergamon Press, Oxford, United Kingdom.
6. **Burke, D. S., and T. P. Monath.** 2001. Flaviviruses, p. 1043–1125. *In* D. M. Knipe, P. M. Howley, D. E. Griffin, S. R. A. Lamb, M. A. Martin, B. Roizman, and S. E. Straus (ed.), *Fields Virology*, 4th ed. Lippincott Williams and Wilkins, Philadelphia, Pa.
7. **Calisher, C. H.** 1988. Antigenic classification and taxonomy of flaviviruses (family *Flaviviridae*) emphasizing a universal system for the taxonomy of viruses causing tick-borne encephalitis. *Acta Virol.* 32:469–478.
8. **Davidson, M. M., H. Williams, and J. A. Macleod.** 1991. Louping ill in man: a forgotten disease. *J. Infect.* 23:241–249.
9. **Ebel, G. D., E. N. Campbell, H. K. Goethert, A. Spielman, and S. R. Telford III.** 1999. A focus of deer tick virus transmission in the northcentral United States. *Emerg. Infect. Dis.* 5:570–574.
10. **Ebel, G. D., E. N. Campbell, H. K. Goethert, A. Spielman, and S. R. Telford III.** 2000. Enzootic transmission of deer tick virus in New England and Wisconsin sites. *Am. J. Trop. Med. Hyg.* 63:36–42.
11. **Ebel, G. D., A. Spielman, and S. R. Telford III.** 2001. Phylogeny of North American Powassan virus. *J. Gen. Virol.* 82:1657–1665.
12. **Ferlenghi, I., M. Clarke, T. Ruttan, S. I. Allison, J. Schalich, F. X. Heinz, et al.** 2001. Molecular organization of a recombinant subviral particle from tick-borne encephalitis virus. *Mol. Cell* 7:593–602.
13. **Gao, G. F., W. R. Jiang, M. H. Hussain, K. Venugopal, T. S. Gritsun, H. W. Reid, and E. A. Gould.** 1993. Sequencing and antigenic studies of a Norwegian virus isolated from encephalomyelitic sheep confirm the existence of louping ill virus outside Great Britain and Ireland. *J. Gen. Virol.* 74:109–114.
14. **Gholam, B. I., A. S. Puksa, and J. P. Provias.** 1999. Powassan encephalitis: a case report with neuropathology and literature review. *Can. Med. Assoc. J.* 161:1419–1422.
15. **Gould, E. A., X. de Lamballerie, P. M. A. Zanotto, and E. C. Holmes.** 2001. Evolution, epidemiology and dispersal of flaviviruses revealed by molecular phylogenies. *Adv. Virus Res.* 57:71–103.
16. **Gray, J. S.** 1991. The development and seasonal activity of the tick *Ixodes ricinus*: a vector of Lyme borreliosis. *Rev. Med. Vet. Entomol.* 79:323–333.
17. **Gritsun, T. S., E. C. Holmes, and E. A. Gould.** 1995. Analysis of flavivirus envelope proteins reveals variable domains that reflect their antigenicity and may determine their pathogenesis. *Virus Res.* 35:307–321.
18. **Gritsun, T. S., V. A. Lashkevich, and E. A. Gould.** 2003. Tick-borne encephalitis. *Antiviral Res.* 57:129–146.
19. **Gritsun, T. S., P. A. Nuttall, and E. A. Gould.** 2004. Tick-borne flaviviruses. *Adv. Virus Res.* 61:317–371.
20. **Hajnická, V., P. Kocáková, M. Slovák, M. Labuda, N. Fuchsberger, and P. A. Nuttall.** 2000. Inhibition of the antiviral action of interferon by tick salivary gland extract. *Parasite Immunol.* 22:201–206.
21. **Hajnická, V., P. Kocáková, M. Sláviková, M. Slovák, J. Gašperík, N. Fuchsberger, and P. A. Nuttall.** 2001. Anti-interleukin-8 activity of tick salivary gland extracts. *Parasite Immunol.* 23:483–489.
22. **Hajnická, V., I. Vancová, P. Kocáková, M. Slovák, J. Gašperík, M. Sláviková, R. S. Hails, M. Labuda, and P. A. Nuttall.** Manipulation of host cytokine network by ticks: a potential gateway for pathogen transmission. *Parasitology*, in press.
23. **Hannier, S., J. Liversidge, J. M. Sternberg, and A. S. Bowman.** 2003. *Ixodes ricinus* tick salivary gland extract inhibits IL-10 secretion and CD69 expression by mitogen-stimulated murine splenocytes and induces hyporesponsiveness in B lymphocytes. *Parasite Immunol.* 25:27–37.

24. Heinz, F. X. 2003. Molecular aspects of TBE virus research. *Vaccine* **21**(Suppl. 1):S3–S10.

25. Heinz, F. X., M. S. Collett, R. H. Purcell, E. A. Gould, C. R. Howard, M. Houghton, R. J. M. Moormann, C. M. Rice, and H. J. Thiel. 2000. Family Flaviviridae, p. 859–878. *In* M. H. V. Regenmortel, C. M. Fauquet, D. H. L. Bishop, E. Carstens, M. K. Estes, S. Lemon, J. Maniloff, M. A. Mayo, D. Mc-Geoch, C. R. Pringle, and R. B. Wickner (ed.), Virus taxonomy. 7th Report of the International Committee on Taxonomy of Viruses. Academic Press, San Diego, Calif.

26. Hoffmann, A., P. Walsmann, G. Riesener, M. Paintz, and F. Markwardt. 1991. Isolation and characterization of a thrombin inhibitor from the tick *Ixodes ricinus*. *Pharmazie* **46**:209–212.

27. Holzmann, H. 2003. Diagnosis of tick-borne encephalitis. *Vaccine* **21**(Suppl. 1):36–40.

28. Jones, L. D., M. Gaunt, R. S. Hails, K. Laurenson, P. J. Hudson, H. Reid, P. Henbest, and E. A. Gould. 1997. Transmission of louping-ill virus between infected and uninfected ticks co-feeding on mountain hares. *Med. Vet. Entomol.* **11**:172–176.

29. Korenberg, E. I., and T. V. Kovalevskii. 1999. Main features of tick-borne encephalitis eco-epidemiology in Russia. *Zentralbl. Bakteriol.* **289**:525–539.

30. Kuno, G., H. Artsob, N. Karabatsos, K. R. Tsuchiya, and G. J. J. Chang. 2001. Genomic sequencing of deer tick virus and phylogeny of Powassan-related viruses of North America. *Am. J. Trop. Med. Hyg.* **65**:671–676.

31. Kunz, C. 2003. TBE vaccination and the Austrian experience. *Vaccine* **21**:50–55.

32. Labuda, M., V. Danielova, L. D. Jones, and P. A. Nuttall. 1993. Amplification of tick-borne encephalitis virus infection during co-feeding of ticks. *Med. Vet. Entomol.* **7**:339–342.

33. Labuda, M., L. D. Jones, T. Williams, V. Danielova, and P. A. Nuttall. 1993. Efficient transmission of tick-borne encephalitis virus between cofeeding ticks. *J. Med. Entomol.* **30**:295–299.

34. Labuda, M., L. D. Jones, T. Williams, and P. A. Nuttall. 1993. Enhancement of tick-borne encephalitis virus transmission by tick salivary gland extracts. *Med. Vet. Entomol.* **7**:193–196.

35. Labuda, M., P. A. Nuttall, O. Kozuch, E. Eleckova, T. Williams, E. Zuffova, and A. Sabo. 1993. Non-viremic transmission of tick-borne encephalitis virus: a mechanism for arbovirus survival in nature. *Experientia* **49**:802–805.

36. Labuda, M., J. Austyn, E. Zuffova, O. Kozuch, N. Fuchsberger, J. Lysy, and P. Nuttall. 1996. Importance of localized skin infection in tick-borne encephalitis virus transmission. *Virology* **219**:357–366.

37. Labuda, M., O. Kozuch, E. Zuffova, E. Eleckova, R. S. Hails, and P. A. Nuttall. 1997. Tick-borne encephalitis virus transmission between ticks co-feeding on specific immune natural rodent hosts. *Virology* **235**:138–143.

38. Lawrie, C. H., S. E. Randolph, and P. A. Nuttall. 1999. *Ixodes* ticks: serum species sensitivity of anti-complement activity. *Exp. Parasitol.* **93**:207–214.

39. Lawrie, C. H., R. B. Sim, and P. A. Nuttall. 2005. Investigation of the mechanisms of anti-complement activity in *Ixodes* ticks. *Mol. Immunol.* **42**:31–38.

40. Leboulle, G., M. Crippa, Y. Decrem, N. Mejri, M. Brossard, A. Bollen, and E. Godfroid. 2002. Characterization of a novel salivary immunosuppressive protein from *Ixodes ricinus* ticks. *J. Biol. Chem.* **277**:10083–10089.

41. Lindenbach, B. D., and C. M. Rice. 2001. *Flaviviridae*: the viruses and their replication, p. 991–1041. *In* D. M. Knipe, P. M. Howley, D. E. Griffin, R. A. Lamb, M. A. Martin, B. Roizman, and S. E. Straus (ed.), *Fields Virology*, vol. 1, 4th ed. Lippincott Williams and Wilkins, Philadelphia, Pa.

42. Norman, R., D. Ross, M. K. Laurenson, and P. J. Hudson. 2004. The role of non-viraemic transmission on the persistence and dynamics of a tick borne virus—Louping ill in red grouse (*Lagopus lagopus scoticus*) and mountain hares (*Lepus timidus*). *J. Math. Biol.* **48**:119–134.

43. Nuttall, P. A., and M. Labuda. 2003. Dynamics of infection in tick vectors and at the tick-host interface. *Adv. Virus Res.* **60**:233–272.

44. Nuttall, P. A., and M. Labuda. Tick-host interactions: saliva-activated transmission. *Parasitology* (Supplement), in press.

45. Nuttall, P. A., L. D. Jones, M. Labuda, and W. R. Kaufman. 1994. Adaptations of arboviruses to ticks. *J. Med. Entomol.* **31**:1–9.

46. Porterfield, J. S. 1975. The basis of arbovirus classification. *Med. Biol.* **53**:400–405.

47. Randolph, S. E., D. Miklisova, J. Lysy, D. J. Rogers, and M. Labuda. 1999. Incidence from coincidence: patterns of tick infestations on rodents facilitate transmission of tick-borne encephalitis virus. *Parasitology* **118**:177–186.

48. Randolph, S. E., L. Gern, and P. A. Nuttall. 1996. Co-feeding ticks: epidemiological significance for tick-borne pathogen transmission. *Parasitol. Today* **12**:472–479.

49. Řeháček, F. 1962. Transovarial transmission of tick-borne encephalitis virus by ticks. *Acta Virol.* **6**:220–226.

50. Reid, H.W. 1984. Epidemiology of louping-ill, p. 161–178. *In* M. A. Mayo and K. A. Harrap (ed.), *Vectors in Virus Biology*. Academic Press, London, England.

51. Reid, H. W. 1988. Louping-ill, p. 117–135. *In* T. P. Monath (ed.), *The Arboviruses: Epidemiology and Ecology*, vol. 3. CRC Press, Inc., Boca Raton, Fla.

52. Rey, F. A., F. X. Heinz, C. Mandl, C. Kunz, and S. C. Harrison. 1995. The envelope glycoprotein from tick-borne encephalitis virus at 2 A resolution. *Nature* **375**:291–298.

53. Smith, C. E. G., and M. G. R. Varma. 1981. Louping ill, p. 191–200. *In* G. W. Beran (ed.), *CRC Handbook Series in Zoonoses, Section B. Viral Zoonoses*, vol. 1. CRC Press, Inc., Boca Raton, Fla.

54. Süss, J. 2003. Epidemiology and ecology of TBE relevant to the production of effective vaccines. *Vaccine* **21**(Suppl. 1):19–35.

55. Telford, S. R., III, P. M. Armstrong, P. Katavolos, I. Foppa, A. S. Garcia, M. L.Wilson, and A. Spielman. 1997. A new tick-borne encephalitis-like virus infecting New England deer ticks, *Ixodes dammini*. *Emerg. Infect. Dis.* **3**:165–170.

56. Wang, H., and P. A. Nuttall. 1999. Immunoglobulin binding proteins in ticks: new target for vaccine development against a blood-feeding parasite. *Cell. Mol. Life Sci.* **56**:286–295.

57. Zanotto, P. M., G. F. Gao, T. Gritsun, M. S. Marin, W. R. Jiang, K. Venugopal, H. W. Reid, and E. A. Gould. 1995. An arbovirus cline across the northern hemisphere. *Virology* **210**:152–159.

58. Zlobin, V. I., and O. Z. Gorin. 1996. *Tick-Borne Encephalitis: Etiology, Epidemiology and Prophylactics in Siberia*. Nauka, Novosibirsk, Russia.

Tick-Borne Diseases of Humans
Jesse L. Goodman et al.
© 2005 ASM Press, Washington, D.C.

Chapter 10

Crimean-Congo Hemorrhagic Fever

FELICITY J. BURT AND ROBERT SWANEPOEL

HISTORY OF THE VIRUS

Crimean-Congo hemorrhagic fever (CCHF) is a tick-borne viral zoonosis widely distributed in Africa, Asia, and Eastern Europe within the range of ticks belonging to the genus *Hyalomma*. The virus is a member of the *Nairovirus* genus of the family *Bunyaviridae*. It causes mild fever and viremia in cattle, sheep, and small mammals such as hares. Humans become infected by contact with infected blood or other tissues of livestock or human patients or from tick bites. Human infection is usually characterized by a febrile illness with headache, myalgia, and petechial rash, frequently followed by a hemorrhagic state with necrotic hepatitis. The case fatality rate is approximately 30%.

A hemorrhagic disease with symptoms suggestive of CCHF infection was described in Eastern Europe and Asia as far back as the 12th century (39). However, a disease given the name Crimean hemorrhagic fever was first described in people bitten by ticks while harvesting crops and sleeping outdoors on the Crimean Peninsula in 1944. In the following year, it was demonstrated by the inoculation of human subjects that the disease was caused by a filterable agent present in the blood of patients during the acute stage of illness and that the agent was also present in suspensions prepared from ticks, suspected to be the vectors of the agent. The causative virus was finally isolated in a laboratory host, suckling mice, in 1967 (16). In 1968 it was found that the agent of Crimean hemorrhagic fever was identical to a virus named Congo which had been isolated in 1956 from the blood of a febrile child in Stanleyville (now Kisangani) in what was then the Belgian Congo (now Democratic Republic of Congo [DRC]), and since that time the two names have been used in combination (13, 16, 17, 85).

ETIOLOGIC AGENT AND BIOLOGY

Crimean-Congo hemorrhagic fever virus is classified as a member of the genus *Nairovirus*, of the family *Bunyaviridae* (14, 19). The genus, consisting of 33 viruses, is divided into seven serogroups on the basis of antigenic relationships. The CCHF serogroup contains CCHF virus, Hazara virus from Pakistan, and Khasan virus from the former USSR. Apart from CCHF virus, the only members of the genus known to be pathogenic for humans are *Nairobi sheep disease virus* and Dugbe virus. *Nairobi sheep disease virus* of East Africa is believed to be identical to Ganjam virus of India and is a tick-borne pathogen of sheep and goats which sporadically causes benign illness in humans (19). Dugbe virus is a tick-borne virus commonly associated with mild infection of cattle and sheep in West Africa and infrequently causes benign human disease (7, 33, 60). The classification of the nairoviruses was originally based on their antigenic relatedness; however, the groupings have subsequently been substantiated through demonstration of morphological and molecular affinities between the viruses (10).

The nairoviruses are spherical, 90 to 120 nm in diameter, and have a host-cell-derived bilipid envelope incorporating virus-coded glycoproteins which form indistinct surface projections (21, 59). The single-stranded, negative-sense RNA genome consists of three segments: L (large), 4.1×10^6 to 4.9×10^6 Da; M (medium), 1.5×10^6 to 1.9×10^6 Da; and S (small), 0.6×10^6 to 0.7×10^6 Da. Each of the three RNA segments is contained in a separate nucleocapsid within the virion (18). The virions contain three major structural proteins: two envelope glycoproteins (G1 and G2) and a nucleocapsid protein (N) plus minor quantities of viral transcriptase or L (large) protein. Hazara virus is reported to have three glycoproteins (18, 31).

Felicity J. Burt and Robert Swanepoel • Special Pathogens Unit, National Institute for Communicable Diseases, Sandringham 2131, Republic of South Africa.

Relatively few studies have been reported on the coding and replication strategies of the nairoviruses. The S segment of Dugbe virus, the most extensively studied member of this genus, has one open reading frame in the viral complementary strand encoding the nucleoprotein (N) of the virus (97). Alignment of the predicted amino acid sequences from the S segment of CCHF and Hazara viruses with that of the Dugbe virus showed significant homology between the three sequences, providing evidence that the S segment of CCHF and Hazara viruses encode the viral N protein. CCHF S RNA comprises 1,672 nucleotides (isolate C68031; China isolate), and has a single open reading frame, which encodes the N protein (53,966 Da), the major structural protein of the virus (56). The N protein of the CCHF virus is the most antigenic viral protein and appears to be the most conserved. Expressed N protein has been used to prepare recombinant laboratory diagnostic reagents (58).

The synthesis of nairovirus glycoproteins, encoded on M segment RNA, appears to involve a precursor polypeptide, a coding strategy which is quite distinct from that used by other genera of bunyaviruses. The M segment of CCHF virus, which is 5,367 nucleotides long (BA8402; China and Pakistan Matin isolates), has one open reading frame which encodes a precursor polypeptide, with a highly variable amino-terminal domain and a fairly conserved carboxyl-terminal region. The two mature glycoproteins, G2 (37 kDa) and G1 (75 kDa), are derived by cleavage via two nonstructural precursors, designated P140 (140 kDa) and P85 (85 kDa) (66, 71). The order of the coding sequence is the same as for Dugbe virus: 5'-G2-G1-3' (57, 71).

The size of the L segment of nairoviruses is estimated to be between 12 to 14 kb; by analogy with other bunyaviruses, it is believed to encode a large protein with RNA polymerase activity. The nucleotide sequence has been determined for the L segment of Dugbe virus, and they were found to have a single open reading frame that could potentially encode a 459-kDa protein. Analysis of the predicted amino acid sequence revealed the core polymerase motif characteristic of RNA-dependent RNA polymerases (57).

Comparatively little is known about the function of the viral proteins of nairoviruses. By analogy with other genera of the *Bunyaviridae*, it can be assumed that glycoproteins are responsible for recognition of receptor sites on susceptible cells and, consequently, cell tropism and pathogenicity of the virus in humans for the induction of protective immune response. Glycoproteins probably also play a role in tick host selection. Replication of CCHF virus occurs in the cytoplasm of infected cells, with maturation and budding of virus occurring on vesicular membranes (72). Genetic studies have shown that despite a high degree of variability between CCHF isolates from geographically distinct regions, the isolates appear to comprise a single virus species (57, 68).

Little information is available on the stability of the CCHF virus, but once enveloped, it is sensitive to lipid solvents (50), and it is known that its infectivity is destroyed by low concentrations of formalin and β-propriolactone. The virus is labile in infected human tissues after host death (39), but the examination of specimens from human patients appears to show that infectivity is preserved for at least a few days at ambient temperature in separated serum. Infectivity is destroyed by boiling or autoclaving, but the virus is stable at temperatures below −60°C. CCHF virus replicates in a wide variety of primary-cell and line cell cultures, including Vero, CER, and BHK21 cells, but not usually to high titer. The virus is poorly cytopathic, so that titers of infectivity are demonstrated by plaque production or immunofluorescence in infected cells (18, 39, 98). The virus has been isolated and titers have been determined most frequently by intracerebral inoculation of suckling mice (39).

Because of its propensity for human-to-human transmission, its ability to cause infections in laboratory workers, and the severity of the disease in humans, CCHF is placed in biohazard class IV in countries which have relevant biosafety guidelines. This dictates that culture of the virus is permitted only in maximum-security biosafety level 4 (BSL-4) laboratories.

LIFE CYCLE AND ZOONOTIC HOSTS

CCHF virus has been isolated from at least 31 species of ticks of seven genera, including 29 ixodids and 2 argasids, but for most species there is no evidence that they are capable of serving as vectors. In some instances, the virus recovered from engorged ticks may merely have been present in the blood meal imbibed from a viremic host (11, 39, 94, 98, 103). Argasid ticks are unlikely to serve as vectors, since CCHF virus failed to replicate in four species: *Argas walkerae*, *Ornithodoros porcinus porcinus*, *Ornithodoros savignyi*, and *Ornithodoros sonrai*, following attempts to infect them experimentally (25, 79).

Ixodid ticks have three instars in their life cycle, larvae, nymphs, and adults, each of which attaches to a vertebrate host to take a blood meal before molting to the next instar. Infection acquired by larvae from engorging on a viremic host can be transmitted after the molt by the ensuing nymphs to a second host; in turn, infection can be passed from nymphs through the molt to vertebrates by the ensuing adult ticks. In addition to such transstadial transmission of infection, there can also be transovarial transmission, with virus passing through the eggs to infect the succeeding generation of larval ticks. Early investigators of CCHF in the former Soviet Union and Eastern Europe demonstrated the occurrence of transstadial and transovarial transmission of infection in members of three genera of ixodid ticks, *Hyalomma marginatum marginatum*, *Dermacentor marginatus*, and *Rhipicephalus rossicus* (39, 52). In more recent experiments, mainly involving African species of ticks and infection either by direct inoculation of virus or by feeding the ticks on viremic hosts, it was shown that *Hyalomma marginatum rufipes*, *Hyalomma truncatum*, *Hyalomma impeltatum*, *Hyalomma dromedarii*, *Amblyomma variegatum*, *Amblyomma hebraeum*, *Rhipicephalus evertsi evertsi*, *Rhipicephalus evertsi mimeticus*, and *Rhipicephalus appendiculatus*, were all capable of supporting replication of CCHF virus. Most were able to transmit infection to vertebrates (transmission was not attempted with *A. hebraeum*) (20, 27, 28, 35, 53, 54, 55, 61, 79, 83, 100). Higher rates of infection, higher virus titers, and increased rates of transmission were observed for the *Hyalomma* species than for ticks of the *Amblyomma* and *Rhipicephalus* genera. Transovarial transmission of CCHF virus to larvae and the ability of larvae to transmit infection to vertebrates were found to occur in a very small proportion of ticks, and it has been estimated that this probably does not occur with sufficient frequency to ensure indefinite perpetuation of the virus in the absence of amplification of infection in vertebrate hosts (39, 98).

Other modes of transmission of infection that probably play a role in the maintenance of virus in nature include sexual transmission of infection in ticks and the phenomenon of nonviremic transfer of infection between ticks cofeeding on a host. Sexual transmission of CCHF virus from infected male ticks to female ticks has been demonstrated for *H. truncatum* (34). Nonviremic transmission of infection between ticks is believed to be facilitated by factors present in tick saliva (47, 48) and has been demonstrated for CCHF virus with infected adult and noninfected immature *H. truncatum* ticks and *H. impeltatum* ticks fed together on nonviremic mammals (34, 37, 55, 100). Nonviremic transmission of CCHF virus has also been demonstrated with *H. marginatum rufipes* ticks feeding on red-beaked hornbill birds (*Tockus erythrorhynchus*) in west Africa (101).

The coincidence in the distribution of CCHF virus and *Hyalomma* ticks and the evidence from vector competence studies strongly suggest that members of the *Hyalomma* genus are the principal vectors of CCHF virus (39, 92, 98).

The occurrence of viremia has been demonstrated in various small mammals of Eurasia and Africa, such as susliks, hedgehogs, hares, and certain myomorph rodents (mice and rats); in some instances, it has been shown that these hosts are capable of infecting ticks (39, 78, 83, 98). Domestic ruminants also develop demonstrable viremia and are capable of infecting ticks (39, 83, 98). The prevalence of antibody to CCHF in the sera of wild vertebrates in South Africa and Zimbabwe is generally low but is highest in large herbivores with a mass similar to or greater than the kudu antelope, such as the zebra, eland, buffalo, rhinoceros, and giraffe, which are the preferred hosts of adult *Hyalomma* ticks (8, 84). Antibody has also been found in the sera of farmed ostriches, which are parasitized by adult *Hyalomma* ticks, but not in wild passerines or water birds (81). Immature *Hyalomma* ticks feed on small mammals and ground-frequenting birds; among these, antibody is most prevalent in hares but is also found in a low proportion of rodents and guinea fowl (84). Although the results of antibody surveys indicate that high rates of infection occur in livestock, the role of large vertebrates in the perpetuation of CCHF virus is theoretically limited by the fact that they are hosts to adult *Hyalomma* ticks in which transovarial transmission occurs with low frequency. Hence, it is postulated that the acquisition of infection by immature ticks on small vertebrates probably constitutes the most important amplifying mechanism which ensures perpetuation of the virus and, through the mechanism of transstadial transmission to adult ticks, facilitates infection of large vertebrates (98).

In limited observations, passerine birds, domestic chickens, and a few species of wild birds in West Africa were found to be refractory to the virus, while experimentally infected guinea fowl in South Africa developed transient viremia of very low intensity and an antibody response which remained demonstrable only for a few weeks, so it is unlikely that birds are able to infect ticks directly (39, 81, 98, 102). Nevertheless, it was shown that birds can infect ticks through the so-called phenomenon of nonviremic transmission of infection (101). Moreover, birds carry immature ticks and could thus serve to disseminate virus which has been transmitted transovarially in the ticks (41, 42, 101). The relatively high prevalence and titers of antibody found in ostriches, which are hosts to adult *Hyalomma* ticks, suggested that they may be more susceptible to infection than other birds; following an outbreak of CCHF among workers at an ostrich abattoir in South Africa, it was found that experimentally infected ostriches developed a viremia which was demonstrable for up to 4 days and a strong antibody response, without exhibiting overt signs of disease (12, 90).

Humans commonly acquire CCHF virus from tick bites or from contact with blood or other tissues of infected livestock. Although some patients are unable to recall specific incidents constituting exposure to infection, it is invariably found they have lived in or visited an environment where such exposure was possible (15, 30, 92). The majority of patients tend to be adult males engaged in the livestock industry, such as farmers, laborers, slaughterhouse workers, and veterinarians (39, 60, 92, 98). Infection sometimes occurs in town dwellers who have contact with animal tissues or are bitten by ticks while on hunting or hiking trips. It has been observed that humans can also become infected merely by squashing ticks between the fingers (39, 92). The occurrence of disease in animal slaughterers indicates that viremic animals must on occasion arrive at abattoirs, yet in 23 years of monitoring CCHF in South Africa, there has been no evidence that urban consumers acquire infection from meat that has been processed and matured according to standard procedures (88). Within abattoirs, infection tends to occur in those involved in bleeding animals at the beginning of the slaughtering process and in those who handle hides where semiengorged ticks that detach from slaughtered animals indiscriminately attach to the nearest available host (88). On one occasion in South Africa, five individuals who butchered cattle on a farm developed the disease, yet another 42 individuals who consumed the meat failed to seroconvert (93). Thus, infection appears to be limited to those who have contact with fresh blood or other tissues, possibly because infectivity is destroyed by the fall in pH which occurs in tissues after death.

The virus causes inapparent infection or mild fever in livestock (91–93). Young ruminants, including calves and lambs, acquire maternal antibody from colostrum, but it has not been determined whether this is protective, and many animals seroconvert early in life after the occurrence of natural infection. Consequently, humans commonly become infected when they come into contact with the viremic blood of young animals in the course of performing procedures such as castrations, vaccinations, insertion of ear tags, or slaughter of animals (39, 93). The evidence suggests that the infection in humans is acquired through contact of viremic blood with broken skin, and this is consistent with the observation that nosocomial infection in medical personnel usually results from accidental pricks with needles contaminated with the blood of patients or similar mishaps (39, 82, 96, 98).

In view of the serological evidence that infection of livestock occurs on a wide scale in areas infested by *Hyalomma* ticks, it is surprising that so few human infections are diagnosed. This raises the possibility that many human infections are asymptomatic or mild and pass unnoticed, but the low prevalence of antibody generally detected in surveys and the sparse evidence of infection encountered among cohorts of cases of the disease suggest that a high proportion of CCHF infections does, in fact, come to medical attention (30, 91–93). Possible explanations for the low incidence of infection which occurs in humans include the fact that viremia in livestock is short lived and of low intensity compared to that in other zoonotic diseases such as Rift Valley fever, which is more readily acquired from contact with infected tissues. Furthermore, despite the fact that a high proportion of patients acquire infection from ticks, humans are not the preferred hosts of *Hyalomma* ticks and are infrequently bitten in comparison to livestock.

EPIDEMIOLOGY

The distribution of the disease coincides with that of the principal vectors of the virus, ticks of the genus *Hyalomma*. Cases of naturally acquired human infection have been documented in the former Soviet Union, China, Bulgaria, Yugoslavia, Albania, Kosovo (formerly part of Yugoslavia), Pakistan, Iran, Iraq, United Arab Emirates, Saudi Arabia, Oman, Tanzania, Central African Republic, DRC (formerly Zaire), Uganda, Kenya, Mauritania, Burkina Faso, South Africa, and Namibia (R. Swanepoel, unpublished data) (1, 2, 4, 24, 26, 32, 36, 38, 39, 64, 69, 70, 73, 75, 77, 87, 95, 98). In addition, virus has been isolated from ticks or non-human mammals in Madagascar, Senegal, Nigeria, Central African Republic, Ethiopia, Afghanistan, Greece, and Hungary (98). Serological evidence alone has been reported from Zimbabwe and Benin, and limited serological observations have been reported from Portugal, France, Turkey, Egypt, Kuwait, and India (98).

The initial outbreaks of CCHF recognized on the Crimean Peninsula in 1944 and 1945 occurred under conditions of war when large numbers of soldiers and peasant farmers were exposed to tick bites while harvesting crops and sleeping outdoors (39). Subsequent recognition of the presence of the disease in many countries in Eastern Europe and Asia similarly came about through the occurrence of highly visible epidemics or nosocomial outbreaks occasioned by human intervention, resulting in multiple exposures of people to infection. These include the institution of major land reclamation schemes or abrupt changes in animal husbandry practices in the former Soviet Union and Bulgaria in the 1950s and 1960s and in Rostov Province of the Russian Federation in 1999; nosocomial outbreaks of infection in Pakistan in 1976 and in Iraq and Dubai in 1979; large-scale exposure of war refugees to outdoor conditions in Kosovo in 2000, Albania in 2001, and Pakistan in 2001–2002; and multiple exposures of people to blood and ticks from the handling and slaughter of livestock imported from Africa and Asia to Saudi Arabia in 1990, the United Arab Emirates in 1994–1995, and Oman in 1995 (2, 26, 39, 40, 51, 62–65, 75, 76, 77, 87, 88, 99). The occurrence of these epidemics led to the perception that CCHF was an emerging disease. However, in many other countries in Eurasia and Africa the presence of the virus was discovered because prospective laboratory investigations were undertaken, not because a specific clinical entity had been recognized; antibody surveys indicate that there is widespread circulation of virus in nature in many countries that have not yet recognized the occurrence of human disease (39, 92).

In Africa, for instance, only 15 human infections had been identified up to 1979, of which 8 occurred in laboratory personnel (39, 92). The situation changed following recognition of the first case of the disease in South Africa in February 1981 in a child bitten by a *Hyalomma* tick. By the end of 2002 a total of 171 cases, of which 42 (25%) were fatal, had been confirmed in southern Africa. Of the 171 cases, 154 were indigenous to South Africa, 2 were imported (1 from a patient residing in the DRC and 1 from a traveller to Tanzania), and 15 involved patients infected in Namibia (32, 49, 82, 88, 89, 91–94, 96). Antibody to CCHF virus was found to be widely distributed in the sera of livestock and wild vertebrates in South Africa, Zimbabwe, and Namibia, including sera which had been in frozen storage since 1964 (8, 84, 92, 94). This implies that the virus must have been in southern Africa long before its presence was recognized, and it is believed that the regular diagnosis of cases of CCHF in the subcontinent in recent years probably stems from an increased awareness among medical clinicians that resulted from wide publicity given to the disease and from the availability of a specific diagnostic service. CCHF disease in humans has also been recognized in Mauritania, Burkina Faso, and Kenya (24, 69, 70). Thus, it appears that the virus is present throughout Africa and that the disease which occurs in Africa is no less severe than that which occurs in Eastern Europe and Asia.

Hoogstraal (39, 40) pointed out that mechanisms for the dissemination of ticks and hence virus, which include the movement of birds migrating annually on a north-south axis (41, 42), must have operated in Eurasia and Africa for millennia. In addition, ticks can be dispersed between continents by movement of livestock. Although there is evidence that recent outbreaks of CCHF in the Arabian peninsula resulted from trade of tick-infested livestock from Africa and Asia, long-established CCHF endemicity in the region cannot be excluded. Despite the potential for dispersal of the virus between the continents, it appears from phylogenetic analyses of CCHF isolates that the circulation of the virus is largely compartmentalized within the two land masses of Africa and Eurasia where the distribution of strains of the virus is probably related to the distribution and dispersal of the virus's vectors (23, 57, 65, 68, 74). The implication is not that there is continuing spread of CCHF from its present range, but that further investigation would reveal the presence of the virus and disease in the remaining countries of Africa, Eastern Europe, and Asia, which lie within the distribution range of *Hyalomma* ticks.

Although the incidence of recognized cases of human infection is generally extremely low in countries where CCHF is endemic, it should be borne in mind in assessing the socioeconomic impact of the virus that the disease affects particular segments of the population, including those involved in the livestock industry and in health care. Hence, the occurrence of outbreaks can have dire consequences. For instance, the dedication of highly trained staff and expensive facilities and equipment to the intensive care of a single patient in isolation can prove to be very costly and disruptive of normal medical services. Bans imposed on the importation of slaughter livestock can seriously affect the economies of exporting countries.

CLINICAL MANIFESTATIONS

Signs and Symptoms

The incubation period commonly ranges from 1 to 3 days after a person has been infected by a tick bite, but occasionally extends to 7 days. It is usually 5 to 6 days in people exposed to infected blood or other tissues of livestock or human patients but may occasionally extend to 9 days or more (89, 92).

Onset of the disease is usually very sudden, with severe headache often being the first symptom. This is frequently accompanied by dizziness, neck pain and stiffness, sore eyes, photophobia, fever, rigor, and chills. Patients rapidly develop general myalgia and malaise, with intense backache or leg pains. Sore throat, nausea, and vomiting commonly occur early in the illness; patients may experience nonlocalized abdominal pain and diarrhea at this stage. Fever is often intermittent, and patients may undergo sharp changes of mood over the next 2 days with feelings of confusion and aggression. By the second to fourth day of illness, patients may exhibit lassitude, depression, and somnolence and may have a flushed appearance with injected conjunctivae and chemosis. By this time, tenderness may be localized in the right upper quadrant of the abdomen, and hepatomegaly may be discernible. Tachycardia is common, and patients may be slightly hypotensive. There may be lymphadenopathy and exanthema and petechiae of the throat, tonsils, and buccal mucosa.

A petechial rash appears on the trunk and limbs by the third to sixth day of illness, and this may be followed rapidly by the appearance of large bruises and ecchymoses, especially in the antecubital fossae, upper arms, axillae, and groin. Epistaxis, hematemesis, hematuria, melena, gingival bleeding, and bleeding from the vagina or other orifices may commence on the fourth or fifth day of illness, or even earlier. Sometimes a hemorrhagic tendency is evident only from the oozing of blood from injection or venipuncture sites. There may be internal bleeding, including retroperitoneal and intracranial hemorrhage. Severely ill patients may enter a state of hepatorenal and pulmonary failure from about the fifth day onward and become progressively drowsy, stuporous, and comatose. Jaundice may become apparent during the second week of illness. The mortality rate is approximately 30%, and deaths generally occur on days 5 to 14 of illness. Patients who recover usually begin to improve on day 9 or 10, but asthenia, conjunctivitis, slight confusion, and amnesia may continue for a month or longer (89, 92, 96).

Clinical Pathology and Histopathology

Changes in the cellular and chemical composition of blood recorded during the first few days of illness in human patients include leukocytosis or leukopenia and elevated serum aspartate transaminase, alanine transaminase, gamma-glutamyltransferase, lactic dehydrogenase, alkaline phosphatase, and creatine kinase levels, while bilirubin, creatinine, and urea levels increase and serum protein levels decline during the second week (49, 89, 92). Thrombocytopenia, elevation of the prothrombin ratio, activated thromboplastin time, increased thrombin time, and elevated levels of fibrin degradation products, as well as depression of fibrinogen and hemoglobin values, are evident during the first few days of illness.

Complete autopsies are seldom performed on patients who die of CCHF, and examination of tissues is often confined to liver samples taken with biopsy needles. Lesions in the liver vary from disseminated foci of necrosis, mainly midzonal in distribution, to massive necrosis involving over 75% of hepatocytes and a variable degree of hemorrhage (3, 9, 49, 92). Necrotic areas are frequently marked by hemorrhage and cell loss and are associated with eosinophilic change of hepatocytes with formation of prominent Councilman body-type lesions. Inflammatory cell infiltrates in necrotic areas are absent or mild and unrelated to the extent of hepatocellular damage. Common findings include fatty changes, hyperplastic and hypertrophic Kupffer cells containing phagocytosed debris, and portal inflammatory infiltrates (Color Plate 5).

Limited observations of splenic tissue show lymphoid depletion, focal necrosis, and scattered lymphoblasts in periarterial sheaths. In addition, diffuse alveolar damage, intra-alveolar hemorrhage, hyaline membrane formation, and a mononuclear interstitial pneumonitis have been observed in the lungs, and congestion and slight interstitial edema have been noted in the heart. Lesions in other organs include congestion, hemorrhage, and focal necrosis in the central nervous system, kidneys, and adrenal glands, and general depletion of lymphoid tissues. None of the histopathologic features is pathognomonic, and similar features can be seen in other viral, rickettsial, and bacterial infections, as well as in toxic exposures. Hence, a definitive diagnosis can be established only by immunohistochemical (Color Plate 5B) or virological tests.

Pathogenesis

The pathogenesis of the disease is incompletely understood (9, 80, 92), but by analogy with other arthropod-borne virus infections it can be surmised that CCHF virus undergoes some replication at the site of inoculation and that there is hematogeneous and lymph-borne spread of infection to organs such as the liver, which are major sites of replication. Localization of CCHF virus in tissues by immunohistochemistry has shown that mononuclear phagocytes and endothelial cells are also major targets of virus infection (9). A similar tropism is exhibited by many lethal hemorrhagic fever viruses. The mononuclear phagocyte system may constitute a mechanism for viral clearance in some patients, but in others replication of virus in these cells may enhance viremia. Infection of mononuclear phagocytes and depletion of lymphoid cells may protect the virus from phagocytosis and immune inactivation and enhance the spread of virus. In addition, infection of mononuclear phagocytes and endothelial cells may play a role in the pathogenesis of CCHF through the release of physiologically active substances, including cytokines, tumor necrosis factor, and other inflammatory mediators and procoagulants. The occurrence of disseminated intravascular coagulation (DIC) appears to be an early and central event in the pathogenesis of the disease. The hepatocytes are a major target of the virus, and the occurrence of minimal inflammatory infiltration suggests that hepatocellular necrosis may be mediated by a direct viral cytopathic effect. Hepatocellular necrosis leads to further release of tumor necrosis factor and other procoagulants into the circulation, and ultimately to impairment of the synthesis of coagulation factors to replace those which are consumed in DIC. Widespread infection of endothelium with degenerative change rather than necrosis is associated with capillary dysfunction, which contributes to the occurrence of a hemorrhagic diathesis and the generation of a petechial rash.

Diagnosis

A diagnosis of CCHF should be suspected when severe influenza-like illness with sudden onset and short incubation period, usually less than 1 week, occurs in persons exposed to tick bites or fresh blood and other tissues of livestock or human patients. The disease is easier to recognize once a rash appears and there are hemorrhagic signs such as epistaxis, hematemesis, and melena.

Etiologic investigation of suspected CCHF infections should be performed in a BSL-4 laboratory. Confirmation of the diagnosis in the acute phase of illness consists of detection of viral nucleic acid by reverse transcriptase PCR (RT-PCR), demonstration of viral antigen by enzyme-linked immunoassay (ELISA) of serum samples, or isolation of the virus (5, 6, 80, 82, 89, 92). In samples collected later, the diagnosis is confirmed by demonstration of an immune response. RT-PCR using conventional thermocycling or real-time PCR constitutes a rapid and sensitive technique for diagnosing CCHF infection during the early stages of illness before an antibody response is demonstrable or in fatal cases where an antibody response is frequently not demonstrable (6, 22, 68, 74). Virus may be isolated in cell cultures, commonly of Vero cells, or by intracerebral inoculation of 1-day-old mice. The virus is detected and identified in cell cultures by performing an immunofluorescence (IF) test. Isolation of the virus in cell cultures can be achieved in 1 to 5 days, compared to 5 to 8 days in mice, but mouse inoculation is more sensitive for isolating virus that is present at low concentrations.

Nairoviruses in general, including CCHF, induce a weak neutralizing antibody response, and serum samples frequently contain nonspecific inhibitors of virus infectivity. Hence, neutralization tests have found limited application for demonstrating antibody response. Complement fixation and agar gel immunodiffusion tests were used in early investigations but are not sensitive enough to be clinically useful. Technical difficulties in preparing reagents limited the use of hemagglutination inhibition and reversed passive hemagglutination inhibition assays. In contrast, indirect IF has proved to be a rapid and sensitive technique for detecting an immune response to CCHF virus. The ELISA is also a sensitive technique, and both ELISA and IF can distinguish between immunoglobulin G (IgG) and IgM antibodies.

Both IgG and IgM antibodies become demonstrable by IF from about day 5 of illness onwards and are present in the sera of all survivors of the disease by day 9 at the latest. The IgM antibody activity declines to undetectable levels by the fourth month after infection, and IgG titers may begin to decline gradually at this stage but remain demonstrable for at least 5 years. Recent or current infection is confirmed by demonstrating seroconversion, a fourfold or greater increase in antibody activity in paired serum samples, or IgM activity in a single specimen.

Patients who succumb rarely develop a demonstrable antibody response, and the diagnosis is confirmed by isolation of virus or detection of viral nucleic acid in serum samples, liver samples taken after death, or demonstration of CCHF antigen by immunohistochemical techniques with paraffin-embedded liver sections. Virus antigen may sometimes be demonstrated in liver impression smears by IF or in serum or liver homogenate by ELISA. Observation of necrotic lesions compatible with CCHF in sections of liver provides presumptive evidence in support of the diagnosis.

Differential Diagnosis

The vast majority of suspected cases of CCHF prove to be severe infections with more common agents, including bacterial septicemias, malaria, viral hepatitis, rickettsioses, and complications of human immunodeficiency virus-AIDS. In arriving at a diagnosis, it is important to take into account an accurate history of possible exposure to infection, signs and symptoms of illness, and clinical pathology findings.

In Africa, CCHF should be distinguished from other febrile diseases associated with ticks (7) and particularly from tick-borne typhus (*Rickettsia conorii* or *Rickettsia africae* infection, commonly known as tick-bite fever), in which there is often a characteristic necrotic lesion or eschar at the site of the tick bite (Color Plates 13A and 14A). Tick-borne typhus has an incubation period of 7 to 10 days and a more insidious onset than CCHF. Tick-borne typhus is associated with a petechial rash and is capable of causing a fatal disease in humans with hemorrhagic manifestations similar to CCHF, but it is amenable to treatment with appropriate antibiotics. Other tick-borne diseases occurring in Africa which could be considered include Q fever (*Coxiella burnetii* infection) and relapsing fever borreliosis (*Borrelia* spp. infection). In addition, there are a number of tick-borne viruses in Africa apart from CCHF, which have been associated with human disease such as Dugbe and Nairobi sheep disease viruses.

Rift Valley fever can also be acquired from contact with the tissues of livestock in Africa, but it usually occurs in the context of massive epidemics involving abortion and death of sheep and cattle at irregular intervals in years when heavy rains favor the breeding of the mosquito vectors of the virus. Less than 1% of Rift Valley fever infections in humans manifest as fatal hemorrhagic disease.

Particular consideration should be given to the other viral hemorrhagic fevers of Africa. In brief, they include Marburg disease and Ebola fever, caused by members of the family *Filoviridae*, and Lassa fever, caused by a virus of the family *Arenaviridae*. Marburg and Ebola viruses cause sporadic outbreaks of highly lethal disease in tropical Africa, often in association with similar disease in non-human primates, but the source of these viruses in nature remains unknown. Lassa fever virus causes chronic renal infection of *Mastomys* spp. rodents in West Africa, and transmission to humans occurs through contamination of food and house dust with rodent urine.

Another group of rodent-associated viruses which belong to the *Hantavirus* genus of the family *Bunyaviridae* are found in Europe, Asia, and the Americas. Diseases caused by the hantaviruses of Europe and Asia are known collectively as hemorrhagic fever with renal syndrome, and these could conceivably be confused with CCHF on occasion. The hantaviruses of North and South America are associated with the so-called hantavirus pulmonary syndrome, which is less likely to be confused with CCHF. There is inconclusive evidence for the presence of hantaviruses in Africa.

Yellow fever and dengue virus (of which there are four serotypes) are mosquito-borne flaviviruses capable of causing fatal hemorrhagic disease in humans within defined geographic ranges. Chikungunya virus is a mosquito-borne alphavirus which has been associated with hemorrhagic disease in Asia, although in Africa it is reported as a benign febrile illness with severe joint pain. Although not found in Africa, Omsk hemorrhagic fever and Kyasanur Forest disease (tickborne flavivirus infections), as well as various spotted fever rickettsial infections other than those caused by *R. conorii* and *R. africae*, might also be considered in the differential diagnosis in their respective ranges.

Distinguishing between the various possible causes of suspected viral hemorrhagic fever is a specialized task, normally undertaken in laboratories dedicated to the purpose.

PREVENTION, CONTROL, AND TREATMENT

Nosocomial infections have been associated with needle stick injuries or contact of broken skin with infected blood, tissues, and body fluids of patients. Aerosol transmission is not considered a primary mode of transmission. In situations where infection with CCHF virus is suspected, patients should be isolated and subjected to barrier nursing techniques until the diagnosis is confirmed or excluded, to protect health care workers from potential exposure to infection. In brief, the patient should be isolated in a room with an adjoining anteroom, if possible, for storage of supplies required for barrier nursing and patient care. Health care workers should wear protective clothing such as disposable gowns, gloves, masks, goggles, and overshoes, which are discarded on leaving the isolation room via the anteroom. All items removed from the isolation ward should be safely disposed of or suitably disinfected. Blood samples should be wrapped in absorbent material such as paper towels and placed in secondary leak-proof containers such as rigid metal or plastic screw-cap containers or sealed plastic bags for safe transport to the laboratory. Clinical laboratory tests should be kept to a minimum and performed by experienced staff wearing protective clothing, and automated analyzers must be decontaminated after use, commonly with dilute chlorine disinfectants. CCHF virus is classified as a biohazard class IV pathogen; hence, specific diagnostic tests and culture of the virus are undertaken only in BSL-4 laboratories in countries which have relevant biosafety regulations.

The control of CCHF through the application of acaricides to livestock is impractical, particularly under the extensive farming conditions which prevail in the arid areas where *Hyalomma* ticks are most prevalent. Pyrethroid preparations are available that can be used to kill ticks which come into contact with human clothing. Following the outbreak of CCHF in an ostrich abattoir in South Africa in 1996, it was decided that ostriches should be treated for ticks with pyrethroids and kept in a tick-free environment for 2 weeks prior to slaughter to reduce the risk of exposing abattoir workers to infection (12, 90). Veterinarians, slaughtermen, and others involved with livestock should be aware of the disease and take practical steps when appropriate, such as wearing gloves, to limit or avoid exposure of naked skin to fresh blood and other tissues of animals.

Treatment of the disease consists essentially of supportive and replacement therapy with blood products. Immune plasma has been used, but the efficacy of this treatment is not clear, since there has been no systematic investigation with a uniform product of known virus-neutralizing activity. Promising results were obtained in limited trials with the chemotherapeutic drug ribavirin (29, 88), but the disease is often recognized only at a late stage; ideally, treatment should commence before day 5 of illness. Owing to the occurrence of vomiting and hemorrhagic gastroenteritis, oral ribavirin cannot be used in severely ill patients who need treatment most, and the intravenous form of the drug is often difficult to obtain, since it is produced on a limited scale owing to the lack of demand. Oral ribavirin can be used prophylactically in instances of known exposure to infection, such as in needlestick injuries with the blood of patients with a confirmed diagnosis. Inactivated vaccines prepared from infected mouse brain were used for the protection of humans in Eastern Europe and the former USSR in the past, but no vaccines are currently available (39).

REFERENCES

1. Altaf, A., S. Luby, A. J. Ahmed, N. Zaidi, A. J. Khan, S. Mirza, J. McCormick, and S. Fisher-Hoch. 1998. Outbreak of Crimean-Congo haemorrhagic fever in Quetta, Pakistan: contact tracing and risk assessment. *Trop. Med. Int. Health* **3**:878–882.

2. Al Tikriti, S. K., F. Al Ani, F. J. Jurji, H. Tantawi, M. Al Moslih, N. Al Janabi, M. I. Mahmud, A. Al Bana, H. Habib, H. Al Munthri, S. Al Janabi, K. Al Jawahry, M. Yonan, F. Hassan, and D. I. Simpson. 1981. Congo/Crimean haemorrhagic fever in Iraq. *Bull. W. H. O.* **59**:85–90.

3. Baskerville, A., A. Satti, F. A. Murphy, and D. I. Simpson. 1981. Congo-Crimean haemorrhagic fever in Dubai: histopathological studies. *J. Clin. Pathol.* **34**:871–874.

4. Burney, M. I., A. Ghafoor, M. Saleen, P. A. Webb, and J. Casals. 1980. Nosocomial outbreak of viral hemorrhagic fever caused by Crimean hemorrhagic fever-Congo virus in Pakistan, January 1976. *Am. J. Trop. Med. Hyg.* **29**:941–947.

5. Burt, F. J., P. A. Leman, J. C. Abbott, and R. Swanepoel. 1994. Serodiagnosis of Crimean-Congo haemorrhagic fever. *Epidemiol. Infect.* **113**:551–562.

6. Burt, F. J., P. A. Leman, J. F. Smith, and R. Swanepoel. 1998. The use of a reverse transcription-polymerase chain reaction for the detection of viral nucleic acid in the diagnosis of Crimean-Congo haemorrhagic fever. *J. Virol. Methods* **70**:129–137.

7. Burt, F. J., D. C. Spencer, P. A. Leman, B. Patterson, and R. Swanepoel. 1996. Investigation of tick-borne viruses as pathogens of humans in South Africa and evidence of Dugbe virus infection in a patient with prolonged thrombocytopenia. *Epidemiol. Infect.* **116**:353–361.

8. Burt, F. J., R. Swanepoel, and L. E. O. Braack. 1993. Enzyme-linked immunosorbent assays for the detection of antibody to Crimean-Congo haemorrhagic fever virus in the sera of livestock and wild vertebrates. *Epidemiol. Infect.* **111**:547–557.

9. Burt, F. J., R. Swanepoel, W. J. Shieh, J. F. Smith, P. A. Leman, P. W. Greer, L. M. Coffield, P. E. Rollin, T. G. Ksiazek, C. J. Peters, and S. R. Zaki. 1997. Immunohistochemical and in situ localization of Crimean-Congo hemorrhagic fever (CCHF) virus in human tissues and implications for CCHF pathogenesis. *Arch. Pathol. Lab. Med.* **121**:839–846.

10. Calisher, C. H., and N. Karabatsos. 1989. Arbovirus serogroups: definition and geographic distribution, p. 19–57. *In* T. P. Monath (ed.), *The Arboviruses: Epidemiology and Ecology*, vol. 1. CRC Press, Inc., Boca Raton, Fla.

11. Camicas, J. L., M. L. Wilson, J. P. Cornet, J. P. Digoutte, M. A. Calvo, F. Adam, and J. P. Gonzalez. 1991. Ecology of ticks as potential vectors of Crimean-Congo hemorrhagic fever virus in Senegal: epidemiological implications. *Arch. Virol.* **115**(Suppl. 1):303–322.

12. Capua, I. 1998. Crimean-Congo haemorrhagic fever in ostriches: a public health risk for countries of the European Union. *Avian Pathol.* **27**:117–120.

13. Casals, J. 1969. Antigenic similarity between the virus causing Crimean hemorrhagic fever and Congo virus. *Proc. Soc. Exp. Biol. Med.* **131**:233–236.

14. Casals, J., and G. H. Tignor. 1980. The *Nairovirus* genus: serological relationships. *Intervirology* **14**:144–147.

15. Chapman, L. E., M. L. Wilson, D. B. Hall, B. Leguenno, E. A. Dykstra, K. Ba, and S. P. Fisher-Hoch. 1991. Risk factors for Crimean-Congo hemorrhagic fever in rural northern Senegal. *J. Infect. Dis.* **164**:686–692.

16. Chumakov, M. P. 1974. Contribution to 30 years of investigation of Crimean-Congo haemorrhagic fever. *Trudy Inst. Polio. Virus. Enstef. Akad. Med. Nauk SSSR* **22**:5–18. (In Russian.)

17. Chumakov, M. P., S. E. Smirnova, and E. A. Tkachenko. 1970. Relationship between strains of Crimean haemorrhagic fever and Congo viruses. *Acta Virol.* **14**:82–85.

18. Clerx, J. P., J. Casals, and D. H. Bishop. 1981. Structural characteristics of nairoviruses (genus Nairovirus, Bunyaviridae). *J. Gen. Virol.* **55**:165–178.

19. Davies, F. G., J. Casals, D. M. Jesset, and P. Ochieng. 1978. The serological relationships of Nairobi sheep disease virus. *J. Comp. Pathol.* **88**:519–523.

20. Dohm, D. J., T. M. Logan, K. J. Linthicum, C. A. Rossi, and M. J. Turell. 1996. Transmission of Crimean-Congo hemorrhagic fever virus by *Hyalomma impeltatum* (Acari:Ixodidae) after experimental infection. *J. Med. Entomol.* **33**:848–851.

21. Donets, M. A., M. P. Chumakov, M. B. Korolev, and S. G. Rubin. 1977. Physicochemical characteristics, morphology and morphogenesis of virions of the causative agent of Crimean hemorrhagic fever. *Intervirology* **8**:294–308.

22. Drosten, C., S. Gottig, S. Schilling, M. Asper, M. Panning, H. Schmitz, and S. Gunther. 2002. Rapid detection and quantification of RNA of Ebola and Marburg viruses, Lassa virus, dengue virus, and yellow fever virus by real-time reverse transcription-PCR. *J. Clin. Microbiol.* **40**:2323–2330.

23. Drosten, C., D. Minnak, P. Emmerich, H. Schmitz, and T. Reinecke. 2002. Crimean-Congo hemorrhagic fever in Kosovo. *J. Clin. Microbiol.* **40**:1122–1123.

24. Dunster, L., M. Dunster, V. Ofula, D. Beti, F. Kazooba-Voskamp, F. Burt, R. Swanepoel, and K. M. DeCock. 2002. First documentation of human Crimean-Congo hemorrhagic fever, Kenya. *Emerg. Infect. Dis.* **8**:1005–1006.

25. Durden, L. A., T. M. Logan, M. L. Wilson, and K. J. Linthicum. 1993. Experimental vector incompetence of a soft tick, *Ornithodoros sonrai* (Acari:Argasidae), for Crimean-Congo hemorrhagic fever virus. *J. Med. Entomol.* **30**:493–496.

26. El Azazy, O. M., and E. M. Scrimgeour. 1997. Crimean-Congo haemorrhagic fever virus infection in the western province of Saudi Arabia. *Trans. R. Soc. Trop. Med. Hyg.* **91**:275–278.

27. Faye, O., J. P. Cornet, J. L. Camicas, D. Fontenille, and J. P. Gonzalez. 1999. Experimental transmission of Crimean-Congo hemorrhagic fever virus: role of 3 vector species in the maintenance and transmission cycles in Senegal. *Parasite* **6**:27–32. (In French.)

28. Faye, O., D. Fontenille, J. Thonnon, J. P. Gonzalez, J. P. Cornet, and J. L. Camicas. 1999. Experimental transmission of Crimean-Congo hemorrhagic fever virus by *Rhipicephalus evertsi evertsi* (Acarina:Ixodidae). *Bull. Soc. Pathol. Exot.* **92**:143–147. (In French.)

29. Fisher-Hoch, S. P., J. A. Khan, S. Rehman, S. Mirza, M. Khurshid, and J. B. McCormick. 1995. Crimean Congo-

haemorrhagic fever treated with oral ribavirin. *Lancet* **346:** 472–475.

30. Fisher-Hoch, S. P., J. B. McCormick, R. Swanepoel, A. Van Middlekoop, S. Harvey, and H. G. Kustner. 1992. Risk of human infections with Crimean-Congo hemorrhagic fever virus in a South African rural community. *Am. J. Trop. Med. Hyg.* **47:**337–345.

31. Foulke, R. S., R. R. Rosato, and G. R. French. 1981. Structural polypeptides of Hazara virus. *J. Gen. Virol.* **53:**169–172.

32. Gear, J. H., P. D. Thomson, M. Hopp, S. Andronikou, R. J. Cohn, J. Ledger, and F. E. Berkowitz. 1982. Congo-Crimean haemorrhagic fever in South Africa. Report of a fatal case in the Transvaal. *S. Afr. Med. J.* **62:**576–580.

33. Georges, A. J., J. F. Saluzzo, J. P. Gonzalez, and G. V. Dussarat. 1980. Arboviroses en Centrafrique: incidence et aspects diagnostiques chez l'homme. *Med. Trop.* **40:**561–568.

34. Gonzalez, J. P., J. L. Camicas, J. P. Cornet, O. Faye, and M. L. Wilson. 1992. Sexual and transovarian transmission of Crimean-Congo haemorrhagic fever virus in *Hyalomma truncatum* ticks. *Res. Virol.* **143:**23–28.

35. Gonzalez, J. P., J. P. Cornet, M. L. Wilson, and J. L. Camicas. 1991. Crimean-Congo haemorrhagic fever virus replication in adult *Hyalomma truncatum* and *Amblyomma variegatum* ticks. *Res. Virol.* **142:**483–488.

36. Gonzalez, J. P., B. Leguenno, M. Guillaud, and M. L. Wilson. 1990. A fatal case of Crimean-Congo haemorrhagic fever in Mauritania: virological and serological evidence suggesting epidemic transmission. *Trans. R. Soc. Trop. Med. Hyg.* **84:** 573–576.

37. Gordon, S. W., K. J. Linthicum, and J. P. Moulton. 1993. Transmission of Crimean-Congo hemorrhagic fever virus in two species of *Hyalomma* ticks from infected adults to cofeeding immature forms. *Am. J. Trop. Med. Hyg.* **48:**576–580.

38. Hassanein, K. M., O. M. El Azazy, and H. M. Yousef. 1997. Detection of Crimean-Congo haemorrhagic fever virus antibodies in humans and imported livestock in Saudi Arabia. *Trans. R. Soc. Trop. Med. Hyg.* **91:**536–537.

39. Hoogstraal, H. 1979. The epidemiology of tick-borne Crimean-Congo hemorrhagic fever in Asia, Europe, and Africa. *J. Med. Entomol.* **15:**307–417.

40. Hoogstraal, H. 1981. Changing patterns of tick-borne diseases in modern society. *Ann. Rev. Entomol.* **26:**75–99.

41. Hoogstraal, H., M. N. Kaiser, M. A. Traylor, S. Gaber, and E. Guindy. 1961. Ticks (Ixodoidea) on birds migrating from Africa to Europe and Asia. *Bull. W. H. O.* **24:**197–212.

42. Hoogstraal, H., M. N. Kaiser, M. A. Traylor, E. Guindy, and S. Gaber. 1963. Ticks (Ixodoidea) on birds migrating from Europe and Asia to Africa. 1959–61. *Bull. W. H. O.* **28:** 235–262.

43. Reference deleted.

44. Reference deleted.

45. Reference deleted.

46. Reference deleted.

47. Jones, L. D., C. R. Davies, G. M. Steele, and P. A. Nuttall. 1987. A novel mode of arbovirus transmission involving a nonviremic host. *Science* **237:**775–777.

48. Jones, L. D., E. Hodgson, and P. A. Nuttall. 1989. Enhancement of virus by salivary glands. *J. Gen. Virol.* **70:**1895–1898.

49. Joubert, J. R., J. B. King, D. J. Rossouw, and R. Cooper. 1985. A nosocomial outbreak of Crimean-Congo haemorrhagic fever at Tygerberg Hospital. III. Clinical pathology and pathogenesis. *S. Afr. Med. J.* **68:**722–728.

50. Karabatsos, N. 1985. *International Catalogue of Arboviruses (including certain other viruses of vertebrates)*, 3rd ed. Amer-ican Society of Tropical Medicine and Hygiene, San Antonio, Tex.

51. Khan, A. S., G. O. Maupin, P. E. Rollin, A. M. Noor, H. H. Shurie, A. G. Shalabi, S. Wasef, Y. M. Haddad, R. Sadek, K. Ijaz, C. J. Peters, and T. G. Ksiazek. 1997. An outbreak of Crimean-Congo hemorrhagic fever in the United Arab Emirates, 1994–1995. *Am. J. Trop. Med. Hyg.* **57:**519–525.

52. Kondratenko, V. F. 1976. Importance of ixodid ticks in the transmission and preservation of the causative agent of Crimean hemorrhagic fever in foci of the infection. *Parazitologiia* **10:**297–302. (In Russian.)

53. Lee, V. H., and G. E. Kemp. 1970. Congo virus: experimental infection of *Hyalomma rufipes* and transmission to a calf. *Bull. Entomol. Soc. Nigeria* **2:**133–135.

54. Logan, T. M., K. J. Linthicum, C. L. Bailey, D. M. Watts, D. J. Dohm, and J. R. Moulton. 1990. Replication of Crimean-Congo hemorrhagic fever virus in four species of ixodid ticks (Acari) infected experimentally. *J. Med. Entomol.* **27:**537–542.

55. Logan, T. M., K. J. Linthicum, C. L. Bailey, D. M. Watts, and J. R. Moulton. 1989. Experimental transmission of Crimean-Congo hemorrhagic fever virus by *Hyalomma truncatum* Koch. *Am. J. Trop. Med. Hyg.* **40:**207–212.

56. Marriott, A. C., and P. A. Nuttall. 1992. Comparison of the S RNA segments and nucleoprotein sequences of Crimean-Congo hemorrhagic fever, Hazara, and Dugbe viruses. *Virology* **189:**795–799.

57. Marriott, A. C., and P. A. Nuttall. 1996. Molecular biology of nairoviruses, p. 41–104. *In* R. M. Elliott (ed.), The *Bunyaviridae*. Plenum Press, New York, N.Y.

58. Marriott, A. C., T. Polyzoni, A. Antoniadis, and P. A. Nuttall. 1994. Detection of human antibodies to Crimean-Congo haemorrhagic fever virus using expressed viral nucleocapsid protein. *J. Gen. Virol.* **75:**2157–2161.

59. Martin, M. L., H. Lindsey-Regnery, D. R. Sasso, J. B. McCormick, and E. Palmer. 1985. Distinction between Bunyaviridae genera by surface structure and comparison with Hantaan virus using negative-stain electron microscopy. *Acta Virol.* **86:**17–28.

60. Moore, D. L., O. R. Causey, D. E. Carey, S. Raddy, A. R. Cooke, F. M. Akinkugbe, T. S. David-West, and G. E. Kemp. 1975. Arthropod-borne viral infections of man in Nigeria, 1964–1970. *Ann. Trop. Med. Parasitol.* **69:**49–63.

61. Okorie, T. G. 1991. Comparative studies on the vector capacity of the different stages of *Amblyomma variegatum* Fabricius and *Hyalomma rufipes* Koch for Congo virus, after intracoelomic inoculation. *Vet. Parasitol.* **38:**215–223.

62. Onishchenko, G. G., G. T. Aidinov, E. A. Moskvitina, Iu. M. Lomov, N. G. Tikhonov, V. I. Prometnoi, M. M. Shvager, V. Iu. Ryzhkov, P. P. Savchenko, T. A. Dmitrieva, V. V. Batashev, Iu. M. Pukhov, N. L. Pichurina, N. G. Ivanova, S. A. Gavrinev, E. V. Kovalev, V. A. Kipaikin, V. L. Pauk, Z. N. Emel'ianova, I. V. Orekhov, A. D. Lipkovich, V. V. Stakheev, V. G. Trepel, A. V. Usatkin, V. I. Markov, I. V. Borisevich, V. A. Merkulov, A. A. Makhlai, N. T. Vasil'ev, B. N. Mishan'kin, S. O. Vodop'ianov, T. V. Mazrukho, and V. P. Badunenko. 2000. Crimean-Congo hemorrhagic fever in Rostov Province: the epidemiological characteristics of an outbreak. *Zh. Mikrobiol. Epidemiol. Immunobiol.* **2:**36–42. (In Russian.)

63. Onishchenko, G. G., V. I. Markov, V. A. Merkulov, N. T. Vasil'ev, A. M. Berezhnoi, I. A. Androshchuk, and V. A. Maksimov. 2001. Isolation and identification of Crimean-Congo hemorrhagic fever virus in the Stavropol territory. *Zh. Mikrobiol. Epidemiol. Immunobiol.* **6:**7–11.

64. Papa, A., S. Bino, A. Llagami, B. Brahimaj, E. Papadimitriou, V. Pavlidou, E. Velo, G. Cahani, M. Hajdini, A. Pilaca, A. Harxhi, and A. Antoniadis. 2002. Crimean-Congo hemorrhagic fever in Albania, 2001. *Eur. J. Clin. Microbiol. Infect. Dis.* 8:603–606.

65. Papa, A., B. Bosovic, V. Pavlidou, E. Papadimitriou, M. Pelemis, and A. Antoniades. 2002. Genetic detection and isolation of Crimean-Congo hemorrhagic fever virus, Kosovo, Yugoslavia. *Emerg. Infect. Dis.* 8:852–854.

66. Papa, A., B. Ma, S. Kouidou, Q. Tang, C. Hang, and A. Antoniadis. 2002. Genetic characterization of the M RNA segment of Crimean Congo hemorrhagic fever virus strains, China. *Emerg. Infect. Dis.* 8:50–53.

67. Reference deleted.

68. Rodriguez, L. L., G. O. Maupin, T. G. Ksiazek, P. E. Rollin, A. S. Khan, T. F. Schwarz, R. S. Lofts, J. F. Smith, A. M. Noor, C. J. Peters, and S. T. Nichol. 1997. Molecular investigation of a multisource outbreak of Crimean-Congo hemorrhagic fever in the United Arab Emirates. *Am. J. Trop. Med. Hyg.* 57:512–518.

69. Saluzzo, J. F., P. Aubry, J. McCormick, and J. P. Digoutte. 1985. Haemorrhagic fever caused by Crimean Congo haemorrhagic fever virus in Mauritania. *Trans. R. Soc. Trop. Med. Hyg.* 79:268.

70. Saluzzo, J. F., J. P. Digoutte, M. Cornet, D. Baudon, J. Roux, and V. Robert. 1984. Isolation of Crimean-Congo haemorrhagic fever and Rift Valley fever viruses in Upper Volta. *Lancet* 1:1179.

71. Sanchez, A. J., M. J. Vincent, and S. T. Nichol. 2002. Characterization of the glycoproteins of Crimean-Congo hemorrhagic fever virus. *J. Virol.* 76:7263–7275.

72. Schmaljohn, C. S., and J. L. Patterson. 1990. Bunyaviridae and their replication, p. 1175–1194. Part II: replication of Bunyaviridae. *In* B. N. Fields (ed.), *Virology*, 2nd ed. Raven Press Ltd., New York, N.Y.

73. Schwarz, T. F., H. Nitschko, G. Jager, H. Nsanze, M. Longson, R. N. Pugh, and A. K. Abraham. 1995. Crimean-Congo haemorrhagic fever in Oman. *Lancet* 346:1230.

74. Schwarz, T. F., H. Nsanze, M. Longson, H. Nitschko, S. Gilch, H. Shurie, A. Ameen, A. R. Zahir, U. G. Acharya, and G. Jager. 1996. Polymerase chain reaction for diagnosis and identification of distinct variants of Crimean-Congo hemorrhagic fever virus in the United Arab Emirates. *Am. J. Trop. Med. Hyg.* 55:190–196.

75. Scrimgeour, E. M. 1996. Crimean-Congo haemorrhagic fever in Oman. *Lancet* 347:692.

76. Scrimgeour, E. M., F. R. Mehta, and A. J. Suleiman. 1999. Infectious and tropical diseases in Oman: a review. *Am. J. Trop. Med. Hyg.* 61:920–925.

77. Scrimgeour, E. M., A. Zaki, F. R. Mehta, A. K. Abraham, S. Al Busaidy, H. El Khatim, S. F. Al Rawas, A. M. Kamal, and A. J. Mohammed. 1996. Crimean-Congo haemorrhagic fever in Oman. *Trans. R. Soc. Trop. Med. Hyg.* 90:290–291.

78. Shepherd, A. J., P. A. Leman, and R. Swanepoel. 1989. Viraemia and antibody response of small African and laboratory animals to Crimean-Congo hemorrhagic fever virus infection. *Am. J. Trop. Med. Hyg.* 40:541–547.

79. Shepherd, A. J., R. Swanepoel, A. J. Cornel, and O. Mathee. 1989. Experimental studies on the replication and transmission of Crimean-Congo hemorrhagic fever virus in some African tick species. *Am. J. Trop. Med. Hyg.* 40:326–331.

80. Shepherd, A. J., R. Swanepoel, and P. A. Leman. 1989. Antibody response in Crimean-Congo hemorrhagic fever. *Rev. Infect. Dis.* 11(Suppl. 4):S801–S806.

81. Shepherd, A. J., R. Swanepoel, P. A. Leman, and S. P. Shepherd. 1987. Field and laboratory investigation of Crimean-Congo haemorrhagic fever virus (Nairovirus, family Bunyaviridae) infection in birds. *Trans. R. Soc. Trop. Med. Hyg.* 81:1004–1007.

82. Shepherd, A. J., R. Swanepoel, S. P. Shepherd, P. A. Leman, N. K. Blackburn, and A. F. Hallett. 1985. A nosocomial outbreak of Crimean-Congo haemorrhagic fever at Tygerberg Hospital. V. Virological and serological observations. *S. Afr. Med. J.* 68:733–736.

83. Shepherd, A. J., R. Swanepoel, S. P. Shepherd, P. A. Leman, and O. Mathee. 1991. Viraemic transmission of Crimean-Congo haemorrhagic fever virus to ticks. *Epidemiol. Infect.* 106:373–382.

84. Shepherd, A. J., R. Swanepoel, S. P. Shepherd, G. M. McGillivray, and L. A. Searle. 1987. Antibody to Crimean-Congo hemorrhagic fever virus in wild mammals from southern Africa. *Am. J. Trop. Med. Hyg.* 36:133–142.

85. Simpson, D. K. H., E. M. Knight, M. C. G. Courtois, M. P. Weinbren, and J. W. Kibukamusoke. 1967. Congo virus: a hitherto undescribed virus occurring in Africa. I. Human isolations—clinical notes. *E. Afr. Med. J.* 44:87–92.

86. Reference deleted.

87. Suleiman, M. N., J. M. Muscat-Baron, J. R. Harries, A. G. Satti, G. S. Platt, E. T. Bowen, and D. I. Simpson. 1980. Congo/Crimean haemorrhagic fever in Dubai. An outbreak at the Rashid Hospital. *Lancet* 2:939–941.

88. Swanepoel, R. 1981–2002. Unpublished observations.

89. Swanepoel, R., D. E. Gill, A. J. Shepherd, P. A. Leman, J. H. Mynhardt, and S. Harvey. 1989. The clinical pathology of Crimean-Congo hemorrhagic fever. *Rev. Infect. Dis.* 11(Suppl. 4):S794–S800.

90. Swanepoel, R., P. A. Leman, F. J. Burt, J. Jardine, D. J. Verwoerd, I. Capua, G. K. Bruckner, and W. P. Burger. 1998. Experimental infection of ostriches with Crimean-Congo haemorrhagic fever virus. *Epidemiol. Infect.* 121:427–432.

91. Swanepoel, R., A. J. Shepherd, P. A. Leman, and S. P. Shepherd. 1985. Investigations following initial recognition of Crimean-Congo haemorrhagic fever in South Africa and the diagnosis of 2 further cases. *S. Afr. Med. J.* 68:638–641.

92. Swanepoel, R., A. J. Shepherd, P. A. Leman, S. P. Shepherd, G. M. McGillivray, M. J. Erasmus, L. A. Searle, and D. E. Gill. 1987. Epidemiologic and clinical features of Crimean-Congo hemorrhagic fever in southern Africa. *Am. J. Trop. Med. Hyg.* 36:120–132.

93. Swanepoel, R., A. J. Shepherd, P. A. Leman, S. P. Shepherd, and G. B. Miller. 1985. A common-source outbreak of Crimean-Congo haemorrhagic fever on a dairy farm. *S. Afr. Med. J.* 68:635–637.

94. Swanepoel, R., J. K. Struthers, A. J. Shepherd, G. M. McGillivray, M. J. Nel, and P. G. Jupp. 1983. Crimean-Congo hemorrhagic fever in South Africa. *Am. J. Trop. Med. Hyg.* 32:1407–1415.

95. Tantawi, H. H., M. I. Al Moslih, N. Y. Al Janabi, A. S. Al Bana, M. I. Mahmud, F. Jurji, M. S. Yonan, F. Al Ani, and S. K. Al Tikriti. 1980. Crimean-Congo haemorrhagic fever virus in Iraq: isolation, identification and electron microscopy. *Acta Virol.* 24:464–467.

96. Van Eeden, P. J., J. R. Joubert, B. W. van de Wal, J. B. King, A. De Kock, and J. H. Groenewald. 1985. A nosocomial outbreak of Crimean-Congo haemorrhagic fever at Tygerberg Hospital. I. Clinical features. *S. Afr. Med. J.* 68:711–717.

97. Ward, K. W., A. C. Marriott, A. A. El-Ghorr, and P. A. Nuttall. 1990. Coding strategy of the S RNA segment of Dugbe virus (*Nairovirus*; Bunyaviridae). *Virology* 175:518–524.

98. Watts, D. M., T. G. Ksiazek, K. J. Linthicum, and H. Hoogstraal. 1989. Crimean-Congo haemorrhagic fever p. 177– 222. *In* T. P. Monath (ed.), *The Arboviruses: Epi-*

demiology and Ecology, vol. 2. CRC Press, Inc., Boca Raton, Fla.

99. **Williams, R. J., S. Al Busaidy, F. R. Mehta, G. O. Maupin, K. D. Wagoner, S. Al Awaidy, A. J. Suleiman, A. S. Khan, C. J. Peters, and T. G. Ksiazek.** 2000. Crimean-congo haemorrhagic fever: a seroepidemiological and tick survey in the Sultanate of Oman. *Trop. Med. Int. Health* **5:**99–106.

100. **Wilson, M. L., J. P. Gonzalez, J. P. Cornet, and J. L. Camicas.** 1991. Transmission of Crimean-Congo haemorrhagic fever virus from experimentally infected sheep to *Hyalomma truncatum* ticks. *Res. Virol.* **142:**395–404.

101. **Zeller, H. G., J. P. Cornet, and J. L. Camicas.** 1994. Experimental transmission of Crimean-Congo hemorrhagic fever virus by West African wild ground-feeding birds to *Hyalomma marginatum rufipes* ticks. *Am. J. Trop. Med. Hyg.* **50:**676–681.

102. **Zeller, H. G., J. P. Cornet, and J. L. Camicas.** 1994. Crimean-Congo haemorrhagic fever virus infection in birds: field investigations in Senegal. *Res. Virol.* **145:**105–109.

103. **Zeller, H. G., J. P. Cornet, A. Diop, and J. L. Camicas.** 1997. Crimean-Congo hemorrhagic fever in ticks (Acari:Ixodidae) and ruminants: field observations of an epizootic in Bandia, Senegal (1989-1992). *J. Med. Entomol.* **34:**511–516.

Tick-Borne Diseases of Humans
Jesse L. Goodman et al.
© 2005 ASM Press, Washington, D.C.

Chapter 11

Lyme Borreliosis

ALLEN C. STEERE, JENIFER COBURN, AND LISA GLICKSTEIN

HISTORY

Lyme disease was described as a separate entity in 1976 because of geographic clustering of children in Lyme, Connecticut, who were thought to have juvenile rheumatoid arthritis (309). The rural setting of the case clusters, the usual onsets of joint symptoms in the summer and early fall, and the onsets in the same families in different years suggested that the disorder was transmitted by an arthropod. Moreover, some of the initial patients noted an expanding red skin lesion, thought to be an insect bite, before the onset of arthritis. The lesion was most compatible with erythema migrans (EM), which was first described in Europe in the early 20th century (4, 184) and in the United States in the 1970s (204, 277). In Europe, the skin lesion had been associated with the bite of *Ixodes ricinus* ticks and with subsequent neurologic abnormalities (21) but not with arthritis.

During the summer of 1976, 24 patients with EM were identified in the Lyme, Connecticut, area and followed prospectively (308). Days to weeks later, 75% of these patients developed arthralgias or arthritis, confirming the link between this skin lesion and Lyme arthritis. Moreover, some of the patients also developed neurologic or cardiac abnormalities, which showed that Lyme disease was a complex, multisystem illness. During the summer of 1977, further epidemiological studies of patients with EM implicated *Ixodes scapularis* (also called *Ixodes dammini*) ticks, a member of the *I. ricinus* complex (also called the *Ixodes persulcatus* complex) as the vector of Lyme disease (296). Moreover, communities that had a higher incidence of the disease also had a higher frequency of animals carrying *I. scapularis* ticks (328). By 1979, 512 cases of Lyme disease had been identified in the United States, mainly along the northeastern coast and in Wisconsin, Minnesota, and northern California (307). These locations correlated closely with the known distribution of *I. scapularis* ticks in the first two areas and with *Ixodes pacificus* in the last. Thus, both clinical and epidemiological evidence strongly implicated ticks of the *I. ricinus* complex as vectors of the disease.

In 1981, Burgdorfer and colleagues at the Rocky Mountain Laboratory discovered a spirochetal bacterium, later named *Borrelia burgdorferi*, in the midgut of a nymphal *I. scapularis* tick (48). This spirochete was subsequently isolated from EM skin lesions, blood, and cerebrospinal fluid (CSF) of patients with Lyme disease in the United States (31, 302), and from patients with related syndromes in Europe (2, 17, 246). Patients' organism-specific antibody responses were linked conclusively with *B. burgdorferi*, proving the spirochetal etiology of Lyme disease.

CAUSATIVE AGENTS OF LYME BORRELIOSIS

Lyme disease or Lyme borreliosis is now recognized as an important infectious disease in North America, Europe, and Asia (291). The formerly designated *B. burgdorferi* has now been subdivided into multiple *Borrelia* species, including three that cause human infection (Table 1). In the United States, the sole cause of infection is *B. burgdorferi* (147). Although all three pathogenic species are found in Europe, most disease there is caused by *Borrelia afzelii* or *Borrelia garinii*; these two species also seem to be responsible for the illness in Asia (22, 54).

Based on minor differences in the sequences of ribosomal RNA, eight other closely related *Borrelia* species have been identified (Table 1) (104, 157, 178, 198, 205, 243, 329). These borrelial species are found in enzootic cycles in which the tick vector rarely bites humans, if at all, and these species rarely cause human Lyme disease.

Allen C. Steere and Lisa Glickstein • Center for Immunology and Inflammatory Diseases, Division of Rheumatology, Massachusetts General Hospital, Harvard Medical School, Boston, MA 02114.   **Jenifer Coburn** • Division of Geographic Medicine and Infectious Diseases, Tufts-New England Medical Center, Boston, MA 02111.

Table 1. Genomic groups or genospecies of *B. burgdorferi* and related *Borrelia* species

Species (no.)	Location	Reference
Pathogenic (3)		
B. burgdorferi	United States and Europe	18
B. afzelii	Europe and Asia	19
B. garinii	Europe and Asia	20
Minimally pathogenic or nonpathogenic (8)		
Borrelia andersonii sp. nov.	United States	22
B. bissettii sp. nov.	United States	26
Borrelia valaisiana	Europe	24
Borrelia lusitaniae	Europe	25
Borrelia japonica	Asia	21
Borrelia tanukii	Asia	23
Borrelia turdi	Asia	23
Borrelia sinica	Asia	27

BIOLOGY OF *B. BURGDORFERI*

The *Borrelia* species, along with the leptospira and treponema, belong to the eubacterial phylum of spirochetes, a group of vigorously motile, corkscrew-shaped bacteria (Fig. 1) (27). The spirochetal cell wall consists of a cytoplasmic membrane surrounded by peptidoglycan, flagella, and a loosely associated outer membrane. The borrelia are longer and more loosely coiled than the other spirochetes. Of the *Borrelia* species, *B. burgdorferi* is the longest (20 to 30 μm) and narrowest (0.2 to 0.3 μm), and it has fewer flagella (138). Flagellar rotation results in waveform motility (115), whereas mutant organisms without flagella are straight and nonmotile (216).

The genome of *B. burgdorferi* is highly unusual in that the chromosome is linear and has telomeres with covalently closed ends (26). In addition, *B. burgdorferi* has plasmids, or extrachromosomal genetic elements, some of which are indispensable and could be thought of as minichromosomes (137). The chromosome and plasmids of a representative *B. burgdorferi* strain, B31, have been fully sequenced (57, 102). The linear chromosome is just under 1 Mb, among the smallest bacterial chromosomes known. In addition, the organism has 9 circular and 12 linear plasmids that constitute 40% of its total DNA. Although all strains contain the linear chromosome, isolates may differ in plasmid content, and they may lose certain plasmids in culture. For example, after 10 to 15 passages, cultured *B. burgdorferi* commonly loses two small linear plasmids, which appear to be essential for infectivity and immune evasion (172, 253). These are designated lp25, which encodes a nicotinamidase, and lp28-1, which encodes the VlsE lipoprotein.

The most remarkable aspect of the *B. burgdorferi* genome is the large number of sequences encoding predicted or known lipoproteins (57, 102). In fact, its genome encodes approximately 10 times more lipoproteins in proportion to its size than any other known bacterial genome. Lipoproteins are found in the outer leaflet of both the cytoplasmic and outer membranes and within the inner leaflet of the outer membrane. The entire protein content of the outer membrane can move to one end of the cylinder, a phenomenon called capping that may be important in adherence to cells (25). Although the lipoproteins of *B. burgdorferi* provoke an inflammatory response, the outer membrane does not contain lipopolysaccharide (also known as endotoxin), as do classical gram-negative bacterial species.

The genome of *B. burgdorferi* encodes few proteins with recognizable biosynthetic activity (102); therefore, the organism apparently depends on the host for most of its nutritional needs. A very unusual feature of *B. burgdorferi* is that it does not require iron, at least for growth in vitro (242). This may allow the spirochete to circumvent a usual host defense against infection, which is to limit the availability of iron. The *B. burgdorferi* genome contains no recognizable toxins or homologues of systems that specialize in the secretion of toxins or other virulence factors. Instead, *B. burgdorferi* causes chronic infection by adhesion to host cells and tissue matrixes, invasion of tissues, and evasion of immune clearance.

Genetic Manipulation of *B. burgdorferi*

For many pathogens, the role of specific bacterial genes has been delineated by comparing the function of wild-type and mutated organisms. Although it has been difficult to manipulate the *B. burgdorferi* genome, progress has recently been made (36, 51, 266, 267, 318). Utilizing selectable markers driven by constitutive promoters of the spirochete and shuttle vectors between *B. burgdorferi* and *Escherichia coli*, mutants and complemented derivatives have been generated in several noninfectious strains of the spirochete (140, 267). It has been harder to generate specific mutants in infectious strains, probably because the lp25 plasmid, which is required for infectivity, encodes restriction-modification systems that prevent recombination (177). However, with a shuttle vector, the infectivity of a strain lacking lp25 was recently restored by the insertion of a single gene (BBE22) encoded by this plasmid (252). Thus, it may be possible to inactivate genes in noninfectious strains, followed by restoration of infectivity with the BBE22 gene (56, 318, 344).

Another approach involves the use of bacteriophages, the viruses that infect bacteria. Phage particles have been observed in *B. burgdorferi* culture

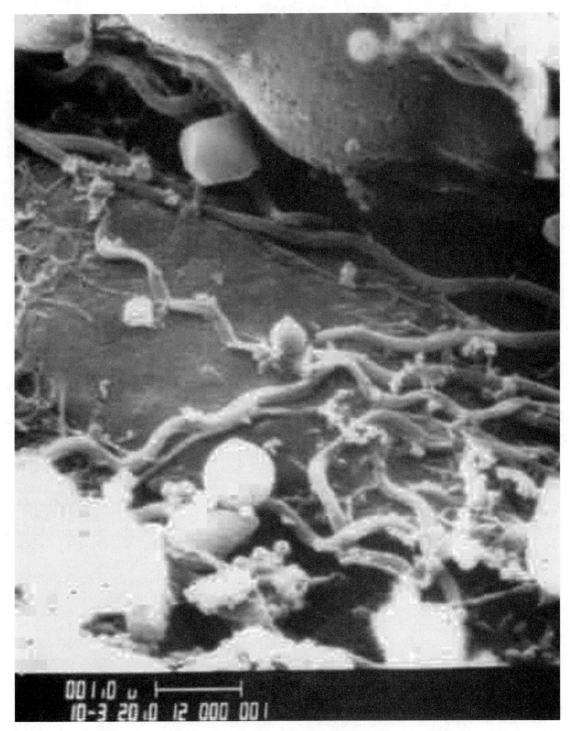

Figure 1. A scanning electron micrograph of *B. burgdorferi* spirochetes in the mid-gut of a nymphal *I. scapularis* tick. The picture was a kind gift of Dr. Willy Burgdorfer.

supernatants (91, 221). When a kanamycin-resistance marker was introduced into one of the 32-kb circular plasmids (cp32) of *B. burgdorferi*, which bears some resemblance to phage genomes, phage-mediated transduction of the antibiotic resistance marker was demonstrated (90).

Cultivation of *B. burgdorferi*

B. burgdorferi spirochetes are fastidious, microaerophilic bacteria that grow best at 33 to 34°C in a complex, liquid medium called Barbour-Stoenner-Kelly medium (24, 245). Bacterial growth is slow, with a doubling time of 12 to 24 h. Colonies of *Borrelia* can also be grown in medium with agarose added at concentrations just sufficient to permit gelation (265). The plating efficiency varies among strains and is generally lower for low-passage, infectious cultures.

ENZOOTIC CYCLES OF *B. BURGDORFERI* AND RELATED *BORRELIA* SPECIES

B. burgdorferi and related *Borrelia* species exist in nature in enzootic cycles primarily involving ticks of the *I. ricinus* complex and a wide range of animal hosts (174, 287). The *I. ricinus* complex consists of four groups of 14 closely related tick species that are nearly identical in appearance (Table 2) (343). However, only some of these ticks bite humans. These include the deer tick, *I. scapularis*, in the northeastern and north-central United States (Color Plate 1C); *I. pacificus* in the western United States; the sheep tick, *I. ricinus*, in Europe; and the taiga tick, *I. persulcatus*, in Asia (Color Map 2). These are the important vectors of human Lyme borreliosis. Although other tick species of the *I. ricinus* complex and their animal hosts may be infected with related *Borrelia* species, these ticks less commonly bite humans; therefore, they are minimally involved, if at all, in disease transmission to humans. *B. burgdorferi* has been demonstrated in other species of ticks (274) and in mosquitoes and deer flies (194), but only ticks of the *I. ricinus* complex have been documented to be important in disease transmission.

Table 2. Ticks of the *I. ricinus* complex[a]

Complex group and species
Group 1
I. pavlovskyi
I. persulcatus
I. nipponensis
I. gibbosus
I. jellisoni
I. pacificus
Group 2
I. pararicinus
I. affinis
I. muris
I. minor
I. ricinus
Group 3
I. scapularis
Group 4
I. granulatus
I. nuttallianus

[a] Based on sequencing of two fragments of 16S rRNA (343).

Ticks of the *I. ricinus* complex have larval, nymphal, and adult stages and feed once during each of the three stages of their usual 2-year cycle. Typically, larval ticks take one blood meal in the late summer, overwinter, and feed as nymphs during the following spring and early summer and as adults during that autumn (336). Except for *I. persulcatus*, in which the adult stage transmits the infection (163), the tiny nymphal ticks are primarily responsible for disease transmission to humans. The risk of infection in a given area depends largely on the density of these ticks, their feeding habits, and their animal hosts, which have evolved differently in different geographic locations.

In the northeastern and north-central United States, the preferred hosts for both the larval and nymphal stages of *I. scapularis* are small rodents, particularly the white-footed mouse, *Peromyscus leucopus*, and chipmunks (189). It is critical for maintenance of *B. burgdorferi* that both the tick's immature stages feed on the same host species because the spirochetal life cycle depends on horizontal transmission: from infected nymphs to mice in early summer, and from infected mice to larvae in late summer. The larvae then molt to become infected nymphs that begin the cycle again in the following year (206). The fact that white-footed mice are tolerant to infection with *B. burgdorferi* is also crucial: they develop neither protective immune responses nor organ pathology (45) and remain spirochetemic throughout the summer (189). This results in high infection rates (from 10 to 50%) in nymphal ticks (37, 197) and in affected animals.

White-tailed deer, which are not necessary for the life cycle of the spirochete itself, are the preferred host for the adult stage of *I. scapularis* (335), and they seem to be critical to the survival of the ticks (337). However, these ticks are not restricted to deer and have also been found on at least 30 types of wild animals and 49 species of birds (12, 195, 196), as well as on domestic animals, including dogs, horses, and cattle (49, 165, 199). Humans are also one of the many incidental hosts for *I. scapularis* ticks, and they have no role in the perpetuation of either the tick or the spirochetal life cycle.

The vector ecology of *B. burgdorferi* is quite different on the west coast of northern California (44), where the frequency of Lyme disease is low (231). There, two intersecting cycles are necessary for disease occurrence. One involves the dusky-footed woodrat and *Ixodes spinipalpis* (also called *Ixodes neotomae*) ticks, which do not bite humans. This cycle maintains high levels of *B. burgdorferi* in nature. The other involves *I. pacificus* ticks, which are less often infected but do bite humans and may transmit the disease to them. Only the relatively few nymphal *I. pacificus* ticks that previously fed in the larval stage on infected woodrats are responsible for spirochetal transmission to humans. In Colorado, *Borrelia bissettii*, one of the nonpathogenic species, is found in an enzootic cycle involving woodrats (*Neotoma mexicana*) and *I. spinipalpis* (271). However, this tick does not bite humans and is not known to transmit human Lyme disease.

In the southeastern United States, nymphal *I. scapularis* ticks feed primarily on lizards, which are resistant to *B. burgdorferi* infection; therefore, Lyme disease is rare in that part of the country. In the southeast, a skin rash resembling erythema migrans, which is not caused by *B. burgdorferi*, has been associated with the bite of the lone star tick, *Amblyomma americanum* (53), but the etiologic agent of that illness is not yet clear.

In Europe, there is still debate about the preferred animal hosts of *I. ricinus* (110). There, several species of mice, voles, rats, shrews, squirrels, and a number of birds have been shown to be competent reservoirs for *Borrelia* species (109). Small rodents are important reservoirs for *B. afzelii* (141), whereas birds are strongly associated with *B. garinii* (229). However, *I. ricinus* ticks feed on more than 300 different animal species, including large and small mammals, birds, and reptiles (11). In Asian Russia, northern China, and Japan, immature *I. persulcatus* ticks commonly feed on voles, shrews, and birds, and adult ticks feed on virtually all larger animals, both wild and domestic, including hares, deer, and cattle (164).

EPIDEMIOLOGY OF HUMAN LYME BORRELIOSIS

Lyme borreliosis is now the most commonly reported arthropod-borne disease in both North America and Europe, accounting for tens of thousands of new cases yearly (80, 226, 231). Since surveillance for Lyme disease was begun in the United States by the Centers for Disease Control and Prevention (CDC) in 1982, the number of reported cases has increased steadily. In recent years, more than 20,000 cases have been reported annually (231).

The disorder occurs primarily in three distinct foci: in the northeast from Maine to Maryland, in the Midwest in Wisconsin and Minnesota, and in the west in northern California (231, 307). In Connecticut, the state with the highest incidence of Lyme disease, the number of reported new cases in 1999 was 98 per 100,000 residents (231). However, most of the cases occurred in only two counties, and even within those counties, some areas were more affected than others. In a Lyme disease vaccine trial sponsored by SmithKline Beecham, which included residents from 10 states where Lyme disease was endemic, the yearly incidence of infec-

tion in high-risk areas was slightly greater than 1 per 100 participants; in these regions, the frequency of seropositivity to *B. burgdorferi* at the time of study entry was as high as 5 per 100 participants (314).

In the northeastern and north-central United States, the infection is most often acquired when nymphal ticks feed between May and July, with the peak period of disease onset around the time of the summer solstice (231). Adult ticks occasionally transmit the disease when they feed in the autumn. Persons of all ages and both sexes are susceptible, but the highest reported incidence is in children less than 15 years of age and in adults 30 to 59 years of age (231).

The earliest documented North American cases occurred only 40 years ago in the 1960s (316). However, *B. burgdorferi* DNA has been identified by PCR in museum specimens of ticks and mice from Long Island dating from the late 19th and early 20th centuries (202, 238), and the infection has probably been present in North America for millennia. During the past 40 years, the infection has spread, and has been responsible for focal outbreaks in some coastal areas of the northeastern United States (126, 176, 316). Such areas have included heavily populated suburban locations near Boston, New York, and Philadelphia (292). The situation in New York State is typical. In 1985, *I. scapularis* ticks and Lyme disease were found in only four counties in the state. By 2002, the ticks had spread to all but 1 of the 62 counties of the state (112).

How does one explain the rapid spread and focal epidemics of Lyme disease in the northeastern United States in recent years? During the European colonization of America, forests were destroyed in New England to make farms, and deer were hunted practically to extinction. By the late 19th century, deer survived in only a few isolated areas, such as Naushon Island near Cape Cod (206, 287). In the 20th century, as farmland in the northeast reverted to new growth woodlands, the habitat for deer improved. Their predators were gone, hunting became a legally restricted activity, the number of deer increased, and the deer migrated to new areas. At the same time, rural and suburban areas where deer and the deer tick lived became heavily populated with suburbanites. Within these settings, Lyme disease continues to flourish and spread.

In Europe, Lyme borreliosis is already widely established in forested areas. The highest reported frequencies of the disease are in central Europe and Scandinavia, particularly in Germany, Austria, Slovenia, and Sweden (80). In a 1-year study of seven counties in southeastern Sweden, the overall incidence of the infection was 69 per 100,000 residents (33). In a report of a 1995 workshop of the World Health Organization, the incidence of the disease was estimated to be 120 per 100,000 residents in Slovenia and 130 per

100,000 residents in Austria (80), similar to the frequency in Connecticut.

CLINICAL CHARACTERISTICS

As with other spirochetal infections, human Lyme borreliosis generally occurs in stages, with remissions, exacerbations, and different clinical manifestations at each stage (290). Early infection consists of stage 1 (localized skin infection), followed within days to weeks by stage 2 (disseminated infection). Late infection, or stage 3 (persistent or progressive infection), usually begins months to years after the disease onset, sometimes following long periods of latent infection. Among individual patients, however, the infection is highly variable, ranging from brief involvement of only one system to chronic, multisystemic involvement of the skin, nerves, and joints for a period of years.

The basic nature of the disease is similar worldwide, but there is regional variation, primarily between the illness found in America and that in Europe and Asia (Table 3). Although infection with any of the three pathogenic *Borrelia* species may occur in the skin, nervous system, or joints, the frequency, severity, or duration of involvement of these systems varies with each species. *B. burgdorferi* seems to be the most arthritogenic and is associated with chronic arthritis, *B. garinii* appears to be the most neurotropic and causes chronic borrelial encephalomyelitis, and *B. afzelii* is most strongly associated with a spectrum of skin manifestations, including acrodermatitis chronica atrophicans (23).

Early Infection: Stage 1 (Localized Skin Infection)

In the United States, EM develops at the site of the tick bite in about 70 to 80%, of patients (Table 4) (313). However, because of the small size of *I. scapularis* nymphs, most patients do not notice or remember the tick bite. During the first several days, the lesion often has a homogeneous red appearance (220, 285). In addition, the centers of early lesions sometimes

Table 3. Comparison of Lyme borreliosis in North America and Eurasia[a]

System(s) affected	Locale, agent, and response	
	North America, *B. burgdorferi*	Eurasia, *B. afzelii* or *B. garinii*
Skin		
Acute	EM faster spreading, more intensely inflamed, and of briefer duration; frequent hematogenous dissemination	EM slower spreading, less intensely inflamed, and of longer duration; less frequent hematogenous dissemination
Chronic	Acrodermatitis rarely reported	Acrodermatitis chronica atrophicans, caused primarily by *B. afzelii*
Nervous system		
Acute	Meningitis, severe headache, mild neck stiffness, less prominent radiculoneuritis	Severe radicular pain and pleocytosis, less prominent headache and neck stiffness, caused particularly by *B. garinii*
Chronic	Subtle sensory polyneuropathy without acrodermatitis	Subtle sensory polyneuropathy within areas affected by acrodermatitis
	Subtle encephalopathy with cognitive disturbance, slight intrathecal antibody production	Severe encephalomyelitis with spasticity, cognitive abnormalities and marked intrathecal antibody production, caused primarily by *B. garinii*
Cardiac		
Acute	Atrioventricular block and subtle myocarditis	Atrioventricular block and subtle myocarditis
Chronic	None reported	Dilated cardiomyopathy
Arthritis		
Acute	More frequent oligoarticular arthritis, more intense joint inflammation	Less frequent oligoarticular arthritis, less intense joint inflammation
Chronic	Antibiotic-refractory arthritis in about 10% of patients probably primarily due to autoimmune mechanism	Persistent arthritis rare, probably rarely due to an autoimmune mechanism
Asymptomatic infection	In ~10%	In >10%
Antibody response	Expansion of response to many spirochetal proteins	Expansion of response to fewer spirochetal proteins

[a] Data from reference 291.

Table 4. Manifestations of Lyme disease by stage[a]

System	Stage and manifestation(s)		
	Early infection		Late infection
	Localized (stage 1)	Disseminated (stage 2)	Persistent (stage 3)
Skin	EM	Secondary annular lesions Malar rash Diffuse erythema or urticaria Evanescent lesions Lymphocytoma	Acrodermatitis chronica atrophicans Localized scleroderma-like lesions
Musculoskeletal		Migratory pain in joints, tendons, bursae, muscle, bone Brief arthritis attacks Myositis Osteomyelitis Panniculitis	Prolonged arthritis attacks Chronic arthritis Peripheral enthesopathy Periostitis or joint subluxations below lesions of acrodermatitis
Neurologic		Meningitis Cranial neuritis, Bell's palsy Motor or sensory radiculoneuritis Subtle encephalitis Mononeuritis multiplex Myelitis Chorea Cerebellar ataxia	Chronic encephalomyelitis Subtle encephalopathy Chronic axonal polyradiculopathy
Lymphatic	Regional lymphadenopathy	Regional or generalized lymphadenopathy Splenomegaly	
Heart		Atrioventricular nodal block Myopericarditis Pancarditis	
Eyes		Conjunctivitis Iritis Choroiditis Retinal hemorrhage or detachment Panophthalmitis	Keratitis
Liver		Mild hepatitis	
Respiratory		Nonexudative sore throat	
Kidney		Microscopic hematuria or proteinuria	
Genitourinary		Orchitis	
Constitutional symptoms	Minor	Severe malaise and fatigue	Fatigue

[a] The staging system provides a guideline for the expected timing of the different manifestations of the illness, but this may vary by individual case. The systems are listed from the most to the least commonly affected. Data are from reference 290.

become intensely erythematous and may become indurated, vesicular, or necrotic. As the area of redness around the center expands, most lesions continue to have bright red outer borders (usually flat, but occasionally raised) and partial central clearing, often resulting in what has been described as a bull's eye appearance (see Color Plates 6A, C, and D) (293). In some instances, developing lesions remain an even, intense red; several red rings are found within the outside one; or the central area turns blue before it clears. Although the lesion can be located anywhere, the thigh, groin, and axilla are particularly common sites. If EM occurs on the head, only a linear streak might be seen to emerge from the hairline. The lesion is hot to the touch. Although the lesion may cause no symptoms, patients often describe it as burning or occasionally as itching or painful.

In Europe, EM is often an indolent, localized infection, whereas in the United States, the lesion is associated with more intense inflammation and signs and symptoms that suggest dissemination of the spirochete (319), probably because of differences between *B. afzelii* and *B. burgdoferi* infection. In one study in the United States, spirochetes were cultured from plasma samples in 50% of patients with EM (339).

Early Infection: Stage 2 (Disseminated Infection)

Within several days to weeks after the onset of the initial EM lesion, patients in the United States may develop multiple annular secondary skin lesions (Table 4) (293), a sign of dissemination. Although their appearance is similar to that of the initial lesions, the lesions are generally smaller, migrate less, and lack indurated centers. Their locations are not associated with previous tick bites. Individual lesions sometimes appear and fade at different times, and their borders sometimes merge. During this period, some patients develop a malar rash on the face, conjunctivitis, or, rarely, diffuse hives. EM and secondary lesions usually fade within 3 to 4 weeks (range, 1 day to 14 months).

Erythema migrans is often accompanied by malaise, fatigue, headache, fever, chills, generalized achiness, or regional lymphadenopathy (290, 293). In about 18% of patients (313), these symptoms are the presenting picture of the infection (297). In addition, patients sometimes develop or present with evidence of meningeal irritation with episodic attacks of excruciating headache, neck pain, mild encephalopathy, and difficulty thinking. However, during the first days of illness, headache and neck stiffness are not associated with a spinal fluid pleocytosis or objective neurologic deficit. Other possible signs and symptoms include generalized lymph node enlargement, migratory musculoskeletal pain, hepatitis, splenomegaly, sore throat, nonproductive cough, or testicular swelling (293). A few patients have had microscopic hematuria (red blood cells in the urine), sometimes with mild proteinuria. Except for fatigue and lethargy, which are often constant, the early signs and symptoms are typically intermittent and changing. For example, a patient might predominantly experience headache and a stiff neck for several days. After a few days of improvement, musculoskeletal pain might begin.

Acute Neuroborreliosis

After several weeks to months, about 15% of untreated patients in the United States develop frank neurologic abnormalities, including meningitis, encephalitis, cranial neuritis (including unilateral or bilateral facial palsy), motor and sensory radiculoneuritis, mononeuritis multiplex, cerebellar ataxia, or myelitis— alone or in various combinations (233, 257). The usual pattern consists of fluctuating symptoms of meningitis with superimposed cranial (particularly facial palsy) or peripheral radiculoneuropathy. On examination, such patients usually have neck stiffness only on extreme flexion. Facial palsy may occur alone (62, 237); in rare instances, it may be the presenting manifestation of the disease. In children, the optic nerve may be affected by inflammation or increased intracranial pressure, which in rare cases may lead to blindness (261). In Europe, the most common neurologic manifestation is Bannwarth's syndrome or meningopolyneuritis, which consists of neuritic pain, a lymphocytic pleocytosis in CSF with minimal headache, and sometimes cranial neuritis (1, 21, 232).

In patients with meningitis, CSF examination typically demonstrates a lymphocytic pleocytosis of about 100 cells/mm^3, often with an elevated protein but typically with a normal glucose level (233). Specific immunoglobulin G (IgG), IgM, or IgA antibody to the spirochete is produced intrathecally (295, 334), and *B. burgdorferi*-specific oligoclonal bands may be present (127, 136). Antibodies to a flagellar antigen of *B. burgdorferi* (FlaB) bind to a component of normal human axons identified as chaperonin-HSP60 (74). However, it is not known whether such autoreactivity causes tissue damage or is a secondary epiphenomenon. Electrophysiologic studies of affected extremities suggest primarily axonal nerve involvement (188). Histologically, the lesions show axonal nerve injury with perivascular infiltration of lymphocytes and plasmocytes around epineural blood vessels (325). Stage 2 neurologic abnormalities usually last for weeks or months, but in untreated patients, they may recur or become chronic.

Lyme Carditis

Within several weeks after the onset of illness, about 5% of untreated patients develop cardiac involvement (294). The most common abnormality is fluctuating degrees of atrioventricular block (first-degree, Wenckebach, or complete heart block). However, some patients have evidence of more diffuse cardiac involvement, including electrocardiographic changes or a radionuclide scan compatible with acute myopericarditis (10), radionuclide evidence of mild left-ventricular dysfunction, or (rarely) cardiomegaly (294). No patients have had heart murmurs clearly ascribed to the infection. The duration of cardiac involvement, which often resolves spontaneously, is usually brief (3 days to 6 weeks), and the insertion of a permanent pacemaker is unnecessary (208). One patient is known to have died of cardiac involvement of Lyme disease (200). At autopsy, that patient had a lympho-plasmacellular infiltrate in the epicardium, myocardium, and endocardium, and a few spirochetes were seen in the myocardium. In Europe, *B. burgdorferi* has been isolated from endomyocardial biopsy samples from several patients with chronic dilated cardiomyopathy (175, 288). However, this complication has not been observed in the United States, nor has there been an association of Lyme disease with cardiac failure in areas where Lyme disease is endemic (286).

Other Stage 2 Manifestations

During stage 2, migratory musculoskeletal pain is common in joints, tendons, bursae, muscle, or bones (293). In addition, a few patients have been described with osteomyelitis (143), myositis (18), panniculitis (168), or borrelial fasciitis (117). Conjunctivitis is the most common eye abnormality in Lyme disease (293), but deeper tissues in the eye may be affected as well (156). There are case reports of iritis followed by panophthalmitis (299), choroiditis with exudative retinal detachment (20), or interstitial keratitis (166), similar to that seen in syphilis.

In Europe, a skin condition called borrelia lymphocytoma, a form of B-cell pseudolymphoma, is a rare manifestation of the infection. Such patients typically present with a solitary bluish-red nodule on the ear lobe or nipple, without extracutaneous signs or symptoms (320).

Late Infection: Stage 3 (Persistent or Progressive Infection)

Lyme arthritis

Months after the onset of the illness, about 60% of untreated patients begin to experience intermittent attacks of joint swelling and pain, primarily in large joints, especially the knee, and usually involving one or two joints at a time (Table 4) (311). Affected knees are commonly more swollen than painful; they are often hot but are rarely red. Baker cysts in the back of the knee, which contain loculated joint fluid, may form and rupture early in the course of the arthritis. However, both large and small joints may be affected. Attacks of arthritis generally last from a few weeks to months, separated by periods of complete remission. Joint fluid white blood cell counts range from 500 to 110,000 cells/mm^3, most of which are polymorphonuclear leukocytes in patients with high white blood

cell counts. Arthritis as the only manifestation of the illness may be more common in children than adults, and joint involvement is usually milder in very young children than in older children or adults (322).

The total number of patients who continue to have recurrent attacks of arthritis decreases by about 10 to 20% each year. However, attacks of knee swelling sometimes become more prolonged during the second or third year of illness. It is usually during this period that approximately 10% of untreated patients develop chronic arthritis, defined as 1 year or more of continuous joint inflammation. However, even in such untreated patients, intermittent or chronic arthritis usually resolves completely within several years.

Antibiotic-refractory Lyme arthritis

Although most patients with Lyme arthritis respond to appropriate antibiotic treatment, about 10% of patients have persistent joint inflammation for months or even several years after ≥2 months of oral antibiotics or ≥1 months of intravenous antibiotics (306). In these patients, synovial histopathology shows synovial cell hyperplasia, vascular proliferation, a heavy infiltration of mononuclear cells, and upregulation of adhesion molecules, findings similar to those found in other forms of chronic inflammatory arthritis, such as rheumatoid arthritis (6, 298).

One hypothesis to explain these findings is that such patients may have persistent infection despite antibiotic therapy (301). *B. burgdorferi* DNA can often be detected in the joint fluid of these patients prior to antibiotic treatment (38, 224), but the results of PCR testing of joint fluid are usually negative after antibiotic therapy of this duration (224). Positive PCR results have been reported in synovial tissue when the results in joint fluid were negative; therefore, negative results in joint fluid do not exclude the possible survival of small numbers of organisms in synovial tissue (248). However, the PCR results for *B. burgdorferi* DNA were negative in synovial tissue samples from all 26 patients with treatment-resistant Lyme arthritis who underwent arthroscopic synovectomy a mean duration of 7 months after the completion of antibiotic therapy (55). Similarly, a few attenuated, noninfectious spirochetes were noted in ticks that fed on mice 3 months after 1-month courses of antibiotic therapy, but no mice had positive results 6 months after treatment (35). Thus, the majority of patients with treatment-resistant Lyme arthritis seem to have persistent synovitis despite the eradication of live spirochetes from the joint with antibiotic therapy.

A related hypothesis is that retained spirochetal antigens may perpetuate synovial inflammation after the eradication of live spirochetes from the joint (301).

However, among the 26 patients with treatment-resistant arthritis who underwent arthroscopic synovectomy, *B. burgdorferi* outer surface proteins (Osps) were not seen in synovial tissue when immunohistochemical techniques were used (55), suggesting that at least large amounts of Osp proteins were not retained in the synovia of these patients.

The alternate hypothesis is that *B. burgdorferi* infection may trigger autoimmunity in the joint because of T-cell epitope mimicry between a spirochetal and host protein or because of bystander activation of autoreactive T cells (301). As with most autoimmune diseases, antibiotic-refractory Lyme arthritis is associated with certain HLA alleles. These include HLA-DRB1*0401, DRB1*0101, and other related alleles, which are also associated with the severity of rheumatoid arthritis (300). In addition, clinical correlations have linked antibiotic-refractory arthritis with cellular and humoral immune responses to OspA of *B. burgdorferi* (60, 149, 150, 179). Among untreated patients with Lyme arthritis followed serially, IgG antibody responses to OspA, which were found in about 70% of patients, often developed near the beginning of prolonged episodes of arthritis (149). Moreover, OspA-specific antibody levels correlated with the severity and duration of arthritis, whereas reactivity with eight other spirochetal proteins tested did not (306). *B. burgdorferi* expresses OspA primarily in the midgut of the tick and not during the early mammalian infection. However, in a mouse model, the spirochete up-regulates OspA expression in inflammatory foci (72), which would appear to be the case in the majority of patients with Lyme arthritis.

According to a computer algorithm, the immunodominant epitope of OspA presented by the DRB1*0401 molecule was predicted to be $OspA_{165-173}$ (118). In an epitope mapping study, 15 of 16 patients with treatment-resistant Lyme arthritis had T-cell reactivity with recombinant OspA, usually with responses to four or five epitopes, compared with only 5 of 14 patients with treatment-responsive arthritis, who usually had reactivity with only one or two epitopes (60). Moreover, all 15 treatment-resistant patients had reactivity with the $OspA_{165-173}$ epitope compared with only 1 of the 5 treatment-responsive patients (303). Thus, an immune response to $OspA_{165-173}$ has been associated with treatment-resistant Lyme arthritis.

In an initial computer search, partial sequence homology was found between this OspA epitope and human lymphocyte function-associated antigen 1 (LFA-$1\alpha_{L332-340}$) (118), an adhesion molecule on leukocytes. An ElisaSpot assay was used to show that synovial fluid mononuclear cells from 10 of 11 patients with treatment-resistant Lyme arthritis produced gamma interferon (IFN-γ) when stimulated with OspA, LFA-1, or both, whereas patients with other chronic inflammatory arthritides, including 5 with rheumatoid arthritis, did not. Moreover, $OspA_{165-173}$-reactive T cells from DRB1*0401-positive patients were expanded in joint fluid compared with peripheral blood (212). However, the LFA-1 peptide was found to act as only a weak, partial agonist for $OspA_{165-173}$-reactive T cells from DRB1*0401-positive patients (324). Furthermore, in direct binding assays, the LFA-1 peptide bound the 0401 molecule well, but it did not bind the 0101 molecule, suggesting that the LFA-1 peptide would be unlikely to serve as an autoantigen in antibiotic-refractory Lyme arthritis (300). Thus, T-cell reactivity with $OspA_{165-173}$ is implicated in antibiotic-refractory arthritis, but a relevant autoantigen has not been identified. Future technologies may allow the identification of spirochetal components or a relevant autoantigen or both in the synovia of these patients.

Chronic neuroborreliosis

Months to years after disease onset, sometimes following long periods of clinically inapparent latent infection, about 5% of untreated patients develop chronic neuroborreliosis (186). In both the United States and Europe, a chronic axonal polyneuropathy may develop, manifested primarily as spinal radicular pain or distal paresthesia (124, 188, 232). Even though sensory symptoms are often localized, electrophysiologic testing frequently shows a diffuse axonal polyneuropathy affecting both proximal and distal nerve segments (188). In Europe, *B. garinii* may cause chronic borrelial encephalomyelitis, characterized by spastic parapareses, ataxia, cognitive impairment, bladder dysfunction, and cranial neuropathy, particularly of the seventh or eighth cranial nerve, accompanied by intrathecal IgG antibody production to *B. burgdorferi* (3, 232).

In the United States, a mild, late neurologic syndrome has been reported in adults and children, called Lyme encephalopathy, manifested primarily by subtle cognitive disturbances (34, 125, 153). Although there are no inflammatory changes in the CSF, intrathecal antibody production to the spirochete can often be demonstrated. Neither neuropsychological tests of memory (153) nor single-photon emission computed tomography scanning of the brain (185) has sufficient specificity to be helpful in diagnosis. Postinfectious phenomena may play a role in the pathogenesis of this syndrome. One unusual case of *B. burgdorferi*-induced meningoencephalitis and cerebral vasculitis has been reported that was unresponsive to antibiotics (135). In this case, a T-cell clone recovered from the CSF responded to both spirochetal epitopes and autoantigens.

Acrodermatitis chronica atrophicans

Acrodermatitis chronica atrophicans, which sometimes follows years after EM, has been observed primarily in Europe in association with *B. afzelii* infection (16). The inflammatory phase begins with red violaceous lesions that gradually become sclerotic or atrophic (see Color Plate 6B). These lesions, which may be the presenting manifestation of the disease, may last for many years, and *B. burgdorferi* has been cultured from such lesions as much as 10 years after their onset (17). Although osseous lesions and peripheral neuropathy have been noted in the area of acrodermatitis skin lesions, systemic symptoms are rare. The inflammatory phase may be treated successfully with antibiotic therapy, but skin atrophy may remain.

Congenital Infection

In the mid-1980s, the transplacental transmission of *B. burgdorferi* was reported in two infants whose mothers had Lyme borreliosis during the first trimester of pregnancy (270, 330). Both infants died during the first week of life. In both, spirochetes were reported to have been visualized in various fetal tissues stained with the Dieterle silver stain, but cultures and serologic testing were not done. In a retrospective review of 19 cases of Lyme disease during pregnancy, 5 cases were associated with adverse fetal outcomes (201). Because all of the outcomes differed, they could not be linked conclusively to maternal Lyme disease. In subsequent retrospective and prospective studies, no cases of congenital infection or birth defects, including congenital heart disease, could be linked to the Lyme disease spirochete (321, 333). Thus, maternal-fetal Lyme disease and adverse pregnancy outcomes related to Lyme disease seem to occur rarely, if at all.

Coinfection

I. scapularis ticks in the United States transmit not only *B. burgdorferi*, the Lyme disease agent, but also other infectious agents, including *Babesia microti* (see Chapter 20) and *Anaplasma phagocytophilum* (formerly referred to as the agent of human granulocytic ehrlichiosis) (see Chapter 13). Each of these pathogens may cause febrile illnesses and other nonspecific systemic symptoms during summer, and coinfection with these tick-borne agents may lead to more severe, acute disease (170).

The frequency of coinfection has been quite variable, depending on geographic location and study methodology. One problem is that anaplasmosis by itself may cause a false-positive IgM Western blot for Lyme disease (340). In one study of 93 patients with culture-proven EM carried out in mainland locations in southern Rhode Island and southeastern Connecticut, two patients (2%) had coinfection with *A. phagocytophilum* and two (2%) had coinfection with *B. microti*, demonstrated by PCR testing or IgG seroconversion (310). In another study, which was done in Nantucket Island, Block Island, and southeastern Connecticut, 75 of 192 patients (39%) had evidence of acute coinfection, most commonly with Lyme disease and babesiosis (169).

In Europe and Asia, *I. ricinus* and *I. persulcatus* ticks, the vectors of *B. burgdorferi* and related *Borrelia* species, also transmit tick-borne encephalitis virus. In a seroprevalence survey of 346 individuals in Liso, southeast of Stockholm, Sweden, 26% had antibodies to *B. burgdorferi*, and half gave a history of symptoms of Lyme borreliosis (123). In addition, 12% had antibody reactivity with tick-borne encephalitis virus, and 3% had symptoms of that infection. Occasionally, patients may be coinfected with both agents.

PATHOGENESIS

Transmission of *B. burgdorferi*

To maintain its complex enzootic cycle, *B. burgdorferi* must adapt to two markedly different environments, the tick and the mammalian host. The spirochete may survive for long periods of time in a dormant state in the tick midgut. When the tick feeds, the expression of a number of spirochetal proteins is altered (227, 276). The best-characterized change involves the expression of the OspA and OspC proteins. In the midgut of the tick, the spirochete expresses OspA but not OspC (214). During tick feeding, spirochetes initially multiply in the midgut and then disseminate throughout the tick via the hemolymph. During dissemination, OspA is no longer detectable in the great majority of spirochetes, and OspC is found instead. Thus, OspC, which is similar to the variable membrane protein (vmp33) of relapsing fever borrelia, would appear to be required for transmission of *B. burgdorferi* from the tick to the mammal (275, 276).

Spread of *B. burgdorferi* within the tick may be facilitated by spirochetal binding of mammalian plasminogen and its activators, which are present in the blood meal of the tick (68, 103, 139). Plasmin, a mammalian protease, is responsible for degrading fibrin clots, but it also dissolves a variety of other substrates, including extracellular matrix proteins. When ticks were fed on plasminogen-deficient mice, spirochetal dissemination to the hemolymph and salivary glands was dramatically reduced (68). Moreover, ticks that fed on plasminogen-deficient mice had significantly fewer spirochetes than ticks that fed on infected wild-type mice, demonstrating the importance of this mechanism for efficient spirochetal transmission.

Dissemination of *B. burgdorferi* within the Mammalian Host

After injection of *B. burgdorferi* by the tick, the spirochete first multiplies locally in the skin at the site of the bite. After an incubation period of 3 to 32 days, EM usually develops at that site. Within days to weeks, the spirochete often disseminates to many sites. During this period, *B. burgdorferi* has been recovered from blood and CSF (31, 155, 302, 339), and it has been seen in small numbers in specimens of myocardium, retina, muscle, bone, spleen, liver, meninges, and brain (88). The organism seems to cross a cell monolayer at intercellular junctions, although it can penetrate through the cytoplasm of a cell (69).

A number of mechanisms may aid in spirochetal dissemination. For example, the sequences of OspC vary considerably among strains, and only a few groups of sequences are associated with disseminated disease (278), probably because they bind as-yet-unidentified host structures. As in the tick, spreading of *B. burgdorferi* through tissue matrixes may be facilitated by the binding of plasminogen and its activators to the surface of the spirochete. Although wild-type and plasminogen-deficient mice still developed *B. burgdorferi* infection in all tissue sites tested, the number of spirochetes in the blood was significantly less in plasminogen-deficient mice (68).

During dissemination and homing to specific sites, *B. burgdorferi* outer membrane proteins bind to a number of host receptors. Three distinct classes of mammalian molecules (integrins, proteoglycans, and glycoproteins) have been characterized as receptors for the spirochete (Table 5). For example, *B. burgdorferi* binds to at least three members of the integrin family of cell surface receptors, including the fibrinogen receptor ($\alpha_{IIb}\beta_3$), the vitronectin receptor ($\alpha_v\beta_3$), and the fibronectin receptor ($\alpha_5\beta_1$) (63, 66, 67). The ligand for the β_3-chain integrins is a 66-kDa spirochetal protein (64, 65), which is expressed on the surface of the organism (46, 249). *B. burgdorferi* attachment to these integrins is likely to be important in the establishment of an initial foothold in the mammalian host and in interactions with the vasculature during dissemination. In addition to integrin binding, a 26-kDa *Borrelia* glycosaminoglycan (GAG)-binding protein (Bgp) binds to the GAG side chains of the proteoglycans heparan sulfate and dermatan sulfate (142, 180, 234). *B. burgdorferi* binds to heparan sulfate on endothelial cells, whereas both heparan sulfate and dermatan sulfate appear to participate in attachment of the organism to glioma and neuronal cells (181).

A differentially expressed 47-kDa fibronectin-binding protein (BBK32) of *B. burgdorferi* binds to fibronectin (98, 250, 251). This protein exists in a soluble form in plasma and in an insoluble form as an extracellular matrix protein. In a clinical study, the highest IgG antibody responses to the BBK32 fibronectin-binding protein were found during early disseminated infection, and higher responses at that time were associated with subsequent arthritis of shorter duration (7). In contrast, there was no association between the early antibody response to the nine other spirochetal proteins tested and the severity and duration of subsequent arthritis. In these patients, antibodies to the BBK32 protein may block adhesion, and fewer organisms may reach and survive in the joint, accounting for the shorter duration of arthritis. Finally, decorin-binding proteins A and B (DbpA and DbpB) of the spirochete bind decorin (100, 120, 121), a proteoglycan that associates with collagen. Spirochetal binding to decorin may explain the alignment of spirochetes with collagen fibrils in the extracellular matrix in the heart, nervous system, or joints (88). In a

Table 5. *B. burgdorferi* proteins involved in adherence or immune evasion

Function and protein name	Genome designation	Specific action	Reference(s)
Adherence to mammalian tissue components			
P66	BB0603	Binds β_3-chain integrins	190, 191
BgP	BB0588	Binds heparan sulfate, dermatan sulfate, GAGs	196
BBK32, fibronectin-binding protein	BBK32	Binds fibronectin	199
DbpA	BBA24	Binds decorin (a dermatan sulfate proteoglycan)	202–205
DbpB	BBA25	Binds decorin	202–205
Immune evasion			
Vls locus (VlsE is expressed gene)	BBF32	Antigenic variation	211, 212
OspE paralogous family members ErpA, ErpP, ErpC	BBP38, BBL39, BBN38	Binds complement factor H and fHL-1	214–217

recent report, decorin-deficient mice had more limited spirochetal colonization of joints and milder arthritis than normal mice of the same strain that expressed decorin (42).

Immune Evasion

Despite a vigorous immune response, the *Borrelia* species may survive for years in certain locations, including the joints, nervous system, or skin. The outer membrane of *B. burgdorferi* has a number of characteristics that enhance immune evasion. The membrane contains few integral proteins (70, 254). Multiple genes encode families of highly homologous lipoproteins, which contributes to antigenic diversity. A number of these proteins, including OspA through OspF, are differentially expressed and may be downregulated during infection (78, 133, 173). During early disseminated infection, one surface-exposed lipoprotein, called VlsE, undergoes extensive antigenic variation (Table 5) (347, 348). The plasmid locus encoding this lipoprotein is capable of generating $>10^{30}$ variants. Finally, *B. afzelii* and, to a lesser degree, *B. burgdorferi* have complement regulator-acquiring surface proteins that bind complement factor H and factor H-like protein 1 (9, 134, 167, 209, 317). These complement factors inactivate C3b, which protects the organism from complement-mediated killing. In contrast, *B. garinii* is efficiently killed by complement. Thus, the organism minimizes or changes antigenic expression of proteins and inhibits certain critical host immune responses.

Although *B. burgdorferi* has multiple mechanisms of potential importance in immune evasion, it does not appear to survive in intracellular locations for long periods of time. In tissue culture systems, intracellular localization of a few spirochetes has been demonstrated in human endothelial cells (192), macrophages (215), or fibroblasts (108). However, in a three-dimensional model of Lyme arthritis, synovial fibroblasts disintegrated after engulfing *B. burgdorferi* or its fragments (101). More importantly, spirochetes have not been seen in intracellular locations in histologic sections from patients with Lyme disease (87) or from infected animals (29).

Host Immunity to *B. burgdorferi*

In most patients, immune cells first encounter *B. burgdorferi* in the skin at the site of the tick bite. On histologic examination, EM skin lesions consist of mild to marked perivascular infiltrates of lymphocytes and macrophages intermingled with small numbers of plasma cells (217). Two distinct subsets of mature, activated dendritic cells are found in the lesions, including both monocytoid (CD11c$^+$) and plasmacy-

toid (CD11c$^-$) subsets (264). Dendritic cells isolated from the dermis readily engulf *B. burgdorferi* in vitro (99). Inflammatory cells in the lesions produce primarily pro-inflammatory responses, particularly IFN-γ (217, 264), and *B. burgdorferi*-stimulated peripheral blood mononuclear cells also produce primarily pro-inflammatory cytokines, especially IFN-γ (114). In a study of 39 patients with culture-proven EM, 72% had antibody responses to at least one of the borrelial antigens tested a median of 4 days after disease onset, and 95% had such responses documented during convalescence (327). Thus, both innate cellular elements and adaptive cellular and humoral immune responses are mobilized to fight the infection.

During disseminated infection, all affected tissues show an infiltration of lymphocytes, macrophages, and plasma cells (87). Some degree of vascular damage, including mild vasculitis or hypervascular occlusion, may be seen in multiple sites, suggesting that spirochetes may have been present in or around blood vessels, particularly arterial walls. Borrelial lipoproteins, which are B-cell mitogens (193), cause polyclonal activation of B cells, resulting in elevated total serum IgM levels (304) and circulating immune complexes (131). Particularly during dissemination, adaptive cellular and humoral immune responses to *B. burgdorferi* lead to the production of antibody against many components of the organism (7, 345). Specific IgM responses peak during the third through the sixth week of infection, and specific IgG responses to an increasing array of spirochetal proteins (7) and nonprotein antigens (332) develop gradually over weeks to months. Spirochetal killing seems to be accomplished primarily by bactericidal B-cell responses (262), which utilize the classical complement pathway (162).

During persistent infection, CD4$^+$ T-helper (Th) cells from patients with Lyme arthritis or neuroborreliosis again preferentially produce the proinflammatory cytokine IFN-γ (119, 228). In patients with Lyme arthritis, *B. burgdorferi*-specific CD8$^+$ T cells are found as well (50), which may also be a significant source of this cytokine. Within the joint, *B. burgdorferi*-specific γδ T cells of the Vδ1 subset may aid in the regulation of these inflammatory responses (111). Patients with Lyme arthritis have very high levels of antibody to many spirochetal proteins, suggestive of hyperimmunization due to recurrent waves of spirochetal growth (7). These immune responses seem to succeed eventually in eradicating *B. burgdorferi* from the joint.

ANIMAL MODELS

To gain a better understanding of pathogenetic mechanisms, animal models of Lyme disease have been developed in mice, hamsters, guinea pigs, dogs, and nonhuman primates. Each animal model is imperfect in that it does not express all features of human Lyme disease. For example, inbred C3H/He mice develop acute arthritis and carditis 2 to 4 weeks after inoculation with *B. burgdorferi*, but they do not develop EM or neurologic abnormalities (28). Even so, the plethora of inbred mouse strains, including genetically modified animals, and the depth of knowledge of the murine immune system have made studies of the mouse particularly valuable.

Mouse Models of Lyme Disease

Inbred strains of mice can be infected with *B. burgdorferi*, but they differ in the severity of arthritis or carditis (Table 6). In mild forms of the disease, anti-inflammatory components of the innate immune response seem to protect C57BL/6 mice from the development of severe arthritis, despite infection of joints with large numbers of organisms (191). In disease of greater severity, *B. burgdorferi*-infected BALB/c mice develop mild to severe joint inflammation, depending on the number of organisms injected, and they require adaptive immune responses for control of the spirochete and resolution of arthritis (191). At the far end of the spectrum, C3H/He mice, which seem to have inadequate innate and adaptive immune responses to the organism, develop severe arthritis and carditis, even with small infectious doses of as few as 100 spirochetes (191).

In C3H mice, macrophages are the primary infiltrating cells in cardiac lesions, and T-cell-mediated immunity is critical for the control of the carditis (263). In contrast, polymorphonuclear leukocytes and then lymphocytes are the prominent infiltrating cells in synovial tissue (28), and antibody responses are crucial for control of the arthritis (95). Despite the resolution of acute lesions, spirochetes persist throughout the life of C3H mice, primarily in the skin. Recurrent waves of spirochetemia may lead to recurrent attacks of arthritis. Although C3H mice provide a good model of the acute, infectious phase of human Lyme arthritis, no currently known mouse strain develops the equivalent of human chronic Lyme arthritis.

These mouse models allow the dissection of the *B. burgdorferi*-induced immune response into its many individual components. Although innate and adaptive immune responses are presented separately here, they occur together in the native infection (264).

Mouse innate immune responses

B. burgdorferi infection induces highly inflammatory innate immune responses. Spirochetal lipoproteins stimulate toll-like receptor 1 (Tlr1) and Tlr2 on macrophages (8, 338) and non-lipopeptide-derived spirochetal signals activate the Fcγ receptors of these cells, leading to the production of proinflammatory cytokines and chemokines (79, 323). These stimuli are mitogenic for both monocytes/macrophages (255) and B cells (81). Macrophages engulf *B. burgdorferi* and degrade the spirochetes in intracellular compartments (214, 215, 258). These cells produce effector molecules, such as nitric oxide (213) and cyclooxygenase 2 (15), which are capable of spirochetal killing, and they produce matrix metalloproteinases, which may also have inflammatory properties (107). Neutrophil extravasation into the joint seems to be a key initial step for the development of experimental Lyme arthritis (39). Thus, these innate inflammatory

Table 6. Infection and arthritis susceptibility in selected strains of mice

Strain	Arthritis	Spirochete burden		Reference (method)[a]
		Joint	Other tissues	
C57BL/6 (B6)				
B6	Minimal or none	High	Dose dependent	241 (*)
B6-rag (no T/B cells)	Minimal or none	Positive	Positive	267 (**)
B6-IL-10 knockout	Moderate	Low	Low	256 (*)
B6-IL-6 knockout	Moderate	ND	ND	257
BALB/c and C.B.17 (congenic)				
BALB/c and C.B.17	Mild to moderate	Dose dependent	Dose dependent	241 (*)
C.B.17-SCID	Severe	Positive	Positive	267 (**)
BALB/c (CD4 depleted)	Severe	High	High	268 (***)
C3H				
C3H	Severe	High	High	241 (*)
C3H-SCID	More severe	Positive	Positive	267 (**)
C3H (CD4 depleted)	More severe	High	High	268 (***)

[a] Assessed by quantitative PCR (*), end-point PCR (**), or culture or microscopy (***). ND, not done.

responses are required for host defense but may also be arthritogenic.

In the mouse model, innate immunity is the primary determinant of susceptibility or resistance to arthritis. Proinflammatory cytokines, such as interleukin-12 (IL-12), enhance macrophage function. In C3H-SCID mice, which lack T and B cells, anti-IL-12 treatment limits innate immunity and further exacerbates arthritis (14). In contrast, IL-10-deficient C57BL/6 mice have 90% fewer spirochetes than infected C57BL/6 control mice, probably due to sustained macrophage activation (43). However, consistent with an anti-inflammatory effect of this cytokine, IL-10-deficient mice develop more severe arthritis. In addition, IL-6-deficient C57BL/6 mice are also more susceptible to arthritis (13), suggesting that this cytokine may also have an anti-inflammatory role. Thus, certain macrophage-derived anti-inflammatory cytokines, secreted as a part of the innate immune response, would appear to protect C57BL/6 mice from the development of severe arthritis despite large numbers of spirochetes in the joint.

A role for γ/δ T cells, which may serve as a bridge from innate to adaptive immune responses, has recently been suggested in the early immune response to OspC (207). Presentation of lipopeptides to γ/δ T cells by the CD1 molecule may be important in this response, as CD1d-deficient mice are more susceptible to arthritis (171).

Mouse adaptive immune responses

As demonstrated in vaccination studies, *B. burgdorferi* lipoproteins, which are strong adjuvants (255), induce T-cell-independent, humoral immune responses that lead to spirochetal killing (97, 222). These responses, which are dependent on Tlr1 and Tlr2 (8), develop without CD40 ligand, major histocompatibility complex class II molecules, CD4$^+$ T cells, or γ/δ T cells (96, 210). In addition, humoral responses to nonlipidated spirochetal proteins, which are likely to be T-cell dependent, may also aid in spirochetal killing (98, 129). Finally, a T-cell-dependent response against a single *B. burgdorferi* protein, arthritis-related protein 1 (Arp-1, also called ErpT) reduces the severity of arthritis, but not infection, when passively transferred to infected C3H-SCID mice (8).

Under normal conditions, antigen-specific T-cell responses participate in control of the spirochete burden, apparently by priming bactericidal B-cell responses. *B. burgdorferi*-infected SCID mice, which lack T and B cells, have large numbers of spirochetes in tissues (30, 41, 268). Depletion of CD4$^+$ T cells in both C3H and BALB/c mice substantially inhibits the early immune response, increasing spirochete burden and

arthritis severity (158). Both mouse strains have equal numbers of *B. burgdorferi*-specific CD8$^+$ T cells (85), which may be a significant source of IFN-γ.

It was originally thought that a Th1 response was pathogenic in C3H mice and that a Th2 response was beneficial in BALB/c mice (158). However, in IFN-γ-deficient C3H mice, severe joint inflammation still developed (40). It is now known that BALB/c mice mount a strong Th1 response early in infection, whereas C3H mice do not (152, 346). Thus, in BALB/c mice, a prominent early Th1 response participates in the reduction of spirochetes, whereas this early response is minimal or lacking in C3H mice.

In 129S mice, which have a level of resistance to Lyme arthritis similar to that of C57BL/6 mice, a Th1 response with IFN-γ production is not necessary to prevent the development of arthritis (113). Osteopontin, which controls IL-12 production and is a potent inducer of Th1 responses, is also dispensable to resistance in 129S mice (244). Thus, Th1 responses to *B. burgdorferi* are not critical for the control of arthritis in mouse strains in which only small numbers of inflammatory cells accumulate in the joint.

Although T cells normally enhance protective B-cell responses, T cells without B cells may be pathogenic. In *B. burgdorferi*-infected C57BL/6-SCID mice, adoptive transfer of T and B cells reduces the severity of arthritis, but adoptive transfer of T cells alone exacerbates arthritis and accelerates its onset (210).

Vaccine-Infection Model of Severe, Destructive Arthritis

Inbred LSH hamsters can be infected with *B. burgdorferi*, but they do not develop arthritis. However, when these hamsters are vaccinated with a whole-cell preparation of *B. burgdorferi* or recombinant OspA followed by challenge with 10^6 viable *B. burgdorferi* cells prior to or after the development of protective immunity, the hamsters develop severe, destructive arthritis (71, 183). The synovia of these animals show hypertrophic villi, focal erosion of articular cartilage, and mononuclear cell infiltrates, the typical findings in chronic inflammatory arthritis. Recently, this same phenomenon was demonstrated in vaccine-sensitized, *B. burgdorferi*-infected, IFN-γ-deficient mice (61). Although the mechanisms involved are incompletely delineated, IL-17, a T-cell-derived proinflammatory cytokine, contributes to the development of arthritis (47).

Neuroborreliosis in Nonhuman Primates

Neuroborreliosis is difficult to study in animal models because this manifestation of *B. burgdorferi* infection seems to occur only in primates and not in rodents. In a rat model, infection with *B. burgdorferi* resulted in increased permeability of the blood-brain barrier and spirochetal invasion of the central nervous system within 24 to 96 h, but this did not lead to neurologic lesions (105). The spread of *B. burgdorferi* in the nervous system and peripheral neuropathy in nonhuman primates have been documented (259). In immunosuppressed monkeys, which had a larger spirochetal burden than did immunocompetent animals, *B. burgdorferi* infiltrated the leptomeninges, motor and sensory nerve roots, and dorsal ganglia but not the brain parenchyma (52). In the peripheral nervous system, spirochetes were seen in the perineurium, the connective tissue sheath surrounding each bundle of peripheral-nerve fibers.

DIAGNOSIS

Culture of *B. burgdorferi* from patient specimens in Barbour-Stoenner-Kelly medium permits definitive diagnosis. However, positive cultures have been obtained only early in the illness, primarily from biopsies of EM skin lesions (32), less often from blood or plasma samples (339), and only occasionally from CSF samples in patients with meningitis. Later in the infection, PCR testing is greatly superior to culture in the detection of *B. burgdorferi* in joint fluid (224). *B. burgdorferi* has not been isolated from the CSF of patients with chronic neuroborreliosis, and *B. burgdorferi* DNA has been detected in CSF samples in only a small number of such patients (223). The Lyme urine antigen test, which has provided grossly unreliable and inconsistent results (161), should not be used to support the diagnosis or manage the treatment of the infection.

In patients in the United States, diagnosis is usually based on the recognition of a characteristic clinical picture, exposure in an area where Lyme disease is endemic, and a positive antibody response to *B. burgdorferi*, except in those with EM in whom seroconversion may not have yet occurred (58). For serologic testing in the United States, done with whole-cell sonicate *B. burgdorferi* antigens, the CDC currently recommends a two-test approach in which samples are first tested by enzyme-linked immunosorbent assay (ELISA) and those with equivocal or positive results are tested by Western blotting (Table 7) (59). According to the CDC criteria, an IgM Western blot is considered positive if two of the following three bands are present: 23, 39, and 41 kDa; however, the combination of the 23- and 41-kDa bands may still be a false-positive result. An IgG blot is considered positive if 5 of the following 10 bands are present: 18, 23, 28, 30, 39, 41, 45, 58, 66, and 93 kDa. About half of the normal population has IgG reactivity with the 41-kDa flagellar antigen of the spirochete, and this response, by itself, has no diagnostic significance. In Europe, where there is less expansion of the antibody response, no single set of criteria for immunoblot interpretation gives high levels of sensitivity and specificity in all countries (260).

Serodiagnosis is insensitive early in the infection. In the United States, approximately 20 to 30% of patients with EM have positive responses in acute-phase samples, usually of the IgM isotype (Fig. 2a) (86, 92), but by convalescence, 2 to 4 weeks after antibiotic treatment, about 70 to 80% have seroreactivity. After 1 month, the great majority of patients with active infection have positive IgG antibody responses, and those with Lyme arthritis usually have reactivity with all 10 bands used for diagnosis (Fig. 2b) (86). In persons with symptoms present for longer than 1 month, a positive IgM response is likely to be a false-positive result if it is not accompanied by a positive IgG response. Therefore, a positive IgM response alone should not be used to support the diagnosis after the first month of infection. In patients with acute neuroborreliosis, especially those with meningitis, intrathecal production of IgM, IgG, or IgA antibody to *B. burgdorferi* may often be demonstrated by antibody capture enzyme immunoassay (128, 295), but this test is less often positive in those with chronic neuroborreliosis.

After antibiotic treatment, antibody titers fall slowly, but IgG and even IgM responses may persist for many years after treatment (151). Thus, a positive IgM response should not be interpreted as indicating recent infection or reinfection unless the appropriate clinical picture is present. *B. burgdorferi* may also cause asymptomatic infection. In a Lyme disease vaccine trial in the United States in which subjects were followed prospectively for 20 months, 7% of those who met diagnostic criteria for definite Lyme disease had IgG seroconversion by Western blot analysis without symptoms of infection (312). In seroprevalence surveys in Europe, more than half of the subjects who were seropositive by ELISA did not remember symptoms of Lyme borreliosis (94, 122). If patients with past or asymptomatic infection who have a positive serologic test for Lyme disease present with new symptoms caused by another illness, the danger is that they may be attributed incorrectly to Lyme disease, potentially resulting in ineffective or harmful treatment.

Several second-generation serologic tests that employ recombinant spirochetal proteins or synthetic peptides have shown promising results (116, 182). Compared with the standard two-test approach of sonicate ELISA and Western blotting, similar results were obtained by using an IgG ELISA that employed a peptide of the sixth invariant region of the VlsE lipoprotein of *B. burgdorferi* (19). However, as with the sonicate tests, the response to the VlsE peptide

Table 7. Lyme Disease National Surveillance Case Definition[a]

Manifestation	Comment
A person with EM, observed by a physician	This skin lesion expands slowly over days to weeks to form a large round lesion, often with central clearing; to be counted for surveillance purposes, a solitary lesion must be at least 5 cm
A person with at least one later manifestation and laboratory evidence of infection	
Nervous system	Lymphocytic meningitis, cranial neuritis, radiculoneuropathy, or rarely, encephalomyelitis, alone or in combination; for encephalomyelitis to be counted for surveillance purposes, there must be evidence of intrathecal antibody production against *B. burgdorferi* in CSF
Cardiovascular system	Acute onset, high-grade (2nd or 3rd degree) atrioventricular conduction defects that resolve in days to weeks and are sometimes associated with myocarditis
Musculoskeletal system	Recurrent, brief attacks (weeks to months) of objective joint swelling in one or a few joints, sometimes followed by chronic arthritis in one or a few joints
Laboratory evidence	Isolation of *B. burgdorferi* from tissue or body fluid or detection of diagnostic levels of antibody to the spirochete by two-test approach of ELISA and Western blotting, interpreted according to CDC/Association of State and Territorial Public Health Laboratory Directors' criteria[b]

[a] Adapted from recommendations made by the CDC (287, 288); also adapted from reference 291.
[b] In a person with acute disease of less than 1 month's duration, IgM and IgG antibody responses should be measured in acute and convalescent serum samples. An IgM Western blot is considered positive if at least two of the following three bands are present: 23, 39, or 41 kDa. An IgG blot is considered positive if at least 5 of the following 10 bands are present: 18, 23, 28, 30, 39, 41, 45, 58, 66, or 93 kDa. Only the IgG response should be used to support the diagnosis after the first month of infection. After that time, an IgM response alone is likely to be a false-positive result.

may persist for months or years after successful antibiotic treatment; therefore, persistence of an anti-VlsE antibody response cannot be equated with spirochetal persistence in Lyme disease (236).

TREATMENT AND OUTCOME

Evidence-based treatment recommendations for Lyme disease have been presented by the Infectious Diseases Society of America (341). In brief, the various manifestations of Lyme disease can usually be treated with oral antibiotic therapy, except for neurologic abnormalities, which seem to require intravenous therapy. For early localized or disseminated infection, doxycycline for 14 to 21 days is recommended in persons aged 8 years or older, except for pregnant women (Table 8). Because the risk of maternal-fetal transmission seems to be very low, standard therapy for the stage and manifestation of the illness may be sufficient for pregnant patients, but doxycycline should be avoided. An advantage of doxycycline is that it is the only antibiotic effective in early Lyme disease that is also known to be active against *A. phagocytophilum*, a possible coinfecting agent. The possibility of coinfection with *A. phagocytophilum* or *babesia* should be carefully considered in patients presenting with severe, febrile illness (see Chapters 5, 13, and 20).

Amoxicillin, the second choice alternative, should be used in children or pregnant women. In case of allergy, cefuroxime axetil is a third-choice alternative. Erythromycin or its cogeners, such as azithromycin, are recommended only for patients who are unable to take doxycycline, amoxicillin, or cefuroxime axetil. Approximately 15% of patients with early disseminated infection experience a Jarisch-Herxheimer-like reaction during the first 24 h of therapy, characterized by an intensification of symptoms, including higher fever (305). In vitro, *B. burgdorferi* is sensitive to tetracycline, penicillin, erythromycin, and their cogeners and to third-generation cephalosporins such as ceftriaxone and cefotaxime, but it is resistant to rifampin, ciprofloxacin, and the aminoglycoside antibiotics (5, 82, 83, 145, 247). Acquired antibiotic resistance, as found with certain other organisms, has not been demonstrated for *B. burgdorferi*.

In multicenter studies of patients with EM, similar results were obtained with doxycycline, amoxicillin, or cefuroxime, and more than 90% of patients had satisfactory outcomes (77, 203, 218). Although some pa-

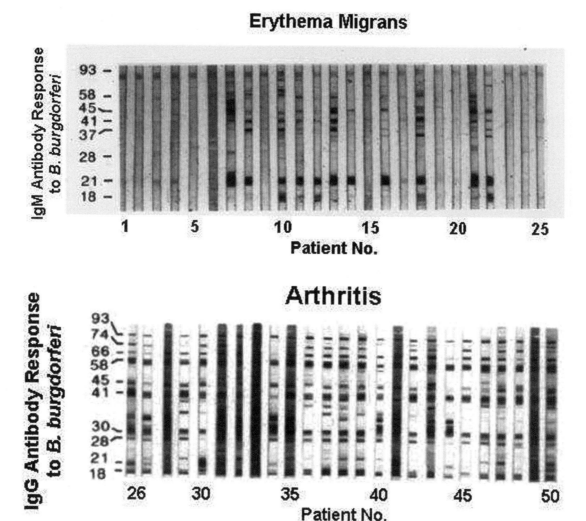

Figure 2. Western blots of the IgM antibody responses to *B. burgdorferi* are shown in 25 patients with EM (a); the IgG responses are demonstrated in 25 patients with Lyme arthritis (b). Patients with EM most commonly had IgM responses to the 23-kDa OspC protein and the 41-kDa flagellar antigen of the spirochete, whereas the patients with Lyme arthritis almost always had IgG reactivity with all 10 bands used for diagnosis with the CDC criteria (86).

tients had subjective symptoms after treatment, objective evidence of persistent infection or relapse was rare, and retreatment was usually not needed. In a recent study, extending treatment with doxycycline from 10 to 20 days or adding one dose of parenteral ceftriaxone to the beginning of a 10-day course of doxycycline did not enhance therapeutic efficacy in patients with EM (289, 342). In another study, significantly more azithromycin recipients than amoxicillin recipients had relapses (190). Intravenous ceftriaxone, although effective, was not superior to oral agents in the absence of objective neurological involvement (76). In contrast with expanded- and broad-spectrum cephalosporin antibiotics, narrow-spectrum cephalosporins, such as cephalexin, were ineffective (225). Although this treatment has not been studied systematically, patients with

asymptomatic infection are often given a course of oral antibiotics.

For patients with objective neurologic abnormalities, 2- to 4-week courses of intravenous ceftriaxone are most commonly given (75, 186, 187). Intravenous therapy with cefotaxime or penicillin G may be a satisfactory alternative (239, 240). In Europe, it has been suggested that oral doxycycline may be adequate therapy for acute neuroborreliosis (154). Although this medication may be used successfully in patients who have only facial palsy in the United States, it is important to assess whether such patients have more diffuse involvement of the nervous system, which is best treated with intravenous therapy. After treatment, the signs and symptoms of acute neuroborreliosis usually resolve within weeks, but those of chronic neuroborreliosis

Table 8. Treatment and vaccination regimens for Lyme disease[a]

Stage or symptom	Regimen
Early infection (local or disseminated)	
Adults	Doxycycline, 100 mg orally twice daily for 14 to 21 days
	Amoxicillin, 500 mg orally three times daily for 14 to 21 days
	Alternatives in case of doxycycline or amoxicillin allergy: cefuroxime axetil, 500 mg orally twice daily for 14 to 21 days, or erythromycin, 250 mg orally 4 times a day for 14 to 21 days
Children (aged 8 or less)	Amoxicillin, 250 mg orally three times a day or 50 mg/kg/day in three divided doses for 14 to 21 days
	Alternatives in case of penicillin allergy: cefuroxime axetil, 125 mg orally twice daily or 30 mg/kg of body wt/day in two divided doses for 14 to 21 days, or erythromycin, 250 mg orally three times a day or 30 mg/kg/day in three divided doses for 14 to 21 days
Neurologic abnormalities (early or late)	
Adults	Ceftriaxone 2 g IV once a day for 14 to 28 days
	Cefotaxime, 2 g IV every 8 h for 14 to 28 days
	Na penicillin G, 3.3 million U IV every 4 h for 14 to 28 days
	Alternative in case of ceftriaxone or penicillin allergy: doxycycline, 100 mg orally three times a day for 30 days, but this regimen may be ineffective for late neuroborreliosis
Facial palsy alone	Oral regimens may be adequate
Children (aged 8 or less)	Ceftriaxone, 75 to 100 mg/kg/day (maximum, 2 g) IV once a day for 14 to 28 days
	Cefotaxime, 150 mg/kg/day in three or four divided doses (maximum, 6 g) for 14 to 28 days
	Na penicillin G, 200,000 to 400,000 U/kg/day in six divided doses for 14 to 28 days
Arthritis (intermittent or chronic)	Oral regimens listed above for 30 to 60 days or
	IV regimens listed above for 14 to 28 days
Cardiac abnormalities	
First-degree AV block	Oral regimens, as for early infection
High-degree AV block (P-R interval >0.3 s)	IV regimens and cardiac monitoring. Once the patient has stabilized, the course may be completed with oral therapy
Pregnant women	Standard therapy for manifestation of the illness. Avoid doxycycline

[a] Antibiotic recommendations are based on the guidelines from the Infectious Diseases Society of America (301); adapted from reference 291. AV, atrioventricular.

improve more slowly over a period of months. Objective evidence of relapse is rare after a 4-week course of therapy. In patients with Lyme carditis and high-degree atrioventricular nodal block, intravenous therapy for at least part of the course and cardiac monitoring are recommended. In some cases, insertion of a temporary pacemaker may be required, However, since the heart block almost always resolves, a permanent pacemaker is not necessary.

Either oral or intravenous regimens are usually effective for the treatment of Lyme arthritis (75, 306). Oral therapy is easier to administer, it is associated with fewer side effects, and it is considerably less expensive (89). Its disadvantages are that spirochetal killing is slower and some patients treated with oral agents have subsequently manifested overt neuroborreliosis, which may require intravenous therapy for

successful treatment (306). Despite treatment with either oral or intravenous antibiotic therapy, about 10% of patients in the United States have persistent joint inflammation for months or even several years after ≥2 months of oral antibiotics or ≥1 month of intravenous antibiotics (306). If patients have persistent arthritis despite this treatment and if the results of PCR testing of joint fluid are negative, such patients may be treated with anti-inflammatory agents or arthroscopic synovectomy (272).

Following appropriate treatment of Lyme disease, a small percentage of patients continue to have subjective symptoms, primarily musculoskeletal pain, neurocognitive difficulties, or fatigue (84, 283, 284, 315). In some instances, disabling symptoms may persist for years. This putative postinfectious syndrome, which is clinically similar to chronic fatigue syndrome or fibromyalgia, occurs more frequently in patients with symptoms suggestive of early dissemination of the spirochete to the nervous system, particularly if treatment is delayed (148, 281). However, in a large study, the frequency of pain and fatigue symptoms was no greater in patients who had Lyme disease than in age-matched subjects who did not have this infection (279).

In a study of patients with post-Lyme disease syndrome who received intravenous ceftriaxone for 30 days followed by oral doxycycline for 60 days or intravenous and oral placebo preparations for the same duration, there were no significant differences between the groups in the treatment outcomes, including the percentage of patients who felt that their symptoms had improved, gotten worse, or stayed the same (160). These patients are best treated symptomatically rather than with prolonged courses of antibiotic therapy. Prolonged antibiotic therapy may be harmful. In studies of patients with unsubstantiated Lyme disease, minor side effects were common (256), ceftriaxone therapy for unsubstantiated Lyme disease resulted in biliary complications (93) or catheter-associated septicemia, and in one reported case, prolonged cefotaxime administration resulted in death (235).

Reinfection may occur in patients who are treated with antibiotics early in the illness (331), but reinfection has not been observed in patients with the expanded immune response associated with Lyme arthritis.

PREVENTION

The risk of tick bite may be reduced by simple measures. When possible, people should avoid tick-infested areas (132). If avoidance is not possible, repellents containing DEET (*N,N*-diethylmetatoluamide) or permethrin effectively deter ticks (273), but permethrin can be applied only on clothing, and in rare instances, DEET may cause side effects with frequent, long-term use (230). Therefore, repellents may be valuable for the occasional hike in the woods but are less helpful for people living in endemic areas who have daily tick exposures.

After potential exposure in tick-infested areas, tick checks are important. Immature *I. scapularis* ticks usually stay within a few inches of the ground; they often transfer to the lower extremities of the host and then migrate to moist parts of the body, such as the groin or axillae. In small children, they may also be found on the head and neck, which are unusual sites for tick attachment in adults. Environmental control of ticks over widespread areas is difficult (132). Methods that may be helpful include application of acaracides (73), landscaping to provide desiccating barriers between tick-infested areas and lawns, and in some set-

tings, removal or exclusion of deer (337). New methods of tick control, including host-targeted acaricides for rodents and deer, are being developed and may provide help in the future (see Chapter 4).

Should *I. scapularis* tick bites be treated with antibiotic prophylaxis? In studies, the frequency of Lyme disease after a recognized tick bite has been only about 1% (282), perhaps because 24 to 72 h of tick attachment is necessary before transmission of the spirochete occurs (241). Thus, if an attached tick is removed quickly, no other treatment is usually necessary. However, if an engorged nymphal *I. scapularis* tick is found, a single 200-mg dose of doxycycline usually prevents Lyme disease when given within 72 h after the tick bite occurs (219).

Vaccination

In 1986, Johnson and his colleagues reported that Syrian hamsters could be immunized successfully against homologous strains of *B. burgdorferi* by using a formalin-inactivated, whole-cell lysate of the spirochete (144, 146). Subsequently, it was shown that immunization of mice with recombinant OspA or passive transfer of a monoclonal antibody to OspA provided protection from infection (97, 269). In the early 1990s, two companies, Pasteur Merieux Connaught (now Aventis Pasteur) and SmithKline Beecham (now Glaxo SmithKline), began the development of recombinant OspA vaccines for human use (159, 326). In December 1998, the vaccine made by GlaxoSmithKline, consisting of recombinant OspA with alum adjuvant, was licensed and sold commercially until February 2002.

In a phase III study of 10,936 patients, vaccine efficacy of the GlaxoSmithKline product in the prevention of definite Lyme disease was 49% after two injections and 76% after three injections (314). The most important factor in protection was the level of antibody response to the protective epitope of OspA. Administration of the vaccine was associated with a mild-to-moderate local or systemic reaction lasting a median of 3 days. Since antibody titers waned rather quickly, it was anticipated that booster injections would likely be needed every 1 to 3 years to maintain protection. Although T-cell responses to OspA in the natural infection have been associated with the severity of Lyme arthritis and with antibiotic-refractory arthritis (60, 118), vaccine or placebo recipients did not differ significantly in the development of arthritis or any other late syndrome after vaccination. Thus, the conditions necessary for the induction of a putative autoimmune response in joints in the natural infection seem not to be duplicated with OspA-based vaccination.

Although the OspA vaccine was shown to be safe and effective, its acceptance by the public and by physicians was limited (130). Some of the reasons included the low risk of Lyme disease in most parts of the country, the anticipated need for booster injections every 1 to 3 years, and the relatively high cost of this preventive approach compared with antibiotic treatment of early infection (211, 280). In addition, there was the theoretical, but never proven, concern that in rare cases, vaccination might trigger autoimmune arthritis.

The OspA Lyme disease vaccines developed in the 1990s should be considered first-generation vaccines (106). A goal for future vaccines should be to provide longer-term protection and perhaps broader protection against variant strains of *B. burgdorferi*. If OspA is a component of the vaccine, alteration of the immunodominant T-cell epitope presented by the DRB1*0401 molecule may be desirable. Nevertheless, experience gained in the last 10 years has proven the feasibility of vaccination for the prevention of this complex, tick-transmitted infection.

REFERENCES

1. **Ackermann, R., P. Horstrup, and R. Schmidt.** 1984. Tick-borne meningopolyneuritis (Garin-Bujadoux, Bannwarth). *Yale J. Biol. Med.* **57:**485–490.
2. **Ackermann, R., J. Kabatzki, H. P. Boisten, A. C. Steere, R. L. Grodzicki, S. Hartung, and U. Runne.** 1984. Spirochaten-Atiologie der Erythema-chronicum-migrans-Krankheit. *Dtsch. Med. Wochenschr.* **109:**92–97.
3. **Ackermann, R., B. Rehse-Kupper, E. Gollmer, and R. Schmidt.** 1988. Chronic neurologic manifestations of erythema migrans borreliosis. *Ann. N. Y. Acad. Sci.* **539:**16–23.
4. **Afzelius, A.** 1921. Erythema chronicum migrans. *Acta Derm. Venereol.* **2:**120–125.
5. **Agger, W. A., S. M. Callister, and D. A. Jobe.** 1992. In vitro susceptibilities of *Borrelia burgdorferi* to five oral cephalosporins and ceftriaxone. *Antimicrob. Agents Chemother.* **36:**1788–1790.
6. **Akin, E., J. Aversa, and A. C. Steere.** 2001. Expression of adhesion molecules in synovia of patients with treatment-resistant Lyme arthritis. *Infect. Immun.* **69:**1774–1780.
7. **Akin, E., G. L. McHugh, R. A. Flavell, E. Fikrig, and A. C. Steere.** 1999. The immunoglobulin (IgG) antibody response to OspA and OspB correlates with severe and prolonged Lyme arthritis and the IgG response to P35 correlates with mild and brief arthritis. *Infect. Immun.* **67:**173–181.
8. **Alexopoulou, L., V. Thomas, M. Schnare, Y. Lobet, J. Anguita, R. T. Schoen, R. Medzhitov, E. Fikrig, and R. A. Flavell.** 2002. Hyporesponsiveness to vaccination with *Borrelia burgdorferi* OspA in humans and in TLR1- and TLR2-deficient mice. *Nat. Med.* **8:**878–884.
9. **Alitalo, A., T. Meri, H. Lankinen, I. Seppala, P. Lahdenne, P. S. Hefty, D. Akins, and S. Meri.** 2002. Complement inhibitor factor H binding to Lyme disease spirochetes is mediated by inducible expression of multiple plasmid-encoded outer surface protein E paralogs. *J. Immunol.* **169:**3847–3853.
10. **Alpert, L. I., P. Welch, and N. Fisher.** 1985. Gallium-positive Lyme disease myocarditis. *Clin. Nucl. Med.* **10:**617.
11. **Anderson, J. F.** 1991. Epizootiology of Lyme borreliosis. *Scand. J. Infect. Dis.* **77:**23–24.
12. **Anderson, J. F.** 1988. Mammalian and avian reservoirs for *Borrelia burgdorferi. Ann. N. Y. Acad. Sci.* **539:**180–191.
13. **Anguita, J., M. Rincon, S. Samanta, S. W. Barthold, R. A. Flavell, and E. Fikrig.** 1998. *Borrelia burgdorferi*-infected, interleukin-6-deficient mice have decreased Th2 responses and increased Lyme arthritis. *J. Infect. Dis.* **178:**1512–1515.
14. **Anguita, J., S. Samanta, S. W. Barthold, and E. Fikrig.** 1997. Ablation of interleukin-12 exacerbates Lyme arthritis in SCID mice. *Infect. Immun.* **65:**4334–4336.
15. **Anguita, J. S., S. K. Samanta, B. Ananthanarayanan, G. P. Revilla, S. W. Geba, S. W. Barthold, and E. Fikrig.** 2002. Cyclooxygenase 2 activity modulates the severity of murine Lyme arthritis. *FEMS Immunol. Med. Microbiol.* **34:**187–191.
16. **Asbrink, E., E. Brehmer-Anderson, and A. Hovmark.** 1986. Acrodermatitis chronica actrophicans—a spirochetosis. *Am. J. Dermatopathol.* **8:**209–219.
17. **Asbrink, E., and A. Hovmark.** 1985. Successful cultivation of spirochetes from skin lesions of patients with erythema chronica migrans afzelius and acrodermatitis chronica atrophicans. *Acta Pathol. Microbiol. Immunol. Scand. B* **93:**161–163.
18. **Atlas, E., S. N. Novak, P. H. Duray, and A. C. Steere.** 1988. Lyme myositis: muscle invasion by *Borrelia burgdorferi. Ann. Intern. Med.* **109:**245–246.
19. **Bacon, R. M., B. J. Biggerstaff, M. E. Schriefer, R. D. Gilmore, M. T. Philipp, A. C. Steere, G. P. Wormser, A. R. Marques, and B. J. B. Johnson.** 2003. Serodiagnosis of Lyme disease by kinetic enzyme-linked immunosorbent assay using recombinant VlsE1 or peptide antigens of *Borrelia burgdorferi* compared with 2-tiered testing using whole-cell lysates. *J. Infect. Dis.* **187:**1187–1199.
20. **Bailasiewicz, A. A., K. W. Ruprecht, G. O. Naumann, and H. Blenk.** 1988. Bilateral diffuse choroiditis and exudate retinal detachments with evidence of Lyme disease. *Am. J. Ophthalmol.* **105:**419–420.
21. **Bannwarth, A.** 1944. Zur Klinik und Pathogenese der "chronischen lymphocytaren Meningitis." *Arch. Psychiatr. Nervenkr.* **117:**161–185.
22. **Baranton, G., D. Postic, I. Saint-Girons, P. Boerlin, J. C. Piffaretti, M. Assous, and P. A. Grimont.** 1992. Delineation of *Borrelia burgdorferi* sensu stricto, *Borrelia garinii* sp. nov., and group VS461 associated with Lyme borreliosis. *Int. J. Syst. Bacteriol.* **42:**378–383.
23. **Baranton, G., G. Seinost, G. Theodore, D. Postic, and D. Dykhuizen.** 2001. Distinct levels of genetic diversity of *Borrelia burgdorferi* are associated with different aspects of pathogenicity. *Res. Microbiol.* **152:**149–156.
24. **Barbour, A. G.** 1984. Isolation and cultivation of Lyme disease spirochetes. *Yale J. Biol. Med.* **57:**521–525.
25. **Barbour, A. G., W. Burgdorfer, E. Grunwaldt, and A. C. Steere.** 1983. Antibodies of patients with Lyme disease to components of the *Ixodes dammini* spirochete. *J. Clin. Investig.* **72:**504–515.
26. **Barbour, A. G., and C. F. Garon.** 1987. Linear plasmids of the bacterium *Borrelia burgdorferi* have covalently closed ends. *Science* **237:**409–411.
27. **Barbour, A. G., and S. F. Hayes.** 1986. Biology of *Borrelia* species. *Microbiol. Rev.* **50:**381–400.
28. **Barthold, S. W., D. S. Beck, G. M. Hansen, G. A. Terwilliger, and K. D. Moody.** 1990. Lyme borreliosis in selected strains and ages of laboratory mice. *J. Infect. Dis.* **162:**133–138.
29. **Barthold, S. W., M. S. DeSouza, J. L. Janotka, A. L. Smith, and D. H. Persing.** 1993. Chronic Lyme borreliosis in the laboratory mouse. *Am. J. Pathol.* **143:**959–971.

30. Barthold, S. W., C. L. Sidman, and A. L. Smith. 1992. Lyme borreliosis in genetically resistant and susceptible mice with severe combined immunodeficiency. *Am. J. Trop. Med. Hyg.* 47:605–613.

31. Benach, J. L., E. M. Bosler, J. P. Hanrahan, J. L. Coleman, G. S. Habicht, T. F. Bast, D. J. Cameron, J. L. Ziegler, A. G. Barbour, W. Burgdorfer, R. Edelman, and R. A. Kaslow. 1983. Spirochetes isolated from the blood of two patients with Lyme disease. *N. Engl. J. Med.* 308:740–742.

32. Berger, B. W., R. C. Johnson, C. Kodner, and L. Coleman. 1992. Cultivation of *Borrelia burgdorferi* from erythema migrans lesions and perilesional skin. *J. Clin. Microbiol.* 30:359–361.

33. Berglund, J., R. Eitrem, K. Ornstein, A. Lindberg, A. Ringner, H. Elmrud, M. Carlsson, A. Runehagen, C. Svanborg, and R. Norrby. 1995. An epidemiologic study of Lyme disease in southern Sweden. *N. Engl. J. Med.* 333:1319–1324.

34. Bloom, B. J., P. M. Wyckoff, H. C. Meissner, and A. C. Steere. 1998. Neurocognitive abnormalities in children after classic manifestions of Lyme disease. *Pediatr. Infect. Dis. J.* 17:189–196.

35. Bockenstedt, L. K., J. Mao, E. Hodzic, S. W. Barthold, and D. Fish. 2002. Detection of attenuated, noninfectious spirochetes in *Borrelia burgdorferi*-infected mice after antibiotic treatment. *J. Infect. Dis.* 186:1430–1437.

36. Bono, J. L., A. F. Elias, J. J. Kupko III, B. Stevenson, K. Tilly, and P. Rosa. 2000. Efficient targeted mutagenesis in *Borrelia burgdorferi*. *J. Bacteriol.* 182:2445–2452.

37. Bosler, E. M., B. G. Ormiston, J. L. Coleman, J. P. Hanrahan, and J. L. Benach. 1984. Prevalence of the Lyme disease spirochete in populations of white-tailed deer and white-footed mice. *Yale J. Biol. Med.* 57:651–659.

38. Bradley, J. F., R. C. Johnson, and J. L. Goodman. 1994. The persistence of spirochetal nucleic acids in active Lyme arthritis. *Ann. Intern. Med.* 120:487–489.

39. Brown, C. R., V. A. Blaho, and C. M. Loiacono. 2003. Susceptibility to experimental Lyme arthritis correlates with KC and monocyte chemoattractant protein-1 production in joints and requires neutrophil recruitment via CXCR2. *J. Immunol.* 171:893–901.

40. Brown, C. R., and S. L. Reiner. 1999. Experimental Lyme arthritis in the absence of interleukin-4 or gamma interferon. *Infect. Immun.* 67:3329–3333.

41. Brown, C. R., and S. L. Reiner. 1999. Genetic control of experimental Lyme arthritis in the absence of specific immunity. *Infect. Immun.* 67:1967–1973.

42. Brown, E. L., R. M. Wooten, B. J. Johnson, R. V. Iozzo, A. Smith, M. C. Dolan, B. P. Guo, J. J. Weis, and M. Hook. 2001. Resistance to Lyme disease in decorin-deficient mice. *J. Clin. Investig.* 107:845–852.

43. Brown, J. P., J. F. Zachary, C. Teuscher, J. J. Weis, and R. M. Wooten. 1999. Dual role of interleukin-10 in murine Lyme disease: regulation of arthritis severity and host defense. *Infect. Immun.* 67:5142–5150.

44. Brown, R. N., and R. S. Lane. 1992. Lyme disease in California: a novel enzootic transmission cycle of *Borrelia burgdorferi*. *Science* 256:1439–1442.

45. Brunet, L. R., C. Sellitto, A. Spielman, and S. R. Telford III. 1995. Antibody response of the mouse reservoir of *Borrelia burgdorferi* in nature. *Infect. Immun.* 63:3030–3036.

46. Bunikis, J., B. Olsen, G. Westman, and S. Bergstroom. 1995. Variable serum immunoglobulin responses against different *Borrelia burgdorferi* sensu lato species in a population at risk for and patients with Lyme disease. *J. Clin. Microbiol.* 33:1473–1478.

47. Burchill, M. A., D. T. Nardelli, D. M. England, D. J. DeCoster, J. A. Christopherson, S. M. Callister, and R. F. Schell. 2003. Inhibition of interleukin-17 prevents the development of arthritis in vaccinated mice challenged with *Borrelia burgdorferi*. *Infect. Immun.* 71:3437–3442.

48. Burgdorfer, W., A. G. Barbour, S. F. Hayes, J. L. Benach, E. Grunwaldt, and J. P. Davis. 1982. Lyme disease—a tick-borne spirochetosis? *Science* 216:1317–1319.

49. Burgess, E. C. 1988. *Borrelia burgdorferi* infection in Wisconsin horses and cows. *Ann. N. Y. Acad. Sci.* 539:235–243.

50. Busch, D. H., C. Jassoy, U. Brinckmann, H. Girschick, and H. I. Huppertz. 1996. Detection of *Borrelia burgdorferi*-specific CD8+ T cytotoxic T cells in patients with Lyme arthritis. *J. Immunol.* 157:3534.

51. Cabello, F. C., M. L. Sartakova, and E. Y. Dobrikova. 2001. Genetic manipulation of spirochetes—light at the end of the tunnel. *Trends Microbiol.* 9:245–248.

52. Cadavid, D., T. O'Neill, H. Schaefer, and A. R. Pachner. 2000. Localization of *Borrelia burgdorferi* in the nervous system and other organs in a nonhuman primate model of Lyme disease. *Lab. Investig.* 80:1043–1054.

53. Campbell, G. L., W. S. Paul, M. E. Schriefer, R. B. Craven, K. E. Robbins, and D. T. Dennis. 1995. Epidemiologic and diagnostic studies of patients with suspected early Lyme disease, Missouri, 1990–1993. *J. Infect. Dis.* 172:470–480.

54. Canica, M. M., F. Nato, L. Du Merle, J. C. Mazie, G. Baranton, and D. Postic. 1993. Monoclonal antibodies for identification of *Borrelia afzelii* sp. nov. associated with late cutaneous manifestations of Lyme borreliosis. *Scand. J. Infect. Dis.* 25:441–448.

55. Carlson, D., J. Hernandez, B. J. Bloom, J. Coburn, J. M. Aversa, and A. C. Steere. 1999. Lack of *Borrelia burgdorferi* DNA in synovial samples in patients with antibiotic treatment-resistant Lyme arthritis. *Arthritis Rheum.* 42:2705–2709.

56. Carroll, J. A., P. E. Stewart, P. Rosa, A. F. Elias, and C. F. Garon. 2003. An enhanced GFP reporter system to monitor gene expression in *Borrelia burgdorferi*. *Microbiology* 149:1819–1828.

57. Casjens, S., N. Palmer, R. Van Vugt, W. Mun Huang, B. Stevenson, P. Rosa, R. Lathigra, G. Sutton, J. Peterson, R. J. Dodson, D. Haft, E. Hickey, M. Gwinn, O. White, and C. M. Fraser. 2000. A bacterial genome in flux: the twelve linear and nine circular extrachromosomal DNAs in an infectious isolate of the Lyme disease spirochete *Borrelia burgdorferi*. *Mol. Microbiol.* 35:490–516.

58. Centers for Disease Control and Prevention. 1990. Case definitions for public health surveillance. *Morb. Mortal. Wkly. Rep.* 39(RR-13):1–43.

59. Centers for Disease Control and Prevention. 1995. Recommendations for test performance and interpretation from the Second International Conference on serologic diagnosis of Lyme disease. *Morb. Mortal. Wkly. Rep.* 44:590–591.

60. Chen, J., J. A. Field, L. Glickstein, P. J. Molloy, B. T. Huber, and A. C. Steere. 1999. Association of antibiotic treatment-resistant Lyme arthritis with T cell responses to dominant epitopes of outer-surface protein A (OspA) of *Borrelia burgdorferi*. *Arthritis Rheum.* 42:1813–1822.

61. Christopherson, J. A., E. L. Munson, D. M. England, C. L. Croke, M. C. Remington, M. L. Molitor, D. J. DeCoster, S. M. Callister, and R. F. Schell. 2003. Destructive arthritis in vaccinated interferon gamma-deficient mice challenged with *Borrelia burgdorferi*: modulation by tumor necrosis factor alpha. *Clin. Diagn. Lab. Immunol.* 10:44–52.

62. Clark, J. R., R. D. Carlson, C. T. Sasaki, A. R. Pachner, and A. C. Steere. 1985. Facial paralysis in Lyme disease. *Laryngoscope* 95:1341–1345.

63. Coburn, J., S. W. Barthold, and J. M. Leong. 1994. Diverse Lyme disease spirochetes bind integrin $\alpha_{IIb}\beta_3$ on human platelets. *Infect. Immun.* **62:**5559–5567.

64. Coburn, J., W. Chege, L. Magoun, S. C. Bodary, and J. M. Leong. 1999. Characterization of a candidate *Borrelia burgdorferi* β_3-chain integrin ligand identified using a phage display library. *Mol. Microbiol.* **34:**926–940.

65. Coburn, J., and C. Cugini. 2003. Targeted mutation of the outer membrane protein P66 disrupts attachment of the Lyme disease agent, *Borrelia burgdorferi*, to integrin $\alpha_v\beta_3$. *Proc. Natl. Acad. Sci. USA* **100:**7301–7306.

66. Coburn, J., J. M. Leong, and J. K. Erban. 1993. Integrin α_{IIb} β_3 mediates binding of the Lyme disease agent *Borrelia burgdorferi* to human platelets. *Proc. Natl. Acad. Sci. USA* **90:** 7059–7063.

67. Coburn, J., L. Magoun, S. C. Bodary, and J. M. Leong. 1998. Integrins $\alpha_v\beta_3$ and $\alpha_5\beta_1$ mediate attachment of Lyme disease spirochetes to human cells. *Infect. Immun.* **66:**1946–1952.

68. Coleman, J. L., J. A. Gebbia, J. Pieman, J. L. Degen, T. H. Bugge, and J. L. Benach. 1997. Plasminogen is required for efficient dissemination of *B. burgdorferi* in ticks and for enhancement of spirochetemia in mice. *Cell* **89:**1111–1119.

69. Comstock, L. E., and D. D. Thomas. 1991. Characterization of *Borrelia burgdorferi* invasion of cultured endothelial cells. *Microb. Pathog.* **10:**137–148.

70. Cox, D. L., D. R. Akins, K. W. Bourell, P. Lahdenne, M. V. Norgard, and J. D. Radolf. 1996. Limited surface exposure of *Borrelia burgdorferi* outer surface lipoproteins. *Proc. Natl. Acad. Sci. USA* **93:**7973–7978.

71. Croke, C. L., E. L. Munson, S. D. Lovrich, J. A. Christopherson, M. C. Remington, D. M. England, S. M. Callister, and R. F. Schell. 2000. Occurrence of severe destructive Lyme arthritis in hamsters vaccinated with outer surface protein A and challenged with *Borrelia burgdorferi*. *Infect. Immun.* **68:** 658–663.

72. Crowley, H., and B. T. Huber. 2003. Host-adapted *Borrelia burgdorferi* in mice expresses OspA during inflammation. *Infect. Immun.* **71:**4003–4010.

73. Curran, K. L., D. Fish, and J. Piesman. 1993. Reduction of nymphal *Ixodes dammini* (Acari: *Ixodidae*) in a residential suburban landscape by area application of insecticides. *J. Med. Entomol.* **30:**107–113.

74. Dai, Z., H. Lackland, S. Stein, Q. Li, R. Radziewicz, S. Williams, and L. H. Sigal. 1993. Molecular mimicry in Lyme disease: monoclonal antibody H9724 to *B. burgdorferi* flagellin specifically detects chaperonin-HSP60. *Biochim. Biophys. Acta* **1181:**97–100.

75. Dattwyler, R. J., J. J. Halperin, D. J. Volkman, and B. J. Luft. 1988. Treatment of late Lyme borreliosis—randomized comparison of ceftriaxone and penicillin. *Lancet* **i:**1191–1194.

76. Dattwyler, R. J., B. J. Luft, M. J. Kunkel, M. F. Finkel, G. P. Wormser, and G. P. Rush. 1997. Ceftriaxone compared with doxycycline for the treatment of acute disseminated Lyme disease. *N. Engl. J. Med.* **337:**289–294.

77. Dattwyler, R. J., D. J. Volkman, S. M. Conaty, S. P. Platkin, and B. J. Luft. 1990. Amoxicillin plus probenecid versus doxycycline for treatment of erythema migrans borreliosis. *Lancet* **336:**1404–1406.

78. de Silva, A. M., and E. Fikrig. 1997. Arthropod- and host-specific gene expression by *Borrelia burgdorferi*. *J. Clin. Investig.* **100:**S3–S5.

79. Defosse, D. L., and R. C. Johnson. 1992. In vitro and in vivo induction of tumor necrosis factor alpha by *Borrelia burgdorferi*. *Infect. Immun.* **60:**1109–1113.

80. Dennis, D. T., and E. B. Hayes. 2002. Epidemiology of Lyme borreliosis, p. 251–280. *In* O. K. J. S. Gray, R. S. Lane, and G. Stanek (ed.), *Lyme Borreliosis: Biology, Epidemiology and Control*. CABI Publishing, Oxford, England.

81. DeSouza, M. S., E. Fikrig, A. L. Smith, R. A. Flavell, and S. W. Barthold. 1992. Nonspecific proliferative responses of murine lymphocytes to *Borrelia burgdorferi* antigens. *J. Infect. Dis.* **165:**471–478.

82. Dever, L. L., J. H. Jorgensen, and A. G. Barbour. 1993. In vitro activity of vancomycin against the spirochete *Borrelia burgdorferi*. *Antimicrob. Agents Chemother.* **37:**1115–1121.

83. Dever, L. L., J. H. Jorgensen, and A. G. Barbour. 1992. In vitro antimicrobial susceptibility testing of *Borrelia burgdorferi*: a microdilution MIC method and time-kill studies. *J. Clin. Microbiol.* **30:**2692–2697.

84. Dinerman, H., and A. C. Steere. 1992. Lyme disease associated with fibromyalgia. *Ann. Intern. Med.* **117:**281–285.

85. Dong, Z., M. Edelstein, and L. J. Glickstein. 1997. CD8$^+$ T cells are activated during the early Th1 and Th2 immune responses in the murine Lyme disease model. *Infect. Immun.* **65:**5334–5337.

86. Dressler, F., J. A. Whalen, B. N. Reinhardt, and A. C. Steere. 1993. Western blotting in the serodiagnosis of Lyme disease. *J. Infect. Dis.* **167:**392–400.

87. Duray, P. H. 1987. The surgical pathology of human Lyme disease: an enlarging picture. *Am. J. Surg. Pathol.* **11:**47–60.

88. Duray, P. H., and A. C. Steere. 1988. Clinical pathologic correlations of Lyme disease by stage. *Ann. N. Y. Acad. Sci.* **539:**65–79.

89. Eckman, M. H., A. C. Steere, R. A. Kalish, and S. G. Pauker. 1997. Cost effectiveness of oral as compared with intravenous antibiotic therapy for patients with early Lyme disease or Lyme arthritis. *N. Engl. J. Med.* **337:**357–363.

90. Eggers, C. H., B. J. Kimmel, J. L. Bono, A. F. Elias, P. Rosa, and D. S. Samuels. 2001. Transduction by phiBB-1, a bacteriophage of *Borrelia burgdorferi*. *J. Bacteriol.* **183:**4771–4778.

91. Eggers, C. H., and D. S. Samuels. 1999. Molecular evidence for a new bacteriophage of *Borrelia burgdorferi*. *J. Bacteriol.* **181:**7308–7313.

92. Engstrom, S. M., E. Shoop, and R. C. Johnson. 1995. Immunoblot interpretation criteria for serodiagnosis of early Lyme disease. *J. Clin. Microbiol.* **33:**419–427.

93. Ettestad, P. J., G. L. Campbell, S. F. Welbel, C. A. Genese, K. C. Spitalny, C. M. Marchetti, and D. T. Dennis. 1995. Biliary complications in the treatment of unsubstantiated Lyme disease. *J. Infect. Dis.* **171:**356–361.

94. Fahrer, H., S. M. Van der Linden, M. J. Sauvain, L. Gern, E. Zhioua, and A. Aeschlimann. 1991. The prevalence and incidence of clinical and asymptomatic Lyme borreliosis in a population at risk. *J. Infect. Dis.* **163:**305–310.

95. Feng, S., E. Hodzic, and S. W. Barthold. 2000. Lyme arthritis resolution with antiserum to a 37-kilodalton *Borrelia burgdorferi* protein. *Infect. Immun.* **68:**4169–4173.

96. Fikrig, E., S. W. Barthold, M. Chen, C. H. Chang, and R. A. Flavell. 1997. Protective antibodies develop, and murine Lyme arthritis regresses, in the absence of MHC class II and CD4+ T cells. *J. Immunol.* **159:**5682–5686.

97. Fikrig, E., S. W. Barthold, F. S. Kantor, and R. A. Flavell. 1990. Protection of mice against the Lyme disease agent by immunizing with recombinant OspA. *Science* **250:**553–556.

98. Fikrig, E., S. W. Barthold, W. Sun, W. Feng, S. R. Telford III, and R. A. Flavell. 1997. *Borrelia burgdorferi* P35 and P37 proteins, expressed in vivo, elicit protective immunity. *Immunity* **6:**531–537.

99. Filgueira, L., F. O. Nestle, M. Rittig, H. I. Joller, and P. Groscurth. 1996. Human dendritic cells phagocytose and process *Borrelia burgdorferi*. *J. Immunol.* **157**:2998–3005.

100. Fischer, J. R., N. Parveen, L. Magoun, and J. M. Leong. 2003. Decorin-binding proteins A and B confer distinct mammalian cell type-specific attachment by *Borrelia burgdorferi*, the Lyme disease spirochete. *Proc. Natl. Acad. Sci. USA* **100**:7307–7312.

101. Franz, J. K., O. Frize, M. Rittig, G. Keyßer, S. Priem, J. Zacher, G. R. Burmester, and A. Krause. 2001. Insights from a novel three-dimensional in vitro model of Lyme arthritis. *Arthritis Rheum.* **44**:151.

102. Fraser, C. M., S. Casjens, W. M. Huang, G. G. Sutton, R. Clayton, R. Lathigra, O. White, K. A. Ketchum, R. Dodson, E. K. Hickey, M. Gwinn, B. Dougherty, J. F. Tomb, R. D. Fleischmann, D. Richardson, J. Peterson, A. R. Kerlavage, J. Quackenbush, S. Salzberg, M. Hanson, R. van Vugt, N. Palmer, M. D. Adams, J. Gocayne, J. C. Venter, et al. 1997. Genomic sequence of a Lyme disease spirochete, *Borrelia burgdorferi*. *Nature* **390**:580–586.

103. Fuchs, H., R. Wallich, M. M. Simon, and M. D. Kramer. 1994. The outer surface protein A of the spirochete *Borrelia burgdorferi* is a plasmin(ogen) receptor. *Proc. Natl. Acad. Sci. USA* **91**:12594–12598.

104. Fukunaga, M., A. Hamase, K. Okada, and M. Nakao. 1996. *Borrelia tanukii* sp. nov. and *Borrelia turdae* sp. nov. found from ixodid ticks in Japan: rapid species identification by 16S rRNA gene-targeted PCR analysis. *Microbiol. Immunol.* **40**:877–881.

105. Garcia-Monco, J. C., B. F. Villar, J. C. Alen, and J. L. Benach. 1990. *Borrelia burgdorferi* in the central nervous system: experimental and clinical evidence for early invasion. *J. Infect. Dis.* **161**:1187.

106. Gardner, P. 1998. Lyme disease vaccines. *Ann. Intern. Med.* **129**:583–585.

107. Gebbia, J. A., J. L. Coleman, and J. L. Benach. 2001. Borrelia spirochetes upregulate release and activation of matrix metalloproteinase gelatinase B (MMP-9) and collagenase 1 (MMP-1) in human cells. *Infect. Immun.* **69**:456–462.

108. Georgilis, K., M. Peacocke, and M. S. Klempner. 1992. Fibroblasts protect the Lyme disease spirochete, *Borrelia burgdorferi*, from ceftriaxone in vitro. *J. Infect. Dis.* **166**:440–444.

109. Gern, L., A. Estrada-Peña, F. Frandsen, J. S. Gray, T. G. Jaenson, F. Jongejan, O. Kahl, E. Korenberg, R. Mehl, and P. A. Nuttall. 1998. European reservoir hosts of *Borrelia burgdorferi* sensu lato. *Zentralbl. Bakteriol.* **287**:196–204.

110. Gern, L., and H. Pierre-Francois. 2002. Ecology of *Borrelia burgdorferi* sensu lato in Europe, p. 149–174. *In* O. K. J. S. Gray, R. S. Lane, and G. Stanek (ed.), *Lyme Borreliosis: Biology, Epidemiology and Control*. CABI Publishing, Oxford, England.

111. Glatzel, A., F. Entschladen, T. M. Zollner, P. Kraiczy, V. Brade, R. Kaufmann, O. Janssen, B. Lengl-Janssen, D. Wesch, and D. Kabelitz. 2002. The responsiveness of human Vδ1 γδ T cells to *Borrelia burgdorferi* is largely restricted to synovial-fluid cells from patients with Lyme arthritis. *J. Infect. Dis.* **186**:1043–1046.

112. Glavanakov, S., D. J. White, T. Caraco, A. Lapenis, G. R. Robinson, B. K. Szymanski, and W. A. Maniatty. 2001. Lyme disease in New York State: spatial pattern at a regional scale. *Am. J. Trop. Med. Hyg.* **65**:538–545.

113. Glickstein, L., M. Edelstein, and J. Z. Dong. 2001. Gamma interferon is not required for arthritis resistance in the murine Lyme disease model. *Infect. Immun.* **69**:3737–3743.

114. Glickstein, L., B. Moore, T. Bledsoe, N. Damle, V. Sikand, and A. C. Steere. 2003. Inflammatory cytokine production predominates in early Lyme disease in patients with erythema migrans. *Infect. Immun.* **71**:6051–6053.

115. Goldstein, S. F., N. W. Charon, and J. A. Kreiling. 1994. *Borrelia burgdorferi* swims with a planar waveform similar to that of eukaryotic flagella. *Proc. Natl. Acad. Sci. USA* **91**: 3433–3437.

116. Gomes-Solecki, M. J., G. P. Wormser, D. H. Persing, B. W. Berger, J. D. Glass, X. Yang, and R. J. Dattwyler. 2001. A first-tier rapid assay for the serodiagnosis of *Borrelia burgdorferi* infection. *Arch. Intern. Med.* **161**:2015–2020.

117. Granter, S. R., R. L. Barnhill, M. E. Hewins, and P. H. Duray. 1994. Identification of *Borrelia burgdorferi* in diffuse fasciitis with peripheral eosinophilia: borrelial fasciitis. *JAMA* **272**:1283–1285.

118. Gross, D. M., T. Forsthuber, M. Tary-Lehman, C. Etling, K. Ito, Z. A. Nagy, J. A. Field, A. C. Steere, and B. T. Huber. 1998. Identification of LFA-1 as a candidate autoantigen in treatment-resistant Lyme arthritis. *Science* **281**:703–706.

119. Gross, D. M., A. C. Steere, and B. T. Huber. 1998. T helper 1 response is dominant and localized to the synovial fluid in patients with Lyme arthritis. *J. Immunol.* **160**:1022–1028.

120. Guo, B. P., E. L. Brown, D. W. Dorward, L. C. Rosenberg, and M. Hook. 1998. Decorin-binding adhesins from *Borrelia burgdorferi*. *Mol. Microbiol.* **30**:711–723.

121. Guo, B. P., S. J. Norris, L. C. Rosenberg, and M. Hook. 1995. Adherence of *Borrelia burgdorferi* to the proteoglycan decorin. *Infect. Immun.* **63**:3467–3472.

122. Gustafson, R., B. Svenungsson, M. Forsgren, A. Gardulf, and M. Granstrom. 1992. Two-year survey of the incidence of Lyme borreliosis and tick-borne encephalitis in a high-risk population in Sweden. *Eur. J. Clin. Microbiol. Infect. Dis.* **11**:894–900.

123. Gustafson, R., B. Svenungsson, A. Gardulf, G. Stiernstedt, and M. Forsgren. 1990. Prevalence of tick-borne encephalitis and Lyme borreliosis in a defined Swedish population. *Scand. J. Infect. Dis.* **22**:297–306.

124. Halperin, J. J., B. W. Little, P. K. Coyle, and R. J. Dattwyler. 1987. Lyme disease: cause of a treatable peripheral neuropathy. *Neurology* **37**:1700–1706.

125. Halperin, J. J., D. J. Volkman, and P. Wu. 1991. Central nervous system abnormalities in Lyme neuroborreliosis. *Neurology* **41**:1571–1582.

126. Hanrahan, J. P., J. L. Benach, J. L. Coleman, E. M. Bosler, D. L. Morse, D. J. Cameron, R. Edelman, and R. A. Kaslow. 1984. Incidence and cumulative frequency of endemic Lyme disease in a community. *J. Infect. Dis.* **150**:489–496.

127. Hansen, K., M. Cruz, and H. Link. 1990. Oligoclonal *Borrelia burgdorferi*-specific IgG antibodies in cerebrospinal fluid in Lyme neuroborreliosis. *J. Infect. Dis.* **161**:1194–1202.

128. Hansen, K., and A. M. Lebech. 1991. Lyme neuroborreliosis: a new sensitive diagnostic assay for intrathecal synthesis of *Borrelia burgdorferi*—specific immunoglobulin G, A, and M. *Ann. Neurol.* **30**:197–205.

129. Hanson, M. S., D. R. Cassatt, B. P. Guo, N. K. Patel, M. P. McCarthy, D. W. Dorward, and M. Hook. 1998. Active and passive immunity against *Borrelia burgdorferi* decorin binding protein A (DbpA) protects against infection. *Infect. Immun.* **66**:2143–2153.

130. Hanson, M. S., and R. Edelman. 2003. Progress and controversy surrounding vaccines against Lyme disease. *Expert Rev. Vaccines* **2**:683–703.

131. Hardin, J. A., A. C. Steere, and S. E. Malawista. 1979. Immune complexes and the evolution of Lyme arthritis: dissemination and localization of abnormal C1q binding activity. *N. Engl. J. Med.* **301**:1358–1363.

132. Hayes, E. B., and J. Piesman. 2003. How can we prevent Lyme disease? *N. Engl. J. Med.* **348**:2424–2430.

133. Hefty, P. S., S. E. Jolliff, M. J. Caimano, S. K. Wikel, and D. R. Akins. 2002. Changes in temporal and spatial patterns of outer surface lipoprotein expression generate population heterogeneity and antigenic diversity in the Lyme disease spirochete, *Borrelia burgdorferi*. *Infect. Immun.* **70:**3468–3478.

134. Hellwage, J., T. Meri, T. Heikkila, A. Alitalo, J. Panelius, P. Lahdenne, I. J. Seppala, and S. Meri. 2001. The complement regulator factor H binds to the surface protein OspE of *Borrelia burgdorferi*. *J. Biol. Chem.* **276:**8427–8435.

135. Hemmer, B., B. Gran, Y. Zhao, A. Marques, J. Pascal, A. Tzou, T. Kondo, I. Cortese, B. Bielekova, S. E. Straus, H. F. McFarland, R. Houghten, R. Simon, C. Pinilla, and R. Martin. 1999. Identification of candidate T-cell epitopes and molecular mimics in chronic Lyme disease. *Nat. Med.* **5:**1375–1382.

136. Henriksson, A., H. Link, M. Cruz, and G. Stiernstedt. 1986. Immunoglobulin abnormalities in cerebrospinal fluid and blood over the course of lymphocytic meningoradiculitis (Bannwarth's syndrome). *Ann. Neurol.* **20:**337–345.

137. Hinnebusch, J., S. Bergstrom, and A. G. Barbour. 1990. Cloning and sequence analysis of linear plasmid telomeres of the bacterium *Borrelia burgdorferi*. *Mol. Microbiol.* **4:** 811–820.

138. Hovind-Hougen, K., E. Asbrink, G. Stiernstedt, A. C. Steere, and A. Hovmark. 1986. Ultrastructural differences among spirochetes isolated from patients with Lyme disease and related disorders, and from *Ixodes ricinus*. *Zentralbl. Bakteriol. Mikrobiol. Hyg. A* **263:**103–111.

139. Hu, L. T., G. Perides, R. Noring, and M. S. Klempner. 1995. Binding of human plasminogen to *Borrelia burgdorferi*. *Infect. Immun.* **63:**3491–3496.

140. Hubner, A., X. Yang, D. M. Nolen, T. G. Popova, F. C. Cabello, and M. V. Norgard. 2001. Expression of *Borrelia burgdorferi* OspC and DbpA is controlled by a RpoN-RpoS regulatory pathway. *Proc. Natl. Acad. Sci. USA* **98:**12724–12729.

141. Humair, P. F., O. Peter, R. Wallich, and L. Gern. 1995. Strain variation of Lyme disease spirochetes isolated from *Ixodes ricinus* ticks and rodents collected in two endemic areas in Switzerland. *J. Med. Entomol.* **32:**433–438.

142. Isaacs, R. D. 1994. *Borrelia burgdorferi* bind to epithelial cell proteoglycans. *J. Clin. Investig.* **93:**809–819.

143. Jacobs, J. C., M. Stevens, and P. H. Duray. 1986. Lyme disease simulating septic arthritis. *JAMA* **256:**1138–1139.

144. Johnson, R. C., C. Kodner, and M. Russell. 1986. Active immunization of hamsters against experimental infection with *Borrelia burgdorferi*. *Infect. Immun.* **54:**887–891.

145. Johnson, R. C., C. Kodner, and M. Russell. 1987. In vitro and in vivo susceptibility of the Lyme disease spirochete, *Borrelia burgdorferi*, to four antimicrobial agents. *Antimicrob. Agents Chemother.* **31:**164–167.

146. Johnson, R. C., C. Kodner, and M. Russell. 1986. Passive immunization of hamsters against experimental infection with *Borrelia burgdorferi*. *Infect. Immun.* **53:**713–715.

147. Johnson, R. C., G. P. Schmid, F. W. Hyde, A. G. Steigerwalt, and D. J. Brenner. 1984. *Borrelia burgdorferi* sp. nov.: etiologic agent of Lyme disease. *Int. J. Syst. Bacteriol.* **34:**496–497.

148. Kalish, R. A., R. F. Kaplan, E. Taylor, L. Jones-Woodward, K. Workman, and A. C. Steere. 2001. Evaluation of study ·patients with Lyme disease, 10–20-year follow-up. *J. Infect. Dis.* **183:**453–460.

149. Kalish, R. A., J. M. Leong, and A. C. Steere. 1993. Association of treatment resistant chronic Lyme arthritis with HLA-DR4 and antibody reactivity to OspA and OspB of *Borrelia burgdorferi*. *Infect. Immun.* **61:**2774–2779.

150. Kalish, R. A., J. M. Leong, and A. C. Steere. 1995. Early and late antibody responses to full-length and truncated constructs of outer-surface protein A of *Borrelia burgdorferi* in Lyme disease. *Infect. Immun.* **63:**2228–2235.

151. Kalish, R. A., G. McHugh, J. Granquist, B. Shea, R. Ruthazer, and A. C. Steere. 2001. Persistence of immunoglobulin M or immunoglobulin G antibody responses to *Borrelia burgdorferi* 10–20 years after active Lyme disease. *Clin. Infect. Dis.* **33:**780–785.

152. Kang, I., S. W. Barthold, D. H. Persing, and L. K. Bockenstedt. 1997. T-helper-cell cytokines in the early evolution of murine Lyme arthritis. *Infect. Immun.* **65:**3107–3111.

153. Kaplan, R. F., and L. Jones-Woodward. 1997. Lyme encephalopathy: a neuropsychological perspective. *Semin. Neurol.* **17:**31–37.

154. Karlsson, M., S. Hammers-Berggren, L. Lindquist, G. Stiernstedt, and B. Svenungsson. 1994. Comparison of intravenous penicillin G and oral doxycycline for treatment of Lyme neuroborreliosis. *Neurology* **44:**1203–1207.

155. Karlsson, M., K. Hovind-Hougen, B. Svenungsson, and G. Stiernstedt. 1990. Cultivation and characterization of spirochetes from cerebrospinal fluid of patients with Lyme borreliosis. *J. Clin. Microbiol.* **28:**473–479.

156. Karma, A., I. Seppala, H. Mikkila, S. Kaakkola, M. Viljanen, and A. Tarkkanen. 1994. Diagnosis and clinical characteristics of ocular Lyme borreliosis. *Am. J. Ophthalmol.* **119:** 127–135.

157. Kawabata, H., T. Masuzawa, and Y. Yanagihara. 1993. Genomic analysis of *Borrelia japonica* sp. nov. isolated from *Ixodes ovatus* in Japan. *Microbiol. Immunol.* **37:**843–848.

158. Keane-Myers, A., and S. P. Nickell. 1995. Role of IL-4 and IFN-gamma in modulation of immunity to *Borrelia burgdorferi* in mice. *J. Immunol.* **155:**2020–2028.

159. Keller, D., F. T. Koster, D. H. Marks, P. Hosbach, L. F. Erdile, and J. P. Mays. 1994. Safety and immunogenicity of a recombinant outer surface protein A Lyme vaccine. *JAMA* **271:**1764–1768.

160. Klempner, M. S., L. T. Hu, J. Evans, C. H. Schmid, G. M. Johnson, R. P. Trevino, D. Norton, L. Levy, D. Wall, J. McCall, M. Kosinski, and A. Weinstein. 2001. Two controlled trials of antibiotic treatment in patients with persistent symptoms and a history of Lyme disease. *N. Engl. J. Med.* **345:**85–92.

161. Klempner, M. S., C. H. Schmid, L. Hu, A. C. Steere, G. Johnson, B. McCloud, R. Noring, and A. Weinstein. 2001. Intralaboratory reliability of serologic and urine testing for Lyme disease. *Am. J. Med.* **110:**217–219.

162. Kochi, S. K., and R. C. Johnson. 1988. Role of immunoglobulin G in killing *Borrelia burgdorferi* by the classical complement pathway. *Infect. Immun.* **56:**314–321.

163. Korenberg, E. I. 1994. Comparative ecology and epidemiology of Lyme disease and tick-borne encephalitis in the former Soviet Union. *Parasitol. Today* **10:**157–160.

164. Korenberg, E. I., N. B. Gorelova, and Y. V. Kovalevskii. 2002. Ecology of *Borrelia burgdorferi* sensu lato in Russia. p. 175–200. *In* O. K. J. S. Gray, R. S. Lane, and G. Stanek (ed.), *Lyme Borreliosis: Biology, Epidemiology and Control.* CABI Publishing, Oxford, England.

165. Kornblatt, A. N., P. H. Urband, and A. C. Steere. 1985. Arthritis caused by *Borrelia burgdorferi* in dogs. *J. Am. Vet. Med. Assoc.* **186:**960–964.

166. Kornmehl, E. W., R. L. Lesser, P. Jaros, E. Rocco, and A. C. Steere. 1989. Bilateral keratitis in Lyme disease. *Ophthalmology* **96:**1194–1197.

167. Kraiczy, P., C. Skerka, M. Kirschfink, V. Brade, and P. F. Zipfel. 2001. Immune evasion of *Borrelia burgdorferi* by acquisition of human complement regulators FHL-1/reconectin and factor H. *Eur. J. Immunol.* **31:**1674–1684.

168. Kramer, N., R. R. Rickert, R. H. Brodkin, and E. D. Rosenstein. 1986. Septal panniculitis as a manifestation of Lyme disease. *Am. J. Med.* **81:**149–152.

169. Krause, P. J., K. McKay, C. A. Thompson, V. K. Sikand, R. Lentz, T. Lepore, L. Closter, D. Christianson, S. R. Telford, D. Persing, J. D. Radolf, and A. Spielman. 2002. Disease-specific diagnosis of coinfecting tickborne zoonoses: babesiosis, human granulocytic ehrlichiosis, and Lyme disease. *Clin. Infect. Dis.* **34:**1184–1191.

170. Krause, P. J., S. R. Telford III, A. Spielman, V. Sikand, R. Ryan, R. N. Christianson, G. Burke, P. Brassard, R. Pollack, J. Peck, and D. H. Persing. 1996. Concurrent Lyme disease and babesiosis: evidence for increased severity and duration of illness. *JAMA* **275:**1657–1660.

171. Kumar, H., A. Belperron, S. W. Barthold, and L. K. Bockenstedt. 2000. Cutting edge: CD1d deficiency impairs murine host defense against the spirochete, *Borrelia burgdorferi*. *J. Immunol.* **165:**4797–4801.

172. Labandeira-Rey, M., and J. T. Skare. 2001. Decreased infectivity in *Borrelia burgdorferi* strain B31 is associated with loss of linear plasmid 25 or 28-1. *Infect. Immun.* **69:**446–455.

173. Lahdenne, P., S. F. Porcella, K. E. Hagman, D. R. Akins, T. G. Popova, D. L. Cox, L. I. Katona, J. D. Radolf, and M. V. Norgard. 1997. Molecular characterization of a 6.6-kilodalton *Borrelia burgdorferi* outer membrane-associated lipoprotein (lp6.6) which appears to be downregulated during mammalian infection. *Infect. Immun.* **65:**412–421.

174. Lane, R. S., J. Piesman, and W. Burgdorfer. 1991. Lyme borreliosis: relation of its causative agent to its vectors and hosts in North America and Europe. *Ann. Rev. Immunol.* **36:**587–609.

175. Lardieri, G., A. Salvi, F. Camerini, M. Cinco, and G. Trevisan. 1993. Isolation of *Borrelia burgdorferi* from myocardium. *Lancet* **342:**8869.

176. Lastavica, C. C., M. L. Wilson, V. P. Berardi, A. Spielman, and R. D. Deblinger. 1989. Rapid emergence of a focal epidemic of Lyme disease in coastal Massachusetts. *N. Engl. J. Med.* **320:**133–137.

177. Lawrenz, M. B., H. Kawabata, J. E. Purser, and S. J. Norris. 2002. Decreased electroporation efficiency in *Borrelia burgdorferi* containing linear plasmids lp25 and lp56: impact on transformation of infectious *B. burgdorferi*. *Infect. Immun.* **70:**4798–4804.

178. Le Fleche, A., D. Postic, K. Girardet, O. Peter, and G. Baranton. 1997. Characterization of *Borrelia lusitaniae* sp. nov. by 16S ribosomal DNA sequence analysis. *Int. J. Syst. Bacteriol.* **47:**921–925.

179. Lengl-Janssen, B., A. F. Strauss, A. C. Steere, and T. Kamradt. 1994. The T helper cell response in Lyme arthritis: differential recognition of *Borrelia burgdorferi* outer surface protein A (OspA) in patients with treatment-resistant or treatment-responsive Lyme arthritis. *J. Exp. Med.* **180:**2069–2078.

180. Leong, J. L., P. E. Morrissey, E. Ortega-Barria, M. E. A. Pereira, and J. Coburn. 1995. Hemagglutination and proteoglycan binding by the Lyme disease spirochete, *Borrelia burgdorferi*. *Infect. Immun.* **63:**874–883.

181. Leong, J. M., H. Wang, L. Magoun, J. A. Field, P. E. Morrissey, D. Robbins, J. B. Tatro, J. Coburn, and N. Parveen. 1998. Different classes of proteoglycans contribute to the attachment of *Borrelia burgdorferi* to cultured endothelial and brain cells. *Infect. Immun.* **66:**994–999.

182. Liang, F. T., A. C. Steere, A. R. Marques, B. J. Johnson, J. N. Miller, and M. T. Philipp. 1999. Sensitive and specific serodiagnosis of Lyme disease by enzyme-linked immunosorbent assay with a peptide based on an immunodominant conserved region of *Borrelia burgdorferi* VlsE. *J. Clin. Microbiol.* **37:**3990–3996.

183. Lim, L. C. L., D. M. England, B. K. DuChateau, N. J. Glowacki, J. R. Creson, S. D. Lovrich, S. M. Callister, D. A. Jobe, and R. F. Schell. 1994. Development of destructive arthritis in vaccinated hamsters challenged with *Borrelia burgdorferi*. *Infect. Immun.* **62:**2825–2833.

184. Lipschutz, B. 1923. Weiterer Beitrag zur Kenntnis des "Erythema chronicum migrans." *Arch. Dermatol.* **143:**365–374.

185. Logigian, E. L. 1997. Peripheral nervous system Lyme borreliosis. *Semin. Neurol.* **17:**25–30.

186. Logigian, E. L., R. F. Kaplan, and A. C. Steere. 1990. Chronic neurologic manifestations of Lyme disease. *N. Engl. J. Med.* **323:**1438–1444.

187. Logigian, E. L., R. F. Kaplan, and A. C. Steere. 1999. Successful treatment of Lyme encephalopathy with intravenous ceftriaxone. *J. Infect. Dis.* **180:**377–383.

188. Logigian, E. L., and A. C. Steere. 1992. Clinical and electrophysiologic findings in chronic neuropathy of Lyme disease. *Neurology* **42:**303–311.

189. LoGiudice, K., R. S. Ostfeld, K. A. Schmidt, and F. Keesing. 2003. The ecology of infectious disease: effects of host diversity and community composition on Lyme disease risk. *Proc. Natl. Acad. Sci. USA* **100:**567–571.

190. Luft, B. J., R. J. Dattwyler, R. C. Johnson, S. W. Luger, E. M. Bosler, D. W. Rahn, E. J. Masters, E. Grunwaldt, and S. D. Gadgil. 1996. Azithromycin compared with amoxicillin in the treatment of erythema migrans: a double-blind, randomized, controlled trial. *Ann. Intern. Med.* **124:**785–791.

191. Ma, Y., K. P. Seiler, E. J. Eichwals, J. H. Weis, C. Teuscher, and J. J. Weiss. 1998. Distinct characteristics of resistance to *Borrelia burgdorferi*-induced arthritis in C57BL/6N mice. *Infect. Immun.* **66:**161–168.

192. Ma, Y., A. Sturrock, and J. J. Weis. 1991. Intracellular localization of *Borrelia burgdorferi* within human endothelial cells. *Infect. Immun.* **59:**671–678.

193. Ma, Y., and J. J. Weis. 1993. *Borrelia burgdorferi* outer surface lipoproteins OspA and OspB possess B cell mitogenic and cytokine stimulatory properties. *Infect. Immun.* **61:**3843–3853.

194. Magnarelli, L. A., and J. F. Anderson. 1988. Ticks and biting insects infected with the etiologic agent of Lyme disease, *Borrelia burgdorferi*. *J. Clin. Microbiol.* **26:**1482–1486.

195. Magnarelli, L. A., J. F. Anderson, C. S. Apperson, D. Fish, R. C. Johnson, and W. C. Chappell. 1986. Spirochetes in ticks and antibodies to *Borrelia burgdorferi* in white-tailed deer from Connecticut, New York State, and North Carolina. *J. Wildlife Dis.* **22:**178–188.

196. Magnarelli, L. A., J. F. Anderson, W. Burgdorfer, and W. A. Chappell. 1984. Parasitism by *Ixodes dammini* (Acari: Ixodidae) and antibodies to spirochetes in mammals in Lyme disease foci in Connecticut, USA. *J. Med. Entomol.* **21:**52–57.

197. Magnarelli, L. A., J. F. Anderson, and W. A. Chappell. 1984. Antibodies to spirochetes in white-tailed deer and prevalence of infected ticks from foci of Lyme disease in Connecticut. *J. Wildlife Dis.* **20:**21–26.

198. Marconi, R. T., D. Liveris, and I. Schwartz. 1995. Identification of novel insertion elements, restriction fragment length polymorphism patterns, and discontinuous 23S rRNA in Lyme disease spirochetes: phylogenetic analyses of rRNA genes and their intergenic spacers in *Borrelia japonica* sp. nov. and genomic group 21038 (*Borrelia andersonii* sp. nov.) isolates. *J. Clin. Microbiol.* **33:**2427–2434.

199. Marcus, L. C., M. M. Patterson, R. E. Gilfillan, and P. H. Urband. 1985. Antibodies to *Borrelia burgdorferi* in New England horses: serologic survey. *Am. J. Vet. Res.* **46:**2570–2571.

200. Marcus, L. C., A. C. Steere, P. H. Duray, A. E. Anderson, and E. B. Mahoney. 1985. Fatal pancarditis in a patient with coexistent Lyme disease and babesiosis: demonstration of spirochetes in the myocardium. *Ann. Intern. Med.* **103**:374–376.

201. Markowitz, L. E., A. C. Steere, J. L. Benach, J. D. Slade, and C. V. Broome. 1986. Lyme disease during pregnancy. *JAMA* **255**:3394–3396.

202. Marshall, W. F., III, S. R. Telford III, P. N. Rys, B. J. Rutledge, D. Mathiesen, S. E. Malawista, A. Spielman, and D. H. Persing. 1994. Detection of *Borrelia burgdorferi* DNA in museum specimens of *Peromyscus leucopus*. *J. Infect. Dis.* **170**:1027–1032.

203. Massarotti, E. M., S. W. Luger, D. W. Rahn, R. P. Messner, J. B. Wong, R. C. Johnson, and A. C. Steere. 1992. Treatment of early Lyme disease. *Am. J. Med.* **92**:396–403.

204. Mast, W. E., and W. M. J. Burrows. 1976. Erythema chronicum migrans in the United States. *JAMA* **236**:859–860.

205. Masuzawa, T., N. Takada, M. Kudeken, T. Fukui, Y. Yano, F. Ishiguro, Y. Kawamura, Y. Imai, and T. Ezaki. 2001. *Borrelia sinica* sp. nov., a Lyme disease-related Borrelia species isolated in China. *Int. J. Syst. Evol. Microbiol.* **51**:1817–1824.

206. Matuschka, F. R., and A. Spielman. 1986. The emergence of Lyme disease in a changing environment in North America and central Europe. *Exp. Appl. Acarol.* **2**:337–353.

207. Mbow, M. L., N. Zeidner, R. D. J. Gilmore, M. Dolan, J. Piesman, and R. G. Titus. 2001. Major histocompatibility complex class II-independent generation of neutralizing antibodies against T-cell-dependent *Borrelia burgdorferi* antigens presented by dendritic cells: regulation of NK and γδ T cells. *Infect. Immun.* **69**:2407–2415.

208. McAlister, H. F., P. T. Klementowicz, C. Andrews, J. D. Fisher, M. Feld, and S. Furman. 1989. Lyme carditis: an important cause of reversible heart block. *Ann. Intern. Med.* **110**:339–345.

209. McDowell, J. V., J. Wolfgang, E. Tran, M. S. Metts, D. Hamilton, and R. T. Marconi. 2003. Comprehensive analysis of the factor H binding capabilities of borrelia species associated with Lyme disease: delineation of two distinct classes of factor H binding proteins. *Infect. Immun.* **71**:3597–3602.

210. McKisic, M. D., and S. W. Barthold. 2000. T-cell-independent responses to *Borrelia burgdorferi* are critical for protective immunity and resolution of Lyme disease. *Infect. Immun.* **68**:5190–5197.

211. Meltzer, M. I., D. T. Dennis, and K. A. Orloski. 1999. The cost effectiveness of vaccinating against Lyme disease. *Emerg. Infect. Dis.* **5**:321–328.

212. Meyer, A. L., C. Trollmo, F. Crawford, P. Marrack, A. C. Steere, B. T. Huber, J. Kappler, and D. A. Hafler. 2000. Direct enumeration of *Borrelia*-reactive CD4+ T cells ex vivo by using MHC class II tetramers. *Proc. Natl. Acad. Sci. USA* **97**:11433–11438.

213. Modolell, M., U. E. Schaible, M. Rittig, and M. M. Simon. 1994. Killing of *Borrelia burgdorferi* by macrophages is dependent on oxygen radicals and nitric oxide and can be enhanced by antibodies to outer surface proteins of the spirochete. *Immunol. Lett.* **40**:139–146.

214. Montgomery, R. R., S. E. Malawista, K. J. M. Feen, and L. K. Bockenstedt. 1996. Direct demonstration of antigenic substitution of *Borrelia burgdorferi* ex vivo: exploration of the paradox of the early immune response to outer surface proteins A and C in Lyme disease. *J. Exp. Med.* **183**:261–269.

215. Montgomery, R. R., M. H. Nathanson, and S. E. Malawista. 1993. The fate of *Borrelia burgdorferi*, the agent for Lyme disease, in mouse macrophages. Destruction, survival, recovery. *J. Immunol.* **150**:909–915.

216. Motaleb, M. A., L. Corum, J. L. Bono, A. F. Elias, P. Rosa, D. S. Samuels, and N. W. Charon. 2000. *Borrelia burgdorferi* periplasmic flagella have both skeletal and motility functions. *Proc. Natl. Acad. Sci. USA* **97**:10899–10904.

217. Mullegger, R. R., G. McHugh, R. Ruthazer, B. Binder, H. Kerl, and A. C. Steere. 2000. Differential expression of cytokine mRNA in skin specimens from patients with erythema migrans or acrodermatitis chronica atrophicans. *J. Investig. Dermatol.* **115**:1115–1123.

218. Nadelman, R. B., S. W. Luger, E. Frank, M. Wisniewski, J. J. Collins, and G. P. Wormser. 1992. Comparison of cefuroxime axetil and doxycycline in the treatment of early Lyme disease. *Ann. Intern. Med.* **117**:273–280.

219. Nadelman, R. B., J. Nowakowski, D. Fish, R. C. Falco, K. Freeman, D. McKenna, P. Welch, R. Marcus, M. E. Aguero-Rosenfeld, D. T. Dennis, and G. P. Wormser. 2001. Prophylaxis with single-dose doxycycline for the prevention of Lyme disease after an *Ixodes scapularis* tick bite. *N. Engl. J. Med.* **345**:79–84.

220. Nadelman, R. B., J. Nowakowski, G. Forseter, N. S. Goldberg, S. Bittker, D. Cooper, M. Aguero-Rosenfeld, and G. Wormser. 1996. The clinical spectrum of early Lyme borreliosis in patients with culture-confirmed erythema migrans. *Am. J. Med.* **100**:502–508.

221. Neubert, U., M. Schaller, E. Januschke, W. Stolz, and H. Schmieger. 1993. Bacteriophages induced by ciprofloxacin in a *Borrelia burgdorferi* skin isolate. *Zentralbl. Bakteriol.* **279**:307–315.

222. Nguyen, T. P., T. T. Lam, S. W. Barthold, S. R. Telford III, R. A. Flavell, and E. Fikrig. 1994. Partial destruction of *Borrelia burgdorferi* within ticks that engorged on OspE- or OspF-immunized mice. *Infect. Immun.* **62**:2079–2084.

223. Nocton, J. J., B. J. Bloom, B. J. Rutledge, D. H. Persing, E. L. Logigian, C. H. Schmid, and A. C. Steere. 1996. Detection of *Borrelia burgdorferi* DNA by polymerase chain reaction in cerebrospinal fluid in patients with Lyme neuroborreliosis. *J. Infect. Dis.* **174**:623–627.

224. Nocton, J. J., F. Dressler, B. J. Rutledge, P. N. Rys, D. H. Persing, and A. C. Steere. 1994. Detection of *Borrelia burgdorferi* DNA by polymerase chain reaction in synovial fluid in Lyme arthritis. *N. Engl. J. Med.* **330**:229–234.

225. Nowakowski, J., D. McKenna, R. B. Nadelman, D. Cooper, S. Bittker, D. Holmgren, C. Pavia, R. C. Johnson, and G. P. Wormser. 2000. Failure of treatment with cephalexin for Lyme disease. *Arch. Fam. Med.* **9**:563–567.

226. O'Connell, S., M. Granstrom, J. S. Gray, and G. Stanek. 1998. Epidemiology of European Lyme borreliosis. *Zentralbl. Bakteriol.* **287**:229–240.

227. Ohnishi, J., J. Piesman, and A. M. de Silva. 2001. Antigenic and genetic heterogeneity of *Borrelia burgdorferi* populations transmitted by ticks. *Proc. Natl. Acad. Sci. USA* **98**:670–675.

228. Oksi, J., J. Savolainen, J. Pene, J. Bousqet, P. Laippala, and M. K. Viljanen. 1996. Decreased interleukin-4 and increased gamma interferon production by peripheral blood mononuclear cells of patients with Lyme borreliosis. *Infect. Immun.* **64**:3620–3623.

229. Olsen, B., T. G. Jaenson, and S. Bergstrom. 1995. Prevalence of *Borrelia burgdorferi* sensu lato-infected ticks on migrating birds. *Appl. Environ. Microbiol.* **61**:3082–3087.

230. Oransky, S., B. Roseman, D. Fish, et al. 1989. Seizures temporarily associated with the use of DEET insect repellent—New York and Connecticut. *Morb. Mortal. Wkly. Rep.* **38**:678.

231. Orloski, K. A., E. B. Hayes, G. L. Campbell, and D. T. Dennis. 2000. Surveillance for Lyme disease—United States, 1992–1998. *Morb. Mortal. Wkly. Rep.* 49:1–11.

232. Oschmann, P., W. Dorndorf, C. Hornig, C. Schafer, H. J. Wellensiek, and K. W. Pflughaupt. 1998. Stages and syndromes of neuroborreliosis. *J. Neurol.* 245:262–272.

233. Pachner, A. R., and A. C. Steere. 1985. The triad of neurologic manifestations of Lyme disease: meningitis, cranial neuritis, and radiculoneuritis. *Neurology* 35:47–53.

234. Parveen, N., and J. M. Leong. 2000. Identification of a candidate glycosaminoglycan-binding adhesin of the Lyme disease spirochete *Borrelia burgdorferi*. *Mol. Microbiol.* 35:1220–1234.

235. Patel, R., K. L. Grogg, W. D. Edwards, A. J. Wright, and N. M. Schwenk. 2000. Death from inappropriate therapy for Lyme disease. *Clin. Infect. Dis.* 31:1107–1109.

236. Peltomaa, M., G. McHugh, and A. C. Steere. 2003. Persistence of antibody response to the VlsE sixth invariant region (IR$_6$) peptide of *Borrelia burgdorferi* after successful antibiotic treatment of Lyme disease. *J. Infect. Dis.* 187:1178–1186.

237. Peltomaa, M., I. Pyykko, I. Seppala, and M. Viljanen. 2002. Lyme borreliosis and facial paralysis—a prospective analysis of risk factors and outcome. *Am. J. Otolaryngol.* 23:125–132.

238. Persing, D. H., S. R. Telford III, P. N. Rys, D. E. Dodge, T. J. White, S. E. Malawista, and A. Spielman. 1990. Detection of *Borrelia burgdorferi* DNA in museum specimens of *Ixodes dammini* ticks. *Science* 249:1420–1423.

239. Pfister, H. W., V. Preac-Mursic, B. Wilske, and K. M. Einhaupl. 1989. Cefotaxime vs penicillin G for acute neurologic manifestations of Lyme borreliosis: a prospective randomized study. *Arch. Neurol.* 46:1190–1194.

240. Pfister, H. W., V. Preac-Mursic, B. Wilske, E. Schielke, F. Sorgel, and K. M. Einhaupl. 1991. Randomized comparison of ceftriaxone and cefotaxime in Lyme neuroborreliosis. *J. Infect. Dis.* 163:311–318.

241. Piesman, J., T. N. Mather, R. J. Sinsky, and A. Spielman. 1987. Duration of tick attachment and *Borrelia burgdorferi* transmission. *J. Clin. Microbiol.* 25:557–558.

242. Posey, J. E., and F. C. Gherardini. 2000. Lack of a role for iron in the Lyme disease pathogen. *Science* 288:1651–1653.

243. Postic, D., N. M. Ras, R. S. Lane, M. Hendson, and G. Baranton. 1998. Expanded diversity among California borrelia isolates and description of *Borrelia bissettii* sp. nov. (formerly *Borrelia* group DN127). *J. Clin. Microbiol.* 36:3497–3504.

244. Potter, M. R., S. R. Rittling, D. T. Denhardt, R. J. Roper, J. H. Weis, C. Teuscher, and J. J. Weis. 2002. Role of osteopontin in murine Lyme arthritis and host defense against *Borrelia burgdorferi*. *Infect. Immun.* 70:1372–1381.

245. Preac-Mursic, V., B. Wilske, and G. Schierz. 1986. European *Borrelia burgdorferi* isolated from humans and ticks: culture conditions and antibiotic sensitivities. *Zentralbl. Bakteriol. Mikrobiol. Hyg. A* 263:112–118.

246. Preac-Mursic, V., B. Wilske, G. Schierz, H. W. Pfister, and K. Einhaupl. 1984. Repeated isolation of spirochetes from the cerebrospinal fluid of a patient with meningoradiculitis Bannwarth. *Eur. J. Clin. Microbiol. Infect. Dis.* 3:564–565.

247. Preac-Mursic, V., B. Wilske, G. Schierz, E. Suss, and B. Gross. 1989. Comparative antimicrobial activity of the new macrolides against *Borrelia burgdorferi*. *Eur. J. Clin. Microbiol. Infect. Dis.* 8:651–653.

248. Priem, S., G. R. Burmester, T. Kamradt, K. Wolbart, M. G. Rittig, and A. Krause. 1998. Detection of *Borrelia burgdorferi* by polymerase chain reaction in synovial membrane, but not in synovial fluid from patients with persisting Lyme arthritis after antibiotic therapy. *Ann. Rheum. Dis.* 57:118–121.

249. Probert, W. S., K. M. Allsup, and R. B. LeFebvre. 1995. Identification and characterization of a surface-exposed, 66-kilodalton protein from *Borrelia burgdorferi*. *Infect. Immun.* 63:1933–1939.

250. Probert, W. S., and B. J. B. Johnson. 1998. Identification of a 47 kDa fibronectin-binding protein expressed by *Borrelia burgdorferi* isolate B31. *Mol. Microbiol.* 30:1003–1015.

251. Probert, W. S., J. H. Kim, M. Höök, and B. J. B. Johnson. 2001. Mapping the ligand-binding region of *Borrelia burgdorferi* fibronectin-binding protein BBK32. *Infect. Immun.* 69:4129–4133.

252. Purser, J. E., M. B. Lawrenz, M. J. Caimano, J. K. Howell, J. D. Radolf, and S. J. Norris. 2003. A plasmid-encoded nicotinamidase (PncA) is essential for infectivity of *Borrelia burgdorferi* in a mammalian host. *Mol. Microbiol.* 48:753–764.

253. Purser, J. E., and S. J. Norris. 2000. Correlation between plasmid content and infectivity in *Borrelia burgdorferi*. *Proc. Natl. Acad. Sci. USA* 97:13865–13870.

254. Radolf, J. D. 1994. Role of outer membrane architecture in immune evasion by *Treponema pallidum* and *Borrelia burgdorferi*. *Trends Microbiol.* 2:307–311.

255. Radolf, J. D., L. L. Arndt, D. R. Akins, L. L. Curetty, M. E. Levi, Y. Shen, L. S. Davis, and M. V. Norgard. 1995. *Treponema pallidum* and *Borrelia burgdorferi* lipoproteins and synthetic lipopeptides activate monocytes/macrophages. *J. Immunol.* 154:2866–2877.

256. Reid, M. C., R. T. Schoen, J. Evans, J. C. Rosenberg, and R. I. Horwitz. 1998. The consequences of overdiagnosis and overtreatment of Lyme disease: an observational study. *Ann. Intern. Med.* 128:354–362.

257. Reik, L., A. C. Steere, N. H. Bartenhagen, R. E. Shope, and S. E. Malawista. 1979. Neurologic abnormalities of Lyme disease. *Medicine (Baltimore)* 58:281–294.

258. Rittig, M. G., A. Krause, T. Haupl, U. E. Schaible, M. Modolell, M. D. Kramer, E. Lutjen-Drecoll, M. M. Simon, and G. R. Burmester. 1992. Coiling phagocytosis is the preferential phagocytic mechanism for *Borrelia burgdorferi*. *Infect. Immun.* 60:4205–4212.

259. Roberts, E. D., R. P. J. Bohm, R. C. J. Lowrie, L. Katona, J. Piesman, and M. T. Philipp. 1998. Pathogenesis of Lyme neuroborreliosis in the rhesus monkey: the early disseminated and chronic phases of disease in the peripheral nervous system. *J. Infect. Dis.* 178:722–732.

260. Robertson, J., E. Guy, N. Andrews, B. Wilske, P. Anda, M. Granstrom, U. Hauser, Y. Moosmann, V. Sambri, J. Schellekens, G. Stanek, and J. Gray. 2000. A European multicenter study of immunoblotting in serodiagnosis of Lyme borreliosis. *J. Clin. Microbiol.* 38:2097–2102.

261. Rothermel, H., T. R. Hedges III, and A. C. Steere. 2001. Optic neuropathy in children with Lyme disease. *Pediatrics* 108:477–481.

262. Rousselle, J. C., S. M. Callister, R. F. Schell, S. D. Lovrich, D. A. Jobe, J. A. Marks, and C. A. Wieneke. 1998. Borreliacidal antibody production against outer surface protein C of *Borrelia burgdorferi*. *J. Infect. Dis.* 178:733–741.

263. Ruderman, E. M., J. S. Kerr, S. R. Telford III, A. Spielman, L. H. Glimcher, and E. M. Gravallese. 1995. Early murine Lyme carditis has a macrophage predominance and is independent of major histocompatibility complex class II-CD4+ T cell interactions. *J. Infect. Dis.* 171:362–370.

264. Salazar, J. C., C. D. Pope, T. J. Sellati, H. M. J. Feder, T. G. Kiely, K. R. Dardick, R. L. Buckman, M. W. Moore, M. J. Caimano, J. G. Pope, P. J. Krause, and J. D. Radolf. 2003. Coevolution of markers of innate and adaptive immunity in skin and peripheral blood of patients with erythema migrans. *J. Immunol.* 171:2660–2670.

265. Samuels, D. S. 1995. Electrotransformation of the spirochete *Borrelia burgdorferi. Methods Mol. Biol.* **47**:253–259.

266. Sartakova, M., E. Dobrikova, and F. C. Cabello. 2000. Development of an extrachromosomal cloning vector system for use in *Borrelia burgdorferi. Proc. Natl. Acad. Sci. USA* **97**:4850–4855.

267. Sartakova, M. L., E. Y. Dobrikova, M. A. Motaleb, H. P. Godfrey, N. W. Charon, and F. C. Cabello. 2001. Complementation of a nonmotile flaB mutant of *Borrelia burgdorferi* by chromosomal integration of a plasmid containing a wild-type flaB allele. *J. Bacteriol.* **183**:6558–6564.

268. Schaible, U. E., S. Gay, C. Museteanu, M. D. Kramer, G. Zimmer, K. Eichmann, U. Museteanu, and M. M. Simon. 1990. Lyme borreliosis in the severe combined immunodeficiency (SCID) mouse manifests predominantly in the joints, heart, and liver. *Am. J. Pathol.* **137**:811–820.

269. Schaible, U. E., M. D. Kramer, K. Eichmann, M. Modolell, C. Museteanu, and M. M. Simon. 1990. Monoclonal antibodies specific for the outer surface protein A (OspA) of *Borrelia burgdorferi* prevent Lyme borreliosis in severe combined immunodeficiency (scid) mice. *Proc. Natl. Acad. Sci. USA* **87**:3768–3772.

270. Schlesinger, P. A., P. H. Duray, B. A. Burke, A. C. Steere, and M. T. Stillman. 1985. Maternal-fetal transmission of the Lyme disease spirochete, *Borrelia burgdorferi. Ann. Intern. Med.* **103**:67–69.

271. Schneider, B. S., N. S. Zeidner, T. R. Burkot, G. O. Maupin, and J. Piesman. 2000. *Borrelia* isolates in northern Colorado identifies *Borrelia bissettii. J. Clin. Microbiol.* **38**:3103–3105.

272. Schoen, R. T., J. M. Aversa, D. W. Rahn, and A. C. Steere. 1991. Treatment of refractory chronic Lyme arthritis with arthroscopic synovectomy. *Arthritis Rheum.* **34**:1056–1060.

273. Schreck, C. E., E. L. Snoddy, and A. Spielman. 1986. Pressurized sprays of permethrin or DEET on military clothing for personal protection against *Ixodes dammini* (Acari: *Ixodidae*). *J. Med. Entomol.* **23**:396–399.

274. Schulze, T. L., G. S. Bowen, E. M. Bosler, M. F. Lakat, W. E. Parkin, R. Altman, B. G. Ormiston, and J. K. Shisler. 1984. *Amblyomma americanum*: a potential vector of Lyme disease in New Jersey. *Science* **224**:601–603.

275. Schwan, T. G., and J. Piesman. 2002. Vector interactions and molecular adaptations of Lyme disease and relapsing fever spirochetes associated with transmission by ticks. *Emerg. Infect. Dis.* **8**:115–121.

276. Schwan, T. G., J. Piesman, W. T. Golde, M. C. Dolan, and P. A. Rosa. 1995. Induction of an outer surface protein on *Borrelia burgdorferi* during tick feeding. *Proc. Natl. Acad. Sci. USA* **92**:2909–2913.

277. Scrimenti, R. J. 1970. Erythema chronicum migrans. *Arch. Derm.* **102**:104–105.

278. Seinost, G., D. E. Dykhuizen, R. J. Dattwyler, W. T. Golde, J. J. Dunn, I. N. Wang, G. P. Wormser, M. E. Schriefer, and B. J. Luft. 1999. Four clones of *Borrelia burgdorferi* sensu stricto cause invasive infection in humans. *Infect. Immun.* **67**:3518–3524.

279. Seltzer, E. G., M. A. Gerber, M. L. Cartter, K. Freudigman, and E. D. Shapiro. 2000. Long-term outcomes of persons with Lyme disease. *JAMA* **283**:609–616.

280. Shadick, N. A., M. H. Liang, C. B. Phillips, K. Fossel, and K. M. Kuntz. 2001. The cost-effectiveness of vaccination against Lyme disease. *Arch. Intern. Med.* **161**:554–561.

281. Shadick, N. A., C. B. Phillips, O. Sangha, E. L. Logigian, R. F. Kaplan, E. A. Wright, A. H. Fossel, K. Fossel, V. Berardi, R. A. Lew, and M. H. Liang. 1999. Musculoskeletal and neurologic outcomes in patients with previously treated Lyme disease. *Ann. Intern. Med.* **131**:919–926.

282. Shapiro, E. D., M. A. Gerber, N. B. Holabird, A. T. Berg, H. M. J. Feder, G. L. Bell, P. N. Rys, and D. H. Persing. 1992. A controlled trial of antimicrobial prophylaxis for Lyme disease after deer-tick bites. *N. Engl. J. Med.* **327**:1769–1773.

283. Sigal, L. H. 1990. Summary of the first 100 patients seen at a Lyme disease referral center. *Am. J. Med.* **88**:577–581.

284. Sigal, L. H., and S. J. Patella. 1992. Lyme arthritis as the incorrect diagnosis in pediatric and adolescent fibromyalgia. *Pediatrics* **90**:523–528.

285. Smith, R. P., R. T. Schoen, D. W. Rahn, V. K. Sikand, J. Nowakowski, D. L. Parenti, M. S. Holman, D. H. Persing, and A. C. Steere. 2002. Clinical characteristics and treatment outcome of early Lyme disease in patients with microbiologically confirmed erythema migrans. *Ann. Intern. Med.* **136**:421–428.

286. Sonnesyn, S. W., S. C. Diehl, R. C. Johnson, S. H. Kubo, and J. L. Goodman. 1995. A prospective study of the seroprevalence of *Borrelia burgdorferi* infection in patients with severe heart failure. *Am. J. Cardiol.* **76**:97–100.

287. Spielman, A. 1994. The emergence of Lyme disease and human babesiosis in a changing environment. *Ann. N. Y. Acad. Sci.* **740**:146–156.

288. Stanek, G., J. Klein, R. Bittner, and D. Glogar. 1990. Isolation of *Borrelia burgdorferi* from the myocardium of a patient with longstanding cardiomyopathy. *N. Engl. J. Med.* **322**:249–252.

289. Steere, A. C. 2003. Duration of antibiotic therapy for Lyme disease. *Ann. Intern. Med.* **138**:761–762.

290. Steere, A. C. 1989. Lyme disease. *N. Engl. J. Med.* **321**:586–596.

291. Steere, A. C. 2001. Lyme disease. *N. Engl. J. Med.* **345**:115–125.

292. Steere, A. C., J. Coburn, and L. Glickstein 2004. The emergence of Lyme disease. *J. Clin. Investig.* **113**:1093–1101.

293. Steere, A. C., N. H. Bartenhagen, J. E. Craft, G. J. Hutchinson, J. H. Newman, D. W. Rahn, L. H. Sigal, P. H. Spieler, K. S. Stenn, and S. E. Malawista. 1983. The early clinical manifestations of Lyme disease. *Ann. Intern. Med.* **99**:76–82.

294. Steere, A. C., W. P. Batsford, M. Weinberg, J. Alexander, H. J. Berger, S. Wolfson, and S. E. Malawista. 1980. Lyme carditis: cardiac abnormalities of Lyme disease. *Ann. Intern. Med.* **93**:8–16.

295. Steere, A. C., V. P. Berardi, K. E. Weeks, E. L. Logigian, and R. Ackermann. 1990. Evaluation of the intrathecal antibody response to *Borrelia burgdorferi* as a diagnostic test for Lyme neuroborreliosis. *J. Infect. Dis.* **161**:1203–1209.

296. Steere, A. C., T. F. Broderick, and S. E. Malawista. 1978. Erythema chronicum migrans and Lyme arthritis: epidemiologic evidence for a tick vector. *Am. J. Epidemiol.* **108**:312–321.

297. Steere, A. C., A. Dhar, J. Hernandez, P. A. Fischer, V. K. Sikand, R. T. Schoen, J. Nowakowski, G. McHugh, and D. H. Persing. 2003. Systemic symptoms without erythema migrans as the presenting picture of early Lyme disease. *Am. J. Med.* **114**:58–62.

298. Steere, A. C., P. H. Duray, and E. C. Butcher. 1988. Spirochetal antigens and lymphoid cell surface markers in Lyme synovitis: comparison with rheumatoid synovium and tonsillar lymphoid tissue. *Arthritis Rheum.* **31**:487–495.

299. Steere, A. C., P. H. Duray, D. J. H. Kauffmann, and G. P. Wormser. 1985. Unilateral blindness caused by infection with the Lyme disease spirochete, *Borrelia burgdorferi. Ann. Intern. Med.* **103**:382–384.

300. Steere, A. C., B. Falk, E. E. Drouin, L. A. Baxter-Lowe, J. Hammer, and G. T. Nepom. 2003. Binding of outer surface protein A and human lymphocyte function-associated

antigen 1 peptides to HLA-DR molecules associated with antibiotic treatment-resistant Lyme arthritis. *Arthritis Rheum.* 48:534–540.

301. Steere, A. C., and L. Glickstein. 2004. Elucidation of Lyme arthritis. *Nature Rev. Immunol.* 4:143–152.

302. Steere, A. C., R. L. Grodzicki, A. N. Kornblatt, J. E. Craft, A. G. Barbour, W. Burgdorfer, G. P. Schmid, E. Johnson, and S. E. Malawista. 1983. The spirochetal etiology of Lyme disease. *N. Engl. J. Med.* 308:733–740.

303. Steere, A. C., D. Gross, A. L. Meyer, and B. T. Huber. 2001. Autoimmune mechanisms in antibiotic treatment-resistant Lyme arthritis. *J. Autoimmun.* 16:263–268.

304. Steere, A. C., J. A. Hardin, S. Ruddy, J. G. Mummaw, and S. E. Malawista. 1979. Lyme arthritis: correlation of serum and cryoglobulin IgM with activity, and serum IgG with remission. *Arthritis Rheum.* 22:471–483.

305. Steere, A. C., G. J. Hutchinson, D. W. Rahn, L. H. Sigal, J. E. Craft, E. T. DeSanna, and S. E. Malawista. 1983. Treatment of the early manifestations of Lyme disease. *Ann. Intern. Med.* 99:22–26.

306. Steere, A. C., R. E. Levin, P. J. Molloy, R. A. Kalish, J. H. Abraham III, N. Y. Liu, and C. H. Schmid. 1994. Treatment of Lyme arthritis. *Arthritis Rheum.* 37:878–888.

307. Steere, A. C., and S. E. Malawista. 1979. Cases of Lyme disease in the United States: locations correlated with distribution of *Ixodes dammini*. *Ann. Intern. Med.* 91:730–733.

308. Steere, A. C., S. E. Malawista, J. A. Hardin, S. Ruddy, W. Askenase, and W. A. Andiman. 1977. Erythema chronicum migrans and Lyme arthritis: the enlarging clinical spectrum. *Ann. Intern. Med.* 86:685–698.

309. Steere, A. C., S. E. Malawista, D. R. Snydman, R. E. Shope, W. A. Andiman, M. R. Ross, and F. M. Steele. 1977. Lyme arthritis: an epidemic of oligoarticular arthritis in children and adults in three Connecticut communities. *Arthritis Rheum.* 20:7–17.

310. Steere, A. C., G. McHugh, C. Suarez, J. Hoitt, N. Damle, and V. J. Sikand. 2003. Prospective study of coinfection in patients with erythema migrans. *Clin. Infect. Dis.* 36:1078–1081.

311. Steere, A. C., R. T. Schoen, and E. Taylor. 1987. The clinical evolution of Lyme arthritis. *Ann. Intern. Med.* 107:725–731.

312. Steere, A. C., V. J. Sikand, R. T. Schoen, and J. Nowakowski. 2003. Asymptomatic infection with *Borrelia burgdorferi*. *Clin. Infect. Dis.* 37:528–532.

313. Steere, A. C., and V. K. Sikand. 2003. The presenting manifestations of Lyme disease and the outcomes of treatment. *N. Engl. J. Med.* 348:2472–2474.

314. Steere, A. C., V. K. Sikand, F. Meurice, D. L. Parenti, E. Fikrig, R. T. Schoen, J. Nowakowski, C. H. Schmid, S. Laukamp, C. Buscarino, and D. S. Krause. 1998. Vaccination against Lyme disease with recombinant *Borrelia burgdorferi* outer-surface lipoprotein A with adjuvant. *N. Engl. J. Med.* 339:209–215.

315. Steere, A. C., E. Taylor, G. L. McHugh, and E. L. Logigian. 1993. The overdiagnosis of Lyme disease. *JAMA* 269:1812–1816.

316. Steere, A. C., E. Taylor, M. L. Wilson, J. F. Levine, and A. Spielman. 1986. A longitudinal assessment of the clinical and epidemiological features of Lyme disease in a defined population. *J. Infect. Dis.* 154:295–300.

317. Stevenson, B., N. El-Hage, M. A. Hines, J. C. Miller, and K. Babb. 2002. Differential binding of host complement inhibitor factor H by *Borrelia burgdorferi* Erp surface proteins: a possible mechanism underlying the expansive host range of Lyme disease spirochetes. *Infect. Immun.* 70:491–497.

318. Stewart, P. E., R. Thalken, J. L. Bono, and P. Rosa. 2001. Isolation of a circular plasmid region sufficient for auton-omous replication and transformation of infectious *Borrelia burgdorferi*. *Mol. Microbiol.* 39:714–721.

319. Strle, F., R. B. Nadelman, J. Cimperman, J. Nowakowski, R. N. Picken, I. Schwartz, V. Maraspin, M. E. Aguero-Rosenfeld, S. Varde, S. Lotric-Furlan, and G. P. Wormser. 1999. Comparison of culture-confirmed erythema migrans caused by *Borrelia burgdorferi* sensu stricto in New York State and by *Borrelia afzelii* in Slovenia. *Ann. Intern. Med.* 130:32–36.

320. Strle, F., D. Pleterski-Rigler, G. Stanek, A. Pejovnik-Pustinek, E. Ruzic, and J. Cimperman. 1992. Solitary borrelial lymphocytoma: report of 36 cases. *Infection* 20:201–206.

321. Strobino, B., S. Abid, and M. Gewitz. 1999. Maternal Lyme disease and congenital heart disease: a case-control study in an endemic area. *Am. J. Obstet. Gynecol.* 180:711–716.

322. Szer, I. S., E. Taylor, and A. C. Steere. 1991. The long-term course of children with Lyme arthritis. *N. Engl. J. Med.* 325:159–163.

323. Talkington, J., and S. P. Nickell. 2001. Role of Fc gamma receptors in triggering host cell activation and cytokine release by *Borrelia burgdorferi*. *Infect. Immun.* 69:413–419.

324. Trollmo, C., A. L. Meyer, A. C. Steere, D. A. Hafler, and B. T. Huber. 2001. Molecular mimicry in Lyme arthritis demonstrated at the single cell level: LFA-1αL is a partial agonist for outer surface protein A-reactive T cells. *J. Immunol.* 166:5286–5291.

325. Vallat, J. M., M. J. Leboutet, A. Loubet, P. Dumas, J. Hugon, and N. Corvisier. 1984. Tick bite neuropathy: an analysis of nerve biopsies from seven cases. *Neurology* 34:180.

326. Van Hoecke, C., M. Comberbach, D. De Grave, P. Desmons, D. Fu, P. Hauser, E. Lebacq, Y. Lobet, and P. Voet. 1996. Evaluation of the safety, reactogenicity and immunogenicity of three recombinant outer surface protein (OspA) lyme vaccines in healthy adults. *Vaccine* 14:1620–1626.

327. Vaz, A., L. Glickstein, J. A. Field, G. McHugh, V. K. Sikand, N. Damle, and A. C. Steere. 2001. Cellular and humoral immune responses to *Borrelia burgdorferi* antigens in patients with culture-positive early Lyme disease. *Infect. Immun.* 69:7437–7444.

328. Wallis, R. C., S. E. Brown, K. O. Kloter, and A. J. J. Main. 1978. Erythema chronicum migrans and Lyme arthritis: field study of ticks. *Am. J. Epidemiol.* 108:322–327.

329. Wang, G., A. P. van Dam, A. Le Fleche, D. Postic, O. Peter, G. Baranton, R. de Boer, L. Spanjaard, and J. Dankert. 1997. Genetic and phenotypic analysis of *Borrelia valaisiana* sp. nov. (*Borrelia* genomic groups VS116 and M19). *Int. J. Syst. Bacteriol.* 47:926–932.

330. Weber, K., H. J. Bratzke, U. Neubert, B. Wilske, and P. H. Duray. 1988. *Borrelia burgdorferi* in a newborn despite oral penicillin for Lyme borreliosis during pregnancy. *Pediatr. Infect. Dis.* 7:286–289.

331. Weber, K., G. Schierz, B. Wilske, U. Neubert, H. E. Krampitz, A. G. Barbour, and W. Burgdorfer. 1986. Reinfection in erythema migrans disease. *Infection* 14:32–35.

332. Wheeler, C. M., J. C. Garcia Monco, J. L. Benach, M. G. Golightly, G. S. Habicht, and A. C. Steere. 1993. Nonprotein antigens of *Borrelia burgdorferi*. *J. Infect. Dis.* 167:665–674.

333. Williams, C. L., B. Strobino, A. Weinstein, P. Spierling, and F. Medici. 1995. Maternal Lyme disease and congenital malformations: a cord blood serosurvey in endemic and control areas. *Paediatr. Perinat. Epidemiol.* 9:320–330.

334. Wilske, B., G. Schierz, V. Preac-Mursic, K. Von Busch, R. Kuhbeck, H. W. Pfister, and K. Einhaupl. 1986. Intrathecal production of specific antibodies against *Borrelia burgdorferi* in patients with lymphocytic meningoradiculitis (Bannwarth's syndrome). *J. Infect. Dis.* 153:304–314.

335. Wilson, M. L., G. H. Adler, and A. Spielman. 1985. Correlation between abundance of deer and that of the deer tick, *Ixodes dammini* (Acari: *Ixodidae*). *Ann. Entomol. Soc. Am.* **78:**172–176.

336. Wilson, M. L., and A. Spielman. 1985. Seasonal activity of immature *Ixodes dammini* (Acari: *Ixodidae*). *J. Med. Entomol.* **22:**408–414.

337. Wilson, M. L., S. R. Telford III, J. Piesman, and A. Spielman. 1988. Reduced abundance of immature *Ixodes dammini* (Acari: *Ixodidae*) following elimination of deer. *J. Med. Entomol.* **25:**224–228.

338. Wooten, R. M., Y. Ma, R. A. Yoder, J. P. Brown, J. H. Weis, J. F. Zachary, C. J. Kirschning, and J. J. Weis. 2002. Toll-like receptor 2 is required for innate, but not acquired, host defense to *Borrelia burgdorferi*. *J. Immunol.* **168:**348–355.

339. Wormser, G. P., S. Bittker, D. Cooper, J. Nowakowski, R. B. Nadelman, and C. Pavia. 2000. Comparison of the yields of blood cultures using serum or plasma from patients with early Lyme disease. *J. Clin. Microbiol.* **38:**1648–1650.

340. Wormser, G. P., H. W. Horowitz, J. Nowakowski, D. McKenna, J. S. Dumler, S. Varde, I. Schwartz, C. Carbonaro, and M. Aguero-Rosenfeld. 1997. Positive Lyme disease serology in patients with clinical and laboratory evidence of human granulocytic ehrlichiosis. *Am. J. Clin. Pathol.* **107:**142–147.

341. Wormser, G. P., R. B. Nadelman, R. J. Dattwyler, D. T. Dennis, E. D. Shapiro, A. C. Steere, T. J. Rush, D. W. Rahn, P. K. Coyle, D. H. Persing, D. Fish, and B. J. Luft. 2000. Practice guidelines for the treatment of Lyme disease. *Clin. Infect. Dis.* **31**(Suppl. 1):S1–S14.

342. Wormser, G. P., R. Ramanathan, J. Nowakowski, D. McKenna, D. Holmgren, P. Visintainer, R. Dornbush, B. Singh, and R. B. Nadelman. 2003. Duration of antibiotic therapy for early Lyme disease. A randomized, double-blind, placebo-controlled trial. *Ann. Intern. Med.* **138:**697–704.

343. Xu, G., Q. Q. Fang, J. E. Keirans, and L. A. Durden. 2003. Molecular phylogenetic analyses indicate that the *Ixodes ricinus* complex is a paraphyletic group. *J. Parasitol.* **89:**452–457.

344. Yang, X. F., S. M. Alani, and M. V. Norgard. 2003. The response regulator Rrp2 is essential for the expression of major membrane lipoproteins in *Borrelia burgdorferi*. *Proc. Natl. Acad. Sci. USA* **100:**11001–11006.

345. Yoshinari, N. H., B. N. Reinhardt, and A. C. Steere. 1991. T cell responses to polypeptide fractions of *Borrelia burgdorferi* in patients with Lyme arthritis. *Arthritis Rheum.* **34:**707–713.

346. Zeider, N., M. L. Mbow, M. Dolan, R. Massung, E. Baca, and J. Piesman. 1997. Effects of *Ixodes scapularis* and *Borrelia burgdorferi* on modulation of the host immune response: induction of a TH2 cytokine response in Lyme disease-susceptible (C3H/HeJ) mice but not in disease-resistant (BALB/c) mice. *Infect. Immun.* **65:**3100–3106.

347. Zhang, J. R., J. M. Hardham, A. G. Barbour, and S. J. Norris. 1997. Antigenic variation in Lyme disease borreliae by promiscuous recombination of VMP-like sequence cassettes. *Cell* **89:**275–285.

348. Zhang, J.-R., and S. J. Norris. 1998. Genetic variation of the *Borrelia burgdorferi* gene vlsE involves cassette-specific, segmental gene conversion. *Infect. Immun.* **66:**3698–3704.

Tick-Borne Diseases of Humans
Edited by Jesse L. Goodman et al.
© 2005 ASM Press, Washington, D.C.

Chapter 12

Tularemia

EDWARD B. HAYES

INTRODUCTION

Tularemia is a disease caused by infection with the bacterium *Francisella tularensis*. The disease is manifested by a broad range of signs and symptoms that include one or more of the following: an ulcer at the initial site of infection, regional lymphadenopathy, fever, chills, headache, malaise, sore throat, cough, abdominal pain, vomiting, diarrhea, and, in severe forms, dyspnea and septic shock (13). Primary or secondary pneumonia may occur following inhalation of *F. tularensis* or after dissemination to the lung from other infected sites, respectively. Cases of probable tularemia were described in both Japan and Norway in the 19th century, but the causative agent was not identified until 1911 when McCoy and Chapin isolated a bacterium, which they named *Bacterium tularense*, from squirrels with a plague-like illness in Tulare County, California. The first link of this agent to human disease came in 1914, when Wherry and Lamb reported the isolation of *B. tularense* from scrapings of a conjunctival ulcer of an Ohio meat cutter (73). Several years later, Francis of the U.S. Public Health Service isolated the organism from blood of patients with an ulcero-glandular illness following deerfly bites in Utah; he named the illness tularemia (25). Shortly thereafter, a Japanese physician, Ohara, described a febrile illness occurring in persons after skinning rabbits and subsequently produced the disease in his wife by rubbing infected rabbit hearts on her skin. Francis later showed that Ohara's disease was tularemia. Francis continued to make major contributions to the understanding of tularemia and the etiologic agent was renamed *Francisella tularensis* in his honor in 1959.

The role of ticks in transmitting tularemia was described by Parker and colleagues in 1924 (56) and subsequently by many other investigators (7, 8, 29, 34, 36, 51, 57, 60, 65, 72). Soviet scientists investigated the epidemiology of tularemia in rural agricul-tural areas, described transmission of the bacteria through contaminated water and through contact with aquatic rodents, and developed a live attenuated vaccine (16, 45, 58). Attenuated strains of *F. tularensis* were transferred to the United States in 1956 and used to produce a live vaccine for use in this country (67). Virulent strains of *F. tularensis* were studied by Japan, the former Soviet Union, and the United States for potential use as biological weapons, and prophylaxis and treatment of airborne transmission of the bacteria were studied directly through experiments with human volunteers (17, 61, 63). In recent years, modern molecular biological techniques have been applied to develop improved diagnostic tests and to better describe the genetic, antigenic, and pathogenic properties of *F. tularensis* (11, 19, 30), and novel mechanisms of transmission have been described (3, 23). *F. tularensis* is a designated category A select agent with potential for misuse as a weapon of terrorism (17).

ETIOLOGIC AGENT AND BIOLOGY

F. tularensis is a pleomorphic, non-spore-forming, nonmotile coccobacillus that can be easily aerosolized in the laboratory and therefore represents a high risk of laboratory-acquired infection (6, 11). Although it is gram negative, its small size (0.2×0.2 to 0.2×0.7 μm) and poor staining qualities make it difficult to see on Gram stain. Most strains of *F. tularensis* require cysteine or cystine in the growth medium for optimal growth at 35 to 37°C and may not grow at all on common growth media that lack these or similar sulfhydryl compounds. The bacterium will grow on Thayer-Martin agar, chocolate agar, buffered chocolate yeast extract agar, cysteine heart agar supplemented with chocolatized sheep blood, thioglycolate broth, and tryptic soy or Mueller-Hinton medium when supplemented with IsoVitaleX, with prolonged (48-h) aerobic incubation (11). Competing bacteria

Edward B. Hayes • Division of Vector-Borne Infectious Diseases, National Center for Infectious Diseases, Centers for Disease Control and Prevention, P.O. Box 2087, Fort Collins, CO 80522.

from clinical specimens can be suppressed by incorporating penicillin, polymyxin B sulfate, or cycloheximide into the medium. In specialized reference laboratories, the organism can be cultured by inoculation into live laboratory animals. Bacteria in the genus *Francisella* are weakly catalase positive and have a unique fatty acid content (11).

There are four subspecies of *F. tularensis* (11, 19). The most common pathogens are *Francisella tularensis* subsp. *tularensis*, or type A, which ferments glycerol and contains citrulline ureidase, and *Francisella tularensis* subsp. *holoarctica*, or type B, which neither ferments glycerol nor contains citrulline ureidase. These two subspecies can also be distinguished by their 16S rRNA genetic sequences. Type A is more virulent in rabbits and is believed to cause a more severe disease in humans than type B does, but the denominators to accurately determine rates of severe and milder infections by infecting type have not been available (51). The other two subspecies are *Francisella tularensis* subsp. *mediasiatica*, which is found in Central Asia but is not known to cause human illness, and *F. tularensis* subsp. *novicida*, which, although it is genetically more similar to type A than type B, is believed to be of low virulence and has been isolated from a few patients in North America with illnesses compatible with tularemia (11, 16, 19). Projects are underway to sequence the genomes of the virulent Schu S4 and the attenuated live vaccine strain (19). Preliminary results of sequencing indicate a small total genome size of <2 Mbp and the presence of two distinct cryptic plasmids.

A distinct pathogenic *Francisella* species, *Francisella philomiragia*, differs biochemically from *F. tularensis* and can be distinguished by genetic typing (19). While *F. tularensis* is oxidase negative, *F. philomiragia* is oxidase positive by Kovac's test (11). It has been isolated from a total of 14 patients in North America and 1 in Switzerland, most of whom had immunodeficiency states such as chronic granulomatous disease or tularemia-like illness following near-drowning in salt water (11, 16, 19).

F. tularensis is an intracellular pathogen. It has a lipopolysaccharide capsule and outer membrane proteins that elicit humoral and cellular immune responses, but it is not known to produce potent toxins (13, 67). The organism survives in macrophages and appears to synthesize chaperone proteins in response to intracellular stress (21, 28). Serum antibodies recognize carbohydrate antigens of the organism's capsule, whereas cellular immune responses appear to be directed against membrane proteins located beneath the capsule (67). *F. tularensis* produces β-lactamase and can survive freezing, but the bacterium is sensitive to water chlorination and heat and can be killed by cooking at 56°C for at least 10 min (13, 16). Within the host, the bacterium appears to be an obligate intracellular parasite (67). It has been suggested that the organism's virulence may be enhanced by parasitizing amoebae, and in vitro studies of the interactions between *F. tularensis* and amoebae indicate that protozoa might be an important environmental reservoir for *F. tularensis* (1, 4).

ECOLOGY

F. tularensis is found in nature from 20° north of the equator to the Arctic Circle (38). Infection has been reported in over 100 species of wild mammals and other vertebrates, including domestic mammals (cats and sheep), birds (grouse, pheasants, quail, and mallards), reptiles, amphibians, and fish. However, the animals most important in maintaining enzootic cycles and transmission to humans are rodents (voles, beavers, muskrats, and mice) and lagomorphs (hares and rabbits) (13, 16, 38). Different rodents and lagomorphs may vary in their resistance to tularemia. Cottontail rabbits (*Sylvilagus* species) are highly susceptible to and usually killed by infection (16). Hornick states that the snowshoe hare, *Lepus americanus*, is resistant and relatively unimportant as a source of human infection (39); however, Hopla and Hopla cite this hare as being a highly important source but state that the Old World rabbit, *Oryctolagus cuniculus*, is resistant and not an important source of infection for people (38). The prevalence of infection in any given species and the importance of that species as an infection source may vary, depending on geographic location and local ecological factors. Arthropods, including hard ticks, tabanid flies, mosquitoes, and possibly fleas, are considered important vectors of infection among vertebrates (37, 38). Animal hosts are thought to acquire infection by various other modes, including ingestion of infected tissues, infective bites and scratches, and ingestion or direct inoculation of con-taminated environmental sources such as vegetation, water, or soil.

The Role of Ticks in Transmission of *F. tularensis*

Parker first identified *F. tularensis* within ticks and showed that *Dermacentor andersoni* could transmit infection to vertebrates (56). Ticks are biological vectors and maintenance hosts of *F. tularensis*, and the bacterium may be inoculated into mammals from tick saliva or feces (38). Infection is commonly transmitted transstadially in ticks, but transovarial transmission is rare and probably unimportant in maintaining natural cycles of infection (36, 38). In the United States, *Dermacentor*, *Ixodes*, and *Amblyomma* ticks are important as vectors of *F. tularensis*; along with *Haemaphysalis* ticks, they help maintain enzootic tularemia cycles by transmitting the bacteria among lagomorphs and rodents (38). The dog tick, *D. variabilis*, is considered a principal vector of *F. tularensis* to humans in the United States, and collections of infected *D. variabilis* ticks have been made during investigations of tularemia outbreaks in South Dakota and Montana (51, 60, 65). *A. americanum* is an important vector in the south-central United States (37). In 1974, Jellison stated that *D. andersoni* was the most important tick vector of tularemia in the Rocky Mountain region, but he noted that *H. leporispalustris* and *H. chordeilis* had been found infected with the bacteria (42). Parker and colleagues isolated *F. tularensis* from *D. occidentalis* (55). Hopla found that both *I. pacificus* and *I. scapularis* were infected with *F. tularensis* and stated that *I. scapularis* was an efficient vector (37). Jellison cited experiments by Burgdorfer and others indicating that *Ornithodoros* ticks were able to transmit *F. tularensis*, but he did not believe that these argasid ticks were important vectors in nature (42).

In Europe, *F. tularensis* has been isolated from *I. ricinus* in Norway; from *D. reticulatus*, *I. ricinus*, and *H. concinna*, found in an area of tularemia endemicity in western Slovakia; from *D. reticulatus*, found in Austria; and from *D. reticulatus* and *I. ricinus*, found in South Moravia in the Czech Republic (32, 33, 48, 70). *H. concinna* ticks found in south-central Siberia were also determined to be infected with *F. tularensis* (46). Burgdorfer cites Kamil and Bilal's experimental transmission of *F. tularensis* by *O. lahorensis* in Turkey (5). In a review of tularemia in the Soviet Union, Pollitzer cites findings that *F. tularensis* was isolated from *D. marginatus*, *I. laguri*, and *Rhipicephalus rossicus* in Stalingrad Oblast and that *I. ricinus*, *D. pictus*, *D. marginatus*, *H. plumbeum*, *R. rossicus*, and *H. punctata* played a role in tularemia transmission in Ukraine (58). Other ticks cited by Pollitzer as involved in transmission of tularemia in the Soviet Union include *R. pumilio*, *R. rossicus*, *I. apronophorus*, *I. laguri*, and *I. trianguliceps*.

EPIDEMIOLOGY

Tularemia has been found throughout North America, Europe (including Scandinavia), and Russia and in parts of the Middle East, central Asia, China, Japan, and the north coast of Africa (2, 38). It has been reported as far south as Guadalajara, Mexico, but is not known to occur in the tropics or the southern hemisphere.

Transmission to Humans and Disease Outbreaks

Tularemia is notable among infectious diseases for its high infectivity and many routes of transmission, yet surprisingly it is not contagious between people. Humans can acquire tularemia by handling, skinning, eating, or being scratched or bitten by infected vertebrates; handling or being bitten by infected arthropods; drinking contaminated water; making skin contact with contaminated mud or water; or inhaling infective aerosols. Person-to-person transmission apparently does not occur, and the reasons for this are not clear (13, 39).

The initial descriptions of tularemia in the United States reported mostly patients who either had been bitten by deerflies (*Chrysops discalis*) or had dressed, skinned, or otherwise handled infected rabbits (26). Since then, individual cases and outbreaks of tularemia have been associated with the manifold routes of exposure mentioned above. A few of the more notable outbreaks are described here.

In 1936, Karpov and Antonoff published the first description of an outbreak of tularemia associated with drinking contaminated water (45). Forty-three patients suffered a sudden onset of fever, headache, and myalgias 2 to 8 days after mowing hay alongside a contaminated brook. Most developed dysphagia, pharyngitis, and cervical lymphadenopathy. There were no deaths, but after defervescence many patients had prolonged weakness. Two groups of workers drank from different streams. All of the workers who drank from one of the streams became ill, whereas all members of the other group remained healthy. The tularemia agent was isolated from the implicated stream water by inoculation into guinea pigs.

In 1919, 1936, 1937, and 1973, outbreaks of tularemia associated with deerfly bites were reported in the United States (25, 35, 39, 47). In the most recent of these, 19 of 39 people who contracted tularemia in Utah during a 3-month period in 1971 reported deerfly bites, and 9 others had bites that were characteristic of deerfly bites. *F. tularensis* was isolated from deerflies (*C. discalis*) and from jackrabbits (*Lepus californicus*) in the area of the outbreak.

Warring and Ruffin described an outbreak of tick-borne tularemia among soldiers on maneuvers in Tennessee in 1946 (72). Of 50 cases of soldiers with symptomatic and serologic evidence of tularemia, 35 were ulceroglandular, 11 were pulmonic, 3 were glandular, and 1 was described as mixed ulceroglandular and pulmonic. Patients were treated only with oxygen and supportive measures; one patient died after developing severe pneumonia. Thirty-two patients reported a tick bite prior to the onset of illness, 5 reported direct contact with rabbits, and 13 had no history of tick bite but were bivouacked in an area where ticks were prevalent. All ticks collected from the area were *A. americanum*. Bacterial agglutination titers in serum were usually elevated in the second or third week of illness and ranged from 1:320 to 1:10,240. The highest titers were observed between the third and eighth week of illness. In some patients, symptoms lasted for over 6 months.

In 1968, Saliba and colleagues reported an outbreak of tularemia associated with exposure to *D. variabilis* on Indian reservations in South Dakota (60). Seven of 12 cases had ticks attached at the site of tularemic ulcers, and *F. tularensis* was isolated from *D. variabilis* ticks collected from dogs and vegetation. The investigators concluded that both highly and moderately pathogenic strains were present.

In 1983, Schmid and colleagues described an outbreak of 12 cases of tularemia on an Indian reservation in Montana (65). All cases had cervical or occipital adenopathy, and four recalled tick bites on the head and neck. *F. tularensis* was isolated from *D. variabilis* ticks collected from dogs.

In 1985, Markowitz and coworkers reported 20 cases of tularemia that occurred on Indian reservations in South Dakota (at sites different from those where the cases described by Saliba had occurred) (51). A case control study showed that cases were more likely than controls to report a tick bite in the week prior to illness. Both type A and type B *F. tularensis* organisms were isolated from *D. variabilis* collected from dogs.

In 1968, Young and colleagues reported 47 cases of tularemia related to contact with muskrats in a stream in Vermont (74). All but one of the cases had elevated serum agglutination titers against *F. tularensis*, and 16 of these had fourfold rises in titers between paired specimens. Eight patients had no symptoms but had elevated agglutination titers ranging from 1:1,280 to 1:10,240; seven of these had fourfold increases in titers between paired sera. None of the cases died, but 14 had severely prostrating disease. Twelve of the symptomatic patients improved without antibiotic treatment. Of the remaining symptomatic patients, 18 were treated with tetracycline, 9 were treated with penicillin, and 2 were treated with streptomycin. Penicillin apparently had no effect. All but one of the patients who received tetracycline improved within 6 days of treatment, but four had relapses. The two patients treated with streptomycin showed a dramatic resolution of symptoms within 24 h of treatment. Of 18 muskrats captured along the stream and examined

for ectoparasites, none had evidence of ticks or fleas. *F. tularensis* was isolated by animal inoculation from muskrats and from the stream's water and mud.

In 1984, Christenson described an outbreak of 529 cases of tularemia that had occurred during the summer of 1981 in north-central Sweden (10). Four hundred cases had laboratory evidence of tularemia. Most cases were ulceroglandular, and most were believed to have been acquired from exposure to mosquitoes.

In 2002, Eliasson and colleagues published a case control study of an outbreak involving 270 tularemia cases that occurred in Sweden in 2000 (18). All the patients were ill during the summer or early autumn. Tularemia was confirmed by serology or culture in 86% of the cases. In all, 218 cases and 414 controls were enrolled in the case-control study. The majority of cases had glandular or ulceroglandular manifestations, but 39 patients were reported to have a cough and 10 patients had pneumonia diagnosed by a physician. After other variables were controlled, cases were significantly more likely than controls to have been bitten by mosquitoes, owned a cat, or participated in farming. The outbreak occurred in both an area where tularemia was previously endemic and an area where tularemia had only rarely occurred. Cases of pneumonic tularemia were more likely to be reported from the area where tularemia was previously endemic.

Contamination of sugar beets by voles apparently caused outbreaks of pneumonic tularemia in Austria as a result of aerosolization when the beets were washed in a sugar factory (39). In 1966, an outbreak of hundreds of cases of tularemia occurred in northern Sweden (15). A large increase in the vole population resulted in the contamination of hay that was stored in field barns. *F. tularensis* was isolated from voles, hares, and contaminated hay. While there were several possible sources of exposure for the cases in this outbreak, including direct contact with hares, voles, and vole feces and consumption of contaminated water, the investigators presented a cogent argument that at least some cases, and perhaps a majority, were the result of direct inhalation of the bacteria from hay dust.

Only two outbreaks of pneumonic tularemia have been described in North America; both occurred on Martha's Vineyard, an island off the coast of Massachusetts. Teutsch and coworkers described seven people who developed pneumonic tularemia after staying together in a single cottage on the island in 1978 (69). The cause of the outbreak was not definitively determined, but the investigators speculated that all the cases might have inhaled *F. tularensis* after a wet dog shook itself inside the cottage, presumably aerosolizing the organism. In 2000, Feldman and colleagues investigated an outbreak of 15 people with pneumonic tularemia on Martha's Vineyard (23). *F. tularensis* subsp. *tularensis* was isolated from blood and lung tissue of the one patient who died. A case control study indicated that cases were more likely than controls to have mowed lawns or cut brush in the 2 weeks before their illness. Only one patient reported being exposed to a rabbit carcass while cutting brush. Presumably *F. tularensis* was aerosolized during the mowing process in all or most of these cases, but the source of the aerosolized bacteria and the ecological determinants that resulted in these two pneumonic tularemia outbreaks remain unknown. A serosurvey of landscapers on Martha's Vineyard found that 9 percent of landscapers had antibody to *F. tularensis* compared with less than 1 percent of nonlandscaper island residents (24). Landscapers who used a power blower were nine times more likely to be seropositive than those who did not use a power blower.

Thousands of cases of tularemia occurred in Eastern Europe during World War II (39). One former Soviet Union biological weapons scientist has suggested that some of these cases could have resulted from intentional release of *F. tularensis* (17). The social disruption of war contributed to an outbreak of tularemia in Kosovo in 2000 that was linked to an explosion in rodent populations and rodent contamination of human food and water stores (59). In a case control study of affected and unaffected households, households with cases of tularemia were more likely to have reported contamination of food stores with rodent feces and to have seen large numbers of field mice around their homes and less likely to have a water supply that was protected from rodents.

Descriptive Epidemiology from Reported Case Series

In 1976, Guerrant and colleagues reviewed 106 cases of tularemia that had occurred over 13 years in Virginia in the United States. They reported a bimodal peak in incidence during winter and summer and associations with vectors in 77% of cases (31). Lopez and colleagues reviewed 177 cases of tularemia that occurred in Georgia in the United States from 1960 to 1979 (49). Eight (5%) of the cases resulted from tick bite, while 91 (51%) were associated with direct contact with rabbits. Uhari and colleagues reviewed 67 cases of tularemia in children that had occurred in Finland from 1967 to 1986 (71). Most cases occurred during the summer and early fall, presumably from exposure to infected mosquitoes, and most had ulceroglandular presentations. Taylor and colleagues reviewed 1,041 cases of tularemia reported during the years 1981 through 1987 from Arkansas, Kansas, Louisiana, Missouri, Oklahoma, and Texas (68). Of 1,026 cases with epidemiologic data, 52%

had an onset during May, June, or July. Of those with known exposure history, 63% reported having had an attached tick, and 23% had rabbit exposure. Ohara and colleagues reviewed 1,274 tularemia cases that occurred in Japan between 1924 and 1996 (54). About 1% of these were reported to be due to arthropod exposure. The authors noted a bimodal peak in annual incidence with increased numbers of cases occurring during winter, associated with contact with hares, and during the summer, associated with arthropod exposure. They also reported that the proportion of cases caused by arthropods increased during the later years of the reviewed period.

In the United States, the incidence of tularemia reached a peak in 1939, when 2,291 cases were reported, and then declined substantially during the 1950s and 1960s to the current average of fewer than 150 cases per year (9). From 1990 to 2000, 1,368 cases were reported; 70% of these occurred from May through August. The age distribution of reported cases was bimodal, with the highest incidence in persons aged 5 to 9 years and over 74 years. Males had a higher incidence than females in all age categories. Incidence was substantially higher among American Indians and Alaskan Natives than among other racial groups. The highest numbers of cases were reported from counties in Arkansas, Missouri, Oklahoma, Kansas, South Dakota, Montana, and Massachusetts (Fig. 1). Before 1950, most cases of tularemia in the United States were associated with hunting and handling rabbits for food, and there was a resultant bimodal peak in reported cases from arthropod exposure in summer and rabbit exposure during the winter hunting months (16). However, the winter increase in incidence is no longer seen, apparently because of a decrease in rabbit hunting, and the spring and summer peak continues to reflect the months of highest human exposure to ticks and other arthropods. In addition, increased use of antimicrobials after 1950 may have resulted in earlier treatment of tularemia and reduced reporting.

CLINICAL MANIFESTATIONS

The clinical manifestations of tularemia depend on the route and mechanism of inoculation, the virulence of the infecting bacterial strain, and the host response of the infected person. As few as 10 to 50 of highly pathogenic type A bacteria regularly cause disease if directly inoculated into the skin or inhaled, but the number required to cause disease after ingestion is orders of magnitude higher (13, 61, 62). About 3 to 6 days after inoculation (the incubation period may be as short as 1 day but is rarely longer than 14 days),

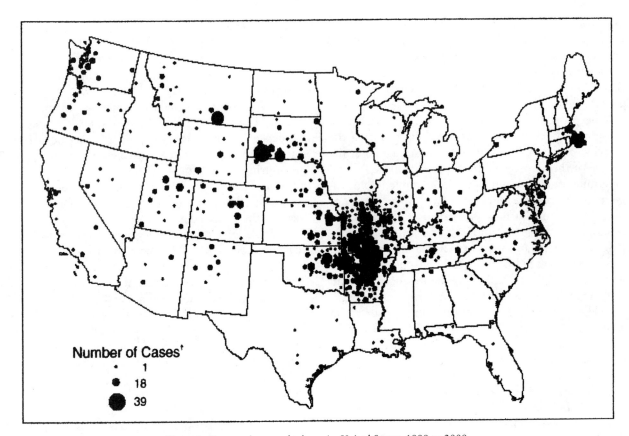

Figure 1. Reported cases of tularemia, United States, 1999 to 2000.

signs and symptoms develop as the bacteria spread through blood and lymphatics to regional lymph nodes and other organs, particularly lungs, pleura, spleen, liver, and kidneys. Infection causes follicular hyperplasia in lymph nodes and focal suppurative necrosis, followed by granuloma formation. Granulomas in the lungs, spleen, lymph nodes, and bone marrow have been found at autopsies of humans. The caseating granulomas of tularemia are grossly indistinguishable from those caused by tuberculosis (67). Based on these pathologic changes and limited evidence from experimental infections with animals and cell cultures, it appears that *F. tularensis* is an obligate intracellular parasite that probably replicates within human macrophages (67).

Six primary clinical syndromes of tularemia have been described: ulceroglandular, glandular, oculoglandular, oropharyngeal, pneumonic, and typhoidal (used to describe tularemia without localizing signs) (13, 16). The onset of tularemia tends to be sudden, and symptoms that may occur with any of the syndromes include fever, fatigue, chills, headache, malaise, myalgias, chest pain, sore throat, abdominal pain, vomiting, diarrhea, and arthralgia (15, 22, 41). Several types of rashes have been reported to occur with

tularemia, including vesiculopapular eruptions, erythema nodosum, and erythema multiforme (13, 15, 22, 66).

Ulceroglandular Tularemia

Ulceroglandular tularemia is the most common syndrome and develops following cutaneous or mucous membrane inoculation, either through direct contact with infected material or through the bite of an arthropod. An ulcer develops at the site of inoculation (see Color Plate 7A), followed by regional lymphadenopathy, usually accompanied by fever, malaise, and any of the other symptoms described above.

When the site of inoculation is the conjunctiva, the syndrome is called oculoglandular tularemia. Many of the first patients described with tularemia had oculoglandular disease, but this presentation occurred in less than 5% of cases reported in recent years (16, 26). The oculoglandular syndrome typically occurs when a person handles an infected animal and then touches his or her eye. Ocular inoculation is followed by conjunctivitis, palpebral edema, the development of small, yellowish ulcers on the palpebral conjunctivae, and preauricular adenopathy (73).

Secondary pneumonia can develop from ulceroglandular or other primary tularemia syndromes and may sometimes be clinically silent but evident on chest radiography (22). Ulceroglandular tularemia may be confused with bubonic plague, sporotrichosis, chancroid, anthrax, tick typhus, and lymphadenitis from other bacterial infections.

Glandular Tularemia

Glandular tularemia is similar to ulceroglandular disease, but without the presence of the cutaneous ulcer. In addition to the diseases mentioned above, this syndrome may need to be differentiated from cat-scratch disease, tuberculosis, toxoplasmosis, and lymphogranuloma venereum.

Oropharyngeal Tularemia

Oropharyngeal tularemia typically develops after ingestion of undercooked, infected animal meat or contaminated water or food (13, 26, 59). Occasionally this syndrome may be seen after inhalation of infectious particles. Patients typically have pharyngitis, which may be exudative, and cervical adenopathy (Color Plate 7B), which may progress to prominent inflammation and suppuration. Differential diagnoses include viral and streptococcal pharyngitis, diphtheria, mumps, and the conditions mentioned above that may mimic cervical glandular tularemia.

Pneumonic Tularemia

Pneumonic tularemia can be either primary, following the inhalation of infectious aerosols, or secondary, following hematogenous or lymphatic spread to the lungs from other infected tissues. Patients with pneumonic tularemia usually develop generalized influenza-like symptoms followed by cough, pleuritic or retrosternal pain, and dyspnea. Chest radiographs show single or multiple infiltrates and often pleural effusions and hilar adenopathy. From 25 to 30% of patients may have infiltrates on radiographs without any clinical signs or symptoms of pneumonia (13, 22). Prior to the development of antibiotics, the mortality rate for pneumonic tularemia was estimated at 30 to 60%, but with early and appropriate antibiotic treatment mortality is 5% or less (17, 22, 53). Pneumonic tularemia must be differentiated from other community-acquired pneumonias including those caused by *Mycoplasma*, *Chlamydia*, *Legionella*, and *Histoplasma* spp. and by common bacterial and viral agents. Other differential diagnoses include Q fever, inhalational anthrax, pneumonic plague, and tuberculosis.

Typhoidal Tularemia

Typhoidal tularemia presents as undifferentiated febrile illness or sepsis without localizing signs. Many of these patients have or develop pneumonia. Patients may present with a mild influenza-like febrile illness or, in more severe cases, with prostration and hypotension. Diarrhea occurs more commonly in typhoidal tularemia than in other tularemia syndromes (13). Typhoidal tularemia may be confused with any other cause of fever without localizing signs, including typhoid fever, brucellosis, Q fever and other rickettsial infections, babesiosis, malaria, and bacterial endocarditis.

Other Uncommon Clinical Forms

F. tularensis infection can also cause meningitis, pericarditis, endocarditis, and septic arthritis (13, 16, 50).

DIAGNOSIS

Tularemia may be suspected on clinical grounds when a patient presents with typical ulceroglandular manifestations after obvious exposure to a potentially infected animal or arthropod bite. Other presentations are less specific, however. In any case, laboratory tests are needed to definitively establish the diagnosis. Because of the potentially severe course of pneumonic illness, tularemia should be considered early in the differential diagnosis of any patient with community-acquired pneumonia of unknown etiology. In any severe presentation of suspected tularemia, appropriate antibiotic treatment should be started without waiting for definitive diagnostic tests.

The most conclusive diagnostic test for infection is isolation of the organism from a clinical specimen. However, the sensitivity of culture in most clinical cases is low. *F. tularensis* may be difficult to grow on routine bacterial culture media, and cystine- or cysteine-enriched medium may be required (11). Laboratory personnel should always be notified when tularemia is suspected because of the high risk of laboratory-acquired infection when working with live cultures. Gram staining of clinical specimens can be useful to rule out other obvious pathogens, but because of its small size, *F. tularensis* is difficult to identify by light microscopy.

F. tularensis antigens or nucleic acids can be detected in clinical specimens by direct fluorescent antibody testing, immunohistochemical staining, and PCR. Immunohistochemical staining can be done on either fresh or formalin-fixed specimens (Color Plate 7E) (11).

Capture enzyme-linked immunosorbent assay, a rapid immunochromatographic antigen detection test, and PCR tests have been developed and are being evaluated but are not yet widely available (11, 19, 30).

Antibody to *F. tularensis* is usually first detectable in patient serum about 2 weeks after the onset of illness. The most commonly used assay is a bacterial agglutination test, but enzyme-linked immunosorbent assay and hemagglutination tests have also been used. A titer of 1:160 or higher by tube agglutination or 1:128 or higher by microagglutination is strong presumptive evidence of acute infection, but serologic confirmation requires a fourfold change in titer in two separate serum samples (11, 13, 17). Cross-reactions with antibody to *Brucella*, *Legionella*, *Yersinia*, and *Mycoplasma* species have been described (13, 39).

TREATMENT

F. tularensis infection can be effectively treated with several classes of antibiotics. Streptomycin is considered by many to be the drug of choice, but gentamicin is more widely available and is also effective; both are bactericidal. An appropriate dose of streptomycin for an adult is 1 g intramuscularly twice daily; for a child, the dose is 15 mg/kg of body weight twice daily (up to a maximum daily dose of 2 g) (13, 17). Gentamicin can be given intramuscularly or intravenously in a dose of 5 mg/kg/day for adults and 7.5 mg/kg/day in children, usually in divided doses (14, 17). Several case reports indicate that ciprofloxacin is also effective (43, 44); ciprofloxacin can be given in a dose of 400 mg intravenously or 500 mg orally twice a day for adults; for children, it can be given at a dose of 15 mg/kg twice daily either intravenously or orally to a maximum daily dose of 1 g per day (17). Johansson and colleagues evaluated 12 children, aged 1 to 10 years, who were treated with ciprofloxacin for 10 to 14 days (43). Treatment was interrupted in two patients because they developed a rash. In one of these cases, ciprofloxacin was initially given for 7 days, withdrawn for 10 days, and then restarted and given for an additional 10 days. All children recovered from their illness without complications. Streptomycin, gentami-cin, and ciprofloxacin should generally be given for 10 days (13, 17). Oral or intravenous doxycycline is an effective alternative for adults and children 8 years of age or older; it is recommended to be given for 14 to 21 days in a dose of 100 mg twice a day for adults and 2.2 mg twice a day up to a maximum daily dose of 200 mg for children (16, 17). Enderlin and colleagues reviewed published outcomes of tularemia treatment and concluded that

97% of patients treated with streptomycin were cured with no relapses, compared to 86% of patients treated with gentamicin and 88% of patients treated with tetracycline (20). The authors felt that delay of initiation and short duration of treatment may have adversely affected the outcome in some patients treated with gentamicin, a conclusion that seems to be supported by several other case reports (22, 27, 50). Seventy-seven percent of patients treated with chloramphenicol and 50% of patients treated with tobramycin were cured. Cross and Jacobs reported treatment failure in eight patients treated with ceftriaxone (12).

Scheel and colleagues evaluated the antimicrobial susceptibility of *F. tularensis* isolates obtained from hares, rodents, and humans in Scandinavia (64). All strains were susceptible to streptomycin, gentamicin, doxycycline, chloramphenicol, and four quinalones including ciprofloxacin but were resistant to many β-lactams including penicillin, cefuroxime, and imipenem. An evaluation by Ikaheimo and colleagues also found that *F. tularensis* strains were resistant to β-lactams but sensitive to streptomycin, gentamicin, tobramycin, and the quinalones ciprofloxacin, levofloxacin, grepafloxacin, and trovafloxacin (40). Maurin and colleagues found good bactericidal activity of aminoglycosides, tetracyclines, and fluoroquinolones against *F. tularensis* (52).

PREVENTION

Strategies for preventing tularemia depend on the anticipated route of exposure. People who hunt, trap, skin, butcher, or otherwise handle potentially infected animals such as rabbits, hares, or rodents should wear gloves to avoid acquiring the bacteria through cuts or scrapes on their hands. Meat from potentially infected animals should be thoroughly cooked before ingestion. Meat that has been frozen can remain infectious after being thawed. Food and water supplies should be kept free from any potential contact with rodents or other potentially infected animals. Chlorination of water supplies will also reduce risk of tularemia transmission.

To avoid exposure to tularemia by infected ticks and other arthropods, persons should avoid arthropod-infested habitat or use protective clothing, repellents (such as *N,N*-dimethyl-metatoluamide [DEET]) on their clothing and skin, and pesticides such as permethrin on their clothing.

To avoid exposure to aerosols of *F. tularensis*, people should avoid vigorous handling, shaking, or maceration of infected animals or their tissue and avoid creating aerosols from hay or other material that is potentially contaminated by infected animals or their excreta. Persons who mow lawns or cut brush in areas where tularemia is endemic should survey the areas for any animal carcasses or excreta before beginning work and use appropriate protective skirting and collection bags on mowing or cutting machines. There is little if any good data on the efficacy of various masks or respirators for preventing tularemia, but high-efficiency respirators should afford at least some protection against infectious aerosols. Laboratory workers should be notified when potentially infective samples are sent to their laboratories, should use at least biologic safety level 2 facilities with equipment for diagnostic procedures that are not likely to cause aerosolization of the bacteria, and should use level 3 facilities for manipulation of cultures or any activity that could potentially create an aerosol. If *F. tularensis* has been identified or presumptively identified in a level 2 laboratory, the cultures should be transferred to a level 3 laboratory for any further study (11). Persons who have had obvious exposure to *F. tularensis* (e.g., from a centrifuge accident, inoculation, or spill of culture material) should immediately begin antimicrobial prophylaxis with either ciprofloxacin or doxycycline for 14 days (17). Laboratory workers exposed to *F. tularensis* cultures under routine level 2 circumstances can be carefully observed for any fever or other signs of illness for 2 weeks after the exposure and promptly treated if they develop any signs or symptoms of tularemia.

Infected humans do not appear to present any risk of infection to other people, and standard hospital infection control precautions are indicated in managing patients with tularemia (17).

A live attenuated vaccine against tularemia became available in the United States in the 1960s (19). Over the first 10 years of its use among laboratory workers, it appeared to reduce the risk of typhoidal tularemia and to ameliorate but not decrease the incidence of ulceroglandular tularemia (6). Until recently, this vaccine could be obtained for reference laboratory workers and others with high occupational risk of tularemia exposure through the U.S. Department of Defense. The vaccine is now under review by the Food and Drug Administration and is not currently available.

Because of the concern regarding the potential use of *F. tularensis* as an agent of bioterrorism, guidelines for responding to an intentional release of this bacterium have been published and include recommendations for management and prophylaxis in both contained and mass casualty situations (17). Health care providers and public health officials should con-

sider tularemia when confronted with clusters of unexplained acute febrile respiratory illness.

REFERENCES

1. Abd, H., T. Johansson, I. Golovliov, G. Sandstrom, and M. Forsman. 2003. Survival and growth of *Francisella tularensis* in *Acanthamoeba castellanii*. *Appl. Environ. Microbiol.* **69:**600–606.

2. Acha, P. N., and B. Szyfres. 2003. *Zoonoses and Communicable Diseases Common to Man and Animals,* 3rd ed., vol. 1. *Bacterioses and Mycoses.* Pan American Health Organization, Washington, D.C.

3. Anda, P., J. Segura Del Pozo, J. M. Diaz Garcia, R. Escudero, F. J. Garcia Pena, M. C. Lopez Velasco, R. E. Sellek, M. R. Jimenez Chillaron, L. P. Sanchez Serrano, and J. F. Martinez Navarro. 2001. Waterborne outbreak of tularemia associated with crayfish fishing. *Emerg. Infect. Dis.* **7:**575–582.

4. Berdal, B. P., R. Mehl, N. K. Meidell, A. M. Lorentzen-Styr, and O. Scheel. 1996. Field investigations of tularemia in Norway. *FEMS Immunol. Med. Microbiol.* **13:**191–195.

5. Burgdorfer, W., and C. Owen. 1956. Experimental studies on argasid ticks as possible vectors of tularemia. *J. Infect. Dis.* **98:** 67–74.

6. Burke, D. S. 1977. Immunization against tularemia: analysis of the effectiveness of live *Francisella tularensis* vaccine in prevention of laboratory-acquired tularemia. *J. Infect. Dis.* **135:**55–60.

7. Byfield, G. U., L. Breslow, R. R. Cross, Jr., and N. J. Hershey. 1945. Tick borne tularemia. Report of fifteen cases. *JAMA* **127:**191–196.

8. Calhoun, E. L. 1954. Natural occurrence of tularemia in the lone star tick, *Ambylomma americanum* (Linn.), and in dogs in Arkansas. *Am. J. Trop. Med. Hyg.* **3:**360–366.

9. Centers for Disease Control and Prevention. 2002. Tularemia—United States, 1990–2000. *Morb. Mortal. Wkly. Rep.* **51:**181–184.

10. Christenson, B. 1984. An outbreak of tularemia in the northern part of central Sweden. *Scand. J. Infect. Dis.* **16:**285–290.

11. Chu, M. C., and R. S. Weyant. 2003. *Francisella* and *Brucella,* p. 789–808. *In* K. V. Forrest, J. H. Jorgensen, and P. R. Murray (ed.), *Manual of Clinical Microbiology,* 8th ed. American Society for Microbiology, Washington, D.C.

12. Cross, J. T., and R. F. Jacobs. 1993. Tularemia: treatment failures with outpatient use of ceftriaxone. *Clin. Infect. Dis.* **17:** 976–980.

13. Cross, J. T., and R. L. Penn. 2000. *Francisella tularensis* (Tularemia), p. 2393–2402. *In* G. L. Mandell, J. E. Bennett, and R. Dolan (ed.), *Mandell's Principles and Practice of Infectious Diseases,* 5th ed. Churchill Livingstone, Inc., New York, N.Y.

14. Cross, J. T., Jr., G. E. Schutze, and R. F. Jacobs. 1995. Treatment of tularemia with gentamicin in pediatric patients. *Pediatr. Infect. Dis. J.* **14:**151–152.

15. Dahlstrand, S., O. Ringertz, and B. Zetterberg. 1971. Airborne tularemia in Sweden. *Scand. J. Infect. Dis.* **3:**7–16.

16. Dennis, D. T. 2004. Tularemia, p. 1446–1451. *In* S. L. Gorbach, J. G. Bartlett, and N. R. Blacklow (ed.), *Infectious Disease,* 3rd ed. Lippincott Williams and Wilkins, New York, N.Y.

17. Dennis, D. T., T. V. Inglesby, D. A. Henderson, J. G. Bartlett, M. S. Ascher, E. Eitzen, A. D. Fine, A. M. Friedlander, J. Hauer, M. Layton, S. R. Lillibridge, J. E. McDade, M. T. Osterholm, T. O'Toole, G. Parker, T. M. Perl, P. K. Russell, and K. Tonat. 2001. Tularemia as a biological weapon: medical and public health management. *JAMA* **285:**2763–2773.

18. Eliasson, H., J. Linback, J. Nuorti, M. Arneborn, J. Giesecke, and A. Tegnell. 2002. The 2000 tularemia outbreak: a case-control study of risk factors in disease-endemic and emergent areas, Sweden. *Emerg. Infect. Dis.* **8:**956–960.

19. Ellis, J., P. C. F. Oyston, M. Green, and R. W. Titball. 2002. Tularemia. *Clin. Microbiol. Rev.* **15:**631–646.

20. Enderlin, G., L. Morales, R. F. Jacobs, and J. T. Cross. 1994. Streptomycin and alternative agents for the treatment of tularemia: review of the literature. *Clin. Infect. Dis.* **19:**42–47.

21. Ericsson, M., A. Tarnvik, K. Kuoppa, G. Sandstrom, and A. Sjostedt. 1994. Increased synthesis of DnaK, GroEL, and GroES homologs by *Francisella tularensis* LVS in response to heat and hydrogen peroxide. *Infect. Immun.* **62:**178–183.

22. Evans, M. E., D. W. Gregory, W. Schaffner, and Z. A. McGee. 1985. Tularemia: a 30-year experience with 88 cases. *Medicine* **64:**251–269.

23. Feldman, K. A., R. E. Enscore, S. L. Lathrop, B. T. Matyas, M. McGuill, M. E. Schriefer, D. Stiles-Enos, D. T. Dennis, L. R. Petersen, and E. B. Hayes. 2001. An outbreak of primary pneumonic tularemia on Martha's Vineyard. *N. Engl. J. Med.* **345:**1601–1606.

24. Feldman, K. A., D. Stiles-Enos, K. Julian, B. T. Matyas, S. R. Telford III, M. C. Chu, L. R. Petersen, and E. B. Hayes. 2003. Tularemia on Martha's Vineyard: seroprevalence and occupational risk. *Emerg. Infect. Dis.* **9:**350–354.

25. Francis, E. 1921. The occurrence of tularemia in nature as a disease of man. *Public Health Rep.* **36:**1731–1751.

26. Francis, E. 1925. Tularemia. *JAMA* **84:**1243–1250.

27. Gallivan, M. V., W. A. Davis II, V. F. Garagusi, A. L. Paris, and E. E. Lack. 1980. Fatal cat-transmitted tularemia: demonstration of the organism in tissue. *South. Med. J.* **73:**240–242.

28. Golovliov, I., M. Ericsson, G. Sandstrom, A. Tarnvik, and A. Sjostedt. 1997. Identification of proteins of *Francisella tularensis* induced during growth in macrophages and cloning of the gene encoding a prominently induced 23-kilodalton protein. *Infect. Immun.* **65:**2183–2189.

29. Green, R. G. 1931. The occurrence of *Bacterium tularense* in the Eastern wood tick, *Dermacentor variabilis.* *Am. J. Hyg.* **14:**600–613.

30. Grunow, R., W. Splettstoesser, S. McDonald, C. Otterbein, T. O'Brien, C. Morgan, J. Aldrich, E. Hofer, E. J. Finke, and H. Meyer. 2000. Detection of *Francisella tularensis* in biological specimens using a capture enzyme-linked immunosorbent assay, an immunochromatographic handheld assay, and a PCR. *Clin. Diagn. Lab. Immunol.* **7:**86–90.

31. Guerrant, R. L., M. K. Humphries, Jr., J. E. Butler, and R. S. Jackson. 1976. Tickborne oculoglandular tularemia: case report and review of seasonal and vectorial associations in 106 cases. *Arch. Intern. Med.* **136:**811–813.

32. Gurycova, D., E. Kocianova, V. Vyrostekova, and J. Rehacek. 1995. Prevalence of ticks infected with *Francisella tularensis* in natural foci of tularemia in western Slovakia. *Eur. J. Epidemiol.* **11:**469–474.

33. Gurycova, D., V. Vyrostekova, G. Khanakah, E. Kocianova, and G. Stanek. 2001. Importance of surveillance of tularemia natural foci in the known endemic area of central Europe, 1991–1997. *Wien. Klin. Wochenschr.* **113:**433–438.

34. Hansen, E. C., and R. S. Green. 1929. Tularemia in Minnesota. *JAMA* **92:**1920–1923.

35. Hillman, C. C., and M. T. Morgan. 1937. Tularemia: report of a fulminant epidemic transmitted by the deerfly. *JAMA* **108:**538–540.

36. Hopla, C. E. 1953. Experimental studies on tick transmission of tularemia organisms. *Am. J. Hyg.* **58:**101–118.

37. Hopla, C. E. 1960. The transmission of tularemia organisms by ticks in the southern states. *South. Med. J.* **53:**92–97.

38. Hopla, C. E., and A. K. Hopla. 1994. Tularemia, p. 113–126. *In* G. W. Beran (ed.), *CRC Handbook of Zoonoses, Section A,* 2nd ed. CRC Press, Boca Raton, Fla.

39. Hornick, R. B. 1998. Tularemia, p. 823–837. *In* A. S. Evans and P. S. Brachman (ed.), *Bacterial Infections of Humans: Epidemiology and Control,* 3rd ed. Plenum Medical Book Company, New York, N.Y.

40. Ikaheimo, I., H. Syrjala, J. Karhukorpi, R. Schildt, and M. Koskela. 2000. In vitro antibiotic susceptibility of *Francisella tularensis* isolated from humans and animals. *J. Antimicrob. Chemother.* **46:**287–290.

41. Jacobs, R. F., Y. M. Condrey, and T. Yamaguchi. 1985. Tularemia in adults and children: a changing presentation. *Pediatrics* **76:**818–822.

42. Jellison, W. L. 1974. Tularemia in North America, 1930–1974. University of Montana, Missoula, Mont.

43. Johansson, A., L. Berglund, L. Gothefors, A. Sjostedt, and A. Tarnvik. 2000. Ciprofloxacin for treatment of tularemia in children. *Pediatr. Infect. Dis. J.* **19:**449–453.

44. Johansson, A. L., L. Berglund, A. Sjostedt, and A. Tarnvik. 2001. Ciprofloxacin for treatment of tularemia. *Clin. Infect. Dis.* **33:**267–268.

45. Karpov, S. P., and N. I. Antonoff. 1936. The spread of tularemia through water, as a new factor in its epidemiology. *J. Bacteriol.* **32:**243–258.

46. Khazova, T. G., and V. K. Iastrebov. 2001. Combined focus of tick-borne encephalitis, tick-borne rickettsiosis and tularemia in the habitat of *Haemaphysalis concinna* in south-central Siberia. *Zh. Mikrobiol. Epidemiol. Immunobiol.* **2001:**78–80. (In Russian.)

47. Klock, L. E., P. F. Olsen, and T. Fukushima. 1973. Tularemia epidemic associated with the deerfly. *JAMA* **226:**149–152.

48. Kohls, G. M., and B. Locker. 1954. Isolation of *Pasteurella tularensis* from the tick *Ixodes ricinus* in Norway. *Nord. Vet. Med.* **6:**883–884.

49. Lopez, C. E., A. N. Kornblatt, R. K. Sikes, and O. E. Hanes. 1982. Tularemia: review of eight cases of tick-borne infection and the epidemiology of the disease in Georgia. *South. Med. J.* **75:**405–407.

50. Lovell, V. M., C. T. Cho, N. J. Lindsey, and P. L. Nelson. 1986. *Francisella tularensis* meningitis: a rare clinical entity. *J. Infect. Dis.* **154:**916–918.

51. Markowitz, L. E., N. A. Hynes, P. de la Cruz, E. Campos, J. M. Barbaree, B. D. Plikaytis, D. Mosier, and A. F. Kaufmann. 1985. Tick-borne tularemia. An outbreak of lymphadenopathy in children. *JAMA* **254:**2922–2925.

52. Maurin, M., N. F. Mersali, and D. Raoult. 2000. Bactericidal activities of antibiotics against intracellular *Francisella tularensis.* *Antimicrob. Agents Chemother.* **44:**3428–3431.

53. Miller, R. P., and J. H. Bates. 1969. Pleuropulmonary tularemia. A review of 29 patients. *Am. Rev. Respir. Dis.* **99:**31–41.

54. Ohara, Y., T. Sato, and M. Homma. 1998. Arthropod-borne tularemia in Japan: clinical analysis of 1,374 cases observed between 1924 and 1996. *J. Med. Entomol.* **35:**471–473.

55. Parker, R. R., C. S. Brooks, and H. Marsh. 1929. The occurrence of *Bacterium tularense* in the wood tick (*Dermacentor occidentalis*) in California. *Public Health Rep.* **44:**1299–1300.

56. Parker, R. R., R. R. Spencer, and E. Francis. 1924. Tularemia XI: tularemia infection in ticks of the species *Dermacentor andersonii stiles* in the Bitter Root Valley, Montana. *Public Health Rep.* **39:**1057–1073.

57. Philip, C. B., and W. L. Jellison. 1934. The American dog tick, *Dermacentor variabilis* as a host of *Bacterium tularense.* *Public Health Rep.* **49.**

58. Pollitzer, R. 1967. History and incidence of tularemia in the Soviet Union. Institute of Contemporary Russian Studies, Fordham University, Bronx, N.Y.

59. Reintjes, R., I. Dedushaj, A. Gjini, T. R. Jorgensen, B. Cotter, A. Lieftucht, F. D'Ancona, D. T. Dennis, M. A. Kosoy, G. Mulliqi-Osmani, R. Grunow, A. Kalaveshi, L. Gashi, and I. Humoli. 2002. Tularemia outbreak investigation in Kosovo: case control and environmental studies. *Emerg. Infect. Dis.* 8: 69–73.

60. Saliba, G. S., F. C. Harmston, B. E. Diamond, C. L. Zymet, M. I. Goldenberg, and T. D. Chin. 1966. An outbreak of human tularemia associated with the American dog tick, *Dermacentor variabilis*. *Am. J. Trop. Med. Hyg.* 15:531–538.

61. Saslaw, S., H. T. Eigelsbach, J. A. Prior, H. E. Wilson, and S. Carhart. 1961. Tularemia vaccine study. II. Respiratory challenge. *Arch. Intern. Med.* 107:702–714.

62. Saslaw, S., H. T. Eigelsbach, H. E. Wilson, J. A. Prior, and S. Carhart. 1961. Tularemia vaccine study. I. Intracutaneous challenge. *Arch. Intern. Med.* 107:689–701.

63. Sawyer, W. D., H. G. Dangerfield, A. L. Hogge, and D. Crozier. 1966. Antibiotic prophylaxis and therapy of airborne tularemia. *Bacteriol. Rev.* 30:542–550.

64. Scheel, O., T. Hoel, T. Sandvik, and B. P. Berdal. 1993. Susceptibility pattern of Scandinavian *Francisella tularensis* isolates with regard to oral and parenteral antimicrobial agents. *APMIS* 101:33–36.

65. Schmid, G. P., A. N. Kornblatt, C. A. Connors, C. Patton, J. Carney, J. Hobbs, and A. F. Kaufmann. 1983. Clinically mild tularemia associated with tick-borne *Francisella tularensis*. *J. Infect. Dis.* 148:63–67.

66. Syrjala, H., J. Karvonen, and A. Salminen. 1984. Skin manifestations of tularemia: a study of 88 cases in northern Finland during 16 years (1967–1983). *Acta Derm. Venereol. (Stockholm)* 64:513–516.

67. Tarnvik, A. 1989. Nature of protective immunity to *Francisella tularensis*. *Rev. Infect. Dis.* 11:440–451.

68. Taylor, J. P., G. R. Istre, T. C. McChesney, F. T. Satalowich, R. L. Parker, and L. M. McFarland. 1991. Epidemiologic characteristics of human tularemia in the southwest-central states, 1981–1987. *Am. J. Epidemiol.* 133:1032–1038.

69. Teutsch, S. M., W. J. Martone, E. W. Brink, M. E. Potter, G. Eliot, R. Hoxsie, R. B. Craven, and A. F. Kaufmann. 1979. Pneumonic tularemia on Martha's Vineyard. *N. Engl. J. Med.* 301:826–828.

70. Treml, F., Z. Hubalek, J. Halouzka, Z. Juricova, M. Hunady, and V. Janik. 2001. Analysis of the incidence of tularemia in the Breclav district 1994–1999. *Epidemiol. Mikrobiol. Imunol.* 50:4–9. (In Czech.)

71. Uhari, M., H. Syrjala, and A. Salminen. 1990. Tularemia in children caused by *Francisella tularensis* biovar *palaearctica*. *Pediatr. Infect. Dis. J.* 9:80–83.

72. Warring, W. B., and J. S. Ruffin. 1946. A tick-borne epidemic of tularemia. *N. Engl. J. Med.* 234:137–140.

73. Weinberg, A. N. 2004. Commentary: Wherry W. B., Lamb B. H. Infection of man with *Bacterium tularense*. *J. Infect. Dis.* 1914; 15:331–40. *J. Infect. Dis.* 189:1317–1331.

74. Young, L. S., D. S. Bickness, B. G. Archer, J. M. Clinton, L. J. Leavens, J. C. Feeley, and P. S. Brachman. 1969. Tularemia epidemic: Vermont, 1968. Forty-seven cases linked to contact with muskrats. *N. Engl. J. Med.* 280:1253–1260.

Chapter 13

Human Granulocytic Anaplasmosis (Ehrlichiosis)

JESSE L. GOODMAN

OVERVIEW

Human granulocytic anaplasmosis (HGA) is a recently recognized acute febrile illness caused by *Anaplasma phagocytophilum*. Like Lyme disease, its causative agent is transmitted by ixodid ticks, and small mammals likely serve as reservoir hosts. The pathogen is noteworthy in its preferential targeting and intracellular infection of neutrophils. Its range is still being defined, but it has been documented in geographic areas in North America and Europe similar to those of Lyme disease, and coinfections with *Borrelia burgdorferi* can occur. The illness is characterized by high fever, myalgias, arthralgias, and headache, often with accompanying thrombocytopenia and leukopenia. Intracellular colonies of bacteria (morulae) may be seen in peripheral blood neutrophils but are often absent early in the course of infection. If the disease is suspected and appropriate therapy (usually doxycycline) is promptly initiated, the outcome is excellent. However, delayed diagnosis and treatment may result in organ failure and even death.

(In this chapter, the disease caused by *A. phagocytophilum* [see "Etiologic Agent and Biology," below] is referred to as human granulocytic anaplasmosis [HGA] due to the recent reclassification of the causative agent as an anaplasma. The disease has also been referred to as human granulocytic ehrlichiosis [HGE] and is clinically similar to the human ehrlichial infections caused by *Ehrlichia chaffeensis* and *Ehrlichia ewingii*.)

HISTORY

In 1994, several cases of an acute, often severe, febrile clinical illness resembling human monocytic ehrlichiosis were reported from the upper midwestern United States in which intracellular organisms were observed within blood neutrophils rather than mono-cytes (10). PCR amplification with 16S ribosomal RNA primers of blood samples from such patients (40) identified DNA sequences suggesting an infecting organism with genetic similarity to *Ehrlichia equi*, an agent causing a febrile illness with intragranulocytic inclusions in horses, and *Ehrlichia phagocytophila*, which similarly infects ruminants. Evidence suggested that ixodid ticks are the vectors of the disease (114), and it was shown that experimentally infected mice could transmit the agent to larval ixodid ticks. These ticks, in turn, could transmit infection to other mice by feeding (130). The causative agent was then isolated (57), allowing further genetic and ecological studies, the development of diagnostics, determination of antibiotic susceptibility, and studies of the organism's cellular interactions, including identification of roles for specific neutrophil carbohydrates and glycoproteins as cellular receptor components.

ETIOLOGIC AGENT AND BIOLOGY

Phylogeny and Nature of the Etiologic Agent

While the agent was initially considered to be a member of the genus *Ehrlichia*, together with the other major pathogen causing a similar human disease, *E. chaffeensis*, recent analysis of available DNA sequences (particularly 16S and *groEL* genes) from a variety of members of what was previously classified as the family *Rickettsiaceae* have led to the reclassification and renaming of the HGE agent (which has also been referred to as the agent of HGE [aoHGE], and *E. phagocytophilum*) as an *Anaplasma* species, *A. phagocytophilum* (49). In this proposal, grouped in the genus of *Anaplasma* with *A. phagocytophilum* are several other organisms, primarily infecting ruminants, including *Anaplasma marginale, Anaplasma centrale, Anaplasma ovis*, and the former *Ehrlichia bovis, E. phagocytophilum*, and *E. equi*, the latter two of which are now

---

Jesse L. Goodman • Center for Biologics Evaluation and Research, U.S. Food and Drug Administration, 1401 Rockville Pike, Suite 200N, HFM-1, Rockville, MD 20852. Dr. Goodman's affiliation is provided for identification purposes. The views expressed in this book are those of the author and do not necessarily reflect those of the Food and Drug Administration or of the U.S. Department of Health and Human Services.

considered conspecific with *A. phagocytophilum*. In contrast, under this revised classification, the genus *Ehrlichia* now includes *E. chaffeensis*, the agent of human monocytic ehrlichiosis (see Chapter 14); *E. ewingii*, an occasional cause of clinical ehrlichiosis (see Chapter 15) that, like *A. phagocytophilum*, infects neutrophils; as well as the veterinary pathogens *Ehrlichia canis* and *Ehrlichia* (formerly *Cowdria*) *ruminatum*. Members of both the *Ehrlichia* and the *Anaplasma* are tick transmitted, and although genetically divergent, they present similarities in their biology and in the human illnesses that some of the species cause. Two other genera, which are not tick transmitted, are now combined with these *Ehrlichia* and *Anaplasma* species to make up the family *Anaplasmataceae*. First are the *Neorickettsia*, which are transmitted by flukes infecting aquatic snails, insects, or fish: this genus also can infect some mammalian monocytes. Among the *Neorickettsia*, *Ehrlichia sennetsu* is a rare cause of a mononucleosis-like syndrome in humans so far described only in parts of Asia, and *Ehrlichia risticii* causes equine monocytic ehrlichiosis (also known as Potomac horse fever). Second are the *Wolbachia*, primarily pathogens of arthropods and helminths, which although not yet known to directly infect mammals may play a role in the pathogenesis of onchocerciasis (122). It is likely that continued identification and sequence analysis of new species and further understanding of the biological and ecological properties of these intracellular pathogens will result in additions to and amendments of this current phylogenic understanding.

A. phagocytophilum, like the other species now included in the genera *Anaplasma* and *Ehrlichia*, are small, gram-negative bacteria that, so far as is known, are all also obligate intracellular organisms that reside within cellular endosomes. All of these organisms appear to have both arthropod vectors and one or more animals that can serve as reservoir hosts in nature.

Pathogenesis of Infection and Host Response

The earliest events in infection following a tick bite have not been well characterized. The organism has a tropism for cells of neutrophil lineage, normally the very host cells best armed and most resistant to invading bacterial organisms. This remarkable fact immediately implies that the organism utilizes a variety of specific adaptive strategies to allow targeting of and survival within such cells. Our laboratory has shown that *A. phagocytophilum* infects mature polymorphonuclear neutrophils (PMN) and susceptible cell lines (e.g., HL60 promyelocytic leukemia cells) utilizing α-1-3 fucose (termed CD15s or sLe^x) glycosylated and sialyated P-selectin glycoprotein ligand 1 (PSGL-1) as receptor components (58, 63).

Thus, in binding to PSGL-1, the organism appears to functionally partially mimic P-selectin, a protein normally expressed on platelets and endothelium, important in early PMN adhesion to endothelium and resultant inflammatory processes. Binding through CD15s/PSGL-1 is likely responsible both for the bacterium's tropism for PMN and for allowing it to escape the normally voracious PMN phagocytic pathways. The adhesin on the organism that binds to CD15s/PSGL-1 is currently unknown. Cells so far shown susceptible to infection include PMN, their bone marrow precursors, and cell lines with leukocytic characteristics, including expression of CD15s-modified PSGL-1. However, we have also shown that variants of *A. phagocytophilum* can be selected that are capable of binding to cells without this receptor (58). In addition, both tick-derived cells (108) and a variety of endothelial cells (109) can be infected in vitro, although neither of these cell types is known to express PSGL-1. Binding to murine PMN, while similar to binding to human PMN in depending upon CD15s, has also been reported to occur in the absence of PSGL-1 (33). Recent evidence (143) suggests differences in the biochemical requirements for *A. phagocytophilum* versus P-selectin binding to PSGL-1. It therefore appears that the organism targets and infects its major cellular reservoirs through CD15s/PSGL-1 while maintaining a capacity to both potentially adapt to and infect some PSGL-1 nonexpressing cells. Thus, in common with many pathogens, *A. phagocytophilum* likely possesses more than one potential adhesin. Not surprisingly, given both the direct infection of PMN through cell adhesion molecules and the rapid elaboration of a variety of cytokines (see below), infection also affects expression of other surface molecules involved in cell-cell interactions. Such changes may play a pathogenic role during infection. For example, β_2 integrins, which can be upregulated by cytokines and through PSGL-1 engagement, are upregulated during murine infection, and β_2 integrin-deficient mice have higher levels of bacteremia (23). It is thus possible that integrin upregulation allows more rapid clearance of infected cells. It is also possible that integrin upregulation, in promoting adhesion to endothelial cells, may facilitate trafficking of infected PMN to these susceptible cells and, potentially, thence to nonvascular sites.

Like many microorganisms, *A. phagocytophilum* is a potent inducer of a variety of cytokines in vitro and in vivo. However, the pattern of cytokine induction has some unusual features likely related to its being nonendotoxin mediated (78). In particular, there is dramatic upregulation of CXC (interleukin-8 [IL-8]) and CC chemokines, including monocyte chemoattractant protein 1, macrophage inflammatory proteins 1α

and 1β, and RANTES (78). The production of these chemokines probably plays important pathogenic roles in the unique interactions of the organism with granulocytes and their precursors, such as increased IL-8 production in attraction and activation of neutrophilic target cells to propagate infection from cell to cell. These chemokines may also suppress hematopoeisis. Studies of IL-8 in a murine receptor knockout model support its importance in chemotaxis and enhancement of infection, and IL-8 elevation has been observed in infected patients (5). Elevation of proinflammatory cytokines typically seen in systemic bacterial infections (IL-1, IL-6, and tumor necrosis factor alpha) was not observed in some culture systems (78) or in infected patients' sera (50), but was reported in vitro when monocytes were present, where the immunodominant bacterial protein p44 major surface protein 2 (MSP2) may modulate the effect (76). Studies of the TH1 cytokine response have also produced somewhat variable results. Gamma interferon (IFN-γ) was not elevated in one in vitro study (76), but elevated levels were noted in patients' serum (50). In murine models, they were associated with both pathologic changes (100) and early host-mediated limitation of infection, although infection could still be cleared by IFN-γ-deficient mice (4). In human infection, where these cytokines likely appear early before the presence of antibodies, they may play a role both in host defense and in the production of some of the disease's symptoms, such as fevers, myalgias, and arthralgias. During recovery of infected mice and humans, elevated levels of IL-10 have been observed (50, 100) and may down-modulate the inflammatory effects of IFN-γ. One study using toll receptor-expressing cell lines (41) suggested that A. phagocytophilum induces cytokines through signal transduction by the toll-like receptor 2 (TLR2). However, another study showed that mice deficient in TLR2 and TLR4 responsiveness are capable of clearing infection (135).

Following cell surface binding (Fig. 1a), the organism is rapidly internalized (Fig. 1b and c) (61), apparently through receptor-mediated endocytosis. It then resides and replicates within a unique endosomal compartment, often surrounded by lysosomal granules (Fig. 1c) and at times colocalizing with major histocompatibility complex class I (MHC-I) and MHC-II molecules and containing vesicle-associated membrane protein 2; but unlike E. chaffeensis vacuoles, it does not contain lysosomal markers, transferrin receptor, or other early endosomal markers (107, 138). These A. phagocytophilum-infected endosomes fail to fuse with the lysosomal compartment and do not become acidified, allowing continued proliferation of the organism, filling the infected cell (Fig. 1d) and ultimately resulting in cell lysis and release of organisms. While both lysis and apoptosis are apparently promoted in HL60 cells in vitro, a unique survival strategy of A. phagocytophilum appears to be its ability to specifically inhibit PMN apoptosis, possibly due to a preformed bacterial protein and seemingly mediated at least in part through bacterial adhesion to PSGL-1 (56, 144). Recent studies suggest engagement of multiple antiapoptotic signaling pathways, including BCL (85a). This strategy makes a great deal of sense when one considers the normal half-life of only hours for PMN in the circulation, and it presumably allows time for protected intracellular replication and spread of the organism.

A number of studies have shown that A. phagocytophilum shuts down the normally microbiocidal toxic PMN oxidative response soon after infection, inhibiting superoxide generation through interference with transcription and assembly of specific components of the NADPH oxidase complex, phox (15, 34, 35). In addition, studies of experimentally A. phagocytophilum-infected sheep show reduced PMN phagocytosis and oxidative activity compared to that for controls (139). However, preservation of superoxide generation in A. phagocytophilum-exposed PMN in vitro has been noted (J. L. Goodman and M. J. Herron, unpublished data), and mice deficient in phox clear their infection normally (14, 135), suggesting that such effects may be variable, transient, methodology dependent, or complex and may not be a major determinant of the outcome of infection. My laboratory reported that A. phagocytophilum reoxidizes cytochrome C, an ability that may allow itself to directly and continuously detoxify reactive oxygen molecules that are generated by PMN (62).

Little is known about how the infection spreads from the initial tick bite site, what cells or tissues are involved, what causes signs of illness, and, when evident in severe cases, how tissue damage occurs. Mice, guinea pigs, dogs, sheep, cows, horses, and primates have all been experimentally infected with A. phagocytophilum isolates of either human or veterinary origin. Horses (60), dogs (59), and sheep (140) may experience clinical illness with fever and hematologic alterations. Chronic infection, immunosuppression, secondary infection, and abortion may be seen in sheep (112); ataxia, limb swelling, and lameness often occur in horses (95). Experimental infection of a variety of immune-competent mouse strains results in asymptomatic infection, usually resolving within 2 to 4 weeks, with little evidence to support significant infection of cell types other than myeloid cells. Mononuclear cell inflammatory aggregates may be seen in some organs, most commonly the liver. The results of four patient autopsies have been reported (86). These autopsies showed evidence of splenic lymphoid depletion, hepatic

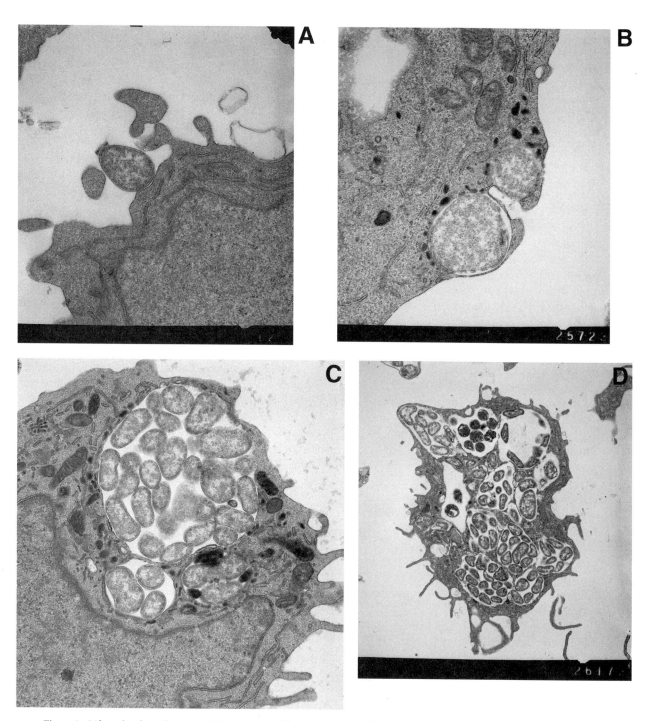

Figure 1. Life cycle of *A. phagocytophilum* in infected human (HL60) cells. (A) Binding to the cell surface; (B) internalization; (C) replication within the endosome with failure of fusion with lysosomal granules; (D) cell filled with multiple infected endosomes, near lysis (61).

macrophage aggregates and focal apoptosis (Color Plate 8B), and normocellular to hypercellular bone marrow with lymphoid aggregates. One patient also had mild pulmonary inflammation; another had myocarditis. Two autopsies showed evidence of superimposed opportunistic infections (Color Plate 8C).

Such infections complicating severe HGA may result from neutrophil hypofunction, prolonged hospitalization with antimicrobial therapy, or both.

Experimentally infected horses have similar pathological findings. Although infected organ parenchymal cells were not documented, splenic sinusoids and small vessels of organs, particularly the lung, were not uncommonly noted to contain infected leukocytes. We have observed infected myeloid progenitor cells containing morulae in the bone marrow of patients who subsequently were treated and recovered from infection (56). These findings suggest that most symptoms, signs, and laboratory findings of disease are not due to direct tissue infection but to factors such as systemic and local cytokine production and/or tissue injury related to the presence of inflammatory cells, some of which may be infected.

At present, the host response components required for control of *A. phagocytophilum* infection are not well understood. As mentioned, IFN-γ production is a prominent response to infection, and the TH-1 cellular responses that IFN-γ normally stimulates likely play an important role in the control and elimination of the organisms. IFN-γ may also play an important role in responding to infection because of its effects on macrophages whose state of differentiation and activation seems critical in determining whether they can control *A. phagocytophilum* replication. We have shown that some bone marrow cells expressing CD14, a marker for monocytic differentiation, can support growth of the organism (79). In addition, infected peripheral blood and bone marrow macrophages have been observed in patients, albeit rarely. However, monocytic differentiation of HL60 cells by IFN-γ stimulation results in the development of resistance to infection through two mechanisms, downregulation of CD15s expression and resultant reduced bacterial binding and (importantly) acquisition by the stimulated cells of the ability to kill intracellular organisms (77). Evidence from knockout mouse models shows that deficiencies in IFN-γ result in a prolonged and increased level of bacteremia, but clearance of the organism can occur nonetheless (4, 100).

Although innate effector mechanisms would appear to be critical in the host response before either antibodies or antigen-specific T cells are present, as described above, recent evidence from some knockout mouse models suggests that neither nitric oxide nor superoxide-mediated killing plays a determinative role (135). However, this evidence is limited, and some studies suggest that nitric oxide may be important (14). NK cells and macrophages may also have effector roles through different pathways (e.g., GTPase) (129), and/or nutritional factors, such as intracellular iron or other nutrient deficiencies, may have a role, as seen in intracellular bacteria that interact with macrophages. The critical role of adaptive immunity in eliminating infection is illustrated by the failure of SCID mice to clear infection (31, 130, 135).

Within 1 to 2 weeks, specific immunoglobulin M (IgM) and then IgG antibody becomes measurable,

and is largely directed against a limited repertoire of bacterial antigens, most notably against antigens in the p44 multigene family (MSP2). These genes are closely related to highly variable MSPs of *A. marginale*, which apparently utilizes them in binding to host erythrocytes (104) and which employs shifts in antigenic expression to escape the immune response, including antigen-specific CD4 T helper. It has been shown that p44 is downregulated in tick cells and that expression upregulates after transfer to mammalian cells or mice and vice versa (73). Furthermore, the profile of differential expression among p44 gene family members shifts during tick feeding and during the evolution of infection of mice. These findings suggest that p44 downregulation in ticks may be a protective mechanism that masks the most immunogenic antigens of the organism and that following infection, variation in expression of different isoforms may help delay an effective immune response. However, limited studies to date have not shown that antibody to p44 can be neutralizing or that recombinant p44 can be an effective vaccinogen. In contrast, preadministration of polyclonal immune serum does appear to reduce but not eliminate infection via either infected ticks or a syringe (127). It is also unclear if and how antibody may help in clearance once infected cells are present, although such effects have been observed with intracellular *Listeria monocytogenes* (52). Opsonization or targeting of antigen-expressing cells is possible, as is antibody interference during cell-to-cell transfer of organisms. However, the general limitations in antibody effectiveness for intracellular infections and the contribution of CD4^{+} T cells to host defense against *A. marginale* (28) suggest that T cells are likely to contribute to the control of *A. phagocytophilum* infection, although, surprisingly, no such experimental evidence has yet been provided.

Considering and summarizing the above available information, it is likely that following tick inoculation the organism infects either local capillary endothelial cells, neutrophils present in or drawn to tissues by chemokines such as IL-8, or both. The infection is likely then spread through the bloodstream within cells of neutrophilic lineage, inducing cytokines systemically and within specific organs such as liver, spleen, and lungs, where the infected cells traffic and marginate. Lodging in the bone marrow and spleen likely allows cell-cell transmission of the organism to uninfected cells of leukocytic origin. Most clinical and pathological manifestations are likely initiated by soluble cytokines and chemokines. Although endothelial infection is not clinically or pathologically prominent, the endothelium may play a role both in transfer of infection among susceptible cells and, in severe disease, in tissue injury.

LIFE CYCLE, TRANSMISSION, AND ZOONOTIC HOSTS

A. phagocytophilum is transmitted by ixodid ticks of the *Ixodes persulcatus* complex (see Color Map 2 for range), including *Ixodes scapularis* (Color Plate 1C) (46, 65, 99, 114) in the eastern and midwestern United States, *Ixodes pacificus* (83, 119, 120) and *Ixodes spinipalpis* (32, 145) in western coastal and mountain areas, respectively, and *Ixodes ricinus* (43, 54) in Europe. The prevalence of nymphal tick infection with *A. phagocytophilum* varies widely, even in areas of endemicity, but is typically in the 3 to 25% range (38, 85, 106, 134). As for *B. burgdorferi*, it appears that transstadial transmission (e.g., from larva to nymph to adult forms) occurs within the tick but that the organism is not transmitted transovarially. Thus, larval and nymphal ticks acquire infection from feeding on a variety of wild zoonotic hosts. In the United States, infection of wild mice (especially *Peromyscus leucopus*) (137), chipmunks, voles, raccoons, opossums, skunks, rabbits, squirrels, wild canids, raccoons, grey squirrels (88), and rabbits have all been reported. While *P. leucopus* is likely the dominant small mammal reservoir, infection is usually transient, unlike the chronic infection observed with *B. burgdorferi*. Also unlike *B. burgdorferi*, *A. phagocytophilum* is more common in ticks collected from vegetation than in ticks collected from mice (87). Such observations suggest either that *A. phagocytophilum* is a less-successful zoonotic pathogen than *B. burgdorferi* or that *P. leucopus* does not play as central a role in maintaining it in nature. While both white-tailed and roe deer may be seropositive and/or PCR positive (18, 90), studies of the potential role of deer in the organism's life cycle have been complicated by the presence of a distinct *Anaplasma* species (to date called WTD for white-tailed deer agent) that may be confused with *A. phagocytophilum* by some serologic and PCR assays (6, 24, 89). Thus, while deer are clearly critical for the livelihood of the ticks, what other role they may have in the life cycle of *A. phagocytophilum* is currently unclear. Lesser reservoir competencies may in part explain the apparent lower incidence of HGA than of Lyme disease. It may also be that the definitive reservoir host(s) for *A. phagocytophilum* remains to be defined. In any event, it is possible that other wild zoonotic hosts and livestock such as cattle and sheep play roles in maintaining the organism in nature. As has been observed with *B. burgdorferi*, larval ticks infected with *A. phagocytophilum* have been found on migratory birds and thus could play a role in disease transmission and geographic spread (45).

As seen with *B. burgdorferi*, the life cycle of *I. pacificus* and its transmission of *A. phagocytophilum*

in a different ecosystem rely on different zoonotic hosts, including the dusky-footed woodrat, *Neotoma fuscipes* (111). Also similar to what has been described for Lyme disease, *I. spinipalpis* appears to transmit *A. phagocytophilum* through *Neotoma mexicana* in Colorado (145). However, little transmission of disease to humans appears to occur, likely related to the feeding habits of *I. spinipalpis*.

Because the same tick vectors described here for *A. phagocytophilum* are also involved in the transmission of the agents of Lyme disease and babesiosis throughout their range and tick-borne encephalitis (TBE) in Eurasia and occasionally in North America, coinfection of vectors (as well as zoonotic hosts and humans) with various combinations of these organisms can and does occur. A number of studies using a variety of methods have examined the frequency of coinfection of ticks in various geographic areas. The incidence of finding multiple pathogens in ticks has varied widely from 1 to 60%, with similar ranges in zoonotic hosts. It appears that tick infection rates are independent for the different pathogens, e.g., the presence of *A. phagocytophilum* in a tick does not make it more likely to acquire *B. burgdorferi* than an uninfected tick and vice versa. While the prevalence of tick coinfection with *B. burgdorferi* and *A. phagocytophilum* is typically <10%, a 26% rate as determined by PCR was reported in one study performed in Westchester County, N.Y., an area of intense transmission to humans of both pathogens (123). In addition, in such areas, up to one-third of *A. phagocytophilum*-carrying ticks may also have *B. burgdorferi* present (134).

Human infection occurs from ixodid tick bites, usually from ticks in the nymphal stage. The exposure is often unnoticed due to the small size of the tick, the painless nature of the bite, and the absence of a rash unless there is coinfection with *B. burgdorferi* or a local hypersensitivity reaction. It is likely, as with Lyme disease, that at least 24 h of tick attachment are required for transmission of *A. phagocytophilum* (47, 75). Given the presence of transient bacteremia in humans, transfusion transmission is a possibility but has not yet been documented. However, lessening the possibility of such transmission becoming a major blood safety issue, it is unlikely that there is more than a very brief period of asymptomatic bacteremia, and acutely ill donors are routinely deferred from blood donation even if they seek to donate. However, if the disease became widespread, such cases could be expected to occur (the experience with West Nile virus and blood donation is instructive in this regard); one study has shown that the organism can survive under storage conditions typically used for red blood cell transfusion (74). One case of perinatal transmission in humans has been documented (69).

EPIDEMIOLOGY

In the United States, ehrlichia infections and HGA have been reportable to the Centers for Disease Control and Prevention (CDC) since 1998. It is certain that significant underdiagnosis and underreporting both occur. A total of 654 confirmed and 434 probable cases of HGA were reported from 1997 to 2001 from 21 states (55). Most cases were from the northeastern and upper-midwestern United States, with the highest total number of cases reported from New York and the highest incidences (cases per million population) in Connecticut (22.3), Minnesota (16.2), Rhode Island (12.7), and New York (4.7). Of interest, while they are not areas endemic for HGA, only Missouri and Tennessee reported cases of both HGA and monocytic ehrlichiosis at rates of >1/1,000,000. Although west-central Wisconsin is not included in the states reporting to the CDC from 1999 to 2001, HGA is also clearly quite common there, particularly in the St. Croix River valley bordering Minnesota, where many of the initially described cases occurred and where 8.79 cases/million were reported in another survey (105). In 2002, 511

cases were reported: the distribution of these cases by state reporting is shown in Fig. 2 (37) and included 4 cases from Wisconsin. States reporting more than 10 cases included New York (176 cases, including 17 from New York City), Minnesota (149 cases), Rhode Island (65 cases), Connecticut (49 cases), Massachusetts (29 cases), and Missouri (19 cases).

That such figures likely underestimate the occurrence of the disease at least in areas of intense transmission is borne out by more-focused studies. In some Wisconsin counties, rates as high as 16 cases/100,000 have been described (13). The most comprehensive study, a 4-year active surveillance program in 12 towns around Old Lyme, Conn., yielded an average annual confirmed case incidence of 42 per 100,000 population (39). During the same time period, there were 234 Lyme disease cases per 100,000. This study confirms the general clinical impression in areas where the disease is endemic that transmission can be intense but that HGA is generally less common than Lyme disease. In addition, this study used geographic information system mapping to document that within areas where A. phagocytophilum infection is most in-

EHRLICHIOSIS, HUMAN GRANULOCYTIC. Reported cases—United States and U.S. territories, 2002

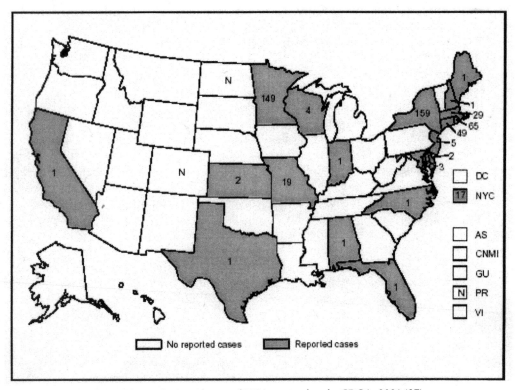

Figure 2. Distribution of cases of HGA reported to the CDC in 2001 (37).

tense, nonhomogeneity of distribution with clustering of cases can occur, in this case around the mouth of the Connecticut River.

The median age of patients in the 2003 CDC report was 51 years. A total of 57% of patients were male, and 97% were Caucasian. While no studies have addressed the issue scientifically, the predominance of male patients may reflect outdoor activity and occupations that increase opportunities for tick exposure. The reason for the relative paucity of reported cases in children is unknown and differs from what is seen with Lyme disease. Given that both infections are transmitted by the same ticks, it appears likely that children either are less susceptible to infection and/or less commonly develop clinical symptoms. Cases occurred throughout the year, with the highest incidence from April through August, corresponding to nymphal tick feeding activity.

Probable human *A. phagocytophilum* infection has been reported widely outside of the United States throughout the range of ixodid tick populations. The case reporting and methods used are variable and likely reflect not only incidence of infection but also local interest and clinical and diagnostic expertise. Published studies include both clinical reports and seroepidemiological surveys; they have used various laboratory methodologies, most commonly serology and, in some cases, PCR of blood or identification of morulae in patients' blood granulocytes. From the reports to date, human infection appears to occur widely across Europe (125), particularly in central and eastern Europe and Scandinavia. European studies suggest that *A. phagocytophilum* is an important tickborne pathogen in Slovenia (93), Denmark (124), and Sweden (22). Serologic studies also support the presence of HGA infection, much of which may be asymptomatic, in potentially exposed adults in Germany (53), Bulgaria (42), Spain (113), Italy (121), Estonia (115), and Greece (44). For example, in our study in Germany (53), only 1.4% of healthy urban blood donors were seropositive while 14% of healthy forestry workers and 11% of Lyme disease patients had antibodies against *A. phagocytophilum*. Of interest, despite widespread seropositivity, there have been only a small number of well-documented, clinically consistent human cases, and the organism has not yet been isolated from European patients. Whether this means that HGA in Europe is generally milder, possibly representing a difference in the biology of the strains involved, whether some infections ascribed to *A. phagocytophilum* on the basis of serologic studies may be due to the presence of cross-reacting pathogens, or whether our knowledge is incomplete simply due to the early stage of clinical studies is not presently known. There are also scattered reports of seropositive individuals elsewhere, for example, in Israel (25).

A limited number of studies have evaluated the potential contribution of HGA as a cause of unexplained febrile illnesses in areas of endemicity either in summer or following tick bite. One prospective study of an area of Lyme disease and HGA endemicity in Wisconsin (20) evaluated 62 patients with undiagnosed summer febrile illness but without a localized rash. The study found similar numbers of patients who had acute Lyme disease without erythema migrans (11%) and HGA (13%) as the cause of their illness. In a similar series (21) from Sweden of 27 patients with fever after tick exposure, 4 patients (~15%) had HGA. In Slovenia (7), a retrospective analysis of patients referred for fever after tick bite resulted in an etiologic diagnosis in half of the patients; TBE and Lyme disease accounted for the majority of diagnoses, with HGA making up approximately 10%. Taken together, these studies suggest that among tick-exposed individuals in areas of endemicity, HGA is a significant cause of unexplained febrile illness, which has important implications for empiric therapy (see "Treatment," below).

CLINICAL MANIFESTATIONS

HGA ranges in severity from asymptomatic seroconversion to a mild febrile illness to a severe acute febrile illness that may, in rare instances, be complicated by organ failure and death. Case series (especially earlier ones, which were nearly all blood smear positive) and case reports have mostly been driven by the stage and severity of the clinical illness itself and therefore tend to overrepresent the more severe end of the disease spectrum. As mentioned (see "Epidemiology," above), older males predominate among infected individuals, infections occur predominantly in areas where and in individuals for whom ixodid tick exposure is common (often areas with known Lyme disease), and most infections occur in spring or summer. However, it is important to recognize that patients of all ages can be infected and that there may not be a prominent exposure history. Where there is a defined history of tick bite or exposure, symptom onset typically develops from 2 days to 3 weeks afterwards, most often in a 5- to 10-day window. Given the unremarkable nature of symptoms, several days often elapse before a patient seeks medical attention and until the diagnosis is suspected or proven.

Even in severe infection, the symptoms and signs of HGA are nonspecific and therefore seldom distinctive. Table 1 lists reported symptoms and their frequency from published case series (3, 9, 10, 13, 17, 20, 36, 48, 57, 67, 94). Again, the range of frequency of these findings and of laboratory abnormalities typically correlates with the variation in the overall severity

Table 1. History, signs, and symptoms of HGA infection

Symptom or sign	Frequency (%)	Additional comment(s)
Fever of >38.5°C	94–100	
Rigors	30–90	
Headache	65–90	Nuchal rigidity uncommon
Myalgia	40–100	
Arthralgia	25–60	True arthritis not seen
Nausea, anorexia	10–50	
Cough, dyspnea	20–50	Nonproductive
Mental status changes	40	Meningitis not seen
Rash	1–10	Erythematous, nonspecific; unless concomitant Lyme disease is present
Malaise	40–98	
Antecedent tick bite	40–90	

of illness in various reports and may also reflect the varying availability of detailed clinical data. As mentioned, limited information suggests that clinical and laboratory manifestations may be less severe in patients infected in Europe (22).

At the time of clinical presentation, the majority of patients describe an acute onset febrile illness, usually with rigors, headache, myalgias, and malaise. The symptoms may be severe and debilitating. Arthralgias are quite common, but true arthritis (e.g., joint swelling, redness, or limitation of motion) should suggest another diagnosis or concomitant Lyme disease (although arthritis is uncommon in early Lyme disease). Nonspecific gastrointestinal symptoms, such as nausea and anorexia, occur in half, or fewer, of HGA patients. Confusion and other mental status changes have been noted in less than half of the patients and may be subtle at times. While often described as a flu-like illness, HGA does not usually present with symptoms such as rhinorrhea. Of course, influenza is typically a winter illness in the Northern hemisphere, while HGA is usually an illness of spring and summer. Nonetheless, nonspecific cough and dyspnea have been reported in a variable proportion of HGA cases, and pneumonia or respiratory failure apparently due to acute lung injury (so-called respiratory distress syndrome) may in rare cases be a dominant feature at the time of presentation. In the absence of Lyme disease, skin rash is not a characteristic manifestation of HGA, although a nonspecific maculopapular erythematous rash has been noted in less than 10% of patients.

It is clear from serologic surveys and clinical experience that *A. phagocytophilum* infection and even clinically significant illness may resolve spontaneously

without treatment. Early recognition and initiation of appropriate treatment in an outpatient setting typically result in rapid resolution of infection. However, in undiagnosed and untreated patients or in patients treated with inappropriate or suboptimal antibiotics (see below), fever typically persists or recurs, lasting 1 to 4 weeks, and the patient worsens. Reflecting difficulties in diagnosis and treatment and the overrepresentation of more serious infections in published series, most case series report that at least half of the patients are hospitalized. In these instances, response to treatment may be less rapid or favorable, complications may develop, and severe morbidity and, in rare cases, death may occur. The death rate in reported case series ranges from 0 to 5%, although it is most likely <1% overall, even in cases of clinically evident disease.

Reported complications (Table 2) include secondary and opportunistic infections (see, for example, *Candida* esophagitis in Color Plate 8C) that may be due to the contribution of underlying diseases (e.g., leukemia and steroid therapy) (10), changes in patient immune status (e.g., lymphocyte numbers and neutrophil function) related to the HGA infection, or hospitalization and other iatrogenic factors. In addition, cases of respiratory failure of uncertain etiology clinically consistent with acute lung injury (e.g., adult respiratory distress syndrome) have occurred, as has renal failure. Cases of fatal myocarditis (72) and pericardial effusion and tamponade with infection of the pericardial fluid (57) have been reported. Isolated cases of peripheral nerve and plexus damage have also been documented (11, 70).

A few patients with underlying immune dysfunction, such as that related to pancreas and renal transplantation (1, 131, 133) or splenectomy (116) have also been noted. Such patients, while typically responding well to treatment, may have more severe disease with a higher percentage of infected neutrophils and may more frequently develop complications. In addition, treating physicians may fail to consider the possibility of tick-borne infections in such patients, given the apparent lack of exposure, the propensity for infections with more typical opportunistic pathogens with very similar manifestations (e.g., cytomegalovirus

Table 2. Reported complications of HGA

Complication	Comments
Pneumonia	No purulent secretions
Respiratory failure	
Opportunistic infection	Viral, fungal
Myocarditis	
Pericarditis	
Renal failure	
Neuropathy, plexopathy	

or Epstein-Barr virus infection, which may also be present during HGA infection), transplant organ rejection, or drug toxicity. Complicating the failure to consider HGA is the fact that the antibiotics commonly used to empirically treat fever in such patients do not typically include those active against *A. phagocytophilum*, and antivirals commonly employed have no such activity.

While apparently uncommon, a single case of reinfection with *A. phagocytophilum* has been reported (66). This patient was appropriately treated for documented infection and developed high antibody titers against the organism. However, antibody levels waned, and she developed clinically and culture-proven HGA and Lyme disease 2 years later after a tick bite, again with a robust antibody response to *A. phagocytophilum*. Possible explanations for recurrent infections include such waning antibody levels, strain variations that prevent cross-protection, and host-specific defects in immune responsiveness.

LABORATORY AND PATHOLOGIC FINDINGS

The majority of patients with HGA have nonspecific, often mild, laboratory abnormalities (Table 3) noted at the time of their clinical presentation. The frequency and intensity of such abnormalities generally increase with the severity and duration of infection until treatment or spontaneous resolution. Hematologic abnormalities, particularly mild to moderate thrombocytopenia and mild leukopenia, are common (8) and typically reach a nadir from days 5 to 7 of illness. Thrombocytopenia (as defined in published series as platelet counts of $<150 \times 10^8$/liter) is noted in ~60% of patients at presentation and ~80% of patients at some time during the course of illness. It is usually mild to moderate and is seldom associated with bleeding but can be profound. Reduced total

mean leukocyte counts (defined as $<4 \times 10^8$ cells/liter) may be noted in one-fourth of patients at presentation and in up to 70% of patients at some time during the illness. Elevated total white blood cell (WBC) counts occur in only ~5% of patients and if present should suggest another diagnosis such as a typical bacterial process. Total granulocyte counts are typically in the low-normal range with moderate elevation in the proportion of immature bands (e.g., 10 to 20% of WBCs) and total lymphocyte numbers (but not their percentage) are usually low early in illness. Atypical lymphocytes may also be noted, particularly in the second week of illness (8). As with other infectious diseases, the development of mild anemia is not uncommon after the first week of illness. Approximately one-fourth of reported patients have no hematologic abnormalities during their illness: this number would undoubtedly be higher among patients with very mild illness and those treated at an early stage.

Mild increases (e.g., up to fourfold higher than normal) in serum hepatic transaminase (aspartate aminotransferase or alanine transaminase) or lactic dehydrogenase (LDH) levels have been noted in approximately one-half of patients with confirmed HGA. Although not evaluated in large case series, nonspecific indicators of inflammation such as C-reactive protein (CRP) and the erythrocyte sedimentation rate (ESR) may be elevated; limited data suggest that the CRP is increased more often than the ESR. While the overall frequency of renal involvement is unknown, mild abnormalities in urinary sediment (e.g., proteinuria) or decreases in renal function have been reported in a variable number of patients, particularly among those with more severe or untreated infection. Although *A. phagocytophilum* can stimulate the elaboration of procoagulant tissue factor (16), significant clotting abnormalities and disseminated intravascular coagulation have rarely been reported.

Because few patients with HGA have localized disease manifestations, materials for pathological studies have been limited. Bone marrow examinations may be performed because of depressed leukocyte or platelet counts and to rule out other causes of fever. When performed, they typically show normal or increased cellularity, suggesting increased peripheral cellular destruction or sequestration of granulocytes and platelets as the major contributing factor(s) in the cytopenias. As discussed above ("Pathogenesis of Infection and Host Response"), animal models and human autopsies generally show little to no direct infection of tissues, other than among leukocytes that appear to be trafficking through them, although inflammatory changes such as hepatitis may be seen (Color Plate 8B). These findings suggest that the end organ damage in severe to fatal cases results primarily from indirect effects.

Table 3. Laboratory findings in HGA

Finding	Frequency at presentation (%)[b]	Frequency at any time in course (%)[b]
Thrombocytopenia	50–75	80
Leukopenia	10–25	50–70
Elevated hepatic transaminase(s) or LDH[a]	25–50	?
Abnormal urinalysis[a]	?	?
Elevated CRP[a]	75–100	?
ESR[a]	~50	?
Elevated creatinine[a]	Unknown	?

[a] Not systematically evaluated; information was from small numbers of sicker patients.
[b] ?, frequency not well defined.

Such effects could range from those due to *A. phago-cytophilum*-induced cytokines and/or other other effects of sepsis to local disturbances due to inflammation or vascular changes provoked by the presence of infected cells.

DIFFERENTIAL DIAGNOSIS

The differential diagnosis of fever following tick exposure is discussed in detail elsewhere (Chapter 5, "The Clinical Approach to the Patient with a Possible Tick-Borne Illness"). Tick-borne infectious diseases, including HGA, babesiosis, human monocytotropic ehrlichiosis (HME), *E. ewingii* ehrlichiosis, and other rickettsial infections (e.g., spotted fevers), must be considered in all patients with an unexplained acute febrile illness who live in or have traveled recently to areas where tick exposure is possible, even with no known tick bites. In the case of HGA, the areas of Lyme disease endemicity of the northeastern and midwestern United States are currently the major disease hotspots. As described elsewhere, HME is more common in the southeastern and central United States, while spotted fever rickettsial infections are more common in the south-central and southeast coastal regions and can also occur in the west.

The diagnosis of HGA should be suggested when a potentially tick-exposed patient presents with high fever of acute onset, chills, myalgias, and headache without another clear-cut etiology. The differential diagnosis of such a syndrome is very broad and includes a variety of rickettsial infections, early disseminated Lyme disease, relapsing fever spirochetosis, sepsis with gram-negative or gram-positive bacteria, and several noninfectious diseases. In severely ill patients and in the absence of the specific diagnostic finding of intragranulocytic morulae, general clinical evaluation should almost always include blood and urine cultures and chest radiography. Fever without localizing symptoms that persists despite broad-spectrum antibiotic regimens (not including tetracyclines) should also always raise the possibility of ehrlichial, rickettsial, or babesial infection in tick-exposed individuals. Approximately 15 to 25% of *B. burgdorferi* infections occur without a typical erythema migrans rash at the tick bite site; in this setting, early Lyme disease may present as an undifferentiated febrile syndrome with or without lymphocytic meningitis. In HGA, symptoms such as coryza, conjunctivitis, rhinorrhea, or productive cough are usually not present and are more suggestive of a primary respiratory tract infection, although nonproductive cough and dyspnea may occur in HGA. Similarly, while nausea and anorexia are not uncommon, prominent vomiting or diarrhea is more suggestive of a primary gastrointestinal process. The presence of a petechial or purpuric rash is distinctly unusual in HGA and should suggest spotted fever infection or relapsing fever as possible tick-borne causes and a variety of other possibilities, such as sepsis (particularly meningococcemia or endocarditis) or a vasculitic or hematologic disorder (such as thrombotic thrombocytopenic purpura, idiopathic thrombocytopenic purpura, or leukemia) (Chapter 5, Table 3). Initial laboratory evaluation of the patient with HGA may be normal, but the presence of thrombocytopenia, leukopenia, and/or elevated hepatic transaminase levels are suggestive of HGA, ehrlichial infection, or other rickettsial diseases. However, similar findings may occur in other forms of sepsis, vasculitis, or leukemia. While mild nonfocal central nervous system manifestations are not uncommon in HGA, a predominantly neurologic presentation or focal findings should always prompt careful evaluation for other processes, particularly bacterial meningitis, viral encephalitis, and brain abscess, and may necessitate brain imaging and lumbar puncture. HME, unlike HGA but like Lyme disease, can cause a lymphocytic meningitis syndrome and associated spinal fluid findings.

In areas where TBE occurs (also transmitted by ixodid species) (Chapter 9, "Tick-Borne Encephalitis"), the differential diagnosis of a febrile illness after tick exposure should include the early phase of TBE, in which neurological findings may be absent or nonspecific, and leukopenia and thrombocytopenia also can occur. The presence of arthralgia or of elevated CRP levels may be more common in HGA than in TBE (92). Focal findings and ataxia are more suggestive of TBE.

DIAGNOSTIC TESTING (SEE TABLE 4)

Stained Blood Smears

All patients in whom HGA is suspected should have a careful, manual evaluation of a Wright- or Giemsa-stained peripheral blood smear. This can usually be performed almost immediately at the site of care and may reveal typical intragranulocytic morulae, the raspberry-like basophilic staining colonies of *A. phagocytophilum* growing within the neutrophil's cytoplasm, usually singly (Color Plate 8A). These inclusions have been noted in 20 to 80% of patients. It is important that clinicians be aware that currently available automated blood counting and differential methods cannot detect morulae. The frequency and intensity of visibly detectable organisms are highly dependent on the duration and severity of disease; detection is also dependent on the experience and vigilance of the examiner. In very early, mild infection, only a

Table 4. Currently available HGA-specific diagnostic laboratory tests

Test	Sensitivity at presentation (%)	Sensitivity during convalescence	Comment
Peripheral blood or buffy coat smear (stained)	20–80	0	Dependent on severity, stage, and duration of infection and examiner experience and diligence; repeated smears more sensitive
Serology	30–60	70–95	Should use specific *A. phagocytophilum*-based cell culture or recombinant derived antigen(s)
			IgM may remain elevated for months and IgG may remain elevated for years; documented seroconversion or fourfold increase supports acute infection
PCR	60 to >90	0	Turns negative within 1–3 days of appropriate treatment; false positives and negatives may occur
Cultivation	40 to >90	0	Not detected by routine bacterial blood cultures; requires specialized cell culture methods and experience; turns rapidly negative once treatment initiated

small minority of patient samples may have bacteria visualized (19), whereas smears are positive in samples from most untreated patients, with severe infection evaluated several days after the onset of fever (10). Although some patients have high numbers of infected neutrophils (10 to 20%) that are easily noted, inclusions are more typically present in less than 0.1% of neutrophils. Prolonged examination and, in some cases, the use of buffy coat-enriched blood may be extremely helpful. Morulae typically rapidly diminish in number in the face of effective treatment, disappearing from the blood within 24 to 72 h. Other phenomena seen on stained blood smears may be erroneously ascribed to ehrlichial or anaplasma infection. These include crystal stain artifacts (typically refractile, needle-like, or crystalloid and present outside of or on top of cells), bacterial contamination of the stain solution (contaminating organisms typically have a coccoid or bacillary form and are also evident on control slides or slides from other patients), platelets (which have typical morphology and occur singly or in small clumps), and toxic granulations or Dohle bodies (which do not have the complex fine-stippled structure of clusters of organisms).

Serologic Testing

Serologic testing is not reliable for timely diagnosis of HGA primarily because, as in most rickettsial infections, an antibody response has usually not yet developed at the time a patient presents with acute infection. Prior to isolation of the causative organism,

assays depended on reactivity of human serum against morulae in granulocytes obtained from horses with equine granulocytic ehrlichiosis. Such cells were difficult both to obtain and use, yielding variable results. Since isolation of the organism, a variety of serologic tests have been described to detect antibodies against *A. phagocytophilum* for diagnostic purposes. Indirect immunofluorescence utilizes in vitro-infected HL60 promyelocytic leukemia cells (see "Cultivation," below) as the substrate (118) for detection of IgM and IgG antibodies, together or individually. Using cutoff values of 1:64 to 1:80, studies indicate that half or fewer of patients later proven to have HGA will be seroreactive at the time of presentation. A detectable antibody response typically develops within 2 weeks of symptom onset, and over 90% of patients with PCR- or culture-proven infection ultimately seroconvert: a fourfold rise in titer between acute and convalescent sera or an increase from titers that are undetectable to values of 1:128 or higher are usually considered diagnostic (128). Of note, seropositivity (including persistent elevation in IgM antibody in some patients), while waning in titer, typically lasts for months and sometimes years (12). Therefore, a single positive antibody titer must be interpreted in the complete clinical context and should not by itself be considered proof of the diagnosis.

Cross-reactivity in immunofluorescence assays (IFAs) has been noted between sera from patients infected with *E. chaffeensis* and *A. phagocytophilum*. This is not usually of immediate clinical importance, as both infections are similar in clinical presentation and treatment. Comparative determination of titers by IFA with the two antigens will usually yield higher values against the infecting organism. In addition, serum from HME patients will usually react against the p30 or p120 protein of *E. chaffeensis* in Western blot or recombinant protein assays but not against *A. phagocytophilum* Western blot antigens or recombinant MSP proteins (96, 118, 132). Conversely, sera from HGA but not HME patients react in Western blotting against immunogenic proteins of *A. phagocytophilum* (such as the immunodominant MSP proteins from 40 to 44 kDa and antigens at 20, 21, 28, 30, and 60 kDa) (118) or recombinant MSP (71, 146). Cross-reactivity in *A. phagocytophilum* IFAs has also been seen with sera from patients with *Bartonella* endocarditis (27). Cross-reactivity between assays for antibodies to *A. phagocytophilum* and *B. burgdorferi* has been described in some studies (141) but not others (30, 96, 98, 118); the significance and potential frequency of such cross-reactivity need to be better defined.

Several recombinant MSP2 protein-based serologic assays have been described and appear to have sensitivities similar to that of infected-cell IFAs and enhanced specificity (71, 97) as does a cell-based enzyme-based immunoassay (EIA) (118). Both a recombinant protein assay and EIA have the advantage of being adaptable to automated methods, although such methods require specialized equipment that may not always be available. One group (91) has reported that combining the analysis of results from individual EIAs or IFAs for seven different recombinant peptides, including MSP2 and several other immunoreactive antigens, further enhanced sensitivity in acute-phase sera to 85 to 95%. It would be highly desirable to improve the sensitivity of acute-phase serology to >90%. Further study and prospective evaluation of these and other recombinant-based assays are awaited.

PCR

Direct detection of *A. phagocytophilum* nucleic acids in the blood of acutely infected patients is currently the most sensitive tool for the diagnosis of acute HGA. A large number of primer sets and related techniques for a variety of gene targets (such as 16S rRNA, *groESL*, and MSP2 genes) have been described (102). Depending on the sequences used, these detect either *A. phagocytophilum* or closely related organisms (for example, *E. chaffeensis* and/or *E. ewingii*). An example of the use of broader-spectrum PCR that also detects *E. chaffeensis* in the diagnosis of acute HGA is shown in Fig. 3, which shows amplification of a

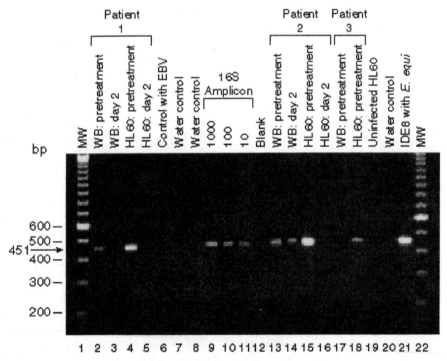

Figure 3. PCR amplification of 16S rRNA sequence from the blood of the first patients from whom the organism was isolated (57). The pretreatment detection of pathogen DNA is seen, as well as the reduction in signal soon after treatment. WB, sample of whole blood; HL60, same sample(s) following cultivation in HL60 cells. The 16S amplicon was a positive control standard with the described numbers of DNA copies used in the PCR. Tick cell line IDE infected with an equine isolate (*E. equi*, likely conspecific with *A. phagocytophilum*) is another positive control. The assay is sensitive to ~10 organisms or fewer. (Reprinted with permission from the *New England Journal of Medicine*.)

451-bp sequence from the 16S rRNA gene from the blood of the first patients from whom the organism was isolated (57). The pretreatment detection of pathogen nucleic acid is seen, as well as the reduction in signal soon after treatment. Note also that the assay is sensitive to ~10 organisms or fewer and the presence of multiple simultaneous negative controls (including water and two types of uninfected cells) included to rule out contamination of the PCR processing steps or reaction mixtures.

The diagnostic sensitivity of PCR testing of samples from patients with acute HGA has ranged from 40 to >90%, though the more-sensitive assays appear to be capable of detecting at least 80% of cases (51, 57, 126). As also seen with blood smears, patients with more severe or longstanding infection typically have higher levels of bacteremia that are easier to detect. Whole blood (EDTA or citrate preserved only, as heparin can inhibit the PCR) is the proper sample for assays in this setting; our experience indicates that serum is less sensitive and unreliable. Because of the very low numbers of organisms that are present in many patients, especially at the time of presentation, laboratories should extract DNA from at least 0.5 ml of whole blood and use an assay that attains a sensitivity of detection in the range of 1 to 10 copies. In addition, the use of gene targets that are multicopy (e.g., some MSP gene [101] or ankyrin [136] repeats) may also be advantageous, although it is important to ensure that primers for such sequences are in regions sufficiently conserved to allow their detection in multiple relevant strains of the organism. While so-called nested PCR assays (one round of initial amplification followed by another round with internal primers) may also increase sensitivity, such assays are highly prone to contamination and resultant false-positive reactions, already a significant problem with PCR, especially in laboratories that do not exercise stringent precautions. A. phagocytophilum DNA rapidly disappears with effective treatment; for this reason, PCR should generally be used only prior to therapy except in circumstances where failure of clinical response raises questions. Because even the most sensitive PCR cannot be assumed to be 100% sensitive, a negative PCR test in a seriously ill patient suspected of having HGA should not be a reason to withhold treatment (see Treatment, below). Similarly, as described, due to the extreme sensitivity of PCR assays, false positives may occur due to faulty laboratory practices. Multiple negative controls, including those taken through sample extraction steps, must be run with all clinical samples in order to ensure that contamination will be detected and positive PCR results should be interpreted carefully and in the complete clinical context.

Cultivation

The promyelocytic leukemia cell line HL60 has been used to successfully isolate A. phagocytophilum from the blood of patients with HGA (57). Because the use of this technique requires specialized cell culture facilities and expertise and because detection in cultures usually takes 2 days or more, it is not generally available or useful for clinical diagnosis. However, our laboratory's experience (56) and that of others (2) is that the technique can result in isolation of A. phagocytophilum from the blood of >90% of patients with acute infection, provided they have not received antimicrobials. HL60 cells are highly polymorphic and undergo changes in biology during passage in culture. Thus, certain sublines or highly passaged cultures may not adequately support growth of the organism. We have found (Goodman et al., unpublished data) that HL60 cell surface expression of CD15s (which we have shown to be an important carbohydrate component of the A. phagocytophilum receptor) (58, 63) correlates with cellular susceptibility and the ability to isolate organisms in vitro. Growth of the organism is typically detectable within 2 to 7 days and multiple morulae may be present in infected cells (Color Plate 8D). In addition to HL60 cells, my colleagues and I have shown that BJAB lymphoblastoid leukemia cells transfected to express CD15s and PSGL-1 are susceptible (63), as well as a variety of tick cells (108) and primary and continuous endothelial cells (109).

TREATMENT

Doxycycline, typically administered orally for 7 days (but also available for intravenous administration), is the treatment of choice for HGA and should generally be used in all patients 8 years of age or older in whom the disease is suspected, unless pregnant or if there is a documented history of severe allergy or other severe adverse reaction to doxycycline or tetracyclines (Table 5). Doxycycline is highly active against A. phagocytophilum in vitro (68, 80, 103), and there has been no documented inherent or acquired antimicrobial resistance to doxycycline among anaplasmas or in other rickettsial or ehrlichial pathogens. It is also worth emphasizing that doxycycline has the important attribute of being highly active against B. burgdorferi, a frequent coinfecting agent, although longer courses of doxycycline (e.g., 14 to 21 days) should be given if B. burgdorferi coinfection is clinically suspected. In areas where Lyme disease is endemic, coinfection of patients with HGA with B. burgdorferi may occur in up to one-fourth to one-third of individuals. For this reason, many clinicians

Table 5. Treatment of *A. phagocytophilum* infection

Patient category	Recommended treatment and dosage[a]	Potential alternatives[a]	Comments and warnings
Adults, children 8 yrs or older	Doxycycline 100 mg BID p.o. or i.v. for 7 days; treat for 14–21 days if coinfection with Lyme disease is prevalent or clinically suspected	Rifampin 300 mg p.o. BID or levofloxacin 500 mg p.o. daily for 7 days (no reported clinical experience)	Efficacy of other antibiotics compared to doxycycline is unproven; use only if doxycycline contraindicated (e.g., documented severe allergy or, potentially, pregnant women or children of <8 yrs with mild disease)
Children of <8 yrs; severe illness	Consult specialist; doxycycline 4 mg/kg of body wt/day for 7 days may be preferred (see Comments and Warnings)	Consult specialist; rifampin 10 mg/kg/day p.o. BID for 7 days	See text; doxycycline may cause dental staining in children of <8 yrs; efficacy of rifampin compared to doxycycline unproven
Children of <8 yrs; mild illness	Consult specialist; rifampin 10 mg/kg p.o. BID for 7 days	Consult specialist; doxycycline 4 mg/kg/day for 7 days (see Comments and Warnings)	Efficacy of rifampin compared to doxycycline unproven; if patient worsens or fails to respond in 24 h and diagnosis confirmed, change to doxycycline; doxycycline may cause staining of permanent teeth and affect bones (see text)
Pregnant women Severe disease — Mild to moderate disease	Consult specialist Doxycycline 100 mg BID p.o. or i.v. for 7 days Rifampin 300 mg p.o. BID	(See Comments and Warnings)	Efficacy of rifampin compared to doxycycline unproven; if patient worsens or fails to respond in 24 h and diagnosis confirmed, change to doxycycline; doxycycline may cause staining of permanent teeth and affect bones (see text)

[a] p.o., orally; i.v., intravenously; BID, twice a day.

choose to treat all HGA patients with at least 2 weeks of doxycycline. In addition, doxycycline is active against many other infections that may occur following tick exposure and have similar clinical manifestations that could be confused with HGA, including rickettsiosis, ehrlichiosis, and tick-borne relapsing fever. A notable exception is babesiosis, which is not susceptible to doxycycline and is usually treated with clindamycin and quinine (Chapter 20).

The clinical response of HGA to doxycycline is usually dramatic, with marked improvement in both well being and fever within 24 to 48 h, typically accompanied by a reduction in the number of infected blood neutrophils. The absence of such a response should suggest another diagnosis, a complicating tick-borne coinfection (such as babesiosis), or a secondary nosocomial infection that is not doxycycline susceptible. Organ dysfunction complicating untreated severe HGA, such as pulmonary, renal, or nervous system involvement, may take longer to respond and may require continuing supportive care.

In vitro susceptibility testing for infectious disease agents and, particularly, for intracellular pathogens can be technically challenging and may not always predict clinical response. It is particularly important that an antibiotic used against intracellular organisms be able to rapidly and easily enter into infected cells and their relevant subcellular compartments and that the antibiotic then kill the organism rather than simply inhibit its growth. Methods used for *A. phagocytophilum* susceptibility testing have been based on determining antibiotic effects on growth of the organism in HL60 cells (68, 80, 103). MICs and, in two studies, minimum bactericidal concentrations (MBCs) required for killing have been determined for a variety of *A. phagocytophilum* strains and anti-infective agents. These studies have yielded generally consistent results with excellent activity (both MICs and MBCs well below recommended cutoffs) against the organism for doxycycline (MIC, ≤ 0.25 μg/ml), rifampin (≤ 0.125 μg/ml), rifabutin (< 0.125 μg/ml), and some newer generation fluoroquinolones including levofloxacin (≤1 μg/ml), and trovafloxacin (no longer generally available; MIC, ≤0.032 μg/ml). The activity of other fluoroquinolones, ofloxacin, and ciprofloxacin was examined in only one study but was significantly less, with a MIC of ofloxacin (2 μg/ml) or ciprofloxacin (2 μg/ml) at or above the recommended cutoffs for susceptibility. *A. phagocytophilum* was found to be resistant to a broad variety of other antimicrobials tested and commonly used in clinical practice, including β-lactam agents (amoxicillin, ampicillin, ceftriaxone, and imipenam-cilastatin), macrolides (erythromycin, azithromycin, and clarithromycin), clindamycin, trimethoprim-sulfamethoxazole, and aminoglycosides (amikacin and gentamicin). Of interest, chloramphenicol, an agent commonly used for the treatment of rickettsial infections but not highly active against *E. chaffeensis* (26), was not generally active with variable MICs that generally exceeded the recommended achievable concentrations.

Some patients cannot receive doxycycline due to severe allergy or intolerance. Furthermore, the use of tetracyclines (including doxycycline) is not generally recommended in children younger than 8 years old or in pregnant women, due to the risk of dental staining and possible adverse effects on bone growth. Potential alternatives to doxycycline include rifampin, which is not only highly active in vitro but has apparently been effective in four cases, including two in pregnancy (29) (the doses employed were not specified) and two in young children (84). As described above, levofloxacin is active in vitro, but there are no reported data concerning its clinical effectiveness. In addition, the use of fluoroquinolones in pregnant women and young children is not generally recommended, due to concerns about articular toxicity. Given the limited experience with alternative agents for severely ill individuals proven or highly likely to have HGA, the benefits of therapy with doxycycline may outweigh the potential risks. Consultation with a pediatric infectious diseases specialist or the CDC is recommended to assist in evaluation. In early, mild, and non-life-threatening infections of pregnant women and children younger than 8 years old, it may be reasonable to consider a trial of initial therapy with rifampin.

As described, initiation of therapy with doxycycline is typically followed by dramatic clinical improvement within 24 to 48 h; the absence of such a clinical response must lead to careful reconsideration of the diagnosis and a search for other or additional disease processes. In general, patients treated early do not require hospitalization; patients without severe end-organ damage or complications of hospitalization do well and fully recover. At this time, there are no well-documented cases of failure of appropriate antibiotics to treat the infection itself or of persistent infection

with *A. phagocytophilum*. One study (117) found that, when compared to matched controls, patients who recovered from HGA reported more fever, sweats, and fatigue in subsequent months. The cause of such persistent symptoms is unclear but may be related to the severity and resultant postinfectious aftermath of the acute infection.

PREVENTION

There is currently no simple approach to prevention of *A. phagocytophilum* infection. As with other tick-borne pathogens, avoidance of areas of high tick density and efforts to cover exposed skin to prevent tick attachment are simple but difficult-to-achieve approaches (Chapter 4). Recommendations include wearing long sleeves and long pants tucked into socks, but this approach is very difficult in warm weather, particularly for people with active lifestyles. Because *Ixodes* ticks may often be relatively easily dislodged early on and because infection transmission usually does not occur until at least 24 h after attachment, measures to detect and/or detach ticks are advised. These include showering and briskly toweling off after outside activity, and careful inspection of skin for ticks, particularly of children. Prophylactic use of doxycycline after a known tick bite has been studied for prevention of Lyme disease. A single dose is effective in preventing Lyme disease, but the incidence of side effects typically exceeds the incidence of Lyme disease transmission, even in areas of endemicity (110). This approach would likely produce similar results in HGA prevention but is not generally recommended even for Lyme disease (142), which is generally more common in ticks, due to the fact that only a very small proportion of recognized tick bites are likely to transmit infection, typically ~1 to 4% even for *B. burgdorferi*. Thus, large numbers of individuals would be exposed to antibiotic therapy, presumably requiring multiple treatments during each tick season, to provide limited benefit. Undesirable outcomes could include not only direct ones (e.g., adverse effects) but also the development of antimicrobial resistance in other organisms both in treated individuals and in the community.

There are currently no known effective vaccines to prevent HGA disease in humans. Both the relatively low number of cases currently reported and the availability of simple and effective treatment for the disease make it unlikely that a human vaccine will be commercially developed for routine use in the near future. As described earlier, immune serum can reduce infection rates after challenge in mouse models. This suggests that a vaccine producing a robust and long-lived antibody response could have at least some efficacy. As previously discussed, antibody alone may not be fully protective against an infection that is generally relatively protected within an intracellular compartment. Induction of effective cellular responses, both innate and specific, may be needed to totally prevent or control infection. Development of a cell culture-based vaccine will also be affected by the challenge of finding a suitable well-characterized cell substrate for commercial vaccine production. An additional concern that will need to be overcome in developing a vaccine, whether based on culture-derived organisms or recombinant DNA or protein technologies, is that antigenic variation may make cross-protection among multiple strains difficult to achieve.

The veterinary experience (81) with vaccines for bovine anaplasmosis caused by the closely related *A. marginale* suggests that such considerations may apply. In general, vaccines, derived in the past from infected bovine erythrocytes and more recently from infected tick cells (82), and whether live attenuated, killed, or more recently recombinant protein or DNA based, provide only partial protection and may not always offer cross-protection against diverse strains. Because veterinary *Anaplasma* infections can be of considerable economic importance, it is possible that both a better understanding of critical components of host immunity, including specific protective antibody and cellular immune responses, and the successful development of effective vaccine strategies will first be accomplished through studies in livestock, the results of which can then help inform approaches to preventing human infection with *A. phagocytophilum*.

Acknowledgments. I thank Gary Wormser and Ulrike Munderloh for their helpful reviews and comments.

This work has been supported by the National Institute of Allergy and Infectious Diseases (NIH) and by the Center for Biologics Evaluation and Research (FDA).

REFERENCES

1. Adachi, J. A., E. M. Grimm, P. Johnson, M. Uthman, B. Kaplan, and R. M. Rakita. 1997. Human granulocytic ehrlichiosis in a renal transplant patient: case report and review of the literature. *Transplantation* 64:1139–1142.

2. Aguero-Rosenfeld, M. E. 2003. Laboratory aspects of tick-borne diseases: Lyme, human granulocytic ehrlichiosis and babesiosis. *Mt. Sinai J. Med.* 70:197–206.

3. Aguero-Rosenfeld, M. E., H. W. Horowitz, G. P. Wormser, D. F. McKenna, J. Nowakowski, J. Munoz, and J. S. Dumler. 1996. Human granulocytic ehrlichiosis: a case series from a medical center in New York State. *Ann. Intern. Med.* 125:904–908.

4. Akkoyunlu, M., and E. Fikrig. 2000. Gamma interferon dominates the murine cytokine response to the agent of human granulocytic ehrlichiosis and helps to control the degree of early rickettsemia. *Infect. Immun.* 68:1827–1833.

5. Akkoyunlu, M., S. E. Malawista, J. Anguita, and E. Fikrig. 2001. Exploitation of interleukin-8-induced neutrophil chemotaxis by the agent of human granulocytic ehrlichiosis. *Infect. Immun.* 69:5577–5588.

6. Arens, M. Q., A. M. Liddell, G. Buening, M. Gaudreault-Keener, J. W. Sumner, J. A. Comer, R. S. Buller, and G. A. Storch. 2003. Detection of Ehrlichia spp. in the blood of wild white-tailed deer in Missouri by PCR assay and serologic analysis. *J. Clin. Microbiol.* 41:1263–1265.

7. Arnez, M., T. Luznik-Bufon, T. Avsic-Zupanc, E. Ruzic-Sabljic, M. Petrovec, S. Lotric-Furlan, and F. Strle. 2003. Causes of febrile illnesses after a tick bite in Slovenian children. *Pediatr. Infect. Dis. J.* 22:1078–1083.

8. Bakken, J. S., M. E. Aguero-Rosenfeld, R. L. Tilden, G. P. Wormser, H. W. Horowitz, J. T. Raffalli, M. Baluch, D. Riddell, J. J. Walls, and J. S. Dumler. 2001. Serial measurements of hematologic counts during the active phase of human granulocytic ehrlichiosis. *Clin. Infect. Dis.* 32:862–870.

9. Bakken, J. S., and J. S. Dumler. 2000. Human granulocytic ehrlichiosis. *Clin. Infect. Dis.* 31:554–560.

10. Bakken, J. S., J. S. Dumler, S. M. Chen, M. R. Eckman, L. L. Van Etta, and D. H. Walker. 1994. Human granulocytic ehrlichiosis in the upper Midwest United States. A new species emerging? *JAMA* 272:212–218.

11. Bakken, J. S., S. A. Erlemeyer, R. J. Kanoff, T. C. Silvestrini, D. D. Goodwin, and J. S. Dumler. 1998. Demyelinating polyneuropathy associated with human granulocytic ehrlichiosis. *Clin. Infect. Dis.* 27:1323–1324.

12. Bakken, J. S., I. Haller, D. Riddell, J. J. Walls, and J. S. Dumler. 2002. The serological response of patients infected with the agent of human granulocytic ehrlichiosis. *Clin. Infect. Dis.* 34:22–27.

13. Bakken, J. S., J. Krueth, C. Wilson-Nordskog, R. L. Tilden, K. Asanovich, and J. S. Dumler. 1996. Clinical and laboratory characteristics of human granulocytic ehrlichiosis. *JAMA* 275:199–205.

14. Banerjee, R., J. Anguita, and E. Fikrig. 2000. Granulocytic ehrlichiosis in mice deficient in phagocyte oxidase or inducible nitric oxide synthase. *Infect. Immun.* 68:4361–4362.

15. Banerjee, R., J. Anguita, D. Roos, and E. Fikrig. 2000. Cutting edge: infection by the agent of human granulocytic ehrlichiosis prevents the respiratory burst by down-regulating gp91phox. *J. Immunol.* 164:3946–3949.

16. Behl, R., M. B. Klein, L. Dandelet, R. R. Bach, J. L. Goodman, and N. S. Key. 2000. Induction of tissue factor procoagulant activity in myelomonocytic cells inoculated by the agent of human granulocytic ehrlichiosis. *Thromb. Haemost.* 83:114–118.

17. Belongia, E. A., K. D. Reed, P. D. Mitchell, P. H. Chyou, N. Mueller-Rizner, M. F. Finkel, and M. E. Schriefer. 1999. Clinical and epidemiological features of early Lyme disease and human granulocytic ehrlichiosis in Wisconsin. *Clin. Infect. Dis.* 29:1472–1477.

18. Belongia, E. A., K. D. Reed, P. D. Mitchell, C. P. Kolbert, D. H. Persing, J. S. Gill, and J. J. Kazmierczak. 1997. Prevalence of granulocytic Ehrlichia infection among white-tailed deer in Wisconsin. *J. Clin. Microbiol.* 35:1465–1468.

19. Belongia, E. A., K. D. Reed, P. D. Mitchell, N. Mueller-Rizner, M. Vandermause, M. F. Finkel, and J. J. Kazmierczak. 2001. Tickborne infections as a cause of nonspecific febrile illness in Wisconsin. *Clin. Infect. Dis.* 32:1434–1439.

20. Bjoersdorff, A., J. Berglund, B. E. Kristiansen, C. Soderstrom, and I. Eliasson. 1999. Varying clinical picture and course of human granulocytic ehrlichiosis. Twelve Scandinavian cases of the new tick-borne zoonosis are presented. *Lakartidningen* 96:4200–4204. (In Swedish.)

21. Bjoersdorff, A., B. Wittesjo, J. Berglun, R. F. Massung, and I. Eliasson. 2002. Human granulocytic ehrlichiosis as a common cause of tick-associated fever in southeast Sweden: report from a prospective clinical study. *Scand. J. Infect. Dis.* 34:187–191.

22. Blanco, J. R., and J. A. Oteo. 2002. Human granulocytic ehrlichiosis in Europe. *Clin. Microbiol. Infect.* 8:763–772.

23. Borjesson, D. L., S. I. Simon, E. Hodzic, C. M. Ballantyne, and S. W. Barthold. 2002. Kinetics of CD11b/CD18 up-regulation during infection with the agent of human granulocytic ehrlichiosis in mice. *Lab. Investig.* 82:303–311.

24. Brandsma, A. R., S. E. Little, J. M. Lockhart, W. R. Davidson, D. E. Stallknecht, and J. E. Dawson. 1999. Novel Ehrlichia organism (Rickettsiales: Ehrlichieae) in white-tailed deer associated with lone star tick (Acari: Ixodidae) parasitism. *J. Med. Entomol.* 36:190–194.

25. Brouqui, P., and J. S. Dumler. 2000. Serologic evidence of human monocytic and granulocytic ehrlichiosis in Israel. *Emerg. Infect. Dis.* 6:314–315.

26. Brouqui, P., and D. Raoult. 1992. In vitro antibiotic susceptibility of the newly recognized agent of ehrlichiosis in humans, *Ehrlichia chaffeensis*. *Antimicrob. Agents Chemother.* 36:2799–2803.

27. Brouqui, P., E. Salvo, J. S. Dumler, and D. Raoult. 2001. Diagnosis of granulocytic ehrlichiosis in humans by immunofluorescence assay. *Clin. Diagn. Lab. Immunol.* 8:199–202.

28. Brown, W. C., V. Shkap, D. Zhu, T. C. McGuire, W. Tuo, T. F. McElwain, and G. H. Palmer. 1998. CD4$^+$ T-lymphocyte and immunoglobulin G2 responses in calves immunized with *Anaplasma marginale* outer membranes and protected against homologous challenge. *Infect. Immun.* 66:5406–5413.

29. Buitrago, M. I., J. W. Ijdo, P. Rinaudo, H. Simon, J. Copel, J. Gadbaw, R. Heimer, E. Fikrig, and F. J. Bia. 1998. Human granulocytic ehrlichiosis during pregnancy treated successfully with rifampin. *Clin. Infect. Dis.* 27:213–215.

30. Bunnell, J. E., L. A. Magnarelli, and J. S. Dumler. 1999. Infection of laboratory mice with the human granulocytic ehrlichiosis agent does not induce antibodies to diagnostically significant Borrelia burgdorferi antigens. *J. Clin. Microbiol.* 37:2077–2079.

31. Bunnell, J. E., E. R. Trigiani, S. R. Srinivas, and J. S. Dumler. 1999. Development and distribution of pathologic lesions are related to immune status and tissue deposition of human granulocytic ehrlichiosis agent-infected cells in a murine model system. *J. Infect. Dis.* 180:546–550.

32. Burkot, T. R., G. O. Maupin, B. S. Schneider, C. Denatale, C. M. Happ, J. S. Rutherford, and N. S. Zeidner. 2001. Use of a sentinel host system to study the questing behavior of *Ixodes spinipalpis* and its role in the transmission of *Borrelia bissettii*, human granulocytic ehrlichiosis, and *Babesia microti*. *Am. J. Trop. Med. Hyg.* 65:293–299.

33. Carlyon, J. A., M. Akkoyunlu, L. Xia, T. Yago, T. Wang, R. D. Cummings, R. P. McEver, and E. Fikrig. 2003. Murine neutrophils require α1,3-fucosylation but not PSGL-1 for productive infection with *Anaplasma phagocytophilum*. *Blood* 102:3387–3395.

34. Carlyon, J. A., W. T. Chan, J. Galan, D. Roos, and E. Fikrig. 2002. Repression of rac2 mRNA expression by *Anaplasma phagocytophila* is essential to the inhibition of superoxide production and bacterial proliferation. *J. Immunol.* 169:7009–7018.

35. Carlyon, J. A., D. A. Latif, M. Pypaert, P. Lacy, and E. Fikrig. 2004. *Anaplasma phagocytophilum* utilizes multiple host evasion mechanisms to thwart NADPH oxidase-mediated killing during neutrophil infection. *Infect. Immun.* 72:4772–4783.

36. Centers for Disease Control and Prevention. 1995. Human granulocytic ehrlichiosis—New York, 1995. *JAMA* 274:867.

37. Centers for Disease Control and Prevention. 2004. Summary of notifiable diseases—United States 2002. *Morb. Mortal. Wkly. Rep.* 51:1–84.

38. Chang, Y. F., V. Novosel, C. F. Chang, J. B. Kim, S. J. Shin, and D. H. Lein. 1998. Detection of human granulocytic ehrlichiosis agent and *Borrelia burgdorferi* in ticks by polymerase chain reaction. *J. Vet. Diagn. Investig.* 10:56–59.

39. Chaput, E. K., J. I. Meek, and R. Heimer. 2002. Spatial analysis of human granulocytic ehrlichiosis near Lyme, Connecticut. *Emerg. Infect. Dis.* 8:943–948.

40. Chen, S. M., J. S. Dumler, J. S. Bakken, and D. H. Walker. 1994. Identification of a granulocytotropic *Ehrlichia* species as the etiologic agent of human disease. *J. Clin. Microbiol.* 32:589–595.

41. Choi, K. S., D. G. Scorpio, and J. S. Dumler. 2004. *Anaplasma phagocytophilum* ligation to toll-like receptor (TLR) 2, but not to TLR4, activates macrophages for nuclear factor-kappa B nuclear translocation. *J. Infect. Dis.* 189:1921–1925.

42. Christova, I. S., and J. S. Dumler. 1999. Human granulocytic ehrlichiosis in Bulgaria. *Am. J. Trop. Med. Hyg.* 60:58–61.

43. Cinco, M., D. Padovan, R. Murgia, M. Heldtander, and E. O. Engvall. 1998. Detection of HGE agent-like *Ehrlichia* in *Ixodes ricinus* ticks in northern Italy by PCR. *Wien. Klin. Wochenschr.* 110:898–900.

44. Daniel, S. A., K. Manika, M. Arvanitidou, E. Diza, N. Symeonidis, and A. Antoniadis. 2002. Serologic evidence of human granulocytic ehrlichiosis, Greece. *Emerg. Infect. Dis.* 8:643–644.

45. Daniels, T. J., G. R. Battaly, D. Liveris, R. C. Falco, and I. Schwartz. 2002. Avian reservoirs of the agent of human granulocytic ehrlichiosis? *Emerg. Infect. Dis.* 8:1524–1525.

46. des Vignes, F., and D. Fish. 1997. Transmission of the agent of human granulocytic ehrlichiosis by host-seeking *Ixodes scapularis* (Acari: Ixodidae) in southern New York state. *J. Med. Entomol.* 34:379–382.

47. des Vignes, F., J. Piesman, R. Heffernan, T. L. Schulze, K. C. Stafford III, and D. Fish. 2001. Effect of tick removal on transmission of *Borrelia burgdorferi* and *Ehrlichia phagocytophila* by *Ixodes scapularis* nymphs. *J. Infect. Dis.* 183:773–778.

48. Dumler, J. S., and J. S. Bakken. 1996. Human granulocytic ehrlichiosis in Wisconsin and Minnesota: a frequent infection with the potential for persistence. *J. Infect. Dis.* 173:1027–1030.

49. Dumler, J. S., A. F. Barbet, C. P. Bekker, G. A. Dasch, G. H. Palmer, S. C. Ray, Y. Rikihisa, and F. R. Rurangirwa. 2001. Reorganization of genera in the families *Rickettsiaceae* and *Anaplasmataceae* in the order *Rickettsiales*: unification of some species of *Ehrlichia* with *Anaplasma*, *Cowdria* with *Ehrlichia* and *Ehrlichia* with *Neorickettsia*, descriptions of six new species combinations and designation of *Ehrlichia equi* and 'HGE agent' as subjective synonyms of *Ehrlichia phagocytophila*. *Int. J. Syst. Evol. Microbiol.* 51:2145–2165.

50. Dumler, J. S., E. R. Trigiani, J. S. Bakken, M. E. Aguero-Rosenfeld, and G. P. Wormser. 2000. Serum cytokine responses during acute human granulocytic ehrlichiosis. *Clin. Diagn. Lab. Immunol.* 7:6–8.

51. Edelman, D. C., and J. S. Dumler. 1996. Evaluation of an improved PCR diagnostic assay for human granulocytic ehrlichiosis. *Mol. Diagn.* 1:41–49.

52. Edelson, B. T., and E. R. Unanue. 2001. Intracellular antibody neutralizes Listeria growth. *Immunity* 14:503–512.

53. Fingerle, V., J. L. Goodman, R. C. Johnson, T. J. Kurtti, U. G. Munderloh, and B. Wilske. 1997. Human granulocytic

ehrlichiosis in southern Germany: increased seroprevalence in high-risk groups. *J. Clin. Microbiol.* **35**:3244–3247.

54. Fingerle, V., U. G. Munderloh, G. Liegl, and B. Wilske. 1999. Coexistence of ehrlichiae of the phagocytophila group with *Borrelia burgdorferi* in *Ixodes ricinus* from southern Germany. *Med. Microbiol. Immunol. (Berlin)* **188**:145–149.

55. Gardner, S. L., R. C. Holman, J. W. Krebs, R. Berkelman, and J. E. Childs. 2003. National surveillance for the human ehrlichioses in the United States, 1997–2001, and proposed methods for evaluation of data quality. *Ann. N. Y. Acad. Sci.* **990**:80–89.

56. Goodman, J. L., and Herron, M. J. Unpublished data.

57. Goodman, J. L., C. Nelson, B. Vitale, J. E. Madigan, J. S. Dumler, T. J. Kurtti, and U. G. Munderloh. 1996. Direct cultivation of the causative agent of human granulocytic ehrlichiosis. *N. Engl. J. Med.* **334**:209–215.

58. Goodman, J. L., C. M. Nelson, M. B. Klein, S. F. Hayes, and B. W. Weston. 1999. Leukocyte infection by the granulocytic ehrlichiosis agent is linked to expression of a selectin ligand. *J. Clin. Investig.* **103**:407–412.

59. Greig, B., K. M. Asanovich, P. J. Armstrong, and J. S. Dumler. 1996. Geographic, clinical, serologic, and molecular evidence of granulocytic ehrlichiosis, a likely zoonotic disease, in Minnesota and Wisconsin dogs. *J. Clin. Microbiol.* **34**:44–48.

60. Gribble, D. H. 1969. Equine ehrlichiosis. *J. Am. Vet. Med. Assoc.* **155**:462–469.

61. Hayes, S. F., C. M. Nelson, and J. L. Goodman. The life cycle of *A. phagocytophilum* in human cells. Unpublished data.

62. Herron, M. J., and J. L. Goodman. 2001. Proceedings, 16th American Society for Rickettsiology Annual Meeting.

63. Herron, M. J., C. M. Nelson, J. Larson, K. R. Snapp, G. S. Kansas, and J. L. Goodman. 2000. Intracellular parasitism by the human granulocytic ehrlichiosis bacterium through the P-selectin ligand, PSGL-1. *Science* **288**:1653–1656.

64. Reference deleted.

65. Hodzic, E., D. Fish, C. M. Maretzki, A. M. De Silva, S. Feng, and S. W. Barthold. 1998. Acquisition and transmission of the agent of human granulocytic ehrlichiosis by *Ixodes scapularis* ticks. *J. Clin. Microbiol.* **36**:3574–3578.

66. Horowitz, H. W., M. Aguero-Rosenfeld, J. S. Dumler, D. F. McKenna, T. C. Hsieh, J. Wu, I. Schwartz, and G. P. Wormser. 1998. Reinfection with the agent of human granulocytic ehrlichiosis. *Ann. Intern. Med.* **129**:461–463.

67. Horowitz, H. W., M. E. Aguero-Rosenfeld, D. F. McKenna, D. Holmgren, T. C. Hsieh, S. A. Varde, S. J. Dumler, J. M. Wu, I. Schwartz, Y. Rikihisa, and G. P. Wormser. 1998. Clinical and laboratory spectrum of culture-proven human granulocytic ehrlichiosis: comparison with culture-negative cases. *Clin. Infect. Dis.* **27**:1314–1317.

68. Horowitz, H. W., T. C. Hsieh, M. E. Aguero-Rosenfeld, F. Kalantarpour, I. Chowdhury, G. P. Wormser, and J. M. Wu. 2001. Antimicrobial susceptibility of Ehrlichia phagocytophila. *Antimicrob. Agents Chemother.* **45**:786–788.

69. Horowitz, H. W., E. Kilchevsky, S. Haber, M. Aguero-Rosenfeld, R. Kranwinkel, E. K. James, S. J. Wong, F. Chu, D. Liveris, and I. Schwartz. 1998. Perinatal transmission of the agent of human granulocytic ehrlichiosis. *N. Engl. J. Med.* **339**:375–378.

70. Horowitz, H. W., S. J. Marks, M. Weintraub, and J. S. Dumler. 1996. Brachial plexopathy associated with human granulocytic ehrlichiosis. *Neurology* **46**:1026–1029.

71. Ijdo, J. W., C. Wu, L. A. Magnarelli, and E. Fikrig. 1999. Serodiagnosis of human granulocytic ehrlichiosis by a recombinant HGE-44-based enzyme-linked immunosorbent assay. *J. Clin. Microbiol.* **37**:3540–3544.

72. Jahangir, A., C. Kolbert, W. Edwards, P. Mitchell, J. S. Dumler, and D. H. Persing. 1998. Fatal pancarditis associated with human granulocytic ehrlichiosis in a 44-year-old man. *Clin. Infect. Dis.* **27**:1424–1427.

73. Jauron, S. D., C. M. Nelson, V. Fingerle, M. D. Ravyn, J. L. Goodman, R. C. Johnson, R. Lobentanzer, B. Wilske, and U. G. Munderloh. 2001. Host cell-specific expression of a p44 epitope by the human granulocytic ehrlichiosis agent. *J. Infect. Dis.* **184**:1445–1450.

74. Kalantarpour, F., I. Chowdhury, G. P. Wormser, and M. E. Aguero-Rosenfeld. 2000. Survival of the human granulocytic ehrlichiosis agent under refrigeration conditions. *J. Clin. Microbiol.* **38**:2398–2399.

75. Katavolos, P., P. M. Armstrong, J. E. Dawson, and S. R. Telford III. 1998. Duration of tick attachment required for transmission of granulocytic ehrlichiosis. *J. Infect. Dis.* **177**:1422–1425.

76. Kim, H. Y., and Y. Rikihisa. 2000. Expression of interleukin-1β, tumor necrosis factor alpha, and interleukin-6 in human peripheral blood leukocytes exposed to human granulocytic ehrlichiosis agent or recombinant major surface protein P44. *Infect. Immun.* **68**:3394–3402.

77. Klein, M. B., S. F. Hayes, and J. L. Goodman. 1998. Monocytic differentiation inhibits infection and granulocytic differentiation potentiates infection by the agent of human granulocytic ehrlichiosis. *Infect. Immun.* **66**:3410–3415.

78. Klein, M. B., S. Hu, C. C. Chao, and J. L. Goodman. 2000. The agent of human granulocytic ehrlichiosis induces the production of myelosuppressing chemokines without induction of proinflammatory cytokines. *J. Infect. Dis.* **182**:200–205.

79. Klein, M. B., J. S. Miller, C. M. Nelson, and J. L. Goodman. 1997. Primary bone marrow progenitors of both granulocytic and monocytic lineages are susceptible to infection with the agent of human granulocytic ehrlichiosis. *J. Infect. Dis.* **176**:1405–1409.

80. Klein, M. B., C. M. Nelson, and J. L. Goodman. 1997. Antibiotic susceptibility of the newly cultivated agent of human granulocytic ehrlichiosis: promising activity of quinolones and rifamycins. *Antimicrob. Agents Chemother.* **41**:76–79.

81. Kocan, K. M., J. de la Fuente, A. A. Guglielmone, and R. D. Melendez. 2003. Antigens and alternatives for control of Anaplasma marginale infection in cattle. *Clin. Microbiol. Rev.* **16**:698–712.

82. Kocan, K. M., T. Halbur, E. F. Blouin, V. Onet, J. de la Fuente, J. C. Garcia-Garcia, and J. T. Saliki. 2001. Immunization of cattle with Anaplasma marginale derived from tick cell culture. *Vet. Parasitol.* **102**:151–161.

83. Kramer, V. L., M. P. Randolph, L. T. Hui, W. E. Irwin, A. G. Gutierrez, and D. J. Vugia. 1999. Detection of the agents of human ehrlichioses in ixodid ticks from California. *Am. J. Trop. Med. Hyg.* **60**:62–65.

84. Krause, P. J., C. L. Corrow, and J. S. Bakken. 2003. Successful treatment of human granulocytic ehrlichiosis in children using rifampin. *Pediatrics* **112**:e252–e253.

85. Layfield, D., and P. Guilfoile. 2002. The prevalence of *Borrelia burgdorferi* (Spirochaetales: spirochaetaceae) and the agent of human granulocytic ehrlichiosis (Rickettsiaceae: Ehrlichieae) in *Ixodes scapularis* (Acari: Ixodidae) collected during 1998 and 1999 from Minnesota. *J. Med. Entomol.* **39**:218–220.

85a. Lee, H. C., J. Han, R. K. Purr, and J. L. Goodman. 2004. *Anaplasma phagocytophilum* inhibits human neutrophil apoptosis through multiple molecular pathways: genomic studies. FDA 2004 Science Forum.

86. Lepidi, H., J. E. Bunnell, M. E. Martin, J. E. Madigan, S. Stuen, and J. S. Dumler. 2000. Comparative pathology,

and immunohistology associated with clinical illness after *Ehrlichia phagocytophila*-group infections. *Am. J. Trop. Med. Hyg.* 62:29–37.

87. Levin, M. L., F. des Vignes, and D. Fish. 1999. Disparity in the natural cycles of *Borrelia burgdorferi* and the agent of human granulocytic ehrlichiosis. *Emerg. Infect. Dis.* 5:204–208.

88. Levin, M. L., W. L. Nicholson, R. F. Massung, J. W. Sumner, and D. Fish. 2002. Comparison of the reservoir competence of medium-sized mammals and *Peromyscus leucopus* for *Anaplasma phagocytophilum* in Connecticut. *Vector Borne Zoonotic Dis.* 2:125–136.

89. Little, S. E., D. E. Stallknecht, J. M. Lockhart, J. E. Dawson, and W. R. Davidson. 1998. Natural coinfection of a white-tailed deer (*Odocoileus virginianus*) population with three *Ehrlichia* spp. *J. Parasitol.* 84:897–901.

90. Liz, J. S., J. W. Sumner, K. Pfister, and M. Brossard. 2002. PCR detection and serological evidence of granulocytic ehrlichial infection in roe deer (*Capreolus capreolus*) and chamois (*Rupicapra rupicapra*). *J. Clin. Microbiol.* 40:892–897.

91. Lodes, M. J., R. Mohamath, L. D. Reynolds, P. McNeill, C. P. Kolbert, E. S. Bruinsma, D. R. Benson, E. Hofmeister, S. G. Reed, R. L. Houghton, and D. H. Persing. 2001. Sero-diagnosis of human granulocytic ehrlichiosis by using novel combinations of immunoreactive recombinant proteins. *J. Clin. Microbiol.* 39:2466–2476.

92. Lotric-Furlan, S., M. Petrovec, T. Avsic-Zupanc, and F. Strle. 2003. Comparison of patients fulfilling criteria for confirmed and probable human granulocytic ehrlichiosis. *Ann. N. Y. Acad. Sci.* 990:344–345.

93. Lotric-Furlan, S., M. Petrovec, T. Avsic-Zupanc, and F. Strle. 2003. Human granulocytic ehrlichiosis in Slovenia. *Ann. N. Y. Acad. Sci.* 990:279–284.

94. Lotric-Furlan, S., M. Petrovec, T. A. Zupanc, W. L. Nicholson, J. W. Sumner, J. E. Childs, and F. Strle. 1998. Human granulocytic ehrlichiosis in Europe: clinical and laboratory findings for four patients from Slovenia. *Clin. Infect. Dis.* 27:424–428.

95. Madigan, J. E., and D. Gribble. 1987. Equine ehrlichiosis in northern California: 49 cases (1968–1981). *J. Am. Vet. Med. Assoc.* 190:445–448.

96. Magnarelli, L., J. Ijdo, C. Wu, and E. Fikrig. 2001. Recombinant protein-44-based class-specific enzyme-linked immunosorbent assays for serologic diagnosis of human granulocytic ehrlichiosis. *Eur. J. Clin. Microbiol. Infect. Dis.* 20:482–485.

97. Magnarelli, L. A., J. W. Ijdo, S. J. Padula, R. A. Flavell, and E. Fikrig. 2000. Serologic diagnosis of Lyme borreliosis by using enzyme-linked immunosorbent assays with recombinant antigens. *J. Clin. Microbiol.* 38:1735–1739.

98. Magnarelli, L. A., K. C. Stafford III, T. N. Mather, M. T. Yeh, K. D. Horn, and J. S. Dumler. 1995. Hemocytic rickettsia-like organisms in ticks: serologic reactivity with antisera to ehrlichiae and detection of DNA of agent of human granulocytic ehrlichiosis by PCR. *J. Clin. Microbiol.* 33:2710–2714.

99. Magnarelli, L. A., K. C. Stafford III, T. N. Mather, M. T. Yeh, K. D. Horn, and J. S. Dumler. 1995. Hemocytic rickettsia-like organisms in ticks: serologic reactivity with antisera to ehrlichiae and detection of DNA of agent of human granulocytic ehrlichiosis by PCR. *J. Clin. Microbiol.* 33:2710–2714.

100. Martin, M. E., K. Caspersen, and J. S. Dumler. 2001. Immunopathology and ehrlichial propagation are regulated by interferon-gamma and interleukin-10 in a murine model of human granulocytic ehrlichiosis. *Am. J. Pathol.* 158:1881–1888.

101. Massung, R. F., K. Slater, J. H. Owens, W. L. Nicholson, T. N. Mather, V. B. Solberg, and J. G. Olson. 1998. Nested PCR assay for detection of granulocytic ehrlichiae. *J. Clin. Microbiol.* 36:1090–1095.

102. Massung, R. F., and K. G. Slater. 2003. Comparison of PCR assays for detection of the agent of human granulocytic ehrlichiosis, *Anaplasma phagocytophilum*. *J. Clin. Microbiol.* 41:717–722.

103. Maurin, M., J. S. Bakken, and J. S. Dumler. 2003. Antibiotic susceptibilities of *Anaplasma* (*Ehrlichia*) *phagocytophilum* strains from various geographic areas in the United States. *Antimicrob. Agents Chemother.* 47:413–415.

104. McGarey, D. J., A. F. Barbet, G. H. Palmer, T. C. McGuire, and D. R. Allred. 1994. Putative adhesins of *Anaplasma marginale*: major surface polypeptides 1a and 1b. *Infect. Immun.* 62:4594–4601.

105. McQuiston, J. H., C. D. Paddock, R. C. Holman, and J. E. Childs. 1999. The human ehrlichioses in the United States. *Emerg. Infect. Dis.* 5:635–642.

106. Morozova, O. V., A. K. Dobrotvorsky, N. N. Livanova, S. E. Tkachev, V. N. Bakhvalova, A. B. Beklemishev, and F. C. Cabello. 2002. PCR detection of *Borrelia burgdorferi* sensu lato, tick-borne encephalitis virus, and the human granulocytic ehrlichiosis agent in *Ixodes persulcatus* ticks from western Siberia, Russia. *J. Clin. Microbiol.* 40:3802–3804.

107. Mott, J., R. E. Barnewall, and Y. Rikihisa. 1999. Human granulocytic ehrlichiosis agent and *Ehrlichia chaffeensis* reside in different cytoplasmic compartments in HL-60 cells. *Infect. Immun.* 67:1368–1378.

108. Munderloh, U. G., S. D. Jauron, V. Fingerle, L. Leitritz, S. F. Hayes, J. M. Hautman, C. M. Nelson, B. W. Huberty, T. J. Kurtti, G. G. Ahlstrand, B. Greig, M. A. Mellencamp, and J. L. Goodman. 1999. Invasion and intracellular development of the human granulocytic ehrlichiosis agent in tick cell culture. *J. Clin. Microbiol.* 37:2518–2524.

109. Munderloh, U. G., M. J. Lynch, M. J. Herron, A. T. Palmer, T. J. Kurtti, R. D. Nelson, and J. L. Goodman. 2004. Infection of endothelial cells with *Anaplasma marginale* and *A. phagocytophilum*. *Vet. Microbiol.* 101:53–64.

110. Nadelman, R. B., J. Nowakowski, D. Fish, R. C. Falco, K. Freeman, D. McKenna, P. Welch, R. Marcus, M. E. Aguero-Rosenfeld, D. T. Dennis, and G. P. Wormser. 2001. Prophylaxis with single-dose doxycycline for the prevention of Lyme disease after an *Ixodes scapularis* tick bite. *N. Engl. J. Med.* 345:79–84.

111. Nicholson, W. L., M. B. Castro, V. L. Kramer, J. W. Sumner, and J. E. Childs. 1999. Dusky-footed wood rats (*Neotoma fuscipes*) as reservoirs of granulocytic ehrlichiae (*Rickettsiales*: *Ehrlichieae*) in northern California. *J. Clin. Microbiol.* 37:3323–3327.

112. Ogden, N. H., Z. Woldehiwet, and C. A. Hart. 1998. Granulocytic ehrlichiosis: an emerging or rediscovered tick-borne disease? *J. Med. Microbiol.* 47:475–482.

113. Oteo, J. A., H. Gil, M. Barral, A. Perez, S. Jimenez, J. R. Blanco, V. Martinez de Artola, V. A. Garcia-Perez, and R. A. Juste. 2001. Presence of granulocytic ehrlichia in ticks and serological evidence of human infection in La Rioja, Spain. *Epidemiol. Infect.* 127:353–358.

114. Pancholi, P., C. P. Kolbert, P. D. Mitchell, K. D. Reed, Jr., J. S. Dumler, J. S. Bakken, S. R. Telford III, and D. H. Persing. 1995. *Ixodes dammini* as a potential vector of human granulocytic ehrlichiosis. *J. Infect. Dis.* 172:1007–1012.

115. Prukk, T., K. Ainsalu, E. Laja, and A. Aigro. 2003. Human granulocytic ehrlichiosis in Estonia. *Emerg. Infect. Dis.* 9:1499–1500.

116. Rabinstein, A., V. Tikhomirov, A. Kaluta, N. Gelfmann, P. Iannini, and L. Edwards. 2000. Recurrent and prolonged fever in asplenic patients with human granulocytic ehrlichiosis. *QJM* 93:198–201.

117. Ramsey, A. H., E. A. Belongia, C. M. Gale, and J. P. Davis. 2002. Outcomes of treated human granulocytic ehrlichiosis cases. *Emerg. Infect. Dis.* 8:398–401.

118. Ravyn, M. D., J. L. Goodman, C. B. Kodner, D. K. Westad, L. A. Coleman, S. M. Engstrom, C. M. Nelson, and R. C. Johnson. 1998. Immunodiagnosis of human granulocytic ehrlichiosis by using culture-derived human isolates. *J. Clin. Microbiol.* 36:1480–1488.

119. Reubel, G. H., R. B. Kimsey, J. E. Barlough, and J. E. Madigan. 1998. Experimental transmission of *Ehrlichia equi* to horses through naturally infected ticks (*Ixodes pacificus*) from northern California. *J. Clin. Microbiol.* 36:2131–2134.

120. Richter, P. J., Jr., R. B. Kimsey, J. E. Madigan, J. E. Barlough, J. S. Dumler, and D. L. Brooks. 1996. *Ixodes pacificus* (Acari: Ixodidae) as a vector of *Ehrlichia equi* (Rickettsiales: Ehrlichieae). *J. Med. Entomol.* 33:1–5.

121. Ruscio, M., and M. Cinco. 2003. Human granulocytic ehrlichiosis in Italy: first report on two confirmed cases. *Ann. N. Y. Acad. Sci.* 990:350–352.

122. Saint, A. A., N. M. Blackwell, L. R. Hall, A. Hoerauf, N. W. Brattig, L. Volkmann, M. J. Taylor, L. Ford, A. G. Hise, J. H. Lass, E. Diaconu, and E. Pearlman. 2002. The role of endosymbiotic *Wolbachia* bacteria in the pathogenesis of river blindness. *Science* 295:1892–1895.

123. Schwartz, I., D. Fish, and T. J. Daniels. 1997. Prevalence of the rickettsial agent of human granulocytic ehrlichiosis in ticks from a hyperendemic focus of Lyme disease. *N. Engl. J. Med.* 337:49–50.

124. Skarphedinsson, S., P. Sogaard, and C. Pedersen. 2001. Seroprevalence of human granulocytic ehrlichiosis in high-risk groups in Denmark. *Scand. J. Infect. Dis.* 33:206–210.

125. Strle, F. 2004. Human granulocytic ehrlichiosis in Europe. *Int. J. Med. Microbiol.* 293(Suppl. 37):27–35.

126. Sumner, J. W., W. L. Nicholson, and R. F. Massung. 1997. PCR amplification and comparison of nucleotide sequences from the *groESL* heat shock operon of *Ehrlichia* species. *J. Clin. Microbiol.* 35:2087–2092.

127. Sun, W., J. W. Ijdo, S. R. Telford III, E. Hodzic, Y. Zhang, S. W. Barthold, and E. Fikrig. 1997. Immunization against the agent of human granulocytic ehrlichiosis in a murine model. *J. Clin. Investig.* 100:3014–3018.

128. Task Force on Consensus Approach for Ehrlichiosis (CAFE). 2000. Diagnosing human ehrlichioses: current status and recommendations. *ASM News* 66:277–280.

129. Taylor, G. A., C. G. Feng, and A. Sher. 2004. p47 GTPases: regulators of immunity to intracellular pathogens. *Nat. Rev. Immunol.* 4:100–109.

130. Telford, S. R., III, J. E. Dawson, P. Katavolos, C. K. Warner, C. P. Kolbert, and D. H. Persing. 1996. Perpetuation of the agent of human granulocytic ehrlichiosis in a deer tick-rodent cycle. *Proc. Natl. Acad. Sci. USA* 93:6209–6214.

131. Trofe, J., K. S. Reddy, R. J. Stratta, S. D. Flax, K. T. Somerville, R. R. Alloway, M. F. Egidi, M. H. Shokouh-Amiri, and A. O. Gaber. 2001. Human granulocytic ehrlichiosis in pancreas transplant recipients. *Transpl. Infect. Dis.* 3:34–39.

132. Unver, A., S. Felek, C. D. Paddock, N. Zhi, H. W. Horowitz, G. P. Wormser, L. C. Cullman, and Y. Rikihisa. 2001. Western blot analysis of sera reactive to human monocytic ehrlichiosis and human granulocytic ehrlichiosis agents. *J. Clin. Microbiol.* 39:3982–3986.

133. Vannorsdall, M. D., S. Thomas, R. P. Smith, R. Zimmerman, R. Christman, and J. P. Vella. 2002. Human granulocytic ehrlichiosis in a renal allograft recipient: review of the clinical spectrum of disease in solid organ transplant patients. *Transpl. Infect. Dis.* 4:97–101.

134. Varde, S., J. Beckley, and I. Schwartz. 1998. Prevalence of tick-borne pathogens in *Ixodes scapularis* in a rural New Jersey county. *Emerg. Infect. Dis.* 4:97–99.

135. Von Loewenich, F. D., D. G. Scorpio, U. Reischl, J. S. Dumler, and C. Bogdan. 2004. Frontline: control of *Anaplasma phagocytophilum*, an obligate intracellular pathogen, in the absence of inducible nitric oxide synthase, phagocyte NADPH oxidase, tumor necrosis factor, Toll-like receptor (TLR) 2 and TLR4, or the TLR adaptor molecule MyD88. *Eur. J. Immunol.* 34:1789–1797.

136. Walls, J. J., P. Caturegli, J. S. Bakken, K. M. Asanovich, and J. S. Dumler. 2000. Improved sensitivity of PCR for diagnosis of human granulocytic ehrlichiosis using *epank1* genes of *Ehrlichia phagocytophila*-group ehrlichiae. *J. Clin. Microbiol.* 38:354–356.

137. Walls, J. J., B. Greig, D. F. Neitzel, and J. S. Dumler. 1997. Natural infection of small mammal species in Minnesota with the agent of human granulocytic ehrlichiosis. *J. Clin. Microbiol.* 35:853–855.

138. Webster, P., J. W. Ijdo, L. M. Chicoine, and E. Fikrig. 1998. The agent of human granulocytic ehrlichiosis resides in an endosomal compartment. *J. Clin. Investig.* 101:1932–1941.

139. Whist, S. K., A. K. Storset, G. M. Johansen, and H. J. Larsen. 2003. Modulation of leukocyte populations and immune responses in sheep experimentally infected with *Anaplasma* (formerly *Ehrlichia*) *phagocytophilum*. *Vet. Immunol. Immunopathol.* 94:163–175.

140. Woldehiwet, Z. 1983. Tick-borne fever: a review. *Vet. Res. Commun.* 6:163–175.

141. Wormser, G. P., H. W. Horowitz, J. Nowakowski, D. McKenna, J. S. Dumler, S. Varde, I. Schwartz, C. Carbonaro, and M. Aguero-Rosenfeld. 1997. Positive Lyme disease serology in patients with clinical and laboratory evidence of human granulocytic ehrlichiosis. *Am. J. Clin. Pathol.* 107:142–147.

142. Wormser, G. P., R. B. Nadelman, R. J. Dattwyler, D. T. Dennis, E. D. Shapiro, A. C. Steere, T. J. Rush, D. W. Rahn, P. K. Coyle, D. H. Persing, D. Fish, and B. J. Luft. 2000. Practice guidelines for the treatment of Lyme disease. Guideline from the Infectious Diseases Society of America. *Clin. Infect. Dis.* 31(Suppl. 1):1–14.

143. Yago, T., A. Leppanen, A. Carlyon, M. Akkoyunlu, S. Karmakar, E. Fikrig, R. D. Cummings, and R. P. McEver. 2003. Structurally distinct requirements for binding of P-selectin glycoprotein ligand-1 and sialyl Lewis x to Anaplasma phagocytophilum and P-selectin. *J. Biol. Chem.* 278:37987–37997.

144. Yoshiie, K., H. Y. Kim, J. Mott, and Y. Rikihisa. 2000. Intracellular infection by the human granulocytic ehrlichiosis agent inhibits human neutrophil apoptosis. *Infect. Immun.* 68:1125–1133.

145. Zeidner, N. S., T. R. Burkot, R. Massung, W. L. Nicholson, M. C. Dolan, J. S. Rutherford, B. J. Biggerstaff, and G. O. Maupin. 2000. Transmission of the agent of human granulocytic ehrlichiosis by *Ixodes spinipalpis* ticks: evidence of an enzootic cycle of dual infection with *Borrelia burgdorferi* in northern Colorado. *J. Infect. Dis.* 182:616–619.

146. Zhi, N., N. Ohashi, Y. Rikihisa, H. W. Horowitz, G. P. Wormser, and K. Hechemy. 1998. Cloning and expression of the 44-kilodalton major outer membrane protein gene of the human granulocytic ehrlichiosis agent and application of the recombinant protein to serodiagnosis. *J. Clin. Microbiol.* 36:1666–1673.

Tick-Borne Diseases of Humans
Edited by Jesse L. Goodman et al.
© 2005 ASM Press, Washington, D.C.

Chapter 14

Human Monocytotropic Ehrlichiosis

J. E. DAWSON, S. A. EWING, W. R. DAVIDSON, J. E. CHILDS, S. E. LITTLE, AND S. M. STANDAERT

HISTORY

Prior to 1987, physicians often referred to patients with undiagnosed febrile illnesses and a history of exposure to ticks as possible victims of "Rocky Mountain spotless fever," an unofficial catchall term that likely included ehrlichiosis (68). The somewhat whimsical name was derived from Rocky Mountain spotted fever (RMSF) caused by *Rickettsia rickettsii*. Other physicians favored regional names for puzzling cases that resembled RMSF, such as "Oklahoma tick fever" (132). When a paper (93) was published in 1987 implicating *Ehrlichia canis* as a human pathogen, wheels were set in motion that led to a sizable body of literature that concerns what is now called human monocytotropic ehrlichiosis (HME), owing to the causative agent's tropism for monocytes. The patient reported by Maeda (93) was from Michigan and had traveled to rural Arkansas, where he had been bitten by ticks in late March 1986. He was critically ill with fever and confusion when hospitalized in mid-April in Michigan. A presumptive diagnosis of RMSF was made even though no rash or petechiae were observed. He was treated with chloramphenicol and, when anemia and thrombocytopenia persisted, switched to doxycycline. The patient was hospitalized for 12 weeks; follow-up after discharge indicated that hematologic, renal, and hepatic parameters returned to normal (93).

Questions were soon raised about the likelihood that *E. canis*, a well-known pathogen of dogs transmitted by the brown dog tick, *Rhipicephalus sanguineus*, was the pathogen involved in this index case of HME (58). Subsequently, an agent genetically closely related to *E. canis* was isolated from a soldier stationed at Fort Chaffee Army Base in northwestern Arkansas and named *Ehrlichia chaffeensis* (3). HME is a zoonotic disease. Thus, although well established in the literature, it is a bit misleading to refer to the disease caused by *E. chaffeensis* in a way that implies that human beings are anything other than minor, dead-end hosts for the causative agent. Like most tick-borne diseases, the life cycle involves ticks and wild vertebrate hosts, and human beings become involved accidentally. Even after HME became well known to the medical community, diagnosis remained problematic due both to its clinical presentation as a nonspecific illness and to its mimicry of RMSF, circumstances that may lead to delays in appropriate therapy.

Soon after *E. chaffeensis* was discovered and recognized as distinct from *E. canis* (1991) efforts were begun to identify its tick vectors and natural vertebrate hosts. Successful culture of *E. chaffeensis* negated the early need to use *E. canis* as a source of surrogate antigen and enabled more refined serologic studies of HME in human beings and candidate vertebrate reservoir hosts (35). These serologic studies implicated white-tailed deer as likely reservoir hosts (39), and evidence of naturally occurring infection of this host was found (90, 91). Experiments were conducted that confirmed that deer were susceptible to experimental infection (40). Previously, dogs had been shown to be susceptible to experimental infection (37); but it had also been determined earlier, before the etiologic agent was isolated and differentiated from *E. canis*, that dogs were not involved in transmitting ehrlichial infection to human beings (68, 133).

Fairly soon after *E. chaffeensis* was isolated, evidence was found that ticks could harbor the bacterium (4). The lone star tick, *Amblyomma americanum* (Acari: Ixodidae), was implicated (5) and its potential to serve as a vector was confirmed experimentally (59). Evidence was then found to implicate this widely

J. E. Dawson • Chelan-Douglas Health District, 200 Valley Mall Pkwy., East Wenatchee, WA 98802.   **S. A. Ewing** • 224 Veterinary Medicine, Oklahoma State University, Stillwater, OK 74078.   **W. R. Davidson** • Southeast Cooperative Wildlife Disease Study, College of Veterinary Medicine, University of Georgia, Athens, GA 30602.   **J. E. Childs** • Department of Biology, 2101 Rollins Basic Science Building, 1510 Clifton Rd. NE, Atlanta, GA 30602.   **S. E. Little** • Department of Microbiology and Parasitology, College of Veterinary Medicine, University of Georgia, Athens, GA 30602.   **S. M. Standaert** • 3525 Ensign Rd. NE, Suite 02, Olympia, WA 98506.

distributed and abundant tick as a vector under natural conditions in the southeastern United States (89).

From this brief history of HME, it is clear that rapid progress in understanding this newly emerged tick-borne zoonosis was facilitated both by its successful cultivation and by experimental studies of ticks linked to field observations. Epidemiological studies were furthered through the use of molecular techniques, and knowledge of HME expanded rapidly in the early to mid-1990s.

BIOLOGY OF THE ETIOLOGIC AGENT

Classification

Recently, a proposal for the reorganization of the order *Rickettsiales* in the families *Rickettsiaceae* and *Anaplasmataceae* was accepted (52). The order was emended by the elimination of the tribes *Rickettsieae*, *Ehrlichieae*, *Wolbachieae*, and *Anaplasmatacieae* (52).

The family *Anaplasmataceae* was broadened to include all species of the α-*Proteobacteria* presently contained in the genera *Ehrlichia*, *Anaplasma*, *Cowdria*, *Wolbachia*, and *Neorickettsia*. The veterinary pathogen *Cowdria ruminantium* was placed in the genus *Ehrlichia* along with the existing species *E. canis*, *E. chaffeensis*, *Ehrlichia ewingii*, and *Ehrlichia muris*.

Cellular Localization and Ultrastructure

Like other bacteria, members of the genus *Ehrlichia* possess a cell wall and plasma membrane (130). The members of this genus are nonmotile gram-negative intracellular bacteria characterized by parasitism of reticuloendothelial cells, especially leukocytes (131). The organisms invade leukocytes but phagolysosomal fusion does not occur; the organisms are protected within cytoplasmic vacuoles (Fig. 1) from lysosomal enzymes and form pleomorphic, coccoid to ellipsoid bodies, which grow to about 0.5 μm in diameter

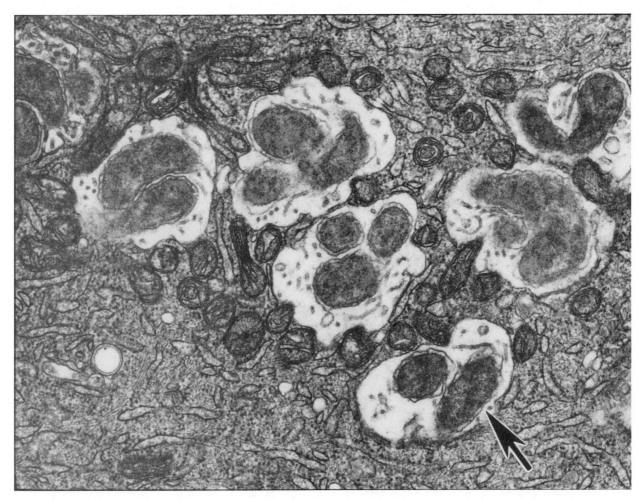

Figure 1. Electron micrograph of *E. chaffeensis* in the cytoplasm of a macrophage. Photograph appears courtesy of Cynthia Goldsmith (CDC).

within 48 h following infection. The elementary bodies divide by binary fission within the phagosome, forming a few tightly packed pleomorphic bodies (immature inclusions) 0.5 to 2.5 μm in diameter. The host leukocyte increases in size during the next 7 to 12 days as the bodies continue to divide. During the late stages of this cycle, some organisms may be visualized when blood smears are examined by Giemsa staining (Color Plate 9A), immunohistochemistry (IHC), or in situ hybridization (ISH) (44). Up to 50 organisms may be found in a mature inclusion, called a morula, and these organisms are released into the bloodstream and/or tissues when the cell lyses. Alternatively, the infected monocyte may divide, retaining morulae in each new cell; in this situation, the organisms may be protected from the extracellular environment (64). Not surprisingly, intracellular division of these organisms alters the function of the host cell with important implications for understanding pathogenesis and for devising therapeutic strategies (51).

Pathogenesis of Infection

Patients usually develop thrombocytopenia, leukopenia, and anemia (55). Bone marrow biopsy samples are usually hypercellular with myeloid hyperplasia and megakaryocytosis (49) and frequently contain noncaseating granulomas (Color Plate 9C). The cytopenias result from peripheral sequestration or destruction rather than bone marrow failure (51).

Another common laboratory finding is elevation of serum hepatic transaminase levels (55). Hepatic pathologic changes have been observed, including scattered lobular lymphohistocytic infiltrates, Kupffer cell hyperplasia with increased phagocytosis, focal necrosis, hepatocyte injury and cell death (Color Plate 9D), bile duct epithelial injury, and microvesicular steatosis (51). In severe cases, autopsies may reveal pulmonary hemorrhage, interstitial pneumonia, focal necrosis not only of the liver but also of the spleen and lymph nodes, multisystem perivascular lymphohistiocytic infiltrates, and extensive hemophagocytosis in the spleen, liver, lymph nodes, and bone marrow (48).

Recovery from infection is associated with the production of antibodies to the surface-exposed 120-kDa glycoprotein and one or more members of the 28-kDa proteins, T-cell lymphocytosis in the blood, and the development of granulomas in infected tissues (51). Gamma interferon (IFN-γ), produced by T-helper cells, cytotoxic lymphocytes, and natural killer (NK) cells, has an important role in the clearance of intracellular bacteria (113). In vitro studies have shown that IFN-γ activates intracellular killing of E. chaffeensis by macrophages in association with the reduction of transferrin receptors (129). If infection of the

cell occurs before IFN-γ activation, this inhibition of E. chaffeensis through iron starvation can be circumvented by the organism through upregulation of cellular transferrin receptor mRNA production (51). IFN-γ has no antiehrlichial effect 24 h after infection because binding of viable E. chaffeensis to macrophages blocks IFN-γ-induced tyrosine phosphorylation of host cell signal transduction pathway proteins by increasing protein kinase A activity, which in turn inhibits several monocyte-macrophage activation pathways (129). Reactive oxygen intermediates generated by activated macrophages have also been proposed as effectors that kill ehrlichia (51). However, E. chaffeensis-infected macrophages become refractory to lipopolysaccharide (LPS)-induced, reactive-oxygen-species-mediated antiehrlichial activity in association with downregulation of NF-κβ (nuclear transcription factor) activation.

Cytokine responses to infection have been investigated in the susceptible THP-1 macrophage-derived cell line. Proinflammatory cytokines such as tumor necrosis factor alpha (TNF-α), interleukin-6 (IL-6), or granulocyte-macrophage colony-stimulating factor mRNA expression are not induced while IL-1β, IL-8, and IL-10, an immunosuppressive cytokine, are (82, 129). However, if antibody against E. chaffeensis is added to the culture system, TNF-α, IL-6, and IL-1β are produced at levels similar to those seen after LPS stimulation (83). These cytokines are activated by sustained degradation of Iκβ-α and activation and nuclear translocation of NF-κβ as occurs with LPS stimulation (83). This result suggests that at later stages of the disease after patients develop antibodies, proinflammatory cytokines may be generated and could contribute to the development of clinical symptoms, pathologic findings, and immune protection (129).

Animal Models

The ideal animal model would use E. chaffeensis or a closely related ehrlichia and produce significant disease in immunocompetent animals with histopathologic findings similar to those observed with HME (144).

Numerous investigators have inoculated E. chaffeensis into immunocompetent mouse strains such as BALB/c, C3H/HeJ, C3H/HeN, C.B.-17, and DBA (92, 153). All have been resistant to development of disease manifestations. A disease model in immunodeficient mice has been developed (164). Severe disease was produced with a fatal outcome. However, histopathologic lesions that differ from those in humans were observed, and immunological studies were not performed. Recently, two animal models were developed using strain HF, an ehrlichial organism closely related to *E. chaffeensis*, that was isolated from *Ixodes ovatus* ticks in Japan (141). C57BL/6 mice became ill on postinoculation day 7 and died on day 9 (144). Confluent necrosis was observed in the liver along with apoptosis, poorly formed granulomas, Kupffer cell hyperplasia, erythrophagocytosis, and microvesicular fatty metamorphosis. Other histologic observations included marked expansion of the marginal zone and infiltration of the red pulp of the spleen by macrophages, interstitial pneumonitis, and increased numbers of immature myeloid cells and areas of necrosis in the bone marrow. Organisms were detected in the liver, lungs, and spleen. The main target cells were macrophages, including Kupffer cells, hepatocytes, and endothelial cells. Apoptosis was detected in Kupffer cells, hepatocytes, and macrophages in the lungs and spleen.

Similarly, BALB/c mice inoculated with the HF strain developed fatal illness (113). On day 9 postinoculation, the liver showed large multifocal necrotic foci around central veins and in the midregion of the lobules. More than half of the liver tissue was necrotic. A few morulae were present in the cytoplasm of endothelial and Kupffer cells, but no morulae were observed in the necrotic lesions. Monocytes were increased in number in the sinuses of the spleens and in lymph nodes. Numerous morulae were present in the cytoplasm of endothelial cells of capillaries of Peyer's patches, in capillaries of solitary follicles of the large intestine, and in veins of perifollicular areas in the spleen. Morulae were also noted in endothelial cells within capillaries in the thymus and bone marrow. Bone marrow cellularity was markedly decreased, and many apoptotic bodies and hemorrhages were found. In the liver and lungs, many monocytes, some adherent to endothelium, were found in central veins and venules, respectively. A few morulae were present in alveolar endothelial cells and macrophages. In the glomerular zone of the adrenal cortex, focal infiltration by lymphocytes and macrophages was seen. Numerous morulae were observed in endothelial cells and in monocytes and macrophages of various tissues, suggesting that intercellular spread of organisms freely occurred between endothelial cells and monocytes and macrophages. The tropism for macrophages and pathologic lesions closely resemble that of HME (44). Although *E. chaffeensis* infection of endothelial cells in humans has not been described, the organism has been cultivated in vitro in an endothelial cell line (38).

NATURAL HISTORY

In the eastern United States, *E. chaffeensis* is maintained in an epizootic cycle involving the lone star tick (*A. americanum*) as the principal vector and the white-tailed deer (*Odocoileus virginianus*) as a major vertebrate reservoir (90, 91). White-tailed deer are the keystone host for *A. americanum* larvae, nymphs, and adults (12, 13, 67, 120). This critical vector-host association places these two species at the core of *E. chaffeensis* epizootiology and strongly influences its geographic distribution and seasonality of transmission. Although lone star ticks and deer are central to the epizootiology of HME, natural exposure to or infection with *E. chaffeensis* may occur in other wild and domestic mammals, and there is some evidence that other tick species may also serve as vectors, albeit in a limited capacity.

Tick Vectors

Soon after the recognition of clinical HME, *A. americanum* (Color Plates 1A and 2A to E) was suggested as a potential vector, based on the geographic distribution of cases (55), and *E. chaffeensis* DNA was then detected in lone star ticks from Kentucky, Missouri, and North Carolina (5). Transstadial transmission of *E. chaffeensis* by both nymph and adult *A. americanum* ticks was confirmed experimentally among white-tailed deer with larvae and nymphs that had been acquisition fed on needle-inoculated deer (59). *E. chaffeensis* infection of *A. americanum* has been verified by PCR detection in nymphs and adults from at least 10 states (Alabama, Arkansas, Connecticut, Georgia, Indiana, Kansas, Kentucky, Maryland, Missouri, North Carolina, New Jersey, Rhode Island, and Virginia) (5, 18, 70, 71, 90, 134, 149, 162, 165). Estimated infection frequencies have ranged from less than 1% to as high as 29% among wild, unfed nymph and adult ticks in these studies. Infection has not been confirmed in unfed *A. americanum* larvae, supporting the assumption that transovarial transmission either does not occur or is rare.

The lone star tick is a prolific, three-host tick, but it generally has only one generation per year (1, 17). Host-seeking adults are most abundant in spring and early summer, nymphs are most abundant in spring through fall, and larvae are most abundant in late summer and early fall, with slight geographic variations in specific timing of activity (32, 120, 138, 143). The spring and summer periods of peak activity of nymphs and adults correlate with the occurrence of human cases (43, 55, 159). Adults and nymphs routinely overwinter, while larvae rarely do so (32). Whether nymphs or adults are more important as sources of human infection is unclear, but both stages probably play roles in transmission among reservoir hosts.

Compared to *A. americanum*, other species of ticks play a very limited role, if any, in *E. chaffeensis* transmission. Attempted experimental transmission by the Gulf Coast tick (*A. maculatum*) was unsuccessful (77), and deer populations parasitized by *A. maculatum*, unlike *A. americanum*, do not have antibodies to *E. chaffeensis* (89). Positive PCR assays for *E. chaffeensis* DNA have been reported from American dog ticks (*Dermacentor variabilis*) collected from either hosts or the environment in Arkansas (4), California (80), and Missouri (134) and from western black-legged ticks (*Ixodes pacificus*) in California (80). Although the PCR primers used in these studies are considered specific for *E. chaffeensis*, none of the products were sequenced or confirmed by other assays, leaving the identity of the organism(s) unconfirmed.

Vertebrate Reservoir Hosts

Serologic surveys have disclosed *E. chaffeensis*-reactive antibodies in white-tailed deer, an animal closely associated with *A. americanum*, across a broad region of the eastern United States (39, 41, 71, 85, 86, 88–91, 109, 148). Antibody prevalences of 50% or higher have been routinely detected. Similarly, PCR-based surveys have detected *E. chaffeensis* DNA in blood and tissues of deer in Arkansas, Georgia, Kentucky, North Carolina, Oklahoma, and South Carolina (85–87, 90, 91, 167). Experimental infection of white-tailed deer by needle inoculation or tick bite (*A. americanum*) has consistently resulted in rickettsemia and seroconversion without clinical illness and in one study caused persistent infection with intermittent bacteremia of several months' duration (34, 40, 59). White-tailed deer were first confirmed as reservoirs hosts when *E. chaffeensis* was isolated from blood of 14% of deer from two populations in Georgia (91). Later, *E. chaffeensis* was isolated from blood or lymph nodes of deer in Arkansas and Georgia (86, 167). Field studies have also disclosed significant temporal (88) and spatial correlations (71, 88–91, 109, 148) between lone star tick infestations and *E. chaffeensis* infection in deer populations.

Lone star ticks and white-tailed deer clearly are critical components in the ecology of *E. chaffeensis*, and both provide mechanisms for persistence of the organism over winter. However, *E. chaffeensis* is not necessarily restricted to this single vector-vertebrate host relationship. All stages of lone star ticks will feed on a variety of wild and domestic animals (1).

Within the recognized enzootic region, serologic surveys have disclosed *E. chaffeensis*-reactive antibodies among other wild and domestic animals commonly parasitized by *A. americanum* including raccoons (*Procyon lotor*) (29, 90), opossums (*Didelphis maruspialis*) (90), red foxes (*Vulpes vulpes*), gray foxes (*Urocyon cinereoargenteus*) (J. E. Dawson, unpublished data),

dogs (42, 79, 110), and goats (47). In contrast, serologic testing of several species of wild rodents and a small number of eastern cottontails (*Sylvilagus floridanus*) from a confirmed enzootic site in Georgia failed to detect *E. chaffeensis*-reactive antibodies (90), although seropositive white-footed mice (11%) were reported from Connecticut (94).

Naturally occurring *E. chaffeensis* infection has been confirmed by PCR in dogs (42, 79, 110) and goats (47), as well as coyotes (*Canis latrans*) (78). Furthermore, experimentally infected dogs (37) and red foxes (33) seroconvert and develop rickettsemia. Interestingly, gray foxes were refractory to experimental infection (33), suggesting that caution should be used in interpreting positive serologic results among wild animals.

Vector-Vertebrate Reservoir-Human Interface

Lone star ticks occur across much of eastern North America, roughly encompassing a region from eastern Mexico to southern Iowa to New Jersey but also including limited portions of New York, Connecticut, Rhode Island, and Massachusetts (Color Map 5) (1). Lone star ticks readily and commonly bite humans (56, 60), and a lone star tick-infested deer population was identified as an important risk factor for human infection (145). A preponderance of HME cases and (based on serologic surveys) relatively high exposure rates occur within the geographic range of *A. americanum* (96, 104).

The distribution of *A. americanum* within this large region of endemicity is discontinuous (89), with considerable portions of several states free of the tick and presumably with lower risk of human infection. Assessment of infection rates in deer to better delineate the distribution of *E. chaffeensis* has been suggested (34, 39, 86, 89, 91). This concept has been applied successfully on a relatively fine (county) scale (71, 109, 148, 168, 169). Monitoring of deer has disclosed that they also harbor and are likely important in the ecology of other zoonotic or potentially zoonotic tick-vectored agents. These include *E. ewingii* (167), an undescribed *Ehrlichia*-like agent (41, 85, 86, 90), and the southern tick-associated rash illness organism, "*Borellia lonestari*" (106), all of which are associated with or known to be transmitted by *A. americanum*. White-tailed deer may also serve as hosts for *Anaplasma phagocytophilum*, the causative agent of human granulocytic anaplasmosis (11, 86, 95, 158). The occurrence of multiple ehrlichiae within deer has important implications for interpreting the results of serologic and molecular testing (85, 167). Additional research on the natural history of *E. chaffeensis* and the constellation of pathogens associated with its vector and vertebrate reservoir hosts will help further the understanding of the health risk from tick-borne diseases to humans in this region.

EPIDEMIOLOGY OF HUMAN DISEASE

HME caused by *E. chaffeensis* is endemic to the United States, with residents in the southeastern and south-central states at highest risk; each of the >20 existing isolates of *E. chaffeensis* was obtained from patients or animals within this region (24, 116, 147). Although human infections ascribed to *E. chaffeensis* have been reported from other countries (e.g., Mali [155] and Korea [69]), most of these reports have relied on serologic diagnostics that lack the specificity to distinguish between infections potentially caused by antigenically related organisms producing cross-reactive antibodies. In addition, there is little serologic or molecular-based evidence of *E. chaffeensis* infection among ticks or animals in countries other than the United States.

National Surveillance for HME

Although *E. chaffeensis* was isolated in the early 1990s, local and national surveillance activities were gradually phased in, and these systems continue to be refined. The Council of State and Territorial Epidemiologists and the Centers for Disease Control and Prevention (CDC) developed formal case definitions for HME and HGE (also commonly termed HGA) in 1996 that included disease classifications (e.g., confirmed, probable) determined by the clinical presentation and specificity of the accompanying diagnostic results (i.e., serology, PCR, or visualization of morulae) (20). HME and human granulocytic ehrlichiosis (HGE) were added to the formal list of nationally notifiable diseases in 1998 (22), and the list of tests considered confirmatory was amended in 2000 to include IHC testing of tissue samples and isolation of ehrlichiae in cell culture. The category of "other or unspecified ehrlichial agent (OE)" was introduced in 2000 for cases where routine diagnostic testing could not unequivocally identify the causative agent, as different ehrlichial pathogens elicit antibodies that may be cross-reactive to multiple antigens (28, 156). Although serologic cross-reactivity has complicated surveillance for specific conditions such as HME, it has also helped find new ehrlichial pathogens. Humans infected with *E. chaffeensis* were first identified by immunofluorescence assay (IFA) with *E. canis* antigen (55), and humans infected with *E. ewingii* often develop high titers of antibody to *E. chaffeensis* antigen (17).

Endemic and Sporadic HME

By the early 1990s, HME had been recognized among residents in the southern United States (55, 65). National surveillance for HME registered case reports from 23 states between 1997 and 2002, and information on the occurrence of disease at the county level is accumulating. The distribution of reports of HME outlines a region of highest risk of disease ranging from central Texas through Oklahoma and Missouri, east to Virginia, and involving all states to the south (Fig. 2). Sporadic cases occur along the Atlantic coastal plain into New England. The geographic range of *A. americanum* is expanding (105), and evidence of *E. chaffeensis* in lone star ticks and other local fauna continues to be accumulated from locations where HME is currently rare or unreported (70). Thus, the distribution map for HME should be considered a work in progress.

Distribution maps of *E. chaffeensis*-positive samples submitted to the CDC for testing (reference 118 and Fig. 4 therein) indicate that HME may be diagnosed in residents from any state. On multiple occasions, persons with a history of travel to areas where HME is known to be endemic have been diagnosed with HME following their return to their state of residence (9, 93, 99, 101, 108, 126). Such cases serve as important reminders that although the risk for acquiring HME may be regionally restricted, a careful travel history is critical in evaluation of any febrile patient and that public health awareness and access to appropriate diagnostic testing are national concerns.

Estimates of the Relative Incidence of HME

Between 1997 and 2001, 482 cases of HME were confirmed and ascribed to the county where the disease was most likely acquired (Fig. 1) (66). The estimated national average annual incidence of HME in the 23 states reporting was 0.7 per million. In ranked order, the states with the highest average incidence of HME were Arkansas, Missouri, Oklahoma, and Tennessee; Missouri reported the largest absolute number ($n = 140$) of cases.

Because of the nonspecific nature of the symptoms that occur, underdiagnosis is likely, and disease recognition and reporting may vary regionally. Incidence estimates for HME have their greatest use as relative indices of disease occurrence among counties within an individual state. In addition, the most commonly used serological test for HME is the IFA, and most acute serum samples acquired during the first 7 to 10 days of illness do not contain diagnostic levels of antibody (25, 26).

In fact, when employed, active surveillance has provided estimates of HME incidence that are on the

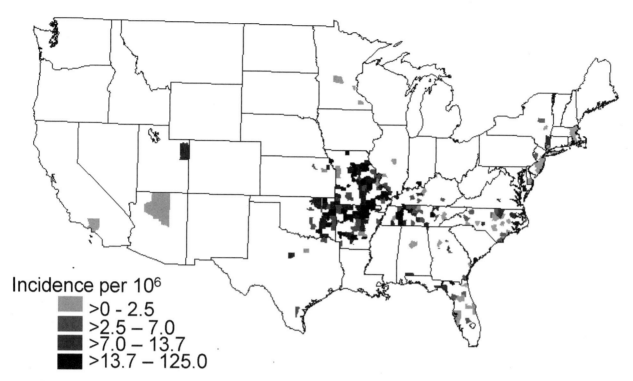

Figure 2. Average annual incidence of HME through 2001, as derived from states reporting cases. The legend indicates incidence values stratified into quartiles.

order of 10-fold higher than those generated by passive means. However, active surveillance efforts have usually targeted sites of high disease incidence. Active surveillance for HME was first conducted among patients with fever presenting to a southeastern Georgia hospital; the estimated annual incidence was 5.5 cases per 100,000, with the IFA test used to confirm infection (63). Active surveillance of patients visiting two medical practices in southeastern Missouri during 1997 and 1998 estimated HME incidence at 8 to 14 cases per 100,000 persons; 43% of the cases required hospitalization. The latter study used several diagnostic tests to confirm HME, including PCR (114). From April to October 1998, *E. chaffeensis* was isolated from 7 of 38 patients in Tennessee with fever and a history of tick bite who were studied; one of the culture-positive patients never seroconverted to *E. chaffeensis*, demonstrating the utility of multiple diagnostic tests. In a similar study (but without attempted cultures), 10 of 35 patients presenting with fever and a history of tick bite over a 2-year period in central North Carolina were diagnosed with ehrlichiosis (likely HME) (19).

Demographics and Seasonality

HME is predominantly a disease of adults (65). National surveillance data are in accord with patient case series (66) and indicate that the highest age-specific incidence of HME occurs among persons of >40 years of age, with a median age of approximately 50 years (Fig. 3a).

a.

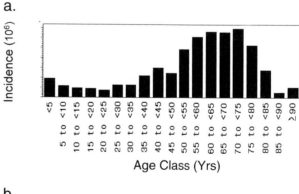

b.

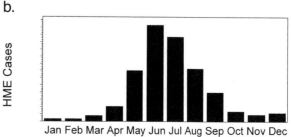

Figure 3. (a) The average age-specific incidence of HME derived from states reporting cases; (b) month of onset for HME.

The rarity of HME cases reported among children has been appreciated since the first 250 cases of human ehrlichiosis in the United States were reviewed, with <10% reported in children aged 2 to 13 years (54, 65). Similar sparing of children has been suggested for HGE but has not been seen with other tick-borne diseases. For example, the pathogens causing Lyme disease and RMSF are transmitted primarily by the genera *Ixodes* and *Dermacentor*, respectively, and both disproportionately affect children aged <15 years (21, 31). Age-related differences in exposure to ticks and tick bite acting preferentially to influence the risk of HME in children are highly unlikely (30). A more likely explanation, discussed below, is that *E. chaffeensis* infection is less severe when it occurs in children (27, 114).

National surveillance data indicate that most HME cases are reported in males (67%) of Caucasian heritage (94%) (66). Males exceed females in all age classes of national surveillance data groups, consistent with previously published estimates reporting a male:female ratio of approximately 2:11 (65, 114).

Approximately 70 to 80% of HME patients recall a tick bite in the weeks preceding the onset of their illness (57, 65, 114, 145). The distribution of month of onset for HME is unimodal, with 70% of cases occurring between May and July (Fig. 3b), a time period that coincides with the peak months of activity by lone star ticks (72).

Risk Factors for Infection and Disease

HME generally occurs sporadically, with only limited evidence for familial or community outbreaks. Many of the outdoor activities that typically place individuals in lone star tick habitats have been linked to the occurrence of HME cases, but except for military training in areas of endemicity, no activity or occupation has been consistently associated with unusually high risk. Military personnel conducting field exercises in New Jersey (123) and Arkansas (8, 170) have repeatedly suffered unusually high attack rates of HME. A soldier returning from training at Fort Chaffee, Ark., provided the sample leading to the first isolate of *E. chaffeensis* (35–36). Interestingly, this site has remained an area of exceptionally high risk for acquiring HME for more than 15 years, indicating the persistence of foci of endemicity (101).

The single account of a nonmilitary outbreak of HME occurred in Tennessee at a retirement facility located adjacent to a golf course. The highest risk of infection was associated with golfers having the worst score, presumably reflecting the amount of exposure time spent searching for balls in the tick-infested rough and woods next to the fairways (145).

Although data are limited, an association between the severity of HME and impaired immune function has been repeatedly identified. Persons with preexisting human immunodeficiency virus (HIV) infection (117) and individuals receiving immunosuppressive drugs following cancer therapy or organ transplantation (6) appear to be at increased risk for severe or fatal HME. Exceptionally high proportions of circulating monocytes harboring morulae have been documented in such cases (116). It is also possible that the high reported incidence of HME among older adults might reflect increasing occurrence of clinical manifestations and increased severity of disease due to natural age-associated declines in immune function, rather than any age-specific differences in exposure to ticks (Fig. 2a). The only serologic survey estimating the prevalence of *E. chaffeensis* antibody among children residing in different southeastern and south-central states found that 13% of approximately 2,000 children aged <17 years had titers of ≥80 (96). Two issues that limit the usefulness of this latter study were that no histories of prior disease compatible with HME were obtained from the children or their parents or guardians and that the serologic methods could not distinguish between infections caused by *E. chaffeensis* and those potentially due to an antigenically related ehrlichiae.

Asymptomatic Infection or Infection by Antigenically Related Ehrlichiae?

Military training exercises have permitted prospective investigation of the relationship between the development of antibodies reactive with *E. chaffeensis* (seroconversion) and the onset of disease consistent with HME (101, 123, 170). Two independent studies found that an illness compatible with HME was identifiable among 33 to 80% of those who seroconverted after field training. The other 20 to 67% of individuals experienced no signs or symptoms consistent with HME, despite seroconversion (101, 170). These findings are consistent with the interpretation that many individuals infected with *E. chaffeensis* do not develop clinical HME. The relative paucity of clinical HME among children is also consistent with this finding and its interpretation and supports a hypothesis of asymptomatic *E. chaffeensis* infection, perhaps occurring even more frequently in children.

However, an alternative interpretation of these findings is that an antigenically related but less virulent organism may cause some asymptomatic infections identified by serologic tests. The recent discovery that *E. ewingii* (see Chapter 15) may routinely cause disease among immune-impaired individuals and that many of the individuals infected produce antibodies cross-reactive with *E. chaffeensis* supports this possibility (17). Only prospective studies using specialized serologic and molecular diagnostic tests will resolve these questions (152, 156).

Coinfections

Because lone star ticks transmit several pathogens, coinfections of humans can be expected to occur naturally. In North Carolina, concurrent infection with *E. chaffeensis* and a spotted fever group rickettsiae has been diagnosed (139), and several seroepidemiologic studies report simultaneous seroconversions to *E. chaffeensis* and spotted fever group rickettsiae among military personnel (101). As *A. americanum* is the likely vector of both *E. chaffeensis* and *E. ewingii* (7, 165), coinfections are likely to be documented. In addition, lone star ticks transmit a spirochete, "*B. lonestari*," which has been suggested to be the cause of a Lyme borreliosis-like disease in several southeastern and south-central states (10, 74). The public health implications of most of these pathogens are poorly understood even when they occur as single infections.

HME through a Glass Darkly

Various factors that contribute to the maintenance of ehrlichial pathogens and affect the frequency and severity of human disease are undergoing or have undergone recent dramatic change. HME shares many of the human, reservoir-host, and vector-tick attributes credited with the rapid emergence of Lyme disease in the eastern United States (154). In addition to environmental factors, changes in the patterns of susceptibility within a population can be critical factors in disease emergence, both in increasing the opportunity for sporadic transmission of pathogens to humans (107) and in the dynamics of infections occurring among reservoir hosts (46). Sociological and demographic changes that influence the size of highly susceptible human subpopulations suggest that conditions favoring an increased incidence of severe HME will be enhanced over the next 25 years. The collective contribution of an aging U.S. population (157), an increasing number of persons receiving immunosuppressive drugs, and improvements in the health and longevity of HIV-infected individuals may substantially increase the incidence of severe and fatal HME. Improvements in awareness, diagnostic capabilities, and national surveillance of HME may aid in efforts to respond to these public health challenges.

CLINICAL MANIFESTATIONS

The clinical recognition of HME can be difficult, since the spectrum of manifestations is broad and nonspecific, ranging from asymptomatic infection to mild self-limited symptoms to rapidly fatal disease. HME typically presents as an uncomplicated, acute, nonspecific febrile illness that resolves rapidly if treated with doxycycline, characteristic of many rickettsial infections. However, not infrequently the illness becomes more severe, and clinical reports have described infections affecting nearly every organ system, potentially leading to a wide variety of clinical presentations. Because of these protean manifestations, a high degree of clinical suspicion in the proper temporal and geographic setting is required to reliably diagnose HME.

Initial Signs and Symptoms

The symptoms of infection usually begin within days to 2 weeks (median, 6 days) following a bite from an infected tick. Although not all patients recall a specific tick bite, a history compatible with exposure to active ticks is usually present (63, 65). The onset of illness is typically quite abrupt with the development of fever, headache, and other nonspecific symptoms, such as myalgias, arthralgias, and chills, which are often attributed to a viral illness. These symptoms may last for 1 to 2 days before progressing to more severe symptoms that may include specific manifestations and organ system involvement (62, 145). Gastrointestinal symptoms of nausea, vomiting, anorexia, and abdominal pain are the most common additional symptoms described. Less-common presenting symptoms include confusion or ataxia, suggestive of meningitis (125, 146), and cough or dyspnea, indicating involvement of the lungs (99, 119, 161). Involvement of other organ systems and tissues, such as cardiac, renal, skin, and skeletal muscle, has been described (48, 98, 140, 163).

The physical examination is often unremarkable, most commonly revealing only fever and mild tachycardia. Pallor and petechiae may result from anemia and thrombocytopenia; delirium, photophobia, and meningismus may occur due to central nervous system (CNS) involvement; and tachypnea and rales may be noted from pneumonia or acute lung injury. Other less-commonly reported findings include hepatomegaly, splenomegaly, and lymphadenopathy. Although diffuse arthralgias are common, frank inflammatory arthritis has not been documented.

Less than 10% of adults have a nonspecific skin rash at the time of presentation, and approximately one-third develop such a rash within the first week of illness. Children with HME develop a skin rash more frequently than adults, perhaps as many as 67%. The rash is usually transient and maculopapular in appearance, commonly involving the trunk and extremities, but petechial rashes may also occur, particularly when thrombocytopenia occurs.

Clinical Course

Most infections with *E. chaffeensis* are mild in nature and resolve rapidly following appropriate therapy, and spontaneous recovery of mild illness without antibiotic therapy has been reported (122, 123). How often asymptomatic infection occurs is currently unresolved, but population-based serologic surveys suggest that subclinical infection is common, perhaps accounting for as many as two-thirds of all infections (146, 170).

Occasionally, more severe illness develops and may include progressive dysfunction of one or more organ systems (55, 61, 97). Among patients with symptomatic HME reported in the literature, 60 to 85% were hospitalized and 15% developed moderate to severe illness, with a mortality rate of 2 to 5% (55, 63, 65). Although reporting bias towards very ill patients in published reports overestimates the proportion of patients with serious illness, it is clear that untreated *E. chaffeensis* infection can be severe. Complications may include meningoencephalitis, acute renal failure, adult respiratory distress syndrome, myocarditis, gastrointestinal hemorrhage, and disseminated intravascular coagulopathy, sometimes occurring in the setting of rapidly fatal overwhelming sepsis syndrome (73, 97). The risk of severe disease and death is highest for patients older than 60 years of age and for the immunocompromised. In addition, delays in diagnosis and in the initiation of appropriate antibiotic therapy are associated with serious complications and death.

Laboratory Findings

During the first week of illness, most patients develop thrombocytopenia, leukopenia, elevated hepatic transaminase levels, and, less frequently, anemia (62, 63, 65, 145). The nadir of the leukopenia is usually >1,000 cells/mm^3. The leukopenia is predominantly due to lymphopenia, although neutropenia may also occur, and is followed during the second week of illness with a reactive lymphocytosis, as the total white blood cell count returns to normal. The platelet count, even though typically reduced, usually remains >50,000/mm^3 and returns to normal after the first week of illness. Rarely, severe thrombocytopenia with ≤20,000 platelets/mm^3 with serious hemorrhage can occur. Although patients with mild HME or those

presenting for evaluation early in the illness may have normal laboratory findings, leukocytosis or thrombocytosis is distinctly unusual and should suggest an alternate diagnosis (147).

Mild to moderate elevations of serum hepatic transaminases (2 to 10 times normal) are very common in patients with HME. Coagulopathy and hyperbilirubinemia are rare in uncomplicated infections but can develop with severe multisystem disease.

Special Clinical Considerations

The most common serious complication of HME is involvement of the CNS, particularly meningitis (Color Plate 9E) or meningoencephalitis, occurring in up to 20% of patients (125, 146). The signs and symptoms range in severity from minor confusion and lethargy, to meningismus, cranial nerve palsies, seizures, and coma. About half of patients with clinical CNS findings will also have abnormal cerebrospinal fluid (CSF) findings, typically a mild lymphocytic pleocytosis (<250 cells/mm^3) and elevated protein levels. A low glucose level is usually not seen, in contrast to bacterial meningitis caused by *Streptococcus pneumoniae*, *Haemophilus influenzae*, and *Neisseria meningitidis*. Long-term sequelae of neurologic involvement are not common, but patients may take weeks to months to fully recover.

Immunocompromised patients with HME have more severe and prolonged illness, as well as increased rates of mortality (117, 137). Most reported cases of *E. chaffeensis* infection among this population have been in patients receiving immunosuppressive medication for inflammatory diseases or organ transplants, patients with asplenia, and those infected with HIV. Among HIV patients with low CD4 lymphocyte counts, the frequency of moderate to severe disease is >70%, and case fatality rates have ranged from 25 to 35%. Although impaired cellular immunity and decreased splenic clearance of infected leukocytes are likely responsible for the more severe illness observed in such patients, delays in diagnosis and treatment because of concern for or confusion with more typical opportunistic infections undoubtedly contribute to worse outcomes.

HME and coincidental infections with other tickborne pathogens, such as *Borrelia burgdorferi* and *Babesia microti*, have been described and may increase the severity of both diseases (75, 139). In the appropriate geographic setting, dual infection should be considered, especially in atypical cases. Transmission through fresh or frozen blood product transfusion is theoretically possible, as *E. chaffeensis* has been shown to survive in frozen blood products (103), but no cases have yet been reported. Persistent infection occurs commonly in dogs from infection with *E. canis*, a closely related ehrlichial organism, but has never been convincingly demonstrated with *E. chaffeensis* infection in humans. A possible persistent infection was reported in a patient who eventually died following a prolonged 2-month illness despite doxycycline therapy and in whom intact ehrlichial morulae were then identified in liver tissue at autopsy (49–50). However, doxycycline was not initiated until day 7 of hospitalization when the patient was quite ill, perhaps demonstrating unremitting progression of infection related to delayed therapy, rather than persistence. Reinfection with two separate strains of *E. chaffeensis* has been reported in a liver transplant recipient receiving immunosuppressive medication (84). Little is known regarding the duration of natural immunity following infection. Experience with other intracellular pathogens and with ehrlichial organisms in other mammals suggests that, in some cases, infection might not confer enduring protective immunity, even in some healthy hosts.

Differential Diagnosis

Because of the nonspecific nature and wide spectrum of manifestations of HME, the illness may be confused with other diseases, contributing to delayed or erroneous diagnosis. Prospective clinical studies demonstrate that rickettsial or ehrlichial infections are suspected initially in only 20% of patients with confirmed HME, even in regions of endemicity (56). Examples of reported erroneous initial diagnoses in patients subsequently found to have HME have included acute appendicitis (142), severe gastroenteritis (45), cholangitis, viral hepatitis (111), bacterial meningitis, pneumonia, acute leukemia, rhabdomyolysis, thrombotic thrombocytopenic purpura, vasculitis (124), toxic shock syndrome, and gram-negative bacterial sepsis. Such reports emphasize the importance of including HME (and, indeed, all rickettsial infections) in the differential diagnosis of patients who present with a compatible clinical and exposure history.

The most important historical clue that should be sought and alert the clinician to consider HME in the differential diagnosis of an acutely ill patient is potential tick exposure. Patients with ehrlichial infection usually reside in rural or suburban regions where tick-borne disease is endemic and/or have occupational and recreational exposures in such areas (146). As would be expected, HME is seasonal, with most cases occurring between April and September. The broad epidemiologic, clinical, and differential diagnostic considerations in evaluation of febrile illnesses occurring after tick exposure are discussed in detail in Chapter 5.

LABORATORY DIAGNOSIS

Direct Visualization of Organisms in the Blood

Classical diagnosis of *E. chaffeensis* infection relied upon direct identification of intracytoplasmic morulae in monocytes or macrophages upon examination of Giemsa, Wright, or Diff-Quik-stained blood smears or buffy coat preparations (65). When stained, the organisms appear as minute, dark blue or purple clusters of cocci within the cytoplasm of monocytes (Color Plate 9A) and macrophages; morulae of *E. chaffeensis* have also been described occasionally in neutrophils (93, 136). Although diagnostic when present, morulae are found in blood or buffy coat smears from clinically ill patients only in a minority of cases (25–26, 147); detection of morulae is more likely in severely immunocompromised patients (65, 117). Therefore, because they are identified only rarely, even by experienced microscopists, the absence of morulae should not be considered evidence against ehrlichial infection.

Cell Culture

Isolation of *E. chaffeensis* in cell culture requires expertise not available in most diagnostic laboratories. Cell lines that have been used successfully include DH82 (canine histiocytes) (Color Plate 9B), HEL299 (human embryonic lung cells), HMEC-1 (human endothelial cells), Vero (green monkey kidney cells), BGM, and L929 cells (15, 23, 24, 35, 38). However, isolation of *E. chaffeensis* is difficult and cumbersome, rendering this approach a poor choice for routine diagnostic use. Evidence of infection may be seen from 2 to 36 days following inoculation of susceptible cells (24, 35, 116, 147). To maximize the likelihood of isolation, cell cultures should be inoculated as soon as possible after collection of the blood sample and monitored for evidence of infection for up to 2 months (147).

Serologic Diagnosis

Serology remains the most commonly used method of confirming a clinical suspicion of HME. As described, *E. canis* antigen was initially used in diagnostic IFA tests for HME until *E. chaffeensis* (Arkansas) was successfully isolated from a patient 5 years later (35, 93). Since that time, the IFA with *E. chaffeensis* antigen has emerged as the preferred method for serologic diagnosis of HME.

A serologic diagnosis of HME can be made when a fourfold change in immunoglobulin G (IgG) antibody titer to *E. chaffeensis* antigen is detected by IFA in paired serum samples obtained 2 to 3 weeks apart

(20). Internal validation of the specific IFA used is essential to determine appropriate cutoff values for individual diagnostic laboratories (115). However, as a general guideline, the Consensus Approach for Ehrlichiosis (CAFÉ) Task Force has suggested that patients with compatible clinical disease and single titers of 1:64 to 1:128 may be considered probable cases of HME, and patients with compatible clinical disease and single titers of greater than 1:256 may be considered confirmed cases of HME (160).

Even when carefully used and interpreted, IFA is not without shortcomings. Antibody titers typically do not develop in the first week of acute clinical disease; IFA tests for IgM or IgG on blood samples drawn less than 7 days after onset have been shown to fail to identify infection in the majority of cases (25–26). Different diagnostic laboratories may use different protocols or isolates of *E. chaffeensis* in their IFAs, making interlaboratory comparison of results difficult. Cross-reactions between *E. chaffeensis* antigens and serum antibodies to other ehrlichial agents can make interpretation of test results problematic (35, 36, 156, 166). For example, infection with *A. phagocytophilum* may stimulate production of antibodies reactive to some *E. chaffeensis* antigens, especially at high anti-*A. phagocytophilum* titers (166).

Although not yet commercially available, immunoblotting techniques or enzyme-linked immunosorbent assays (ELISAs) that target specific *E. chaffeensis* antigens have been developed by several research groups in an effort to improve the specificity of serologic tests. Immunoblotting has been developed to detect antibodies specific to 27- and 29-kDa proteins, a recombinant fusion protein (rP30) apparently specific to *E. chaffeensis*, and a recombinant 120-kDa protein of *E. chaffeensis* (15, 24, 112, 156, 172, 173). An ELISA has been described that detects antibodies reactive to a recombinant major antigenic protein 2 (rMAP2) homologue of *E. chaffeensis* (2).

Molecular Diagnostics

PCR amplification of *E. chaffeensis* DNA sequences from blood or tissues of patients suspected of having HME is a valuable diagnostic tool, especially during the acute phase of infection when antibody titers often have not yet developed. Sensitivity of the PCR assay in patients with HME has been reported to be 80 to 87% (159). When performed by experienced personnel using appropriate controls, PCR assays for *E. chaffeensis* have the added advantage of high specificity as compared to IFA.

Anticoagulated whole blood (EDTA or citrate) collected during the acute phase of infection and before antibiotic therapy is instituted is the most com-

mon and preferred sample tested. However, while sensitivity is unknown and likely far lower, the amplification of *E. chaffeensis* DNA has also been described from serum, CSF, bronchoalveolar lavage fluid, and fresh or formalin-fixed paraffin-embedded tissues, including samples of bone marrow, lymph node, spleen, and liver (28, 44, 53, 117).

The 16S rRNA gene of *E. chaffeensis* was the first gene widely exploited for diagnosis of HME and remains the most commonly used PCR target. Nested amplification of a 16S rRNA gene fragment has also been performed to further enhance sensitivity, and evaluation of resultant amplicons by hybridization to specific probes or direct sequencing has been pursued to confirm specificity (4, 41–42). HME-diagnostic PCR assays have also been designed to amplify fragments of the 120-kDa gene, a variable length PCR target (VLPT), and the *groESL* heat shock operon of *E. chaffeensis*. These genes typically have greater variability than 16S rRNA and thus may prove useful for studies attempting to distinguish between individual *E. chaffeensis* strains (25–26, 116, 147, 150, 151).

Pathologic Identification of the Organism

Diagnosis of *E. chaffeensis* may also be made by means of IHC or ISH to identify organisms in tissue sections. IHC using human anti-*E. chaffeensis* or canine anti-*E. canis* serum has identified morulae within histiocytes and occasionally lymphocytes in bone marrow, spleen, liver, lymph nodes, and various other tissues from infected patients (44, 48–50, 98, 116, 117). Specificity may be enhanced by use of monoclonal antibodies (171). An ISH assay for detection of *E. chaffeensis* rRNA in tissues of infected patients has also been described (44).

Case Definition for Surveillance Purposes

According to the CDC, the diagnosis of HME can be considered confirmed for surveillance purposes when any one of the following is demonstrated: (i) seroconversion or a fourfold change in IgG antibody titer to *E. chaffeensis* antigen by IFA in paired serum samples obtained 2 to 3 weeks apart, (ii) a positive PCR assay confirmed by sequencing to reveal an *E. chaffeensis* gene sequence, (iii) identification of morulae in white blood cells and a positive IFA titer to *E. chaffeensis* antigen based on the values established by the laboratory performing the assay, (iv) positive immunostaining of *E. chaffeensis* antigen in a tissue sample, or (v) culture of *E. chaffeensis* from a clinical specimen (20). These criteria are not intended for use in clinical management of patients; in most clinical settings, presumptive diagnosis and treatment are appropriate when the disease is suspected and in the absence of laboratory confirmation.

Treatment and Prevention

The treatment of ehrlichial infections is based largely upon clinical experience rather than controlled studies. The antibiotics of choice are tetracycline and doxycycline, the latter preferred because of its better tolerability and longer half-life. The dramatic improvement of ill patients within 1 to 2 days following the initiation of appropriate treatment is often striking, leaving no doubt of its effectiveness.

Empiric antibiotic therapy should be given promptly once the diagnosis of HME is considered likely, to avoid the potentially serious consequences of delayed therapy. In the proper geographic and seasonal setting, a significant nonspecific acute febrile illness other than a typical upper respiratory infection with no apparent and reasonable explanation occurring in a patient with a history of potential tick exposure should be empirically treated for a potential tick-borne rickettsial infection. Therapy should not be delayed until diagnosis is confirmed, because such confirmation may take several days to weeks. Even a delay of 24 to 48 h required for diagnosis by PCR, where available, could result in disastrous clinical consequences in severely ill patients. In addition, neither serologic testing nor PCR is sufficiently sensitive such that a negative result excludes ehrlichial infection. The response to treatment is often quite dramatic and is usually apparent within 24 to 48 h. The lack of this characteristic improvement in clinical condition suggests that an alternate diagnosis must be considered.

Doxycycline (100 mg in adults or 1.5 mg/kg of body weight in children, administered twice daily either orally or intravenously) is generally agreed to be the best available agent for HME and should always be used if not contraindicated. The duration of therapy is also based upon empiric observation, and a course of 7 to 14 days is most often recommended. In treatment of pregnant women and children who are <8 years old, a specialist or the CDC should be consulted and, if tetracyclines are used, the total dose should be minimized to avoid bone and dental complications. Doxycycline can be discontinued 2 days following defervescence and clinical recovery.

Tetracycline given at 25 mg/kg/day in four divided doses can be used, but it is often less well tolerated and is not available for intravenous administration. There are only a limited number of alternative antibiotics that have been used successfully in the treatment of HME. Tetracycline should not be given to children younger than 8 years of age because of higher risks of dental staining than with doxycycline.

When therapy with tetracyclines (including doxycycline) is relatively contraindicated, such as with pregnant women, children younger than 8 years of age, or in individuals with severe drug hypersensitivity, rifampin may have benefit as an alternative. Although there are no clinical reports of treating HME with rifampin, it has been used successfully in the treatment of HGE (16), and in vitro susceptibility data with E. chaffeensis also support its activity against the organism (14).

In contrast to some other rickettsial infections, chloramphenicol should not be used to treat HME. In vitro susceptibility studies demonstrate resistance to chloramphenicol by E. chaffeensis, and there are very little clinical data supporting its efficacy (14). The fluoroquinolones were once thought a promising alternative antibiotic therapy for ehrlichial infections, based upon the favorable in vitro susceptibility of several species, including A. phagocytophilum (76). However, naturally occurring DNA gyrase-mediated resistance to fluoroquinolones has recently been demonstrated among members of the E. canis genogroup, of which E. chaffeensis is a member, and A. phagocytophilum is not (100). These results underline the importance of approaching each ehrlichial species infection as unique and not simply as a generic syndrome ehrlichial disease.

Tick avoidance measures are the best method of prevention of HME and are reviewed in detail elsewhere. The development of a vaccine to protect against HME is being investigated but is not likely to be available in the near future, nor would the current incidence of disease likely justify its routine use. No data exist to support prophylactic antibiotic use, either after a tick bite or before a potential exposure, and should be avoided.

REFERENCES

1. **Allan, S. A.** 2001. Ticks (Class Arachnida: Order Acarina), p. 72–106. *In* W. M. Samuel, M. J. Pybus, and A. A. Kocan (ed.), *Parasitic Diseases of Wild Mammals*, 2nd ed. Iowa State University Press, Ames, Iowa.
2. **Alleman, A. R., A. F. Barbet, M. V. Bowie, H. L. Sorenson, S. J. Wong, and M. Belanger.** 2000. Expression of a gene encoding the major antigenic protein 2 homolog of *Ehrlichia chaffeensis* and potential application for serodiagnosis. *J. Clin. Microbiol.* 38:3705–3709.
3. **Anderson, B. E., J. E. Dawson, D. C. Jones, and K. H. Wilson.** 1991. *Ehrlichia chaffeensis*, a new species associated with human ehrlichiosis. *J. Clin. Microbiol.* 29:2838–2842.
4. **Anderson, B. E., J. W. Sumner, J. E. Dawson, T. Tzianabos, C. R. Greene, J. G. Olson, D. B. Fishbein, M. Olsen-Rasmussen, B. P. Holloway, E. H. George, and A. F. Azad.** 1992. Detection of the etiologic agent of human ehrlichiosis by polymerase chain reaction. *J. Clin. Microbiol.* 30:775–780.
5. **Anderson, B. E., K. G. Sims, J. E. Olson, J. E. Childs, J. F. Piesman, C. M. Happ, G. O. Maupin, and B. J. B. Johnson.**

1993. *Amblyomma americanum*: a potential vector of human ehrlichiosis. *Am. J. Trop. Med. Hyg.* **49**:239–244.

6. Antony, S. J., J. S. Dumler, and E. Hunter. 1995. Human ehrlichiosis in a liver transplant recipient. *Transplantation* **60**:879–881.

7. Anziani, O. S., S. A. Ewing, and R. W. Barker. 1990. Experimental transmission of a granulocytic form of the tribe Ehrlichieae by *Dermacentor variabilis* and *Amblyomma americanum* to dogs. *Am. J. Vet. Res.* **51**:929–931.

8. Arguin, P. M., J. Singleton, Jr., L. D. Rotz, E. Marston, T. A. Treadwell, K. Slater, M. Chamberland, A. Schwartz, J. G. Olson, J. E. Childs, and the Transfusion-Associated Tick-Borne Illness Task Force. 1999. An investigation of possible transmission of tick-borne pathogens via blood transfusion. *Transfusion* **39**:828–833.

9. Armstrong, R. W. 1992. Ehrlichiosis in a visitor to West Virginia. *J. Med.* **157**:182–184.

10. Barbour, A. G., G. O. Maupin, G. J. Teltow, C. J. Carter, and J. Piesman. 1996. Identification of an uncultivable *Borrelia* species in the hard tick *Amblyomma americanum*: possible agent of a Lyme disease-like illness. *J. Infect. Dis.* **173**:403–409.

11. Belongia, E. A., K. D. Reed, P. D. Mitchell, C. P. Kolbert, D. H. Persing, J. S. Gill, and J. J. Kazmierczak. 1997. Prevalence of granulocytic Ehrlichia infection among white-tailed deer in Wisconsin. *J. Clin. Microbiol.* **35**:1465–1468.

12. Bloemer, S. R., E. L. Snoddy, J. C. Cooney, and K. Fairbanks. 1986. Influence of deer exclusion on populations of lone star ticks and American dog ticks (Acari:Ixodidae). *J. Econ. Entomol.* **79**:679–683.

13. Bloemer, S. R., R. H. Zimmerman, and K. Fairbanks. 1988. Abundance, attachment sites, and density estimators for lone star ticks (Acari: Ixodidae) infesting white-tailed deer. *J. Med. Entomol.* **25**:295–300.

14. Brouqui, P., and D. Raoult. 1992. In vitro antibiotic susceptibility of the newly recognized agent of ehrlichiosis in humans, *Ehrlichia chaffeensis*. *Antimicrob. Agents Chemother.* **36**:2799–2803.

15. Brouqui, P., M. L. Birg, and D. Raoult. 1994. Cytopathic effect, plaque formation, and lysis of *Ehrlichia chaffeensis* grown on continuous cell lines. *Infect. Immun.* **62**:405–411.

16. Buitrago, M. I., J. W. Ijdo, P. Rinaudo, H. Simon, J. Copel, J. Gadbaw, R. Heimer, E. Fikrig, and F. J. Bia. 1998. Human granulocytic ehrlichiosis during pregnancy treated successfully with rifampin. *Clin. Infect. Dis.* **27**:213–215.

17. Buller, R. S., M. Arens, S. P. Hmiel, C. D. Paddock, J. W. Sumner, Y. Rikihisa, A. Unver, M. Gaudreault-Keener, F. A. Manian, A. M. Liddell, N. Schmulewitz, and G. A. Storch. 1999. *Ehrlichia ewingii*, a newly recognized agent of human ehrlichiosis. *N. Engl. J. Med.* **341**:148–155.

18. Burket, C. T., C. N. Vann, R. R. Pinger, C. L. Chatot, and F. E. Steiner. 1998. Minimum infection rate of *Amblyomma americanum* (Acari: Ixodidae) by *Ehrlichia chaffeensis* (Rickettsiales: Ehrlichieae) in southern Indiana. *J. Med. Entomol.* **35**:653–659.

19. Carpenter, C. F., T. K. Gandhi, L. K. Kong, G. R. Corey, S. M. Chen, D. H. Walker, J. S. Dumler, E. Breitschwerdt, B. Hegarty, and D. J. Sexton. 1999. The incidence of ehrlichial and rickettsial infection in patients with unexplained fever and recent history of tick bite in central North Carolina. *J. Infect. Dis.* **180**:900–903.

20. Centers for Disease Control and Prevention. 1997. Case definitions for infectious conditions under public health surveillance. *Morb. Mortal. Wkly. Rep.* **46**(RR-10):46–47.

21. Centers for Disease Control and Prevention. 2000. Surveillance for Lyme disease—United States, 1992–1998. CDC Surveillance Summaries, April 28, 2000. *Morb. Mortal. Wkly. Rep.* **49**(SS-3):1–11.

22. Centers for Disease Control and Prevention. 2001. Summary of notifiable diseases, United States, 1999. *Morb. Mortal. Wkly. Rep.* **48**:1–104.

23. Chen, S.-M., V. L. Popov, H.-M. Feng, J. Wen, and D. H. Walker. 1995. Cultivation of *Ehrlichia chaffeensis* in mouse embryo, Vero, BGM, and L929 cells and study of *Ehrlichia*-induced cytopathic effect and plaque formation. *Infect. Immun.* **63**:647–655.

24. Chen, S.-M., X.-J. Yu, V. L. Popov, E. L. Westerman, F. G. Hamilton, and D. H. Walker. 1997. Genetic and antigenic diversity of *Ehrlichia chaffeensis*: comparative analysis of a novel human strain from Oklahoma and previously isolated strains. *J. Infect. Dis.* **175**:856–863.

25. Childs, J. E., J. W. Sumner, W. L. Nicholson, R. F. Massung, S. M. Standaert, and C. D. Paddock. 1999. Outcome of diagnostic tests using samples from patients with culture-proven human monocytic ehrlichiosis: implications for surveillance. *J. Clin. Microbiol.* **37**:2997–3000.

26. Childs, J. E., J. H. McQuiston, J. W. Sumner, W. L. Nicholson, J. A. Comer, R. F. Massung, S. M. Standaert, and C. D. Paddock. 1999. Human monocytic ehrlichiosis due to *Ehrlichia chaffeensis*: how do we count the cases? *In* D. Raoult and P. Brouqui (ed.), p. 287–293. *Rickettsiae and Rickettsial Diseases at the Turn of the Third Millennium.* Elsevier, Paris, France.

27. Childs, J. E., and C. D. Paddock. 2002. The ascendancy of *Amblyomma americanum* as a vector of pathogens affecting humans in the United States. *Annu. Rev. Entomol.* **48**:307–337.

28. Comer, J. A., W. L. Nicholson, J. W. Sumner, J. G. Olson, and J. E. Childs. 1999. Diagnosis of human ehrlichiosis by PCR assay of acute-phase serum. *J. Clin. Microbiol.* **37**:31–34.

29. Comer, J. A., W. L. Nicholson, C. D. Paddock, J. W. Sumner, and J. E. Childs. 2000. Detection of antibodies reactive with *Ehrlichia chaffeensis* in the raccoon. *J. Wildlife Dis.* **36**:705–712.

30. Cooley, R. A., and G. M. Kohls. 1944. The genus *Amblyomma* (Ixodidae) in the U. S. *J. Parasitol.* **30**:77–111.

31. Dalton, M. J., M. J. Clarke, R. C. Holman, J. W. Krebs, D. B. Fishbein, J. G. Olson, and J. E. Childs. 1995. National surveillance for Rocky Mountain spotted fever, 1981–1992: epidemiologic summary and evaluation of risk factors for fatal outcome. *Am. J. Trop. Med. Hyg.* **52**:405–413.

32. Davidson, W. R., D. A. Siefken, and L. H. Creekmore. 1994. Seasonal and annual abundance of *Amblyomma americanum* (Acari: Ixodidae) in central Georgia. *J. Med. Entomol.* **31**:67–71.

33. Davidson, W. R., J. M. Lockhart, D. E. Stallknecht, and E. W. Howerth. 1999. Susceptibility of red and gray foxes to infection by *Ehrlichia chaffeensis*. *J. Wildlife Dis.* **35**:696–702.

34. Davidson, W. R., J. M. Lockhart, D. E. Stallknecht, E. W. Howerth, J. E. Dawson, and Y. Rechav. 2001. Persistent *Ehrlichia chaffeensis* infection in white-tailed deer. *J. Wildlife Dis.* **37**:538–546.

35. Dawson, J. E., Y. Rikihisa, S. A. Ewing, and D. B. Fishbein. 1991. Serologic diagnosis of human ehrlichiosis using two *Ehrlichia canis* isolates. *J. Infect. Dis.* **163**:564–567.

36. Dawson, J. E., B. E. Anderson, D. B. Fishbein, J. L. Sanchez, C. S. Goldsmith, K. H. Wilson, and C. W. Duntley. 1991. Isolation and characterization of an *Ehrlichia* sp. from a patient diagnosed with human ehrlichiosis. *J. Clin. Microbiol.* **29**:2741-2745.

37. Dawson, J. E., and S. A. Ewing. 1992. Susceptibility of dogs to infection with *Ehrlichia chaffeensis*, causative agent of human ehrlichiosis. *Am. J. Vet. Res.* **53**:1322–1327.

38. Dawson, J. E., F. J. Candal, V. G. George, and E. W. Ades. 1993. Human endothelial cells as an alternative to DH82 cells for isolation of *Ehrlichia chaffeensis*, *E. canis*, and *Rickettsia rickettsii*. *Pathobiology* **61**:293-296.

39. Dawson, J. E., J. E. Childs, K. L. Biggie, C. Moore, D. E. Stallknecht, J. Shaddock, J. Bouseman, E. Hofmeister, and J. G. Olson. 1994. White-tailed deer as a potential reservoir of *Ehrlichia* spp. *J. Wildlife Dis.* **30**:162–168.

40. Dawson, J. E., D. E. Stallknecht, E. W. Howerth, C. Warner, K. Biggie, W. R. Davidson, J. M. Lockhart, V. F. Nettles, J. G. Olson, and J. E. Childs. 1994. Susceptibility of white-tailed deer (*Odocoileus virginianus*) to infection with *Ehrlichia chaffeensis*, the etiologic agent of human ehrlichiosis. *J. Clin. Microbiol.* **32**:2725–2728.

41. Dawson, J. E., C. K. Warner, V. Baker, S. A. Ewing, D. E. Stallknecht, W. R. Davidson, A. A. Kocan, J. M. Lockhart, and J. G. Olson. 1996. *Ehrlichia*-like 16S rDNA sequence from wild white-tailed deer (*Odocoileus virginianus*). *J. Parasitol.* **82**:52–58.

42. Dawson, J. E., K. L. Biggie, C. K. Warner, K. Cookson, S. Jenkins, J. F. Levine, and J. G. Olson. 1996. Polymerase chain reaction evidence of *Ehrlichia chaffeensis*, an etiologic agent of human ehrlichiosis, in dogs from southeast Virginia. *Am. J. Vet. Res.* **57**:1175–1179.

43. Dawson, J. E., and A. M. Marty. 1997. Ehrlichiosis, p. 49–59. *In* C. R. Horsburgh, Jr., and A. M. Nelson (ed.), *Pathology of Emerging Infections*. American Society for Microbiology, Washington, D.C.

44. Dawson, J. E., C. D. Paddock, C. K. Warner, P. W. Greer, J. H. Bartlett, S. A. Ewing, U. G. Munderloh, and S. R. Zaki. 2001. Tissue diagnosis of *Ehrlichia chaffeensis* in patients with fatal ehrlichiosis by use of immunohistochemistry, in situ hybridization, and polymerase chain reaction. *Am. J. Trop. Med. Hyg.* **65**:603–609.

45. Devereaux, C. E. 1997. Human monocytic ehrlichiosis presenting as febrile diarrhea. *J. Clin. Gastroenterol.* **25**:544–545.

46. Dobson, A., and J. Foufopoulos. 2001. Emerging infectious pathogens of wildlife. *Philos. Trans. R. Soc. Lond. B Biol. Sci.* **356**:1001–1012.

47. Dugan, V. G., S. E. Little, D. E. Stallknecht, and A. D. Beall. 2000. Natural infection of domestic goats with *Ehrlichia chaffeensis*. *J. Clin. Microbiol.* **38**:448–449.

48. Dumler, J. S., P. Brouqui, J. Aronson, J. P. Taylor, and D. H. Walker. 1991. Identification of *Ehrlichia* in human tissue. *N. Engl. J. Med.* **325**:1109–1110. (Letter.)

49. Dumler, J. S., J. E. Dawson, and D. H. Walker. 1993. Human ehrlichiosis: hematopathology and immunohistologic detection of *Ehrlichia chaffeensis*. *Hum. Pathol.* **24**:391–396.

50. Dumler, J. S., W. L. Sutker, and D. H. Walker. 1993. Persistent infection with *Ehrlichia chaffeensis*. *Clin. Infect. Dis.* **17**:903–905.

51. Dumler, J. S., and D. H. Walker. 2001. Tick-borne ehrlichioses. *Lancet Infect. Dis.* **6**:21–28.

52. Dumler, J. S., A. F. Barbet, C. Bekker, G. A. Dasch, G. H. Palmer, S. C. Ray, Y. Rikihisa, and F. R. Rurangirwa. 2001. Reorganization of genera in the families *Rickettsiaceae* and *Anaplasmataceae* in the order Rickettsiales: unification of some species of *Ehrlichia* with *Anaplasma*, *Cowdria* with *Ehrlichia* and *Ehrlichia* with *Neorickettsia*, descriptions of six new species combinations and designations of *Ehrlichia equi* and 'HGE agent' as subjective synonyms of *Ehrlichia phagocytophila*. *Int. J. Syst. Evol. Microbiol.* **51**:2145–2165.

53. Dunn, B. E., T. P. Monson, J. S. Dumler, C. C. Morris, A. B. Westbrook, J. L. Duncan, J. E. Dawson, K. G. Sims, and B. E. Anderson. 1992. Identification of *Ehrlichia chaffeensis* morulae in cerebrospinal fluid mononuclear cells. *J. Clin. Microbiol.* **30**:2207–2210.

54. Edwards, M. S. 1994. Ehrlichiosis in children. *Semin. Ped. Infect. Dis.* **5**:143–147.

55. Eng, T. R., J. R. Harkess, D. B. Fishbein, J. E. Dawson, C. N. Greene, M. A. Redus, and F. T. Satalowich. 1990. Epidemiologic, clinical, and laboratory findings of human ehrlichiosis in the United States, 1988. *JAMA* **264**:2251–2258.

56. Estrada-Peña, A., and F. Jongejan. 1999. Ticks feeding on humans: a review of records on human-biting Ixodoidea with special reference to pathogen transmission. *Exp. Appl. Acarol.* **23**:685–715.

57. Everett, E. D., K. A. Evans, R. B. Henry, and G. McDonald. 1994. Human ehrlichiosis in adults after tick exposure; diagnosis using polymerase chain reaction. *Ann. Intern. Med.* **120**:730–735.

58. Ewing, S. A., E. M. Johnson, and K. M. Kocan. 1987. Human infection with *Ehrlichia canis*. *N. Engl. J. Med.* **317**:899. (Letter.)

59. Ewing, S. A., J. E. Dawson, A. A. Kocan, R. W. Barker, C. K. Warner, R. J. Panciera, J. C. Fox, K. M. Kocan, and E. F. Blouin. 1995. Experimental transmission of *Ehrlichia chaffeensis* (Rickettsiales: Ehrlichieae) among white-tailed deer by *Amblyomma americanum* (Acari: Ixodidae). *J. Med. Entomol.* **32**:368–374.

60. Felz, M. W., and L. A. Durden. 1999. Attachment site of four tick species (Acari: Ixodidae) parasitizing humans in Georgia and South Carolina. *J. Med. Entomol.* **36**:361–364.

61. Fichtenbaum, C. J., L. R. Peterson, and G. J. Weil. 1993. Ehrlichiosis presenting as a life-threatening illness with features of the toxic shock syndrome. *Am. J. Med.* **95**:351–357.

62. Fishbein D. B., L. A. Sawyer, C. J. Holland, E. B. Hayes, W. Okoroanyanwu, D. Williams, K. Sikes, M. Ristic, and J. E. McDade. 1987. Unexplained febrile illnesses after exposure to ticks. Infection with an *Ehrlichia*? *JAMA* **257**:3100–3104.

63. Fishbein, D. B., A. Kemp, J. E. Dawson, N. R. Greene, M. A. Redus, and D. H. Fields. 1989. Human ehrlichiosis: prospective active surveillance in febrile hospitalized patients. *J. Infect. Dis.* **160**:803–809.

64. Fishbein, D. B., and J. E. Dawson. 1991. Ehrlichiae, p. 1054–1058. *In* A. Balows, W. J. Hausler, K. L. Herrmann, H. D. Isenberg, and H. J. Shadomy (ed.), *Manual of Clinical Microbiology*, 5th ed. American Society for Microbiology, Washington, D.C.

65. Fishbein, D. B., J. E. Dawson, and L. E. Robinson. 1994. Human ehrlichiosis in the United States, 1985 to 1990. *Ann. Intern. Med.* **120**:736–743.

66. Gardner, S. L., R. C. Holman, J. W. Krebs, R. Berkelman, and J. E. Childs. 2003. National surveillance for the human ehrlichioses in the United States, 1997–2001, and proposed methods for evaluation of data quality. *Ann. N. Y. Acad. Sci.* **990**:80–89.

67. Haile, D. G., and G. A. Mount. 1987. Computer simulation of population dynamics of the lone star tick, *Amblyomma americanum* (Acari: Ixodidae). *J. Med. Entomol.* **24**:356–369.

68. Harkess, J. R., S. A. Ewing, J. M. Crutcher, J. Kudlac, G. McKee, and G. R. Istre. 1989. Human ehrlichiosis in Oklahoma. *J. Infect. Dis.* **159**:576–579.

69. Heo, E. J., J. H. Park, J. R. Koo, M. S. Park, M. Y. Park, J. S. Dumler, and J. S. Chae. 2002. Serologic and molecular detection of *Ehrlichia chaffeensis* and *Anaplasma phagocytophila* (human granulocytic ehrlichiosis agent) in Korean patients. *J. Clin. Microbiol.* **40**:3082–3085.

70. Ijdo, J. W., C. Wu, L. A. Magnarelli, K. C. Stafford III, J. F. Anderson, and E. Fikrig. 2000. Detection of *Ehrlichia chaffeensis* DNA in *Amblyomma americanum* ticks in Connecticut and Rhode Island. *J. Clin. Microbiol.* 38:4655–4656.

71. Irving, R. P., R. R. Pinger, C. N. Vann, J. B. Olesen, and F. E. Steiner. 2000. Distribution of *Ehrlichia chaffeensis* (Rickettsiales: Rickettsiaeceae) in *Amblyomma americanum* in southern Indiana and prevalence of *E. chaffeensis*-reactive antibodies in white-tailed deer in Indiana and Ohio in 1998. *J. Med. Entomol.* 37:595–600.

72. Jackson, L. K., D. M. Gaydon, and J. Goddard. 1996. Seasonal activity and relative abundance of *Amblyomma americanum* in Mississippi. *J. Med. Entomol.* 33:128–131.

73. Jackson R. T., and J. W. Jackson. 1997. Ehrlichiosis with systemic sepsis syndrome. *Tenn. Med.* 90:185–186.

74. James, A. M., D. Liveris, G. P. Wormser, I. Schwartz, M. A. Monteclavo, and B. J. Johnson. 2001. *Borrelia lonestari* infection after a bite by an *Amblyomma americanum* tick. *J. Infect. Dis.* 183:1810–1814.

75. Javed, M. Z., M. Srivastava, S. Zhang, and M. Kandathil. 2001. Concurrent babesiosis and ehrlichiosis in an elderly host. *Mayo Clin. Proc.* 76:563–565.

76. Klein, M. B., C. M. Nelson, and J. L. Goodman. 1997. Antibiotic susceptibility of the newly cultivated agent of human granulocytic ehrlichiosis: promising activity of quinolones and rifamycins. *Antimicrob. Agents Chemother.* 41:76–79.

77. Kocan, A. A., S. A. Ewing, D. Stallknecht, G. L. Murphy, S. Little, L. C. Whitworth, and R. W. Barker. 2000. Attempted transmission of *Ehrlichia chaffeensis* among white-tailed deer by *Amblyomma maculatum*. *J. Wildlife Dis.* 36:592–594.

78. Kocan, A. A., G. C. Levesque, L. C. Whitworth, G. L. Murphy, S. A. Ewing, and R. W. Barker. 2000. Naturally occurring *Ehrlichia chaffeensis* infection in coyotes from Oklahoma. *Emerg. Infect. Dis.* 6:477–480.

79. Kordick, S. K., E. B. Breitschwerdt, B. C. Hegarty, K. L. Southwick, C. M. Colitz, S. I. Hancock, J. M. Bradley, R. Rumbough, J. T. McPherson, and J. N. MacCormack. 1999. Coinfection with multiple tick-borne pathogens in a Walker hound kennel in North Carolina. *J. Clin. Microbiol.* 37:2631–2638.

80. Kramer, V. L., M. P. Randolph, L. T. Hui, W. E. Irwin, A. G. Gutierrez, and D. J. Vugia. 1999. Detection of the agents of human ehrlichioses in ixodid ticks from California. *Am. J. Trop. Med. Hyg.* 60:62–65.

81. LaBarre, R. 1994. Absence of *Ehrlichia chaffeensis* in West Texas tick vectors and identification of *Rickettsia*-like organism with shared antigenicity, D-37. *Abstr. 94th Gen. Meet. Am. Soc. Microbiol. 1994.* American Society for Microbiology, Washington, D.C.

82. Lee, E., and Y. Rikihisa. 1996. Lack of tumor necrosis factor alpha, interleukin-6 (IL-6), and granulocyte-macrophage colony-stimulating factor expression but presence of IL-1β, IL-8, and IL-10 expression in human monocytes exposed to viable or killed *Ehrlichia chaffeensis*. *Infect. Immun.* 64:4211–4219.

83. Lee, E., and Y. Rikihisa. 1997. Anti-*Ehrlichia chaffeensis* antibody induces potent proinflammatory cytokine mRNA expression in human monocytes exposed to *E. chaffeensis* through sustained reduction of Iκβ-a and activation of NF-κβ. *Infect. Immun.* 65:2890–2897.

84. Liddell, A. M., J. W. Sumner, C. D. Paddock, Y. Rikihisa, A. Unver, R. S. Buller, and G. A. Storch. 2002. Reinfection with *Ehrlichia chaffeensis* in a liver transplant recipient. *Clin. Infect. Dis.* 34:1644–1647.

85. Little, S. E., J. E. Dawson, J. M. Lockhart, D. E. Stallknecht, C. K. Warner, and W. R. Davidson. 1997. Development and use of specific polymerase chain reaction for the detection of an *Ehrlichia*-like organism in white-tailed deer. *J. Parasitol.* 33:246–253.

86. Little, S. E., D. E. Stallknecht, J. M. Lockhart, J. E. Dawson, and W. R. Davidson. 1998. Natural co-infection of a white-tailed deer (*Odocoileus virginianus*) population with three *Ehrlichia* spp. *J. Parasitol.* 84:897–901.

87. Little, S. E., and E. W. Howerth. 1999. *Ehrlichia chaffeensis* in archived tissues of a white-tailed deer. *J. Wildlife Dis.* 35:596–599.

88. Lockhart, J. M., W. R. Davidson, J. E. Dawson, and D. E. Stallknecht. 1995. Temporal association of *Amblyomma americanum* with the presence of *Ehrlichia chaffeensis*-reactive antibodies in white-tailed deer. *J. Wildlife Dis.* 31:119–124.

89. Lockhart, J. M., W. R. Davidson, D. E. Stallknecht, and J. E. Dawson. 1996. Site-specific geographic association between *Amblyomma americanum* (Acari: Ixodidae) infestations and *Ehrlichia chaffeensis*-reactive (Rickettsiales: Ehrlichieae) antibodies in white-tailed deer. *J. Med. Entomol.* 33:153–158.

90. Lockhart J. M., W. R. Davidson, D. E. Stallknecht, J. E. Dawson, and S. E. Little. 1997. Natural history of *Ehrlichia chaffeensis* in the Piedmont physiographic province of Georgia. *J. Parasitol.* 83:887–894.

91. Lockhart, J. M., W. R. Davidson, D. E. Stallknecht, J. E. Dawson, and E. W. Howerth. 1997. Isolation of *Ehrlichia chaffeensis* from white-tailed deer (*Odocoileus virginianus*) confirms their role as natural reservoir hosts. *J. Clin. Microbiol.* 35:1681–1686.

92. Lockhart, J. M., and W. R. Davidson. 1999. Evaluation of C3H/HeJ mice for xenodiagnosis of infection with *Ehrlichia chaffeensis*. *J. Vet. Diag. Investig.* 11:55–59.

93. Maeda, K. M., M. Markowitz, R. C. Hawley, M. Ristic, D. Cox, and J. E. McDade. 1987. Human infection with *Ehrlichia canis*, a leukocytic rickettsia. *N. Engl. J. Med.* 316:853–856.

94. Magnarelli, L. A., J. F. Anderson, K. C. Stafford III, and J. S. Dumler. 1997. Antibodies to multiple tick-borne pathogens of babesiosis, ehrlichiosis, and Lyme borreliosis in white-footed mice. *J. Wildlife Dis.* 33:466–473.

95. Magnarelli, L. A., J. W. Ijdo, K. C. Stafford III, and E. Fikrig. 1999. Infections of granulocytic ehrlichiae and *Borrelia burgdorferi* in white-tailed deer in Connecticut. *J. Wildlife Dis.* 35:266–274.

96. Marshall, G. S., R. F. Jacobs, G. E. Schutze, H. Paxton, S. C. Buckingham, J. P. Devincenzo, M. A. Jackson, V. H. San Joaquin, S. M. Standaert, and C. R. Woods. 2002. *Ehrlichia chaffeensis* seroprevalence among children in the Southeast and south-central regions of the United States. *Arch. Pediatr. Adolesc. Med.* 156:166–170.

97. Martin, G. S., B. W. Christman, and S. M. Standaert. 1999. Rapidly fatal infection with *Ehrlichia chaffeensis*. *N. Engl. J. Med.* 341:763–764.

98. Marty, A. M., J. S. Dumler, G. Imes, H. P. Brusman, L. L. Smrkovski, and D. M. Frisman. 1995. Ehrlichiosis mimicking thrombotic thrombocytopenic purpura. Case report and pathological correlation. *Hum. Pathol.* 26:920–925.

99. Mathisen, G., P. J. Weis, and C. A. Kennedy. 1993. Pneumonia, aseptic meningitis, and leukopenia in a 28-year-old man. *Clin. Infect. Dis.* 16:809–815.

100. Maurin, M., C. Abergel, and D. Raoult. 2001. DNA gyrase-mediated natural resistance to fluoroquinolones in *Ehrlichia* spp. *Antimicrob. Agents Chemother.* 45:2098–2105.

101. McCall, C. L., A. T. Curns, J. S. Singleton, J. A. Comer, J. G. Olson, L. D. Rotz, T. A. Treadwell, P. Arguin, and J. E. Childs. 2001. Fort Chaffee revisited; the epidemiology

of tickborne diseases at a persistent focus. *Vector Borne Zoonotic Dis.* **2:**119–127.

102. **McDade, J. E.** 1990. Ehrlichiosis—a disease of animals and humans. *J. Infect. Dis.* **161:**609–617.

103. **McKechnie, D. B., K. S. Slater, J. E. Childs, R. F. Massung, and C. D. Paddock.** 2000. Survival of *Ehrlichia chaffeensis* in refrigerated, ADSOL-treated RBCs. *Transfusion* **40:**1041–1047.

104. **McQuiston, J. H., C. D. Paddock, R. C. Holman, and J. E. Childs.** 1999. The human ehrlichioses in the United States. *Emerg. Infect. Dis.* **5:**635–642.

105. **Means, R. G., and D. J. White.** 1997. New distribution records of *Amblyomma americanum* (L.) (Acari: Ixodidae) in New York State. *J. Vector Ecol.* **22:**133–145.

106. **Moore, V. A., A. S. Varela, M. J. Yabsley, W. R. Davidson, and S. E. Little.** 2003. Detection of *Borrelia lonestari*, putative agent of STARI (southern tick-associated rash illness), in white-tailed deer (*Odocoileus virginianus*) from the southeastern United States. *J. Clin. Microbiol.* **41:**424–427.

107. **Morris, J. G., Jr., and M. Potter.** 1997. Emergence of new pathogens as a function of changes in host susceptibility. *Emerg. Infect. Dis.* **3:**435–441.

108. **Moskovitz, M., R. Fadden, and T. Min.** 1991. Human ehrlichiosis: a rickettsial disease associated with severe cholestasis and multisystemic disease. *J. Clin. Gastroenterol.* **13:**86–90.

109. **Mueller-Anneling, L., M. J. Gilchrist, and P. S. Thorne.** 2000. *Ehrlichia chaffeensis* antibodies in white-tailed deer, Iowa, 1994 and 1996. *Emerg. Infect. Dis.* **6:**397–400.

110. **Murphy, G. L., S. A. Ewing, L. C. Whitworth, J. C. Fox, and A. A. Kocan.** 1998. A molecular and serologic survey of *Ehrlichia canis*, *E. chaffeensis*, and *E. ewingii* in dogs and ticks from Oklahoma. *Vet. Parasitol.* **79:**325–339.

111. **Nutt, A. K., and J. Raufman.** 1999. Gastrointestinal and hepatic manifestations of human ehrlichiosis: 8 cases and a review of the literature. *Dig. Dis.* **17:**37–43.

112. **Ohashi, N., A. Unver, N. Zhi, and Y. Rikihisa.** 1998. Cloning and characterization of multigenes encoding the immunodominant 30-kilodalton major outer membrane proteins of *Ehrlichia canis* and application of the recombinant protein for serodiagnosis. *J. Clin. Microbiol.* **36:**2671–2680.

113. **Okada, H., T. Tajima, M. Kawahara, and Y. Rikihisa.** 2001. Ehrlichial proliferation and acute hepatocellular necrosis in immunocompetent mice experimentally infected with the HF strain of *Ehrlichia*, closely related to *Ehrlichia chaffeensis*. *J. Comp. Pathol.* **124:**165–171.

114. **Olano, J. P., E. Masters, L. Cullman, W. Hoegrefe, X. J. Yu, and D. H. Walker.** 1999. Human monocytotropic ehrlichiosis (HME): epidemiological, clinical and laboratory diagnosis of a newly emergent infection in the United States, p. 262–268. *In* D. Raoult and P. Brouqui (ed.), *Rickettsiae and Rickettsial Diseases at the Turn of the Third Millennium*. Elsevier, Paris, France.

115. **Olano, J. P., and D. H. Walker.** 2002. Human ehrlichioses. *Med. Clin. North Am.* **86:**375–392.

116. **Paddock, C. D., J. W. Sumner, G. M. Shore, D. C. Bartley, R. C. Elie, J. G. McQuade, C. R. Martin, C. S. Goldsmith, and J. E. Childs.** 1997. Isolation and characterization of *Ehrlichia chaffeensis* strains from patients with fatal ehrlichiosis *J. Clin. Microbiol.* **35:**2496–2502.

117. **Paddock, C. D., S. M. Folk, G. M. Shore, L. J. Machado, M. M. Huycke, L. N. Slater, A. M. Liddell, R. S. Buller, G. A. Storch, T. P. Monson, D. Rimland, J. W. Sumner, J. Singleton, K. C. Bloch, Y. W. Tang, S. M. Standaert, and J. E. Childs.** 2001. Infections with *Ehrlichia chaffeensis* and *Ehrlichia ewingii* in persons coinfected with human immunodeficiency virus. *Clin. Infect. Dis.* **33:**1586–1594.

118. **Paddock, C. D., and J. E. Childs.** 2003. *Ehrlichia chaffeensis*: a prototype emerging pathogen. *Clin. Microbiol. Rev.* **16:**37–64.

119. **Patel, R. G., and M. A. Byrd.** 1999. Near fatal acute respiratory distress syndrome in a patient with human ehrlichiosis. *South Med. J.* **92:**333–335.

120. **Patrick, C. D., and J. A. Hair.** 1977. Seasonal abundance of lone star ticks on white-tailed deer. *Environ. Entomol.* **6:**263–269.

121. **Patrick, C. D.** 1978. White-tailed deer utilization of three different habitats and its influence on lone star tick populations. *J. Parasitol.* **64:**1100–1106.

122. **Pearce, C. J., M. E. Conrad, P. E. Nolan, D. B. Fishbein, and J. E. Dawson.** 1988. Ehrlichiosis: a cause of bone marrow hypoplasia in humans. *Am. J. Hematol.* **28:**53–55.

123. **Petersen, L. R., L. A. Sawyer, D. B. Fishbein, P. W. Kelley, R. J. Thomas, L. A. Magnarelli, M. Redus, and J. E. Dawson.** 1989. An outbreak of ehrlichiosis in members of an Army Reserve unit exposed to ticks. *J. Infect. Dis.* **159:**562–568.

124. **Pick, N., I. Potasman, C. Strenger, A. Keysary, and I. Schwartz.** 2000. Ehrlichiosis associated vasculitis. *J. Intern. Med.* **247:**674–678.

125. **Ratnasamy, N., E. D. Everett, W. E. Roland, G. McDonald, and C. W. Caldwell.** 1996. Central nervous system manifestations of human ehrlichiosis. *Clin. Infect. Dis.* **23:**314–319.

126. **Rawlings, J.** 1996. Human ehrlichiosis in Texas. *J. Spir. Tick-borne Dis.* **3:**94–97.

127. **Reddy, G. R., and C. P. Streck.** 1999. Variability in the 28-kDa surface antigenic protein multigene locus of isolates of the emerging disease agent *Ehrlichia chaffeensis* suggest that it plays a role in immune invasion. *Mol. Cell. Biol. Res. Commun.* **1:**167–175.

128. **Rikihisa, Y.** 1991. The tribe *Ehrlichieae* and ehrlichial diseases. *Clin. Microbiol. Rev.* **4:**286–308.

129. **Rikihisa, Y.** 1999. Clinical and biological aspects of infection caused by *Ehrlichia chaffeensis*. *Microbes Infect.* **1:**367–376.

130. **Ristic, M.** 1986. Pertinent characteristics of leukocytic rickettsiae of humans and animals, p. 182–187. *In* L. Leive (ed.), *Microbiology-1986*. American Society for Microbiology, Washington, D.C.

131. **Ristic, M., and D. L. Huxsoll.** 1984. Ehrlichiae, p. 704–709. *In* N. R. Krieg and J. G. Holt (ed.), *Bergey's Manual of Systematic Bacteriology*, vol. 1. The Williams & Wilkins Co., Baltimore, Md.

132. **Rohrbach, B. W., J. R. Harkess, and J. Kudlac.** 1987. Human ehrlichiosis: a cause of "Oklahoma Tick Fever"? *Okla. St. Dep. Health Commun. Dis. Bull.* **87:**1.

133. **Rohrbach, B. W., J. R. Harkess, S. A. Ewing, J. Kudlac, G. L. McKee, and G. R. Istre.** 1990. Epidemiologic and clinical characteristics of persons with serologic evidence of *E. canis* infection. *Am. J. Public Health* **80:**442–445.

134. **Roland, W. E., E. D. Everett, T. L. Cyr, S. Z. Hasan, C. B. Dommarju, and G. A. McDonald.** 1998. *Ehrlichia chaffeensis* in Missouri ticks. *Am. J. Trop. Med. Hyg.* **59:**641–643.

135. **Rydkina, E., V. Roux, and D. Raoult.** 1999. Determination of the genome size of *Ehrlichia* spp., using pulsed field gel electrophoresis. *FEMS Microbiol. Lett.* **176:**73–78.

136. **Rynkiewicz, D., and L. X. Liu.** 1994. Human ehrlichiosis in New England. *N. Engl. J. Med.* **330:**292. (Letter.)

137. **Safdar, N., R. B. Love, and D. G. Maki.** 2002. Severe *Ehrlichia chaffeensis* infection in a lung transplant recipient: a review of ehrlichiosis in the immunocompromised patient. *Emerg. Infect. Dis.* **8:**320–323.

138. **Semnter, P. J., J. R. Saurer, and J. A. Hair.** 1973. The ecology and behavior of the lone star tick (Acarina: Ixodidae). IV.

Abundance and seasonal distribution in different habitat types. *J. Med. Entomol.* **10**:618–628.

139. Sexton, D. J., G. R. Corey, C. Carpenter, L. Q. Kong, T. Gandhi, E. Breitschwerdt, B. Hegarty, S. M. Chen, H. M. Feng, X. J. Yu, J. Olano, D. H. Walker, and J. S. Dumler. 1998. Dual infection with *Ehrlichia chaffeensis* and a spotted fever group rickettsia: a case report. *Emerg. Infect. Dis.* **4**:311–316.

140. Shea, K. W., A. J. Calio, N. C. Klein, and B. A. Cunha. 1995. Rhabdomyolysis associated with *Ehrlichia chaffeensis* infection. *Clin. Infect. Dis.* **21**:1056–1057.

141. Shibata, S.-I., M. Y. Kawahara, Y. Rikihisa, H. Fujita, Y. Watanabe, C. Suto, and T. Ito. 2000. New ehrlichia species closely related to *Ehrlichia chaffeensis* isolated from *Ixodes ovatus* ticks in Japan. *J. Clin. Microbiol.* **38**:1331–1338.

142. Smith, S., A. E. Sehdev, P. S. Sehdev, R. Jacobs, and J. S. Dumler. 2002. Human monocytic ehrlichiosis presenting as acute appendicitis during pregnancy. *Clin. Infect. Dis.* **35**:99–102.

143. Sonenshine, D. E., and G. J. Levy. 1971. The ecology of the lone star tick *Amblyomma americanum* (L.) in two contrasting habitats in Virginia (Acari: Ixodidae). *J. Med. Entomol.* **8**:623–635.

144. Sotomayor, E. A., V. L. Popov, H. Feng, D. H. Walker, and J. P. Olano. 2001. Animal model of fatal human monocytotropic ehrlichiosis. *Am. J. Pathol.* **158**:757–769.

145. Standaert, S. M., J. E. Dawson, W. Schaffner, J. E. Childs, K. L. Biggie, J. Singleton, Jr., R. R. Gerhardt, M. L. Knight, and R. H. Hutcheson. 1995. Ehrlichiosis in a golf-oriented retirement community. *N. Engl. J. Med.* **333**:420–425.

146. Standaert, S. M., L. A. Clough, W. Schaffner, J. S. Adams, and K. M. Neuzil. 1998. Neurologic manifestations of human monocytic ehrlichiosis. *Infect. Dis. Clin. Pract.* **7**:358–362.

147. Standaert, S. M., T. Yu, M. A. Scott, J. E. Childs, C. D. Paddock, W. Nicholson, J. Singleton, and M. J. Blaser. 2000. Primary isolation of *Ehrlichia chaffeensis* from patients with febrile illnesses: clinical and molecular characteristics. *J. Infect. Dis.* **181**:1082–1088.

148. Steiner, F. E., R. R. Pinger, and C. N. Vann. 1999. Infection rates of *Amblyomma americanum* (Acari: Ixodidae) by *Ehrlichia chaffeensis* (Rickettsiales: Ehrlichieae) and prevalence of *E. chaffeensis*-reactive antibodies in white-tailed deer in southern Indiana, 1997. *J. Med. Entomol.* **36**:715–719.

149. Stromdahl, E. Y., S. R. Evans, J. J. O'Brien, and A. G. Guttierez. 2001. Prevalence of infection in ticks submitted to the human tick test kit program of the U.S. Army Center for Health Promotion and Preventive Medicine. *J. Med. Entomol.* **38**:67–74.

150. Sumner, J. W., W. L. Nicholson, and R. F. Massung. 1997. PCR amplification and comparison of nucleotide sequences from the groESL heat shock operon of *Ehrlichia* species. *J. Clin. Microbiol.* **35**:2087–2092.

151. Sumner, J. W., J. E. Childs, and C. D. Paddock. 1999. Molecular cloning and characterization of the *Ehrlichia chaffeensis* variable-length PCR target: an antigen-expressing gene that exhibits interstrain variation. *J. Clin. Microbiol.* **37**:1447–1453.

152. Sumner, J. W., G. A. Storch, R. S. Buller, A. M. Liddell, S. L. Stockham, Y. Rikihisa, S. Messenger, and C. D. Paddock. 2000. PCR amplification and phylogenetic analysis of groESL operon sequences from *Ehrlichia ewingii* and *Ehrlichia muris*. *J. Clin. Microbiol.* **38**:2746–2749.

153. Telford, S. R. III, and J. E. Dawson. 1996. Persistent infection of C3H/HeJ mice by *Ehrlichia chaffeensis*. *Vet. Microbiol.* **52**:103–112.

154. Thompson, C., A. Spielman, and P. J. Krause. 2001. Coinfecting deer-associated zoonoses: Lyme disease, babesiosis, and ehrlichiosis. *Clin. Infect. Dis.* **33**:676–685.

155. Uhaa, I. J., J. D. Maclean, C. R. Green, and D. B. Fishbein. 1992. A case of human ehrlichiosis acquired in Mali: clinical and laboratory findings. *Am. J. Trop. Med. Hyg.* **46**:161–164.

156. Unver, A., S. Felek, C. D. Paddock, N. Zhi, H. W. Horowitz, G. P. Wormser, L. C. Cullman, and Y. Rikihisa. 2001. Western blot analysis of sera reactive to human monocytic ehrlichiosis and human granulocytic ehrlichiosis agents. *J. Clin. Microbiol.* **39**:3982–3986.

157. U.S. Census Bureau. 2001. Profiles of general demographic characteristics; 2000 census of population and housing, United States. U.S. Department of Commerce, Washington D.C.

158. Walls, J. J., K. M. Asanovich, J. S. Bakken, and J. S. Dumler. 1998. Serologic evidence of a natural infection of white-tailed deer with the agent of human granulocytic ehrlichiosis in Wisconsin and Maryland. *Clin. Diag. Lab. Immunol.* **5**:762–765.

159. Walker, D. H., A. G. Barbour, J. H. Oliver, R. S. Lane, J. S. Dumler, D. T. Dennis, D. H. Persing, A. F. Azad, and E. McSweegan. 1996. Emerging bacterial zoonotic and vector-borne diseases: ecological and epidemiological factors. *JAMA* **275**:463–469.

160. Walker, D. H., and the Task Force on Consensus Approach for Ehrlichiosis (CAFÉ). 2000. Diagnosing human ehrlichioses: current status and recommendations. *ASM News* **66**:287–290.

161. Weaver, R. A., G. Virella, and A. Weaver. 1999. Ehrlichiosis with severe pulmonary manifestations despite early treatment. *South Med. J.* **92**:336–339.

162. Whitlock, J. E., Q. Q. Fang, L. A. Durden, and J. H. Oliver, Jr. 2000. Prevalence of *Ehrlichia chaffeensis* (Rickettsiales: Rickettsiaceae) in *Amblyomma americanum* (Acari: Ixodidae) from the Georgia coast and barrier islands. *J. Med. Entomol.* **37**:276–280.

163. Williams, J. D., R. M. Snow, and J. G. Arciniegas. 1995. Myocardial involvement in a patient with human ehrlichiosis. *Am. J. Med.* **98**:414–415.

164. Winslow, G. M., E. Yager, K. Shilo, D. N. Collins, and F. K. Chu. 1998. Mechanisms of immunity to *Ehrlichia chaffeensis*. *Infect. Immun.* **66**:3892–3899.

165. Wolf, L., T. McPherson, B. Harrison, B. Engber, A. Anderson, and P. Whitt. 2000. Prevalence of *Ehrlichia ewingii* in *Amblyomma americanum* in North Carolina. *J. Clin. Microbiol.* **38**:2795. (Letter.)

166. Wong, S. J., G. S. Brady, and J. S. Dumler. 1997. Serological responses to *Ehrlichia equi*, *Ehrlichia chaffeensis*, and *Borrelia burgdorferi* in patients from New York State. *J. Clin. Microbiol.* **35**:2198–2205.

167. Yabsley, M. J., A. S. Varela, C. M. Tate, V. G. Dugan, D. E. Stallknecht, S. E. Little, and W. R. Davidson. 2002. *Ehrlichia ewingii* infection in white-tailed deer (*Odocoileus virginianus*). *Emerg. Infect. Dis.* **8**:668–671.

168. Yabsley, M. J., V. G. Dugan, D. E. Stallknecht, S. E. Little, J. M. Lockhart, J. E. Dawson, and W. R. Davidson. 2003. Evaluation of a prototype *Ehrlichia chaffeensis* surveillance system using white-tailed deer (*Odocoileus virginianus*) as natural sentinels. *Vector Borne Zoonotic Dis.* **3**:195–207.

169. Yabsley, M. J., S. E. Little, E. J. Sims, V. G. Dugan, D. E. Stallknecht, and W. R. Davidson. 2003. Molecular variation in the variable-length PCR target and 120-kilodalton antigen genes of *Ehrlichia chaffeensis* from white-tailed deer (*Odocoileus virginianus*). *J. Clin. Microbiol.* **41**:5202–5206.

170. Yevich, S. J., J. L. Sanchez, R. F. Defraites, C. C. Rives, J. E. Dawson, I. J. Uhaa, B. J. Johnson, and D. B. Fishbein. 1995.

Seroepidemiology of infections due to spotted fever group rickettsiae and *Ehrlichia* species in military personnel exposed in areas of the United States where such infections are endemic. *J. Infect. Dis.* **171:**1266–1273.

171. **Yu, X., P. Brouqui, J. S. Dumler, and D. Raoult.** 1993. Detection of *Ehrlichia chaffeensis* in human tissue by using a species-specific monoclonal antibody. *J. Clin. Microbiol.* **31:**3284–3288.

172. **Yu, X. J., P. Crocquet-Valdes, L. C. Cullman, and D. H. Walker.** 1996. The recombinant 120-kilodalton protein of *Ehrlichia chaffeensis*, a potential diagnostic tool. *J. Clin. Microbiol.* **34:**2853–2855.

173. **Yu, X. J., J. W. McBride, and D. H. Walker.** 1999. Genetic diversity of the 28-kilodalton outer membrane protein gene in human isolates of *Ehrlichia chaffeensis*. *J. Clin. Microbiol.* **37:**1137–1143.

Tick-Borne Diseases of Humans
Edited by Jesse L. Goodman et al.
© 2005 ASM Press, Washington, D.C.

Chapter 15

Other Causes of Tick-Borne Ehrlichioses, Including *Ehrlichia ewingii*

CHRISTOPHER D. PADDOCK, ALLISON M. LIDDELL, AND GREGORY A. STORCH

INTRODUCTION

At least three species of tick-borne bacteria in the genera *Ehrlichia* (*Ehrlichia chaffeensis* and *Ehrlichia ewingii*) and *Anaplasma* (*Anaplasma phagocytophilum*) cause moderately severe to life-threatening infections in humans, and they are collectively termed human ehrlichioses. None of these diseases was recognized formally before 1986, but several thousand cases of ehrlichioses were identified among patients from the United States, Europe, and Asia during the following 17 years (41). In addition, *Ehrlichia canis*, a pathogen of dogs that was identified more than 70 years ago, was recently isolated from a patient without clinical signs of illness; the role of this pathogen as a cause of human disease remains incompletely defined (42, 55).

For various reasons, the diseases caused by *E. chaffeensis* and *A. phagocytophilum* (discussed in Chapters 13 and 14) have received considerably more attention than ehrlichiosis caused by *E. ewingii*. (i) The infections caused by *E. chaffeensis* (human monocytic ehrlichiosis [HME]) and *A. phagocytophilum* (human granulocytic anaplasmosis [HGA]) were identified several years before the recognition of *E. ewingii* ehrlichiosis. (ii) Cases of *E. ewingii* ehrlichiosis have to date been reported predominantly among individuals with underlying immune suppression. (iii) Extensive cross-reactivity among *Ehrlichia* sp. antigens may complicate definitive identification of the causative agent in given cases; as a result, at least some cases of *E. ewingii* ehrlichiosis are likely misdiagnosed as HME. (iv) Because HGA and Lyme borreliosis are transmitted by the same tick vectors and have substantially overlapping natural histories and geographic distributions, considerable preexisting scientific and public health interest have been brought to bear on the study of *A. phagocytophilum*. In this context, an understanding of the epidemiology and ecology of *E. ewingii* and characterization of the disease it causes are relatively nascent.

E. EWINGII EHRLICHIOSIS

History

Sidney A. Ewing, a veterinary parasitologist and pioneering investigator of ehrlichioses, is credited with the first description of *E. ewingii* in a vertebrate host. In 1970, Ewing observed membrane-bound clusters of bacteria in neutrophils of a febrile dog from Arkansas and considered the pathogen to be a novel strain of *E. canis* because of its growth in granulocytes and because it caused a milder illness than that characteristically associated with *E. canis* (22). The disease in dogs caused by this pathogen was identified as a distinct clinical entity and named canine granulocytic ehrlichiosis (CGE) in 1985 (50). By using sequence analysis of the 16S rRNA gene, the etiologic agent was recognized as a novel species and designated *E. ewingii* in 1992 (3).

It was not until 1999 that *E. ewingii* infection in humans was first reported. Investigators at Washington University in St. Louis, Mo., applied a broad-range PCR assay to blood samples from four patients who appeared to have HME; the samples were negative when tested with a PCR assay specific for *E. chaffeensis* DNA. Subsequent molecular and serologic evaluation identified *E. ewingii* as the cause of disease in these patients (9). In this context, the recognition of *E. ewingii* as a pathogen of humans was facilitated by enhanced clinical awareness of ehrlichioses and by application of assays designed to identify novel ehrlichial pathogens. By 2002, only eight infections in human patients had been reported (9, 40), and these occurred predominantly among patients with underlying immune-suppressing conditions.

Christopher D. Paddock • Infectious Disease Pathology Activity, Centers for Disease Control and Prevention, Atlanta, GA 30333. **Allison M. Liddell** • InfectiousCare, 8320 Walnut Ln., Suite 300 LB3, Dallas, TX 75231. **Gregory A. Storch** • Department of Pediatrics, Washington University School of Medicine, St. Louis, MO 63110.

Etiologic Agent and Biology

E. ewingii is a small, obligate intracellular bacterium of the order *Rickettsiales*, family *Anaplasmataceae*. This organism and the disease it causes in vertebrate hosts share various morphological, genetic, ecological, and clinical features with *E. canis* (the agent of canine monocytic ehrlichiosis), *E. chaffeensis*, *Ehrlichia muris* (an agent of murine ehrlichiosis), and *Ehrlichia* (formerly *Cowdria*) *ruminantium*, the agent of heartwater in ruminants, which collectively define the genus *Ehrlichia*. All of these agents are pathogens of animals or humans. They reside and replicate in cytoplasmic vacuoles in host cells (typically leukocytes or endothelial cells, depending on the particular organism), are at least 97.7% similar in their 16S rRNA gene sequences, and are transmitted to vertebrate hosts by various species of hard ticks (20). Ehrlichiae are maintained in their tick vectors by transstadial transmission (4, 15, 23, 27); transovarial passage of these bacteria has not been demonstrated in the few species investigated (27, 31).

E. ewingii is a gram-negative, nonmotile, coccoid-to-ellipsoidal bacterium that is observed predominantly in neutrophils and occasionally in eosinophils of naturally infected dogs (22, 51) and humans (9, 40) and within neutrophils of experimentally infected deer (59). Compact clusters of ehrlichiae form intracytoplasmic, membrane-bound inclusions termed morulae, a distinctive feature of all *Ehrlichia* spp. (Fig. 1).

Morulae of *E. ewingii* range from 1 to 5 μm in greatest dimension, generally contain 5 to 30 ehrlichiae, and stain light to dark blue-gray on eosin-azure-type stains (Color Plates 9F and 9G). Infected cells typically contain a single morula; rarely, they may contain as many as three (51).

Information about molecular, phenotypic, and biologic characteristics of *E. ewingii* is rudimentary compared with that known about most other pathogenic ehrlichiae because of its novelty as a recognized pathogen of animals and humans, the relatively small number of described cases of disease in humans, and the fact that the agent has eluded attempts at isolation (3, 40). Characterized nucleotide sequences of *E. ewingii* include the 16S rRNA gene (3), the *groESL* operon (53), and a gene homologous to members of multigene families of *E. chaffeensis*, *E. canis*, and *E. ruminantium* that encode major antigenic proteins (e.g., p28, p30, and map1 proteins, respectively) (28).

All 16S rRNA gene sequences obtained from human cases have been identical (9, 40); however, some sequences of this gene obtained from infected ticks and deer have revealed a few nucleotide substitutions (54, 59), suggesting, as expected, that variants of *E. ewingii* may exist, as seen with *E. canis* (55) and *A. phagocytophilum* (20). The discoveries of loci containing multiple, paralogous genes coding for immunodominant antigens in closely related *Ehrlichia* spp. suggest that a multigene locus might also exist in the genome of *E. ewingii* (28). The considerable molecular heterogeneity

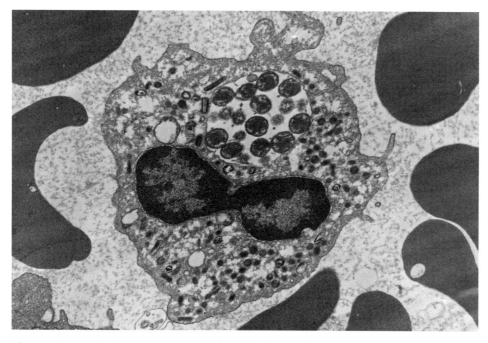

Figure 1. Electron micrograph of a canine neutrophil infected by *E. ewingii* (uranyl acetate-lead citrate stain). This image is provided courtesy of D. A. Kinden and S. L. Stockham (50); it is reprinted with permission from *Veterinary Medical Review*.

observed among individual *p28* alleles and among corresponding alleles of different strains of *E. chaffeensis* (45) suggests that similar genetic variability occurs among strains of *E. ewingii* (28). Differential expression of these genes may play a role in immune evasion by ehrlichiae (12, 45), although this mechanism remains to be demonstrated for *E. ewingii*.

Ecology and Natural History

Amblyomma americanum (the lone star tick) (Color Plate 1A) appears to be the primary vector involved in the natural transmission of *E. ewingii*. *E. ewingii* DNA has been amplified from questing adult and nymphal stage lone star ticks collected from several locations in Florida, Missouri, and North Carolina (Fig. 2), where the aggregate prevalence of infection in adult ticks was 1.6% (of 121 ticks), 5.4% (of 579 ticks), and 0.6% (of 462 ticks), respectively (49, 54, 58). Infection prevalence in nymphal stage ticks appears to be lower: minimum infection estimates determined from pools of nymphal *A. americanum* collected in Missouri and North Carolina were 0.6% (of 115 ticks) and 0.4% (of 1,308 ticks), respectively (49,

58). Transstadial passage of *E. ewingii* from nymphal to adult stage *A. americanum* and successful transmission of the pathogen among dogs by this tick have been demonstrated experimentally (4). Coinfections of adult lone star ticks with *E. ewingii* and *E. chaffeensis* have been described (49).

A. americanum is distributed broadly throughout the southeastern quadrant of the United States, and its range extends northward along coastal New England (Color Map 5). Questing ticks are most abundant from April to June, and the number of nymphs and adults diminishes as summer progresses (13). *A. americanum* is an aggressive and relatively nonspecific feeder, and ticks in all three stages will bite humans. This tick is also the principal tick vector of *E. chaffeensis*, and the range and seasonal activities of *A. americanum* mirror distributions in time and space of HME and *E. ewingii* ehrlichiosis (41). The roles of other tick species in the natural history of *E. ewingii* remain undetermined. DNA of *E. ewingii* has been amplified from adult *Dermacentor variabilis* (the American dog tick) collected from dogs (39) and vegetation (49, 54), although this tick failed to transmit *E. ewingii* to dogs in one study (4). *E. ewingii* DNA

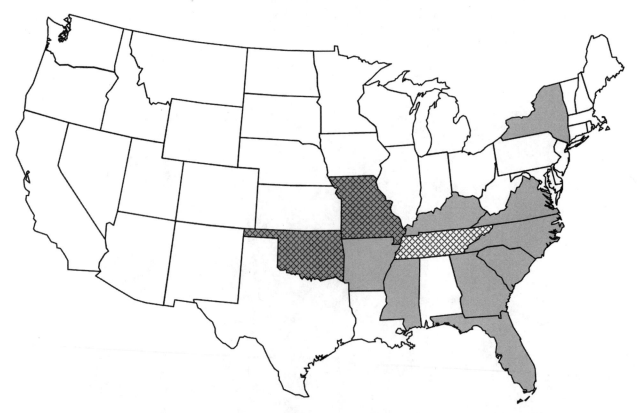

Figure 2. Representative distribution of *E. ewingii* in 2003 in the United States as determined by PCR assay detection of the agent in deer, dogs, and ticks (shaded) and in human patients (cross-hatched). The actual distribution of the pathogen is likely to include many additional states within the range of the vector tick, *A. americanum* (data from references 5, 9, 18, 26, 35, 39, 40, 49, 54, 58, and 59).

has also been amplified from adult *Rhipicephalus sanguineus* (the brown dog tick) removed from canines naturally infected with the pathogen (39).

PCR has been used to identify *E. ewingii* infection in domestic dogs from Mississippi, Missouri, New York, North Carolina, Oklahoma, and Virginia (Fig. 2) (9, 18, 25, 26, 35, 39). Additional CGE cases have been identified presumptively within the range of *A. americanum* by serology or visualization of morulae in granulocytes of dogs in Arkansas and Tennessee (6, 22). Canine disease caused by *E. ewingii* is considered less severe than that caused by *E. canis* (3, 22). CGE is notable for the frequent occurrence of polyarthritis involving one or more limbs, which manifests as acute lameness, generalized stiffness, or stilted gait. CGE-associated arthritis can involve various joints, including the humeroulnar, humeroradial, radiocarpal, antebrachial, and tarsocrural joints, and all limbs. Affected joints often contain effusions characterized by a predominance of neutrophils, occasionally containing morulae (6, 11, 16, 25, 26, 50). The pathogenesis of the arthritis remains undetermined, although immune complex deposition has been proposed as a possible contributing factor (52). Mild to moderately severe thrombocytopenia, anemia, and neutropenia are the most frequently described hematologic abnormalities (6, 26, 50). Morulae are typically detected in 1 to 4% of the peripheral blood granulocytes of ill dogs (6, 11, 16, 51), although percentages of infected granulocytes as high as 26% have been reported (50). Intraleukocytic morulae are occasionally visualized in cerebrospinal fluid of dogs with meningeal signs (38) and in the synovial fluid of dogs with arthritis (6, 11, 16, 26, 50). Coinfections with *E. ewingii* and *E. canis* have been reported (38).

Similar to other ehrlichioses, a continuum of disease severity exists among dogs with CGE: some infected animals develop only mild transient pyrexia (4, 52), while others exhibit profound thrombocytopenia with ecchymotic and petechial hemorrhages, vomiting, diarrhea, icterus, or meningitis (4, 11, 25, 26, 39). Various neurological manifestations, including proprioceptive deficits, paraparesis, ataxia, head tilt, tremors, and anisocoria, have been described in dogs with CGE (26). *E. ewingii* DNA has also been detected in the blood of apparently healthy, asymptomatic dogs, suggesting that such animals might also serve as reservoirs of this agent (9, 25, 26, 35).

E. ewingii DNA has been detected in peripheral blood of wild white-tailed deer (*Odocoileus virginianus*) from Arkansas, Georgia, Kentucky, Missouri, North Carolina, and South Carolina (Fig. 2) (5, 59). PCR testing of whole blood or leukocyte samples from 110 deer collected from eight southeastern states from 1996 through 2001 revealed *E. ewingii* DNA in 6 animals (5.5%); by locale, 0 to 29% of deer were positive (59). Precise regional estimates of infection prevalence are difficult to define when relatively few deer are evaluated at a particular location; however, during a recent investigation of 217 hunter-killed white-tailed deer from Boone County in central Missouri, PCR demonstrated an overall infection prevalence of approximately 20% (Table 1) (5). Because the sensitivities of these assays are not well characterized, infection prevalences may actually be higher. This possibility is suggested by a report in which deer blood that tested negative for *E. ewingii* by PCR subsequently produced infections when inoculated into naïve fawns (59). Simultaneous infections with *E. ewingii* and *E. chaffeensis* in white-tailed deer have been described (5, 59).

There are no data that document clinical features of *E. ewingii* infection in deer, and it is unknown whether deer become ill following infection with this agent. Because white-tailed deer represent a keystone host for all stages of the putative tick vector of *E. ewingii* (i.e., the lone star tick) and may also be an

Table 1. Comparison of prevalences of infection with *E. ewingii* and *E. chaffeensis* in various animal and human cohorts evaluated by PCR assays for both agents

Cohort	No. tested in cohort	Sampling location(s)[b]	No. (%) infected with:		Reference
			E. ewingii	*E. chaffeensis*	
White-tailed deer	110	AR, FL, GA, KY, LA, MS, NC, SC	6 (5.5)	6 (5.5)	59
White-tailed deer	217	MO	44 (20.3)	50 (23.0)	5
Domestic dogs from kennels or animal shelters	38	VA	6 (15.8)	8 (21.0)	18
Domestic dogs infested with ticks	65	OK	4 (6.2)	4 (6.2)	39
Domestic dogs with ehrlichiosis[a]	20	MO	18 (90.0)	1 (5.0)	35
Humans with ehrlichiosis	60	MO	4 (6.7)	56 (93.3)	9

[a] One dog in the series was positive for *A. phagocytophilum*.
[b] Abbreviations: AR, Arkansas; FL, Florida; GA, Georgia; KY, Kentucky; LA, Louisiana; MO, Missouri; MS, Mississippi; NC, North Carolina; OK, Oklahoma; SC, South Carolina; VA, Virginia.

important reservoir host for this pathogen, the ecological dynamics responsible for the emergence of *E. ewingii* ehrlichiosis in humans are likely similar to those described for HME (13, 41). In this context, the remarkable increase in white-tailed deer populations that occurred in the eastern, central, and southern United States during the 20th century created the circumstances by which a threshold of identifiable zoonotic disease in humans was reached (13).

E. ewingii has not been demonstrated conclusively in wildlife other than deer or in domesticated animals other than dogs. Extensive antigenic cross-reactivity exists among various *Ehrlichia* species, and it is possible that serologic surveys that detect antibodies reactive with *E. chaffeensis* in wildlife, including raccoons, red and gray foxes, and opposums (14, 17, 36), may also be recognizing cross-reacting infections with *E. ewingii*. In this context, the roles of these and other wildlife species as reservoir hosts of *E. ewingii* remain unknown.

Epidemiology

National surveillance data for human ehrlichioses do not specifically identify cases of ehrlichiosis caused by *E. ewingii* (http://www.cste.org/ps/2000/2000-id-03.htm); however, *E. ewingii* ehrlichiosis is documented from case series that include patients from Missouri, Oklahoma, and Tennessee (9, 40) (Fig. 2). The paucity of recognized cases in humans and the absence of prospective active surveillance for *E. ewingii* ehrlichiosis preclude broad epidemiologic generaliza-

tions about this disease. Because immune-suppressing conditions are observed frequently with patients with documented *E. ewingii* ehrlichiosis, it is possible that this patient cohort represents a sentinel population for whom disease manifestations are severe enough to merit formal recognition of the disease in humans; however, the total number of cases of infection and the burden of disease attributable to *E. ewingii* in the general population remain unknown.

Selected descriptive epidemiologic data, determined on the basis of 17 cases diagnosed at Washington University School of Medicine or the Centers for Disease Control and Prevention from 1996 through 2001, are summarized in Table 2 (9, 37, 40, 57). Fifteen (88%) patients were male, and the patients ranged in age from 11 to 65 years (median, 49 years). Twelve (70%) patients had underlying medical conditions causing immune suppression at the time of their illness, including solid-organ transplantation (5 patients), infection with human immunodeficiency virus (HIV) (4 patients), methotrexate or corticosteroid therapy (2 patients), or diabetes mellitus (1 patient). The patients became ill from May through August, and all reported a tick bite or known exposure to ticks shortly before disease onset. Twelve (75%) of 16 patients for whom pet ownership data were available owned dogs; DNA of *E. ewingii* was amplified from the blood of two asymptomatic dogs owned by 1 of these patients (9).

Because *E. ewingii* and *E. chaffeensis* share a principal tick vector and perhaps several vertebrate reservoir hosts, it is likely that there is considerable

Table 2. Selected epidemiologic characteristics of tick-exposed patients with ehrlichiosis caused by *E. ewingii*, 1996–2001[a]

Age (yr)/sex[b]	Date of onset (mo yr)	State[c]	Preexisting condition	Dog ownership
11/M	May 1996	MO	Renal transplantation	Yes
49/M	July 1996	MO	Rheumatoid arthritis	Yes
60/M	June 1998	MO	None	Yes
65/M	August 1998	MO	Chronic obstructive pulmonary disease	Yes
35/M	June 1999	MO	Renal transplantation	Yes
45/M	June 1999	OK	HIV infection	Unknown
48/M	June 1999	OK	HIV infection	Yes
52/M	June 1999	MO	Liver transplantation	Yes
38/M	July 1999	MO	None	No
48/M	May 2000	MO	Renal transplantation	No
62/F	May 2000	MO	None	Yes
40/M	June 2000	MO	HIV infection	No
49/M	June 2000	TN	HIV infection	Yes
27/M	July 2000	MO	None	No
49/F	July 2000	MO	Liver transplantation	Yes
53/M	August 2000	MO	Diabetes mellitus	Yes
57/M	June 2001	MO	None	Yes

[a] Data from references 9, 37, 40, and 57.
[b] M, male; F, female.
[c] MO, Missouri; OK, Oklahoma; TN, Tennessee.

overlap in the distribution of these two pathogens (13). Information about *E. ewingii* ehrlichiosis among humans and identification of the agent from ticks, dogs, and deer indicate a distribution of the pathogen in the southeastern and south-central United States that so far resembles the distribution of *E. chaffeensis* (5, 9, 18, 26, 39, 40, 49, 54, 58, 59). In a similar manner, because the diseases caused by these two agents may be indistinguishable clinically and serologically, it is likely that some cases reported as HME represent misidentified cases of *E. ewingii* ehrlichiosis (9).

Data examining the relative prevalence of *E. chaffeensis* and *E. ewingii* in vertebrate hosts in areas where both agents are endemic suggest that *E. ewingii* occurs in canine and deer populations at frequencies similar to, or in some cases greater than, infection with *E. chaffeensis* (Table 1); however, confirmed cases of human disease attributed to *E. ewingii* are uncommon relative to cases of HME (9, 35, 57). It is therefore possible that *E. ewingii* causes a milder illness than *E. chaffeensis* (41), particularly in persons with no underlying immune suppressing conditions, and that fewer *E. ewingii*-infected patients seek medical attention and subsequent laboratory evaluation.

Clinical Manifestations

The clinical manifestations of *E. ewingii* ehrlichiosis resemble those of disease caused by *E. chaffeensis* (9, 40, 57). The typical illness consists of a febrile syndrome accompanied by headache, malaise, and myalgia. In most patients, *E. ewingii* appears to produce milder disease than *E. chaffeensis*, but sufficient overlap of disease manifestations precludes clinical distinction in individual cases. None of the patients diagnosed to date have exhibited syndromes of multisystem organ failure, with or without the disseminated intravascular coagulopathy that is sometimes seen with disease caused by *E. chaffeensis*, and no deaths attributable to human infection with *E. ewingii* have yet been reported. Interestingly, the well-defined manifestations of joint involvement (e.g., arthritis and synovial effusions) described in dogs infected with *E. ewingii* have not been observed in human patients.

Table 3 compares selected clinical findings in *E. ewingii*-infected patients to those of *E. chaffeensis*-infected patients diagnosed at Washington University Medical Center in St. Louis, Mo., from 1999 to 2000 (57). The available clinical laboratory findings of these two patient groups are shown in Table 4. In general, laboratory abnormalities were less pronounced in individuals with *E. ewingii* ehrlichiosis than in patients with HME (57). Infection with *E. ewingii* should be suspected in patients with unexplained fever following tick exposures in regions of the United States

Table 3. Selected clinical manifestations of patients infected with *E. ewingii* or *E. chaffeensis*[a]

Manifestation	No. (%) infected[b] with:	
	E. ewingii	*E. chaffeensis*
Fever	7 (100)	39 (100)
Headache	5 (71)	28 (72)
Stiff neck	2 (29)	2 (5)
Myalgias	5 (71)	18 (46)
Arthralgias	3 (43)	15 (38)
Arthritis	0	1 (3)
Nausea	2 (29)	15 (38)
Vomiting	1 (14)	11 (28)
Diarrhea	2 (29)	10 (26)
Cough	2 (29)	7 (18)
Rash	0	8 (20)

[a] Patients were diagnosed at Washington University Medical Center, St. Louis, Mo., between 1999 and 2000. Data are taken from reference 57.
[b] Seven patients were diagnosed with *E. ewingii* infections, and 39 patients were diagnosed with *E. chaffeensis* infections.

where this agent is endemic, particularly among patients with preexisting immunocompromising conditions who fail to improve clinically while receiving commonly prescribed antibiotics other than tetracyclines (40). See Chapter 5 for further discussion of the general clinical and therapeutic approach to febrile illness in individuals with tick exposure.

Table 4. Selected laboratory findings in patients infected with *E. ewingii* or *E. chaffeensis*[a]

Laboratory value	Patients infected with[b]:	
	E. ewingii	*E. chaffeensis*
No. of patients with[c]:		
Leukopenia (<4,500/mm³)	5/7	28/32
Thrombocytopenia (<140,000/mm³)	4/7	26/30
Anemia (hematocrit, <36%)	4/7	14/24
Elevated serum AST (>47 IU/liter)	5/7	27/31
Additional parameters[d]		
Lowest leukocyte count/mm³	2,900 (7)	2,700 (32)
Lowest platelet count/mm³	128,000 (7)	85,500 (30)
Lowest hematocrit (%)	30 (7)	32 (24)
Highest AST (IU/liter)	52 (7)	130 (31)
CSF leukocyte count/ml	10 (3)	7 (6)
CSF protein level (g/dl)	96 (3)	62 (7)
CSF glucose level (g/dl)	64 (3)	65 (7)

[a] Patients were diagnosed at Washington University Medical Center, St. Louis, Mo., between 1999 and 2000. Data are taken from reference 57.
[b] Seven patients were infected with *E. ewingii* and 39 were infected with *E. chaffeensis*.
[c] Values shown are the number of patients with the manifestation divided by the number of patients for whom data were available. AST, aspartate aminotransferase. CSF, cerebrospinal fluid.
[d] Parameter values shown are median values (number of patients for whom parameter was available).

Laboratory Diagnosis

The laboratory diagnosis of *E. ewingii* ehrlichiosis begins with a careful inspection of the Wright- or Giemsa-stained peripheral blood smear. Although morulae have not been visible in blood smears from most *E. ewingii*-infected patients, their frequency may be greater than in specimens from those infected with *E. chaffeensis*. When noted, morulae were observed in 5 to 50% of circulating granulocytes (9, 40). Morulae have been identified most frequently within peripheral blood neutrophils (Color Plate 9F) and eosinophils, and less commonly in leukocytes in bronchoalveolar lavage fluid (Color Plate 9G) or cerebrospinal fluid (CSF) (9).

The specific laboratory diagnosis of *E. ewingii* infection currently depends on molecular methods. The greatest experience to date has been with assays that amplify a segment of the 16S rRNA gene (3, 9). DNA of *E. ewingii* has been detected in clinical samples, including whole blood and CSF, by a broad-range PCR assay that detects all known pathogenic *Ehrlichia* species (9). Following a positive result with the broad-range assay, individual species can be identified by using species-specific assays with unique primer binding sites in the 16S rRNA gene (56) or in the *groESL* operon (53).

Through 2004, attempts to isolate *E. ewingii* in continuous cell lines have been unsuccessful, which currently precludes the use of isolation as a diagnostic technique. The failure to cultivate *E. ewingii* has also hampered the development of specific reagents for serologic testing. Individuals with *E. ewingii* ehrlichiosis typically have an antibody response that can be detected by an indirect immunofluorescence antibody assay that evaluates cross-reactivity against antigens of *E. canis* or *E. chaffeensis*. Convalescent-phase serum of humans and dogs infected with *E. ewingii* fails to react with the 28- and 30-kDa major antigenic proteins of *E. chaffeensis* and *E. canis*, respectively, which suggests that the cross-reacting antigens that assist in serological diagnosis are proteins of high relative molecular mass (9, 46). Because indirect immunofluorescence antibody assays cannot distinguish between antibodies produced in response to infection with *E. chaffeensis* or *E. ewingii* (9, 40), it is likely that some patients who have been diagnosed with *E. chaffeensis* ehrlichiosis by indirect immunofluorescence antibody assays may have actually been infected with *E. ewingii*.

Treatment and Prevention

Patients with *E. ewingii* ehrlichiosis respond promptly to therapy with doxycycline at the same dosage used to treat HME (i.e., 100 mg given twice a day). There have been no studies that evaluate the optimal duration of therapy, but treatment for 10 to 14 days has been used successfully (9, 40). Relapse of disease has not been described, even though most patients infected with *E. ewingii* have been markedly immunosuppressed.

Because *E. ewingii* appears to be transmitted by *A. americanum*, preventive measures for *E. ewingii* ehrlichiosis are the same as those for *E. chaffeensis*. Standard precautions that reduce the risk of lone star tick bites or minimize the duration of tick attachment following bites should be followed (41). Because *E. ewingii* ehrlichiosis has been described most frequently among persons with compromised immunity, it is particularly important that individuals with diseases that cause immune suppression and persons taking immunosuppressive medications who reside in or travel to areas where ehrlichioses are endemic are well informed about measures to minimize tick exposure. It is also important for all patients to bring possible tick exposure to the attention of health care providers if they develop a febrile illness following visitation to a tick-infested area and that health care professionals be aware of the possibility of tick-borne infections, including *E. ewingii*, as a cause of fever in patients with chronic underlying illnesses.

E. CANIS AND OTHER TICK-BORNE EHRLICHIOSES

E. canis, discovered in 1935 (19), is the prototypical species of the genus *Ehrlichia*. Various animals are susceptible to infection with *E. canis*, including domestic dogs, red and gray foxes, wolves, coyotes, and domestic cats (2, 7, 21, 30). *R. sanguineus* is the principal vector of *E. canis* (27). As with CGE, the recognition of canine ehrlichiosis caused by *E. canis* infection preceded identification of human infection by several decades. The only confirmed *E. canis* infection in a human was reported in 1996 when *E. canis* was isolated from the blood of an asymptomatic individual in Venezuela (42). Molecular analyses of DNA amplified from the isolate and from pools of brown dog ticks and dog blood samples collected from Lara State, Venezuela, revealed 99.9% identity among these sequences with the type strain of *E. canis* (55).

E. canis causes life-threatening and chronic infections in dogs, and considerable data exist on the pathogenesis and immunology of infection in canines (29). However, almost nothing is known about the interaction of this bacterium with human hosts. The patient for whom infection with this agent was reported showed no clinical or laboratory evidence of disease (42); in this context, the relative contribution of *E. canis* as a cause of human ehrlichiosis, if any, is unknown. Given the cosmopolitan distribution of this ehrlichia and its vector, it is curious that additional *E. canis* infections among humans have not been identified. Most populations of *R. sanguineus* in the United States seldom bite humans, perhaps explaining the absence of documented human infections with *E. canis* in this country. However, because of extensive antigenic cross-reactivity of *E. canis* with *E. chaffeensis*, it is also possible that some cases of human ehrlichiosis caused by *E. canis* are classified as HME when group-specific serologic assays are used to diagnose the infection. Geographic foci of increased parasitism of humans by *R. sanguineus* may exist in the United States (10, 24), and other potential tick vectors that frequently bite humans, including *D. variabilis*, could potentially be involved in the natural history of *E. canis* (33). In this context, it is possible that unrecognized human infections occur.

The paradigm exemplified by recent discoveries of novel spotted fever group rickettsioses on several continents (43) may also apply to the human ehrlichioses. Antibodies reactive with *Ehrlichia* spp. have been detected in patients from various locations beyond the recognized geographic range of *E. chaffeensis*, *E. ewingii*, and the lone star tick, including Argentina, Israel, Italy, Portugal, Mali, Mexico, Russia, Japan, and Thailand, suggesting infections with antigenically related agents (34, 41, 44). Various incompletely characterized *Ehrlichia*- and *Anaplasma*-like bacteria have been detected in wildlife and ticks in the United States and elsewhere (1, 5, 8), although data linking any of these agents with specific diseases are currently lacking.

In Japan, at least two recently identified *Ehrlichia* spp. represent potential pathogens of humans. *E. muris*, isolated from a wild mouse (*Eothenomys kageus*) in 1983 and characterized as a distinct species in 1995, causes a mild, transient illness in laboratory mice. This ehrlichia has also been isolated from other rodents, including *Apodemus speciosus* and *Apodemus argenteus*, and from questing nymphal *Haemaphysalis flava* ticks (34). DNA of *E. muris* has also been detected in questing adult *Ixodes persulcatus* ticks collected in the Perm and Baltic regions of Russia (1, 44). Both of these ticks bite humans, and persons with antibodies reactive with *E. muris* have been identified in central Japan (34).

An *Ehrlichia* sp. isolated from questing *Ixodes ovatus* ticks collected in central and northern Japan shows 98.2% similarity to *E. chaffeensis* by 16S rRNA gene sequence analysis (47). This agent (termed *I. ovatus* ehrlichia [IOE]) causes severe disease in laboratory mice. Histopathologic lesions of IOE-infected mice resemble lesions identified in some human patients with fatal HME, including interstitial pneumonitis, hepatocyte apoptosis, and erythrophagocytosis (48). An animal reservoir of IOE has not been identified, although DNA of IOE was detected in a blood sample from a dog in Japan (32). *I. ovatus* is found throughout Japan, and the adult stage tick will bite humans (47); however, cases of disease in humans caused by IOE have not yet been identified.

CONCLUDING COMMENTS

Since 1987, various clinical, epidemiological, and laboratory achievements have facilitated the recognition and characterization of a genus of tick-borne pathogens previously unheard of by most clinicians. In 2004, the term human ehrlichiosis has become conventional parlance for most physicians; however, many aspects of these diseases, particularly infection caused by *E. ewingii*, remain only partially characterized. Areas for future investigation in the natural history of *E. ewingii* include field investigations that define roles of tick species other than *A. americanum* and vertebrate hosts other than dogs and deer. Understanding the frequency and mechanism of asymptomatic canine infection may provide insights to the pathogenesis of *E. ewingii* infections in natural and non-natural hosts. Prospective active surveillance is needed to better identify (i) the numbers of cases of disease in humans caused by *E. ewingii*, (ii) the geographical distribution of disease in humans, and (iii) the spectrum of clinical disease in various human cohorts. More robust laboratory techniques need to be developed, including methods to isolate *E. ewingii* in cell culture and serological techniques to distinguish this infection from HME. It is likely that other tick-borne ehrlichiae will be recognized eventually as additional agents of human ehrlichioses around the world. The key to identifying novel agents lies in the perspicacity of, and cooperation among, clinicians, veterinarians, epidemiologists, and laboratorians.

REFERENCES

1. Alekseev, A. N., H. V. Dubinina, I. van De Pol, and L. M. Schouls. 2001. Identification of *Ehrlichia* spp. and *Borrelia burgdorferi* in *Ixodes* ticks in the Baltic regions of Russia. *J. Clin. Microbiol.* **39:**2237–2242.
2. Amyx, H. L., and D. L. Huxsoll. 1973. Red and gray foxes—potential reservoir for *Ehrlichia canis*. *J. Wildl. Dis.* **9:**47–50.
3. Anderson, B. E., C. R. Greene, D. C. Jones, and J. E. Dawson. 1992. *Ehrlichia ewingii* sp. nov., the etiologic agent of canine granulocytic ehrlichiosis. *Int. J. Syst. Bacteriol.* **42:**299–302.
4. Anziani, O. S., S. A. Ewing, and R. W. Barker. 1990. Experimental transmission of a granulocytic form of the tribe Ehrlichieae by *Dermacentor variabilis* and *Amblyomma americanum* to dogs. *Am. J. Vet. Res.* **51:**929–931.

5. Arens, M. Q., A. M. Liddell, G. Buening, M. Gaudreault-Keener, J. W. Sumner, J. A. Comer, R. S. Buller, and G. A. Storch. 2003. Detection by PCR and serology of *Ehrlichia* spp. in the blood of wild white-tailed deer in Missouri. *J. Clin. Microbiol.* 41:1263–1265.

6. Bellah, J. R., R. M. Shull, and E. V. Shull Selcer. 1986. *Ehrlichia canis*-related polyarthritis in a dog. *J. Am. Vet. Med. Assoc.* 189:922–923.

7. Boulay, R. P., M. R. Lappin, C. H. Holland, M. A. Thrall, D. Baker, and S. O'Neil. 1994. Clinical ehrlichiosis in a cat. *J. Am. Vet. Med. Assoc.* 204:1475–1478.

8. Brandsma, A. R., S. E. Little, J. M. Lockhart, W. R. Davidson, D. E. Stallknecht, and J. E. Dawson. 1999. Novel *Ehrlichia* organism (Rickettsiales: Ehrlichieae) in white-tailed deer associated with lone star tick (Acari: Ixodidae) parasitism. *J. Med. Entomol.* 36:190–194.

9. Buller, R. S., M. Arens, S. P. Hmiel, C. D. Paddock, J. W. Sumner, Y. Rikihisa, A. Unver, M. Gaudreault-Keener, F. A. Manian, A. L. Liddell, N. Schmulewitz, and G. A. Storch. 1999. *Ehrlichia ewingii*, a newly recognized agent of human ehrlichiosis. *N. Engl. J. Med.* 341:148–155.

10. Carpenter, T. I., M. C. McMeans, and C. P. McHugh. 1990. Additional instances of human parasitism by the brown dog tick (Acari: Ixodidae). *J. Med. Entomol.* 27:1065–1066.

11. Carrillo, J. M., and R. A. Green. 1978. A case report of canine ehrlichiosis: neutrophilic strain. *J. Am. Anim. Hosp. Assoc.* 14:100–104.

12. Cheng, C., C. D. Paddock, and R. R. Reddy. 2003. Molecular heterogeneity of *Ehrlichia chaffeensis* isolates determined by sequence analysis of the 28-kilodalton outer membrane protein genes and other regions of the genome. *Infect. Immun.* 71:187–195.

13. Childs, J. E., and C. D. Paddock. 2003. The ascendancy of *Amblyomma americanum* as a vector of pathogens affecting humans in the United States. *Annu. Rev. Entomol.* 48:307–337.

14. Comer, J. A., W. L. Nicholson, C. D. Paddock, J. W. Sumner, and J. E. Childs. 2000. Detection of antibodies reactive with *Ehrlichia chaffeensis* in the raccoon. *J. Wildl. Dis.* 36:705–712.

15. Cowdry, E. V. 1925. Studies on the etiology of heartwater. II. *Rickettsia ruminantium* (n. sp.) in the tissues of ticks transmitting the disease. *J. Exp. Med.* 42:253–274.

16. Cowell, R. L., R. D. Tyler, K. D. Clinkenbeard, and J. H. Meinkoth. 1988. Ehrlichiosis and polyarthritis in three dogs. *J. Am. Vet. Med. Assoc.* 8:1093–1095.

17. Davidson, W. R., J. M. Lockhart, D. E. Stallknecht, and E. W. Howerth. 1999. Susceptibility of red and gray foxes to infection by *Ehrlichia chaffeensis*. *J. Wildl. Dis.* 35:696–702.

18. Dawson, J. E., K. L. Biggie, C. K. Warner, K. Cookson, S. Jenkins, J. F. Levine, and J. G. Olson. 1996. Polymerase chain reaction evidence of *Ehrlichia chaffeensis*, an etiologic agent of human ehrlichiosis, in dogs from southeast Virginia. *Am. J. Vet. Res.* 57:1175–1179.

19. Donatien, A., and F. Lestoquard. 1935. Existence en Algérie d'une *Rickettsia* du chien. *Bull. Soc. Pathol. Exot.* 28:418–419.

20. Dumler, J. S., A. F. Barbet, C. P. J. Bekker, G. A. Dasch, G. H. Palmer, S. C. Ray, Y. Rikihisa, and F. R. Rurangirwa. 2001. Reorganization of genera in the families *Rickettsiaceae* and *Anaplasmataceae* in the order *Rickettsiales*: unification of some species of *Ehrlichia* with *Anaplasma*, *Cowdria* with *Ehrlichia* and *Ehrlichia* with *Neorickettsia*, descriptions of six new species combinations and designation of *Ehrlichia equi* and "HGE agent" as subjective synonyms of *Ehrlichia phagocytophila*. *Int. J. Syst. Evol. Microbiol.* 51:2145–2165.

21. Ewing, S. A., R. G. Buckner, and B. C. Springer. 1964. The coyote, a potential host for *Babesia canis* and *Ehrlichia* sp. *J. Parasitol.* 50:704.

22. Ewing, S. A., W. R. Roberson, R. G. Buckner, and C. S. Hayat. 1971. A new strain of *Ehrlichia canis*. *J. Am. Vet. Med. Assoc.* 159:1771–1774.

23. Ewing, S. A., J. E. Dawson, A. A. Kocan, R. W. Barker, C. K. Warner, R. J. Panciera, J. C. Fox, K. M. Kocan, and E. F. Blouin. 1995. Experimental transmission of *Ehrlichia chaffeensis* (Rickettsiales: Ehrlichieae) among white-tailed deer by *Amblyomma americanum* (Acari: Ixodidae). *J. Med. Entomol.* 32:368–374.

24. Goddard, J. 1989. Focus of human parasitism by the brown dog tick, *Rhipicephalus sanguineus* (Acari: Ixodidae). *J. Med. Entomol.* 26:628–629.

25. Goldman, E. E., E. B. Breitschwerdt, C. B. Grindem, B. C. Hegarty, J. J. Walls, and J. S. Dumler. 1998. Granulocytic ehrlichiosis in dogs from North Carolina and Virginia. *J. Vet. Intern. Med.* 12:61–70.

26. Goodman, R. A., E. C. Hawkins, N. J. Olby, C. B. Grindem, B. Hegarty, and E. B. Breitschwerdt. 2003. Molecular identification of *Ehrlichia ewingii* infection in dogs: 15 cases (1997–2001). *J. Am. Vet. Med. Assoc.* 222:1102–1107.

27. Groves, M. G., G. L. Dennis, H. L. Amyx, and D. L. Huxsoll. 1975. Transmission of *Ehrlichia canis* to dogs by ticks (*Rhipicephalus sanguineus*). *Am. J. Vet. Res.* 36:937–940.

28. Gusa, A. A., R. S. Buller, G. A. Storch, M. M. Huycke, L. J. Machado, L. N. Slater, S. L. Stockham, and R. F. Massung. 2001. Identification of a *p28* gene in *Ehrlichia ewingii*: evaluation of gene for use as a target for a species-specific PCR diagnostic assay. *J. Clin. Microbiol.* 39:3871–3876.

29. Harrus, S., T. Waner, H. Bark, F. Jongejan, and A. W. C. A. Cornelissen. 1999. Recent advances in determining the pathogenesis of canine monocytic ehrlichiosis. *J. Clin. Microbiol.* 37:2745–2749.

30. Harvey, J. W., C. F. Simpson, J. M. Gaskin, and J. H. Sameck. 1979. Ehrlichiosis in wolves, dogs, and wolf-dog crosses. *J. Am. Vet. Med. Assoc.* 175:901–905.

31. Illemobade, A. A., and P. Leeflang. 1978. Experiments on the transmission of *Cowdria ruminantium* by the tick *Amblyomma variegatum*, p. 527–530. *In* J. K. H. Wilde (ed.), *Tick-Borne Diseases and Their Vectors*. Edinburgh University Press, Edinburgh, Scotland.

32. Inokuma, H., K. Ohno, T. Onishi, D. Raoult, and P. Brouqui. 2001. Detection of ehrlichial infection by PCR in dogs from Yamaguchi and Okinawa Prefectures, Japan. *J. Vet. Med. Sci.* 63:815–817.

33. Johnson, E. M., S. A. Ewing, R. W. Barker, J. C. Fox, D. W. Crow, and K. M. Kocan. 1998. Experimental transmission of *Ehrlichia canis* (Rickettsiales: Ehrlichieae) by *Dermacentor variabilis* (Acari: Ixodidae). *Vet. Parasitol.* 74:277–288.

34. Kawahara, M., T. Ito, C. Suto, S. Shibata, Y. Rikihisa, K. Hata, and K. Hirai. 1999. Comparison of *Ehrlichia muris* strains isolated from wild mice and ticks and serologic survey of humans and animals with *E. muris* as antigen. *J. Clin. Microbiol.* 37:1123–1129.

35. Liddell, A. M., S. L. Stockham, M. A. Scott, J. W. Sumner, C. D. Paddock, M. Gaudreault-Keener, M. Q. Arens, and G. A. Storch. 2003. Predominance of *Ehrlichia ewingii* in Missouri dogs. *J. Clin. Microbiol.* 41:4617–4622.

36. Lockhart, J. M., W. R. Davidson, D. E. Stallknecht, J. E. Dawson, and S. E. Little. 1997. Natural history of *Ehrlichia chaffeensis* (Rickettsiales: Ehrlichieae) in the piedmont physiographic province of Georgia. *J. Parasitol.* 83:887–894.

37. Masters, E. J. Personal communication.

38. Meinkoth, J. H., S. A. Ewing, R. L. Cowell, J. E. Dawson, C. K. Warner, J. S. Mathew, M. Bowles, A. E. Thiessen, R. J. Panciera, and C. Fox. 1998. Morphologic and molecular evidence of a dual species ehrlichial infection in a dog presenting

with inflammatory central nervous system disease. *J. Vet. Intern. Med.* **12**:389–393.

39. **Murphy, G. L., S. A. Ewing, L. C. Whitworth, J. C. Fox, and A. A. Kocan.** 1998. A molecular and serologic survey of *Ehrlichia canis*, *E. chaffeensis*, and *E. ewingii* in dogs and ticks from Oklahoma. *Vet. Parasitol.* **79**:325–339.

40. **Paddock, C. D., S. M. Folk, G. M. Shore, L. J. Machado, M. M. Huycke, L. N. Slater, A. M. Liddell, R. S. Buller, G. A. Storch, T. P. Monson, D. Rimland, J. W. Sumner, J. Singleton, K. C. Bloch, Y. Tang, S. M. Standaert, and J. E. Childs.** 2001. Infections with *Ehrlichia chaffeensis* and *Ehrlichia ewingii* in persons coinfected with human immunodeficiency virus. *Clin. Infect. Dis.* **33**:1586–1594.

41. **Paddock, C. D., and J. E. Childs.** 2003. *Ehrlichia chaffeensis*: a prototypical emerging pathogen. *Clin. Microbiol. Rev.* **16**: 37–64.

42. **Perez, M., Y. Rikihisa, and B. Wen.** 1996. *Ehrlichia canis*-like agent isolated from a man in Venezuela: antigenic and genetic characterization. *J. Clin. Microbiol.* **34**:2133–2139.

43. **Raoult, D., and J. G. Olson.** 1999. Emerging rickettsioses, p. 17–36. *In* W. M. Scheld, W. A. Craig, and J. M. Hughes (ed.), *Emerging Infections 3.* American Society for Microbiology, Washington, D.C.

44. **Ravyn, M. D., E. I. Korenberg, J. A. Oeding, Y. V. Kovalevskii, and R. C. Johnson.** 1999. Monocytic *Ehrlichia* in *Ixodes persulcatus* ticks from Perm, Russia. *Lancet* **353**:722–723.

45. **Reddy, G. R., and C. P. Streck.** 1999. Variability in the 28-kDa surface antigen protein multigene locus of isolates of the emerging disease agent *Ehrlichia chaffeensis* suggests that it plays a role in immune evasion. *Mol. Cell Biol. Res. Commun.* **1**:167–175.

46. **Rikihisa, Y., S. A. Ewing, and J. C. Fox.** 1994. Western immunoblot analysis of *Ehrlichia chaffeensis*, *E. canis*, or *E. ewingii* infections in dogs and humans. *J. Clin. Microbiol.* **32**:2107–2112.

47. **Shibata, S.I., M. Kawahara, Y. Rikihisa, H. Fujita, Y. Watanabe, C. Suto, and T. Ito.** 2000. New *Ehrlichia* species closely related to *Ehrlichia chaffeensis* isolated from *Ixodes ovatus* ticks in Japan. *J. Clin. Microbiol.* **38**:1331–1338.

48. **Sotomayor, E. A., V. L. Popov, H. M. Feng, D. H. Walker, and J. P. Olano.** 2001. Animal model of fatal human monocytotropic ehrlichiosis. *Am. J. Pathol.* **158**:757–769.

49. **Steiert, J. G., and F. Gilfoy.** 2002. Infection rates of *Amblyomma americanum* and *Dermacentor variabilis* by *Ehrlichia chaffeensis* and *Ehrlichia ewingii* in southwest Missouri. *Vector Borne Zoonotic Dis.* **2**:53–60.

50. **Stockham, S. L., D. A. Schmidt, and J. W. Tyler.** 1985. Canine granulocytic ehrlichiosis in dogs from central Missouri: a possible cause of polyarthritis. *Vet. Med. Rev.* **6**:3–5.

51. **Stockham, S. L., D. A. Schmidt, K. S. Curtis, B. G. Schauf, J. W. Tyler, and S. T. Simpson.** 1992. Evaluation of granulocytic ehrlichiosis in dogs of Missouri, including serologic status to *Ehrlichia canis*, *Ehrlichia equi*, and *Borrelia burgdorferi*. *Am. J. Vet. Res.* **53**:63–68.

52. **Stockham, S. L., J. W. Tyler, D. A. Schmidt, and K. S. Curtis.** 1990. Experimental transmission of granulocytic ehrlichial organisms in dogs. *Vet. Clin. Pathol.* **19**:99–104.

53. **Sumner, J. W., G. S. Storch, R. S. Buller, A. M. Liddell, S. L. Stockham, Y. Rikihisa, S. Messenger, and C. D. Paddock.** 2000. PCR amplification and phylogenetic analysis of *groESL* operon sequences from *Ehrlichia ewingii* and *Ehrlichia muris*. *J. Clin. Microbiol.* **38**:2746–2749.

54. **Sumner, J. W., D. McKechnie, D. Janowski, and C. D. Paddock.** 2000. Detection of *Ehrlichia ewingii* in field-collected ticks by using PCR amplification of 16S rRNA gene and *groESL* operon sequences, abstr. 72. 15th Meeting of the American Society for Rickettsiology. Captiva Island, Fla.

55. **Unver, A., M. Perez, N. Orellana, H. Huang, and Y. Rikihisa.** 2001. Molecular and antigenic comparison of *Ehrlichia canis* isolates from dogs, ticks, and a human in Venezuela. *J. Clin. Microbiol.* **39**:2788–2793.

56. **Warner, C. K., and J. E. Dawson.** 1996. Genus and species-level identification of *Ehrlichia* species by PCR and sequencing, p. 100–105. *In* D. H. Persing (ed.), *PCR Protocols for Emerging Infectious Diseases: A Supplement to Diagnostic Molecular Microbiology.* ASM Press, Washington, D.C.

57. **Washington University School of Medicine.** 2003. Unpublished data.

58. **Wolf, L., T. McPherson, B. Harrison, B. Engber, A. Anderson, and P. Whitt.** 2000. Prevalence of *Ehrlichia ewingii* in *Amblyomma americanum* in North Carolina. *J. Clin. Microbiol.* **38**:2795.

59. **Yabsley, M. J., A. S. Varela, C. M. Tate, V. G. Dugan, D. E. Stallknecht, S. E. Little, and W. R. Davidson.** 2002. *Ehrlichia ewingii* infection in white-tailed deer (*Odocoileus virginianus*). *Emerg. Infect. Dis.* **8**:668–671.

Chapter 16

Relapsing Fever

ALAN G. BARBOUR

INTRODUCTION AND HISTORY

Relapsing fever is an arthropod-borne infection that occurs in two forms: tick-borne relapsing fever (TBRF) and louse-borne relapsing fever (LBRF) (106). The etiologic agents of relapsing fever are several species of spirochetes in the genus *Borrelia* (15, 27). TBRF is usually a zoonosis and is endemic on most continents, each with a characteristic *Borrelia* species. Examples are *Borrelia hermsii* in North America and *Borrelia duttonii* in Africa. LBRF is caused by a single species, *Borrelia recurrentis*. It is spread from person to person by human lice and can occur in epidemics of hundreds of thousands of cases. The multiple episodes of fever and disease relapses in both TBRF and LBRF are due to antigenic variation by the spirochetes (13).

Relapsing fever's distinctive clinical course has been recognized as an entity since ancient times (106). The large number of spirochetes in the blood at the fever's peak enabled their identification as the etiologic agent in the 19th century, many decades before cultivation in the laboratory (16). For many years after their discovery, *Borrelia* species and relapsing fever were subjects of considerable scientific interest. Ehrlich and other pioneers in immunology recognized that the characteristic pattern of recurrences of the presence of bacteria in the blood during relapsing fever episodes revealed clues about the adaptive immune responses of vertebrates (193). Most of the important features of the biology and immunology of the disease were described at the end of the 19th century and in the first half of the 20th century. But elucidation of the pathogenesis and genetics of relapsing fever agents awaited the developments in the field of molecular biology.

ETIOLOGIC AGENTS

Biology

Like other spirochetal organisms, *Borrelia* are spiral or wavy filaments with inner and outer cell membranes and several flagella that start at each end and overlap in the middle of the cell's periplasmic space (132, 137). Unlike the flagellas of other bacteria, those of spirochetes are not surface exposed and thus are not susceptible to attack by the host's antibodies. *Borrelia* cells are approximately 0.2 μm wide and 10 to 30 μm in length. They can be visualized in wet mounts by dark-field or phase-contrast microscopy but not by standard light microscopy without special stains. In comparison to treponemes and leptospires, motile borrelias exhibit fewer and larger amplitude waves. Known species of *Borrelia* are host-associated microorganisms and are to be found either in an arthropod, usually a tick, or in a mammal or bird, but not free living in the environment. In their hosts, borrelias are usually found outside of cells. *Borrelia* spp. are very susceptible to drying, hypotonic or hypertonic conditions, dilute detergents, and temperatures above 40°C (19).

Borrelia spp. are microaerophilic and have complex nutritional requirements for growth in a cell-free medium under laboratory conditions (27, 139). Cell-free medium contains serum, glucose, albumin, peptides, amino acids, vitamins, and a thickening agent such as gelatin. In addition, N-acetylglucosamine, the building block for an arthropod's chitin exoskeleton, is required for cultivation (18, 144). Some *Borrelia* species have yet to be cultivated in serial passage outside of a natural host or experimental animal. Cocultivation of some *Borrelia* species with either mammalian or tick cell lines can enhance their growth in

Alan G. Barbour • Departments of Medicine and Microbiology and Molecular Genetics, University of California—Irvine, Irvine, CA 92697–4025.

the laboratory (150, 153), and in some cases an otherwise noncultivable isolate can be propagated and maintained by serial passage in immunodeficient mice (204). Even if a relapsing fever species can be grown in cell-free broth medium, it can lose its capacity to infect animals after a few passages in culture medium, and prolonged passage in laboratory mammals may result in loss of infectivity for ticks (26, 27).

The complete genome sequence of another *Borrelia* species, *Borrelia burgdorferi*, an agent of Lyme borreliosis, revealed a limited biosynthetic potential consistent with its parasitic lifestyle and complex nutritional requirements for cultivation (110). Probing a DNA array of the open reading frames of the *B. burgdorferi* genome with relapsing fever *Borrelia* sp. DNA revealed that *B. hermsii* and *Borrelia turicatae* share at least 70% of their genes with *B. burgdorferi* (239).

Spirochetes of the genus *Borrelia* do not have lipopolysaccharides with lipid A (125, 219), and there is little evidence they have potent exotoxins. Relapsing fever *Borrelia* cells do have a large number of lipoproteins anchored in the fluid outer membrane by N-terminal fatty acids (65, 227). These lipoproteins are potent B-cell mitogens and stimulators of monokines, such as tumor necrosis factor (TNF) (205), which is mediated by their recognition by toll-like receptor 2 of vertebrates (131).

Genetics and Phylogeny

The genomes of relapsing fever *Borrelia* species are largely linear (20, 107, 182). In the individual organism, there are 5 to 20 identical genomes distributed along its length (148). Each genome consists of a linear chromosome of about 1,000 kb and one copy each of different types of linear and circular plasmids. The linear plasmids range in size from about 10 to 180 kb, and the circular plasmids are about 8 to 40 kb (107, 126, 147, 218). The telomeres of the linear plasmids are sealed as hairpins (130). *Borrelia* plasmids, both linear and circular, may be of viral origin (27, 66). All *Borrelia* species studied to date have G+C contents of about 30%. Although *Borrelia* spp. carry both bacteriophage and numerous plasmids, Lyme borreliosis and relapsing fever species have a clonal population structure with only rare examples of horizontal gene transfer (49, 101, 129). The repertoire of highly polymorphic antigens of relapsing fever species (see below) probably arose through multiple rounds of gene duplications and intragenic recombinations rather than by acquisition of new genetic information from other strains and species (188, 192).

The genus *Borrelia* represents a deep division among spirochetes (113, 173, 185). On the basis of DNA sequences, members of the genus are more closely related to treponemes, such as *Treponema pallidum*, the agent of syphilis, than they are to leptospires. Characteristics of *Borrelia* organisms that collectively serve to distinguish the genus from other spirochetes are a dependence on arthropods for transmission, G+C contents of about 30%, multiple flagella, and a tolerance of oxygen.

DNA sequence analysis of ribosomal RNA and other genes has established that *Borrelia* spp. fall into two major groups (Fig. 1). One group contains the agents of Lyme borreliosis, such as *B. burgdorferi* in North America and *Borrelia afzelii* in Europe, but also other species, such as *Borrelia andersonii* and *Borrelia valaisiana,* which may overlap Lyme borreliosis agents in their geographic distribution but are not known to be disease agents for humans. The species in this first group are all transmitted by prostriate hard ticks, such as *Ixodes scapularis* in North America, *Ixodes ricinus* in Europe, and *Ixodes persulcatus* in Asia. The second major group includes the relapsing fever agents, which, with the exception of the louse-borne *B. recurrentis*, are transmitted by soft-bodied or argasid ticks (Color Plate 2A to E). This second major group also includes at least three *Borrelia* species, *Borrelia theileri*, *Borrelia miyamotoi*, and "*Borrelia lonestari*," that are found in metastriate ticks such as *Amblyomma americanum* as well as prostriate hard ticks like *I. scapularis* (28, 114, 191, 204).

Phylogenetic classification of the relapsing fever agents based on DNA hybridization and sequencing has generally confirmed previous taxonomies that relied more on the geographic ranges of the microorganisms, the types of ticks capable of transmitting them, and the small mammals that could serve as reservoirs of infection (22, 86, 133). For instance, the susceptibility of the guinea pig was a biological assay to discriminate between *B. duttonii*, which did not infect this species, from other TBRF species, which generally did (10). The several TBRF species in the past were also divided into Old World and New World species, but a more appropriate characterization now is by ecological region (Table 1). The sole LBRF species, *B. recurrentis*, which became global in its distribution in the 19th and 20th centuries, clusters with the Palearctic and Afrotropical species of TBRF agents, such as *Borrelia crocidurae* and *B. duttonii*, rather than with Nearctic species, such as *B. hermsii* (Fig. 1).

Typing and phylogenetic studies of strains within a species of TBRF have revealed that in a given geographic area of transmission, such as the eastern Sierra Mountains in California, there is only one or at most two strains (50). This limited strain diversity is in contrast to what has been observed with two Lyme borreliosis agents, *B. burgdorferi* and *B. afzelii*. In forested areas no larger than a football field there may be

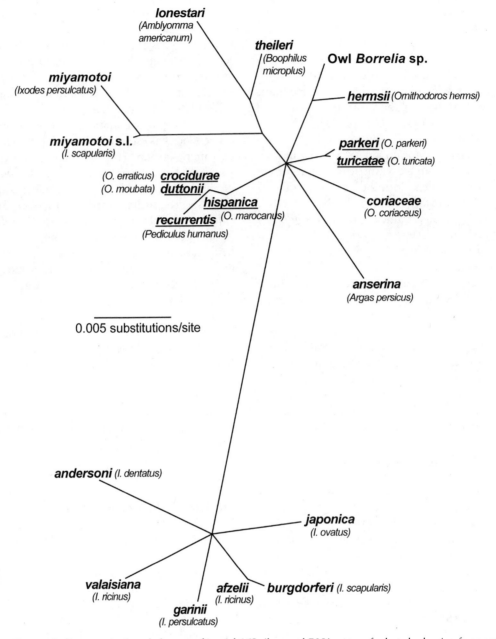

Figure 1. Unrooted, distance criterion phylogram of partial 16S ribosomal RNA genes of selected relapsing fever and other *Borrelia* species (15, 29). The species known to cause relapsing fever of humans are underlined. Representative arthropod vectors are shown in parentheses by each *Borrelia* species; all the vectors are soft ticks (*Ornithodoros* and *Argas*) or hard ticks (*Ixodes*, *Boophilus*, and *Amblyomma*), except for the human louse, *P. humanus*. *B. miyamotoi* of *I. persulcatus* was isolated in Japan (115), and the *B. miyamotoi* sensu lato organism of *I. scapularis* was isolated in the northeastern United States (204). The "Owl" *Borrelia* sp. was isolated from a northern spotted owl in the northwestern United States (221).

maintenance of 10 to 13 different strains of *B. burgdorferi* in North America and *B. afzelii* in northern Europe (49).

Transmission and Pathogenesis

A *Borrelia* infection of humans almost always begins following contact with a tick or louse carrying the spirochetes. Much less commonly the disease is acquired through (i) accidental inoculation of infected blood; (ii) contact of abraded or lacerated skin, mucous membranes, or conjunctiva with infected patient or animal blood (128); or (iii) transplacental or perinatal transmission from mother to fetus (111, 235). Transmission between humans by aerosols, fomites, human saliva, urine, feces, or sexual contact does not

Table 1. *Borrelia* species that cause relapsing fever and related species

Species	DNA[a]	Ecological region	Arthropod vector
Relapsing fever agents			
B. crocidurae	Yes	Palearctic	O. erraticus
B. duttonii	Yes	Afrotropical	O. moubata
B. hermsii	Yes	Nearctic	O. hermsi
B. hispanica	Yes	Palearctic	Ornithodoros marocanus
B. latyschewii	No	Palearctic	O. tartakovskyi
B. mazzottii	No	Nearctic	O. talaje
B. parkeri	Yes	Nearctic	O. parkeri
B. persica	Yes	Palearctic	O. tholozani
B. recurrentis	Yes	Global (?Palearctic origin)	P. humanus
B. turicatae	Yes	Nearctic	O. turicata
B. venezuelensis	No	Neotropical	O. rudis
Related species			
B. anserina	Yes	Global (?Afrotropical origin)	Argas spp.
B. coriaceae	Yes	Nearctic	O. coriaceus
B. lonestari	Yes	Nearctic	A. americanum
B. miyamotoi sensu lato	Yes	Palearctic and Nearctic	Ixodes spp.
B. theileri	Yes	Global (?Afrotropical origin)	Boophilus spp.

[a] DNA, the sequence of one or more genes has been determined.

occur. Although rodents can acquire the infection in the laboratory by feeding on the brains and livers of infected animals, peroral transmission is highly unlikely in humans. The incubation period between exposure and the onset of fever is from 3 to 12 days. Although laboratory-acquired infections are now rare, relapsing fever *Borrelia* spp. are classified as biosafety level 2 pathogens.

Most *Ornithodoros* ticks that transmit relapsing fever feed for less than 30 min and usually at night. As many as half of the individuals with TBRF were not aware of being bitten at the time, but there may be a telltale skin reaction that appears later at the bite site. The argasid tick's usual feeding duration is too short to allow for the migration of the spirochetes from midgut to salivary glands while embedded. The TBRF species spirochetes have already migrated to the salivary glands by the time an *Ornithodoros* tick begins to feed, and consequently, the spirochetes enter the host's skin and blood within minutes of the start of feeding (53). In some species of *Ornithodoros*, such as *Ornithodoros moubata*, there may be transmission at the bite site through entry of infected coxal fluid (225).

LBRF is not acquired from the bite or the saliva of the louse. After entering the midgut of the louse, the spirochetes move to the hemolymph where they may persist for the approximately 3-week life span of the louse. But the spirochetes do not migrate to the salivary glands or appear in the feces of the louse, and there is no regurgitation of the spirochetes from the midgut. Instead, humans become infected with *B. recurrentis* when they crush an infected louse with fin-

gers or pop one with their teeth. The organism is introduced at the bite site, the skin of the crushing fingers, the conjunctivae when people rub their eyes, or through the mucous membranes of the mouth.

A single spirochete of the TBRF species *B. duttonii*, *B. hermsii*, or *B. turicatae* is sufficient to infect experimental animals (35, 198, 215). The bacteria multiply in the blood at an estimated rate of one cell division every 6 to 12 h until they number as many 10^8 per ml of blood at their peak (Color Plate 10). Some spirochetes migrate from the blood through the endothelium to invade the central nervous system, the eye, the liver, and other organs and tissues (57, 59). In tissues, spirochetes are generally found in the interstitial spaces between cells, except when they have been engulfed by phagocytes. Although spirochetes do not completely disappear from the blood between febrile periods, they are uncommon enough to be undetectable by microscopic examination of unconcentrated blood (198, 215). Figure 2 shows a typical temperature curve of a patient with untreated relapsing fever. During relapses of disease, the number of spirochetes in the blood increases again but usually not to the same peak level as during the initial spirochetemia. The interval between relapses in experimental infections is usually 2 to 7 days.

The waxing and waning of the spirochetes in the blood for up to several weeks reflects the spirochetal population's ability to undergo multiphasic antigenic variation. Early investigators of relapsing fever recognized that each new crop of spirochetes differed antigenically from the population it succeeded and the

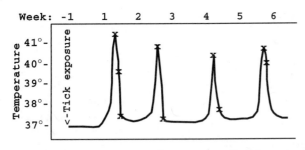

Figure 2. Body temperature (in degrees Centigrade) of a patient with tick-borne relapsing fever over time and in relation to exposure to *O. hermsi* ticks in the northwestern United States. Adapted from Thompson et al. (221).

population that will in turn succeed it (162, 193). The different variants of a given strain are called serotypes. There is little or no antigenic cross-reactivity between serotypes with polyclonal antisera obtained from either infected patients or an immunized animal (74, 215). Early researchers also noted that the same serotype could appear again if the infection was transmitted to an immunologically naïve animal (17).

The most extensive studies of antigenic variation by a relapsing fever agent have been of *B. hermsii* (13). The several known serotypes of one strain of this species can be derived from a single cell injected into a mouse (30, 190, 215). Specific antisera to each of 24 serotypes of this strain were produced and used to study the relapses that occur during experimental infections. With this battery of antisera and an immunofluorescence assay of blood smears from infected animals, Stoenner and his colleagues could identify the serotype of about 90% of the variants that appeared during relapses in hundreds of mice. This finding indicates that the full repertoire of serotypes for a given strain is approximately 30 to 35. The specific antisera were also used to show that order of appearance of serotypes during individual infections of mice is not random: some serotypes are significantly more likely to occur during the first relapse than others, no matter what serotype caused the initial infection (30, 74, 215).

B. hermsii not only changes serotype in infected mammals but also changes to a unique serotype when its cells are taken up from an infected rodent by an *Ornithodoros hermsi* tick (200). Although this tick-associated serotype can circulate in the blood of experimentally infected mice (26), it was not noted in a prospective study of relapses in infected mice by a battery of serotype-specific antisera, including the tick-associated serotype (30, 215). When spirochetes of the tick-associated serotype enter a new mouse host from the tick, they change back to the mammal-associated serotype they last were in the previous mouse (200). The tick and vertebrate environments for the spiro-

chetes differ in several ways, including the absence of an adaptive immune system in ticks and lice and the cooler ambient temperature inside of arthropods.

The phenomenon of neurotropism has been observed in both infected ticks and mammals (57). In *Ornithodoros* ticks, the spirochetes accumulate around the central ganglion cells (51). Among both human cases and in experimental infections of rodents, neurotropism is more common with some species than with others (57). For example, the greater incidence of neurologic involvement in cases of relapsing fever due to *B. duttonii* in Africa and *B. turicatae* in North America has long been noted. A newly described species of relapsing fever borrelia in Spain appears to be particularly neurotropic (118). Neurotropism can also vary within a single strain of some TBRF species. Cadavid et al. demonstrated in an experimental animal model that some serotypes of a *B. turicatae* strain were present in higher numbers in the brain than in other serotypes of the same strain (59–61). Neurotropism is not necessarily associated with other measures of virulence. One of the less neurotropic serotypes of the same strain of *B. turicatae* achieved 10-fold-higher numbers in the brain of infected mice and caused higher mortality of infant mice than did the brain-invasive serotype (61, 177). Further study of the neurotropic serotype of *B. turicatae* revealed that the spirochetes concentrated around the leptomeninges and blood vessels (59).

Attachment to host cells is another factor associated with the pathogenicity of relapsing fever spirochetes. It had long been noted that some relapsing fever spirochetes in the blood of infected animals formed clumps or rosettes with platelets or erythrocytes (106). For *B. crocidurae*, a Palearctic TBRF species, aggregation of spirochetes and erythrocytes into rosettes appears to delay immune clearance (54). In this state, antibodies appear and rise in the blood more slowly than is observed during experimental infection with *Borrelia* spp. that do not aggregate erythrocytes. Erythrocyte and spirochete rosettes activate endothelial cells and cause microvascular thrombi and emboli that lead to pathologic changes in tissues (207–209). Erythrocyte aggregation has also been noted with some serotypes of *B. duttonii* (218), and invasion of the brain and kidneys by *B. crocidurae* is delayed in plasminogen-deficient mice (169).

B. hermsii spirochetes adhere to platelets by binding to an integrin (4, 5). The spirochetes may also attach to host cells through binding to glycosaminoglycans (157, 241). Relapsing fever *Borrelia* spp. may also avoid the innate immune responses through the binding of factor H to its cell surfaces, thereby mediating cleavage of complement component 3b (160).

The pathologic findings of relapsing fever are known mainly from autopsies of fatal human cases and from histologic examinations of experimentally infected animals (47, 57, 213). Extracellular spirochetes were demonstrated in tissues, often in perivascular locations, by silver stain, such as Warthin-Starry or Dieterle (97), or by immunofluorescence with conjugated antibodies (177). The liver and spleen were often enlarged and showed inflammation, with microabscesses in the spleen (7, 142, 220). The microabscesses, areas of necrosis, and petechiae may be consequences, in part, of microemboli of spirochetes and blood cells and transendothelial migration of neutrophils (207, 209). Intracranial hemorrhage has been observed in both LBRF and TBRF (7, 9, 91, 141, 220). When spirochetes in the brain were noted, they were more common around vessels and adjacent to leptomeninges (7, 59, 118). Although cardiac abnormalities are not usually associated with relapsing fever, myocarditis with the presence of numerous spirochetes has been demonstrated in experimental TBRF and LBRF infections (40, 61, 142). Relapsing fever spirochetes have also been observed in the eye and testes (208). In experimental *B. turicatae* infection, the severity of illness correlated with the numbers of spirochetes in the blood (177).

Antigenic Variation during Relapsing Fever

Antigenic variation by relapsing fever *Borrelia* spp. is among the most extensive of any vector-borne bacterial or protozoal parasite (29), and the mechanisms of antigenic variation by *Borrelia* spp. are reviewed in depth elsewhere (12, 13). Its characteristics most closely resemble the antigenic variation manifested by African trypanosomes (93).

Serotype identity is determined by what as a group are called variable major proteins (31). The known set of about 30 variable major proteins are divided about equally between two different families: variable large proteins (Vlp) of about 36 kDa and variable small proteins (Vsp) of about 20 kDa (23, 53, 65, 190). These abundant lipoproteins are anchored in the outer membrane by their lipid moieties. The corresponding *vlp* and *vsp* genes use the same locus for expression (see below) and may have near-identical signal peptides, but after the conserved signal peptide has been cleaved off, the processed Vsp and Vlp proteins are highly polymorphic in sequence. *B. turicatae* (60, 176, 178), *B. recurrentis* (227), *B. crocidurae* (54), and *B. duttonii* (217) have genes that are homologous to *vlp* and *vsp* genes. Serotype 33 of *B. hermsii* HS1 has a Vsp-like protein that has been named Vtp because of its unique signal peptide and because of its association with the tick (65, 200). The Vsp and Vtp proteins of relapsing fever *Borrelia* spp. are homologous to the OspC proteins of Lyme borre-

liosis *Borrelia* spp. (65), and the Vlp proteins are homologous to the Vls proteins of the Lyme borreliosis agents. (238). *B. miyamotoi* also has *vsp*- and *vlp*-like genes (123); thus, the origin of the two families of genes predates the division of *Borrelia* genus into two major groups.

The Vlp family of proteins of *B. hermsii* is further divided into four subfamilies with less than 70% sequence identity between them: α, β, γ, and δ (53, 190). Different strains of *B. hermsii* from distant geographic origins in western North America had the same four subfamilies (129). The *vlp* genes found to date in other relapsing fever *Borrelia* species are most similar to the β and δ subfamily sequences of *B. hermsii*. The Vls protein of *B. burgdorferi* is most like the subfamily δ proteins of *B. hermsii* (238).

Vsp and Vtp proteins, like OspC proteins, are highly α-helical (240). The processed N terminus is acylated similarly to other bacterial lipoproteins (65, 205). The C terminus is not anchored but is also close to the N terminus near the cell's surface. The loops between α-helices are exposed to the environment as ligands or epitopes. Native and recombinant Vsp and OspC proteins exist as dimers in solution and on the surface of the spirochetes (240, 241).

Although there is little discernible homology between the Vlp-Vls family and Vsp-OspC family at the primary sequence level, it is likely that the *vlp-vls* ancestor was the result of a duplication of a *vsp-ospC* ancestor gene before the divergence of Lyme borreliosis and relapsing fever species. The Vlp proteins are about twice the size of Vsp proteins, and both types of proteins have α-helical secondary structures (53, 240). While Vsp and OspC proteins are dimers, Vlp proteins are monomers. Crystallographic studies of a Vls protein and Vlp protein revealed a structure similar to a dimer of Vsp or OspC: the C terminus was close to the N terminus, and surface-exposed loops separated the α-helices in a bundle (102). The display of the variable loops at different points of the protein is consistent with the finding that serotype-specific epitopes for Vlp proteins are distributed throughout the protein (33).

There appears to be a complete or near-complete *vsp* or *vlp* gene for each Vsp or Vlp protein that a spirochete is capable of expressing (13). Although chimeric proteins, which are fusions of parts of two different Vlp or Vsp proteins, can occur (149), this phenomenon has been observed only in immunodeficient animals (215). An immunocompetent animal presumably is still able to clear an organism from the blood that is expressing a variable major protein different from the previously expressed protein but which has retained one or more epitopes of the old variable major protein. Thus, for a genetic switch to provide sufficient antigenic novelty for avoidance of an ongoing adaptive immune response to previous predominant population, all or almost all of the previously expressed gene needs to be replaced by a different sequence. A partial or mosaic replacement, as occurs in some mucosal surface pathogens manifesting antigenic variation, e.g., *Neisseria gonorrhoeae*, is inadequate for immune evasion by blood-borne *Borrelia* spp. (29).

Five other features of the antigenic variation that must be accounted for in any model of the genetic mechanism are the following (13). (i) Only one variable major protein is detectably and stably expressed on the cell's surface at a time. (ii) A copy of the gene for a previously expressed variable major protein is archived in the cell to serve as a potential donor sequence at some point in the future. (iii) The switch is nonreciprocal; that is, no exchange results in the alteration of two different genetic loci. (iv) The effective serotype switch rate is an estimated 10^{-4} to 10^{-3} per cell per generation; that is, by the time a given serotype reaches a population size of 1,000 to 10,000 cells in an animal, it is likely that at least one cell of a different serotype has appeared in the population. (v) The switch appears to be constitutive and not inducible by a change in the environment, such as a change from broth medium to mice.

In *B. hermsii*, two mechanisms can account for all the observed features of antigenic variation (Fig. 3). The first and most common mechanism is a nonreciprocal recombination between a linear plasmid with an array of silent, archived *vsp* and *vlp* genes and another linear plasmid with a transcribed *vsp* or *vlp* gene (147, 161, 182). In *B. hermsii*, as well as in *B. turicatae*, what is effectively a gene conversion results in the replacement of the expressed gene for a variable major protein at a site downstream from a promoter at an expression site (25, 60, 176, 178). An archived *vsp* gene can replace an expressed *vlp* gene or vice versa. The boundaries for the recombination are regions of sequence identity between silent and expression sites around and flanking the extreme 5′ and 3′ ends of the expressed and silent *vsp* or *vlp* genes.

In *B. hermsii*, the longest length of converted sequence that has been observed is about 2 kb (147, 190). In *B. turicatae*, a more extensive gene conversion involving ≥10 kb downstream of the promoter on the expression site plasmid occurs (176). The mechanism of intermolecular recombination between plasmids first demonstrated in New World species, like *B. hermsii*, also seems to occur in Old World species. Rearrangements incorporating long lengths of plasmids have also been noted in *B. duttonii* (218). Silent and expressed versions of *vlp* genes have also been documented in *B. recurrentis* (226).

The second mechanism for expressing a different variable major protein is an intramolecular DNA rearrangement of the plasmid with the expression site (Fig. 3). This mechanism has only been noted when there is another variable major protein gene just downstream of an expressed *vlp* gene (189). The downstream gene is in the same orientation as the expressed gene but is untranscribed. A deletion between short direct repeats at the 5′ ends of each of the tandemly arrayed genes effectively excises the sitting *vlp* gene, and the downstream gene moves up with the deletion to take the place of the deleted gene next to the promoter. After this deletion, the newly expressed gene is susceptible to further small gene conversions that provide further diversity of variable membrane proteins (188).

The activation of the *vtp* gene when *B. hermsii* is in the tick occurs by a mechanism that does not require recombination or transposition: modification of transcripts by expression site switching (Fig. 3). The *vtp* gene is located at another locus on a different plasmid than the expression site; at that location, *vtp* has its own promoter (26, 200). There is only one copy of *vtp* per genome. How differential transcription between the *vtp* locus and the expression site locus is achieved is unknown.

Immunity

Immunity in relapsing fever has been the subject of study since the late 19th century (14, 17). In infected animals, immunoglobulin M antibodies alone are sufficient to limit or eliminate infection in the blood (3, 8, 24, 76, 166, 167). When antibodies are administered intravenously, the spirochetes are cleared from the blood within 1 h (24, 58). Within 24 to 48 h after the spirochetes reach a peak of 10^6 to 10^7 organisms per ml of blood in an immunocompetent animal, they become undetectable by light microscopy of the blood. This neutralizing antibody response is serotype specific; the animal remains susceptible to other serotypes of the same strain or of different strains (14, 17). Up to 10 different relapses have been recorded during experimental infections. Whether recovery is due to the development of antibodies to all or most serotypes during the infection's course or to the eventual rise of cross-protective antibodies directed against antigens expressed by all serotypes is unknown. In areas where relapsing fever is endemic, newcomers or visitors appear to be more at risk of symptomatic TBRF than long-term residents, an indication that long-lasting immunity to the local strain or strains may occur among humans.

Experimental animals with deficient T-cell function, such as nude mice, are as capable of clearing

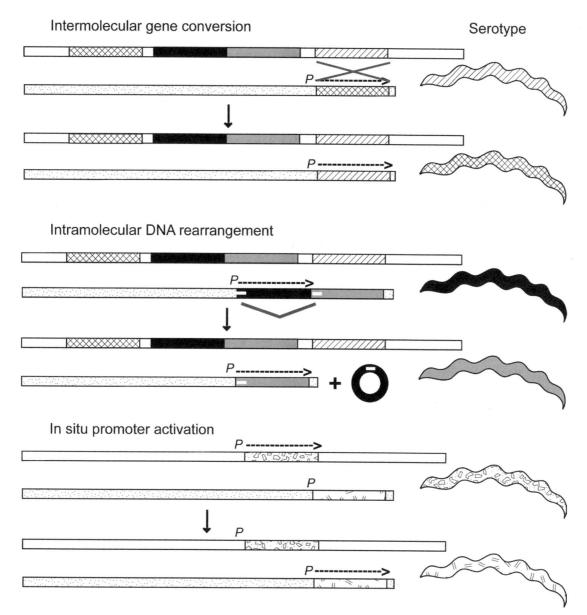

Figure 3. Schematic representation of three mechanisms for changing expression of a variable major protein gene of *B. hermsii* during relapsing fever: intermolecular gene conversion, intramolecular DNA rearrangement, and in situ activation of a promoter. For each mechanism, the states and locations of selected genes on two linear plasmids before and after a change (downward arrow) in a serotype are shown. The genotype of the expressed variable major protein gene, which is downstream of an active promoter (P →), and the serotype phenotype of the spirochete are indicated by the same fill pattern. Other genes are designated by other fill patterns. In the middle, an intramolecular DNA recombination between two direct repeats (short white bars) of tandemly arrayed variable major protein genes is shown. A product of this recombination is a nonreplicative circle (190).

spirochetes from the blood as are their immunocompetent counterparts (24, 167). Whether T cells play a more important role in long-term protection from infection or in control of infection within the central nervous system is not known. Because specific antibodies, even Fab monomers, to outer membrane proteins of *B. hermsii* and *B. burgdorferi* can kill borrelias in the absence of complement or phagocytes (194), deficiencies in the latter immune effectors may not hinder clearance of borrelias from the blood. Those immune deficiencies that do increase susceptibility to more serious manifestations of relapsing fever or result in prolonged disease are absence of the spleen and impaired B-cell function (14, 17), again supporting the importance of antibodies in host defense.

During infection, both experimental animals and human patients develop antibody responses against a number of different spirochetal components, including the periplasmic flagella and heat-shock proteins. However, it appears that only antibody directed against variable major proteins is effective in controlling infection (24, 58, 215). If there are other, less variable antigens that the infected animal or person eventually responds to with neutralizing antibody or cytotoxic T cells, they have not yet been identified. The reduced numbers of fully virulent spirochetes in the blood during relapses in comparison to during the first fever indicate that there may be other factors that limit infection after the initial attack. An antibody response that eradicates the spirochetes of the predominant serotype from the blood is often not successful in clearing borrelias from the brain, cerebrospinal fluid, or eye (17, 57), and relapsing fever spirochetes can persist for years in these locations. Recrudescences of relapsing fever with stress or during another infection, such as typhoid, have been reported in humans. This recrudescent disease phenomenon is similar to the return of spirochetemia with the Lyme borreliosis agent *Borrelia garinii* noted among birds under the stress of migration (122).

LIFE CYCLE AND ECOLOGY

The vectors of TBRF are soft-bodied (argasid) ticks of the genus *Ornithodoros* (77, 106, 134). Some *Ornithodoros* species may feed on just one type of animal during their lifetimes and are usually found in or close to the nests, burrows, or dens of their animal hosts. The hosts either are permanent residents or intermittently or seasonally return to the shelter. Other *Ornithodoros* species may feed on a variety of hosts. The species of *Ornithodoros* ticks that transmit TBRF usually pass through two or more nymphal stages between larval and adult stages (Fig. 4). These ticks may live for up to 10 to 20 years and can survive without a blood meal for several years. Transovarial transmission is frequent, occurring in up to 100% of offspring and in most but not all species (52, 82, 85). The longevity of these ticks and their transovarial trans-

mission allow persistence of the spirochetes in an environment for years despite long periods of absence or low numbers of suitable vertebrate hosts. Hoogstraal proposed that the *Borrelia* lineage began as symbionts of ticks rather than as parasites of vertebrates (134).

The vertebrate reservoir hosts of the TBRF *Borrelia* spp. are usually rodents (168) but may include pigs, goats, sheep, rabbits, bats, opossums, armadillos, foxes, cats, and dogs (106, 133, 175). Although the competence of birds as reservoirs of relapsing fever *Borrelia* spp. has not been established, they can be infected (106, 220), and *Ornithodoros* ticks have been found in the habitats of burrowing owls. While *Ornithodoros* species have been observed to feed on snakes, turtles, toads, and even crabs, these animals probably are not competent reservoirs of *Borrelia* spp. Although the natural reservoir for tick-borne *B. duttonii* has been said to be humans (106), the genetic similarity of this species to *B. crocidurae* (Fig. 1) and the ease with which rodents were infected with *B. duttonii* in one study (120) suggest that there may be a nonprimate alternate reservoir for *B. duttonii*.

LBRF is transmitted from person to person by the body louse, *Pediculus humanus corporis*, and less commonly, by the head louse, *Pediculus humanus capitis*, both of which feed only on humans (47, 55, 105, 195, 213). Lice only become infected with *B. recurrentis* through a blood meal; there is no transovarial transmission. The body louse's niche is clothing; accordingly, it is more likely to thrive in temperate or subarctic regions than in the tropics. Some nonhuman primates can be infected with *B. recurrentis* in the laboratory, and there are reports of experimental infections of newborn rabbits and some rodents (11), but there is no evidence that animals other than humans maintain the infection in nature.

B. theileri is another *Borrelia* species that is transmitted by a vector other than argasid ticks. *B. theileri* produces spirochetemia and mild illness in cattle on different continents now but probably originated in Africa (44, 211, 212). *B. theileri* is transmitted by metastriate ticks of the genus *Boophilus*, mainly

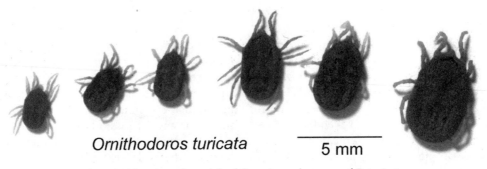

Ornithodoros turicata   5 mm

Figure 4. Nymphs and an adult of *O. turicata*, the vector of *B. turicatae*.

Boophilus microplus and *Boophilus annulatus*. Transovarial transmission of *B. theileri* in *B. microplus* has been documented (212). In the last decade, other species that are genetically related to *B. theileri*, as well as to the TBRF species (Fig. 1), have been discovered to be transmitted by hard ticks. One of the new species is "*B. lonestari*," which has been found in the United States in *A. americanum*, another metastriate tick (28, 191). *B. miyamotoi* was first discovered in *I. persulcatus* ticks in Japan (112), and similar organisms have been found in *I. scapularis* ticks in the northeastern United States (50, 204) and *I. ricinus* ticks in Europe (50, 109). Collectively, these *Ixodes*-associated organisms are called *B. miyamotoi* sensu lato. In enzootic areas, approximately 1 to 5% of the ticks are infected with "*B. lonestari*" or *B. miyamotoi* sensu lato (28, 50). Laboratory mice can be infected with *B. miyamotoi* sensu lato from *I. scapularis*, which transovarially transmits the spirochete (204).

Borrelia anserina and *Borrelia coriaceae* are two additional species in the major group that includes relapsing fever species (Fig. 1). *B. anserina* has long been known as the cause of avian or fowl spirochetosis and is transmitted by *Argas persicus*, a member of another genus of soft ticks, (81, 92, 236). Avian spirochetosis is now a cosmopolitan disease of poultry flocks, but its origin and evolutionary relationship to relapsing fever species remain unclear. *B. anserina* infection of imported poultry fowl may be the source of new infections of wild birds in a given area. *B. coriaceae*, on the other hand, was first identified comparatively recently in *Ornithodoros coriaceus* ticks in California (127, 155). These ticks feed on deer as well as cattle, but the role of these large mammals in maintenance of the infection remains to be determined. *O. coriaceus* has been associated with epizootic bovine abortion in California and Nevada (196), and *B. coriaceae*'s etiological role in this disease has been suggested but not proven (154).

EPIDEMIOLOGY

TBRF of humans occurs in the Palearctic, Nearctic, Afrotropical, and Neotropical ecological regions. It either does not occur or has not been well documented in the Indo-Malayan, Australasian, or Oceanian ecological regions. Reports of relapsing fever from areas with rain forests or monsoon forests may be attributable to louse-borne infection or the importation of infected argasid ticks with livestock. A "*Borrelia queenslandia*" in wild rodents in Australia was reported (64), but there is no apparent association with human disease. Table 1 lists the species that are most commonly described in the literature. Several other

Borrelia species names have been given to relapsing fever agents (106), but these have not been well characterized, and it is likely that many of these are synonymous with known species. Even among the TBRF species in the table, only about half have been genotyped with DNA sequences (185). It is likely that some of the older species designations and associations with different hosts or geographic regions will be revised as species identities are better defined. The emphasis here is on species for which there is convincing genetic evidence of a unique identity.

In the United States and Canada, most cases of autochthonous relapsing fever are attributable to *B. hermsii*, which is transmitted by *O. hermsi*, or to *B. turicatae*, whose vector is *Ornithodoros turicata* (87, 89, 98). Figure 5, based on the work of Cooley and Kohls (77), shows the distribution in the United States of these two Nearctic species, as well of *Borrelia parkeri*. Although the vectors are widely distributed, human disease is highly focal in its occurrence. In a retrospective study of 450 cases of TBRF occurring in the United States from 1977 to 2000, 13 counties of the western United States accounted for half of the cases (100). In this survey, 40% of the cases were diagnosed in residents of states other than the state in which exposure occurred, an indication of the association of TBRF in the United States with recreational activities and tourism.

O. hermsi has been documented in mountainous regions at elevations ranging from 1,000 to 2,700 m, depending on latitude, throughout the western United States and British Columbia, Canada (34, 42, 77, 232) (Fig. 3). *B. hermsii* has been isolated from patients, animals, and ticks from New Mexico, Colorado, Idaho, Montana, Washington, Oregon, California, and British Columbia. The ecological designation for the usual habitat of *O. hermsi* and its hosts is Northwestern Forested Mountains, which typically have ponderosa pine and/or Douglas fir. Common hosts for the ticks are chipmunks and squirrels; *O. hermsi* ticks have been found in nests of these rodents in tree stumps or hollow logs (156). In natural locations away from buildings and during the daytime, humans seldom encounter *O. hermsi*. Instead, most cases of *B. hermsii* infections are acquired at night while humans sleep in or near cabins and houses, in which the rodent hosts reside in the roof, under eaves, in walls, under porches, or in woodpiles (39, 174, 201). Ground burrows may extend beneath the cabin or house. Ticks have been found between the mattresses of beds in the cabins (228). Some of the known outbreaks of relapsing fever from *B. hermsii* have occurred in rustic cabins in the Grand Canyon park in Arizona (39, 174), around Lake Tahoe in the Sierra Nevada mountains (43), in the San Bernardino mountains of southern

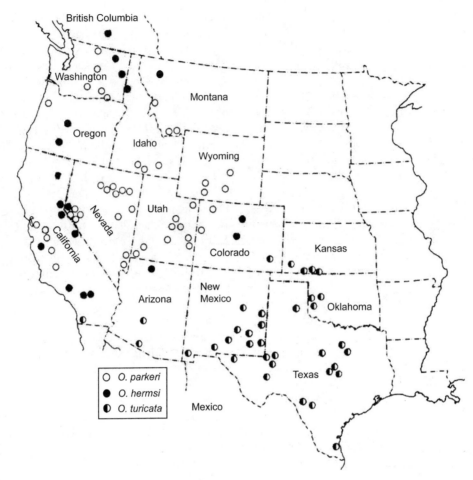

Figure 5. Collection of *O. hermsi*, *O. parkeri*, and *O. turicata* ticks from the western United States and Canada. Figure adapted from Boyer et al. (39), who used the data of Cooley and Kohls (77). The identification of *O. hermsi* in western Montana was reported by Schwan et al. (201).

California (34), and in cabins on an island on a Montana lake (201). Both outbreaks and individual cases usually occur during the summer months when human visits and tick activity are at their highest (99), but some cases have occurred during the winter, such as when a vacation cabin is opened and heated again after an absence (221).

O. turicata ticks are generally found at lower elevations than *B. hermsii* and in desert, semidesert, and scrub landscapes in Texas, Oklahoma, Kansas, Arizona, New Mexico, and California (Fig. 5), as well as in the drier regions of central Mexico (77, 145). The ecological designations for this habitat are North American Deserts and Great Plains, both of which extend into central and northeastern Mexico. The ticks are associated with rodent burrows or with caves and overhanging rock ledges that shelter larger animals. In addition to rodents, armadillos and opossums are naturally infected with *B. turicatae* in Texas (37). In Mexico, *O. turicata* has been found in human habi-

tats, especially in and around pigsties. Humans become infected with *B. turicatae* by entering caves, crawling under houses, or sleeping in structures with walls infested with *O. turicata* (145). The source of an outbreak of *B. turicatae* infections in Texas was a cave that served as a seasonal den for wild boar (186). *B. turicatae* infections can occur during winter as well as summer (100). *O. turicata* has also been reported in a focus in Florida (77), and a *B. turicatae*-like spirochete has been isolated from Florida dogs (41).

Ornithodoros parkeri ticks morphologically resemble *O. turicata* ticks, and hybridization between them has been demonstrated under laboratory conditions (77). *B. parkeri*, likewise, is closely related to *B. turicatae* and arguably may be the same species on the basis of DNA sequences (Fig. 1). However, Davis reported a biological difference between the two ticks: transovarial transmission of spirochetes was observed in *O. turicata* but not *O. parkeri* (82). *O. parkeri* ticks, like *O. turicata* ticks, are found in burrows of prairie dogs, ground squirrels, and burrowing owls. But the geographic distribution of *O. parkeri* is generally northwest of that of *O. turicata* and includes basins and valleys, such as the Great Basin of Utah, Nevada, Wyoming, Montana, Colorado, and Idaho, the San Joaquin Valley in California, and eastern Washington and Oregon (Fig. 5). Although *O. parkeri* feeds readily on humans and has been associated with some human cases (87, 88), *B. parkeri* appears to be a much less common cause of TBRF than *B. hermsii* or *B. turicatae*. Human encounters with the vector *O. parkeri* appear to be uncommon, perhaps because the tick avoids human habitats or because of the sparse human populations in its enzootic areas.

On other continents, enzootic and endemic transmission of TBRF likely continues in its historic patterns (105, 133, 168), but there is less surveillance and study of TBRF than in the past. Most recent reports of the TBRF are from sub-Saharan Africa (96, 115, 121, 222, 223). Most cases are associated with human habitats with thatched roofs and/or mud walls or floors (170). In east, south, and central Africa, most cases have been attributed to *B. duttonii* transmitted by *O. moubata* (133). However, in the same area of Tanzania, both *B. duttonii* and another hitherto-unknown species of *Borrelia* have been identified (146). *B. crocidurae*, a cause of TBRF in West Africa, particularly the arid Sahel region (223), is genetically very similar to *B. duttonii* and *B. recurrentis* (Fig. 1) and is transmitted by *Ornithodoros erraticus*. *B. crocidurae* and *O. erraticus* have also been reported in North Africa (133).

Human infections from less-well-characterized Palearctic species, such *Borrelia persica*, *Borrelia hispanica*, and *Borrelia latyschewii* probably occur in central Asia, Iran, North Africa, and the Middle East (Table 1). The range of *B. persica* extends from the Mediterranean area and the Middle East to Central Asia, up to 45°N, including the former Soviet republics of Tajikistan, Uzbekistan, Turkmenistan, Kyrgyzstan, and Kazakhstan (151). The vector of *B. persica* has commonly been called *Ornithodoros tholozani*, but Russian taxonomists prefer the term *Ornithodoros papillipes* for what they consider a distinct species within a cluster of species under the broad "*O. tholozani*" designation (108). *B. persica*'s vector lives in buildings, burrows, and caves and feeds on a variety of warm-blooded vertebrates (151). In Cyprus, TBRF from *B. persica* was usually acquired in caves that were inhabited by fruit bats (117, 233). In Israel and Palestine, TBRF, probably caused by *B. persica*, has often been attributed to entry into caves (1). Other TBRF *Borrelia* species in central Asia and the Caucasus are less likely to infect humans, because the ticks rarely occur in dwellings (151). These species include *B.*

latyschewii, which is transmitted by *Ornithodoros tartakovskyi*, a tick that infests rodents, small carnivores, reptiles, and birds in their burrows (151, 175). Another species designation, *Borrelia caucasica*, is used for the agent of TBRF in Georgia, Armenia, Azerbaijan, and parts of the Ukraine and southern Russia. The vector for *B. caucasica* is *Ornithodoros verrucosus*, another tick in the "*O. tholozani*" group, but which unlike *O. papillipes* does not have a preference for human buildings (151).

A *Borrelia* sp. that appears to be distinct from *B. crocidurae* in its vector associations has been isolated from *Ornithodoros savignyi* ticks in Egypt (210), but its relationship to other Palearctic species is not known. In the past, *B. hispanica* caused TBRF on the Iberian peninsula and in western North Africa (72, 135). More recently in Spain, endemic relapsing fever has been reported to be caused by a *Borrelia* sp. that is similar to Palearctic species characterized to date but which may be distinct from *B. hispanica* (6).

In the Nearctic region, the distribution of *Ornithodoros talaje* overlaps that of the distribution of *O. turicata* in the southwestern United States but extends as far south as Guatemala (77, 84). This tick is the vector of *Borrelia mazzottii*, which is poorly characterized but does appear to be distinguishable from *B. turicatae* on the basis of tick associations: *B. mazzottii* was experimentally transmitted by *O. talaje* but not *O. turicata* (86). TBRF has been documented in Panama at the interface between the Nearctic and Neotropical ecological regions (62). In Panama, natural hosts include squirrel monkeys, opossums, and armadillos (71); the vector is *Ornithodoros rudis* and/or *O. talaje* (94), and the agent is said to be *Borrelia venezuelensis*. *B. venezuelensis* could be transmitted experimentally by *O. rudis* ticks from Colombia and *O. turicata* ticks from Mexico but not by *O. hermsi* or *O. parkeri* ticks from the United States (159). In South America and the Neotropical region, relapsing fever has mainly been reported from Venezuela and Colombia, where it is attributed to *B. venezuelensis*. In Colombian seaports, ticks associated with relapsing fever were found in the walls of houses and in straw mattresses (95). In Brazil, *Ornithodoros* ticks and a *Borrelia* organism called *Borrelia brasiliensis* were associated with dogs and the soil under houses and animal shelters (83).

If humans are the only reservoir for LBRF, then there is the potential for the eradication of this disease, but this has yet to be achieved. *B. recurrentis* still occurs in the Horn of Africa, particularly in the Ethiopian highland, where it has been endemic and sporadically epidemic for many decades (2, 38, 67, 164, 216). Hundreds to thousands of cases occur every year, and in 1998–1999 there was a large outbreak of

LBRF in neighboring Sudan. The highest incidence of LBRF in this region occurs during the rainy season when the poor gather together in shelters. Lice move from one person to another, spreading infection to new hosts. Predisposing factors for epidemics include famine, war, and the movements and congregations of refugees; thus, the disease has been called famine fever and vagabond fever. Common contributing conditions include crowding, poor hygiene, few changes of clothing, and lack of access to washing. Epidemics of millions of cases of LBRF occurred around both world wars (47).

Human cases of *B. anserina*, *B. theileri*, or *B. coriaceae* infection are possible, but they have not been documented. The vectors of *B. theileri* are one-host hard ticks of the genus *Boophilus*, and these feed on humans very infrequently. The range of the Nearctic *O. coriaceus*, which commonly feeds on deer as well as cattle, overlaps with the range of *O. hermsi* in California and Nevada, but this tick was not competent for transmission of *B. hermsii* (128). The distribution in the southern and eastern United States of *A. americanum*, the vector of "*B. lonestari*," corresponds with the distribution of an illness characterized by a rash resembling erythema migrans of Lyme borreliosis (63). There has also been documentation of "*B. lonestari*" in a rash illness of a patient from North Carolina (138), but little is known of its potential role in human disease beyond this. This uncertainty applies also to Holoarctic *B. miyamotoi* sensu lato, which occurs in the same vectors that transmit Lyme borreliosis agents and in the same areas that are highly endemic for Lyme borreliosis in North America, Europe, and Asia (50). *B. miyamotoi* causes levels of spirochetemia in mice that are comparable to that observed with TBRF *Borrelia* spp. (199), but whether they can cause infections in humans has not been established.

CLINICAL MANIFESTATIONS

The term relapsing fever concisely describes the key clinical feature of the infection (21, 47, 57, 99, 213). No other untreated infection is characterized by periods of 2 to 3 days of fever and constitutional symptoms, separated by 4 to 14 days of relative well-being. Unless there is an ongoing epidemic with cases of fever under surveillance, most patients with relapsing fever present for medical care only after at least two episodes of fever. The first febrile period, which is commonly accompanied by nonspecific symptoms such as headache, arthralgia, myalgia, and nausea, is often dismissed as an uncomplicated viral infection. Less typical of a viral infection, though, is the crisis that heralds the end of the fever. During the crisis,

which lasts about half an hour, there are shaking chills or rigors, a further rise in temperature, and tachycardia. The crisis is followed by profuse diaphoresis, falling temperature, and hypotension that usually persist for several hours. Mortality is highest during the crisis and in its immediate aftermath. The return of fever a few days later usually then prompts medical attention and diagnostic studies.

Untreated LBRF tends to have fewer relapses than TBRF (36, 38, 45, 47, 119, 195, 216). However, the first episode of fever during LBRF may be unremitting for 3 to 6 days, and the illness is more severe, sometimes accompanied by delirium. Hemorrhagic complications, such as epistaxis, are common (90, 179). If a patient with LBRF survives the initial illness, there may be only a single relapse with milder symptoms. In untreated TBRF, there may be multiple febrile episodes lasting from 2 to 3 days each (32, 39, 75, 96, 152, 171, 184, 222, 233). In a survey of 450 cases of TBRF in the United States from 1977 to 2000, about one-quarter of the patients had at least four relapses before diagnosis (100). While LBRF tends to have a more severe course, TBRF caused by *B. duttonii* and *B. turicatae* has a higher frequency of neurologic complications, which may include facial palsy, weakness, radiculopathy, and occasionally stupor or coma (57). These neurologic manifestations are more common during or around the time of the second or third fever episode than during the first. There may also be ocular involvement (124) and occasionally frank myocarditis (231).

During febrile periods the temperature is usually above 39°C and may be as high as 43°C. Fevers during relapses may be lower than in the initial fever episode. With the exception of a small red or violaceous papule with central eschar that sometimes appears at the bite site, a localized rash is not prominent in relapsing fever. During LBRF, petechiae and ecchymoses may occur, and some patients may become jaundiced. A macular rash has been noted during TBRF but is not common. Enlargement of the spleen and/or the liver may be detected. Patients may complain of polyarthralgia, but swollen joints are unusual. Gallops on cardiac auscultation may be a sign of myocarditis.

Stupor, coma, or localizing central nervous system signs, such as aphasia or hemiplegia, indicate meningoencephalitis or subarachnoid hemorrhage. More commonly observed during TBRF than LBRF are unilateral or bilateral Bell's palsy or deafness, due to seventh or eighth cranial nerve involvement, respectively (57). Unilateral or bilateral iridocyclitis or panophthalmitis may also occur, and visual impairment may be permanent. In LBRF, neurologic manifestations such as altered mental state are thought to be the effect of the heavy spirochetemia rather than of direct invasion of organisms into the central nervous system (57).

Laboratory findings in relapsing fever are generally nonspecific. Mild to moderate normocytic anemia is common, but frank hemolysis and hemoglobinuria do not occur. Leukocyte counts are usually in the normal range or only slightly elevated (172). Leukopenia and platelet counts below 50,000/mm^3 may occur during the crisis. The erythrocyte sedimentation rate is typically moderately elevated. There may be laboratory evidence of hepatitis, such as elevated serum concentrations of aminotransferases, and mildly to moderately prolonged prothrombin and partial thromboplastin times may also be noted. Analysis of the cerebrospinal fluid (CSF) is usually indicated when there are signs of meningitis or meningoencephalitis (57). In meningeal inflammation due to relapsing fever, there may be a mononuclear pleocytosis and mildly to moderately elevated protein levels, but glucose levels in the CSF are typically normal.

The mortality rates for untreated LBRF and TBRF range from 10 to 70% and 4 to 10%, respectively. The higher mortality rates observed in some series with LBRF may be attributable in part to the association of LBRF with wars, famine, and refugees, situations in which malnutrition and inadequate health care are common. Nevertheless, the frequent reports of hemorrhagic complications in cases of *B. recurrentis* infection suggest a difference in pathogenesis between the two forms of relapsing fever.

When prompt treatment with appropriate antibiotics is administered, the death rate for LBRF is 2 to 5% and for TBRF is <2%. Predictors of unfavorable outcomes include stupor or coma, severe hemorrhagic complications, myocarditis, and coinfection with typhus, typhoid, or malaria. Infants and pregnant women are at a higher risk of developing severe disease. Relapsing fever during pregnancy frequently leads to abortion or stillbirth (96, 140, 163, 224).

DIAGNOSIS

Differential Diagnosis

Relapsing fever should be considered in any patient with a characteristic fever pattern, especially if the febrile episodes terminate with a crisis and if there is an epidemiologic history of exposure to lice or soft-bodied ticks within 7 to 10 days of the onset of illness. In areas of North America where there is enzootic transmission of TBRF, commonly reported exposures include entry into a cave, sleeping in or next to a rustic cabin or hut, and crawling under a house for inspections or repairs. There may be signs of rodent activity, such as burrows, nests, and sighting of diurnal animals, such as chipmunks, around houses where infection is acquired. Some cases of TBRF occur among visitors or tourists who acquire the infection in an area where TBRF is endemic, such as in a rural area of sub-Saharan Africa or the Sierra Nevada Mountains of California, but who then do not become symptomatic until they return home. Among long-term residents of areas where TBRF is endemic, a high proportion of cases may occur among children. LBRF is very unlikely to occur among tourists or other short-term visitors to areas of transmission. At present, almost all cases of LBRF occur among low-income residents or refugees. However, under conditions of war, famine, and refugee camps, the risk of exposure to LBRF for care workers, military personnel, and visitors may be high.

Human body lice also transmit epidemic typhus, which may be a coinfection or be confused with the first episode of fever during relapsing fever. The conditions that foster transmission of louse-borne diseases also promote the outbreaks of typhoid fever, an infection that may have a remitting course. *Ornithodoros* ticks are known to transmit other infectious agents, particularly viruses, such as the African swine fever virus of livestock, but relapsing fever appears to be the only symptomatic infection commonly transmitted to humans. In areas where both TBRF and malaria are endemic, such as sub-Saharan Africa, fever may be misdiagnosed as a *Plasmodium* infection and be inappropriately managed. In malaria, febrile episodes are generally more closely spaced and more regular in their recurrence; examination of blood smears should allow their differentiation.

Two viral diseases may present with a so-called saddle-back fever pattern that may resemble relapsing fever. These are dengue, whose range overlaps with that of TBRF in some parts of the world, and Colorado tick fever, which may be enzootic in the same mountainous regions of western North America as is TBRF. (The differential diagnosis of recurrent fever is discussed further in Chapter 5, including Table 2.) Depending on the geographic area of exposure, other febrile illnesses that may resemble the clinical features of the initial febrile period of relapsing fever and have somewhat similar epidemiologic features include murine typhus, Rocky Mountain spotted fever, Q fever, granulocytic ehrlichiosis, monocytic ehrlichiosis, babesiosis, tularemia, leptospirosis, rat-bite fever, bartonellosis, boutonneuse fever, North Asian tick-borne rickettsiosis, scrub typhus, and Queensland tick typhus.

Laboratory Diagnostic Procedures

Before the widespread adoption by clinical laboratories of automated instruments for blood cell counts, technicians examining a Wright-stained peripheral blood smear for a white cell differential count sometimes made the diagnosis of relapsing fever before physicians suspected the illness. Now, in many parts of the world the diagnosis must be under active consideration, and a manual examination of a peripheral blood smear must be ordered to detect spirochetes. A thorough examination, i.e., 100 to 200 high-powered fields, of a thin smear will allow detection of the spirochetes, provided their concentration is greater than 10^5 per ml (Color Plate 10). Another order of magnitude of sensitivity can be obtained with a thick smear of the blood. As few as 10^3 spirochetes per ml may be detected if the buffy coat is examined or if a platelet-rich plasma fraction is further centrifuged and the pellet is stained (73, 158). The optimum time period for obtaining blood for microscopy is from when the temperature is on the rise again to just before its peak. Once the body temperature of an untreated patient declines, it is usually not possible to visualize spirochetes, even with concentration of the blood or plasma.

Thin smears are fixed with methanol and then stained with Giemsa or Wright stain. Thick smears are treated with 0.5 to 1.0% acetic acid before fixation and staining. The dehemoglobinization with acetic acid step can be omitted if the smear is stained with acridine orange (203), which binds to nucleic acids and allows microscopic detection of the spirochetes under ultraviolet light. Direct or indirect immunofluorescence to visualize spirochetes is another procedure that can be used with thick or thin smears (178, 215). A fluorescein-labeled polyclonal antibody to B. burgdorferi is commercially available and has sufficient cross-reactivity with other Borrelia spp. to be useful in detecting relapsing fever spirochetes in blood smears and in tissues.

Wet mounts under a cover slip can also be made with blood diluted in saline, the buffy-coat fraction, or uncentrifuged serum from a tube of clotted blood. The wet mounts are immediately examined under high power by phase-contrast or dark-field microscopy and may reveal motile spirochetes (172). Coiling, uncoiling, and bending movements of the spirochetes may be observed as they swim among erythrocytes and serve to distinguish the spirochetes from artifacts, such as fibrin strands, under the influence of Brownian motion.

Inoculation of blood, plasma, or CSF into laboratory rodents may yield a Borrelia sp. from blood even when obtained between fever episodes (69, 70, 78). Most TBRF agents will infect and proliferate in mice, rats, and hamsters; guinea pigs are resistant to some species, such as B. duttonii. B. recurrentis may cause a transient spirochetemia in weanling mice or newborn rabbits. For suspected TBRF, most outbred and in-

bred strains of mice are suitable, with the possible exception of C57BL/6 mice. The initial spirochetemia of mice or rats can be prolonged by sublethal gamma irradiation (23), treatment with cyclophosphamide (215), the severe combined immunodeficiency (SCID) phenotype (61), or splenectomy (162). The blood of immunocompetent mice should be examined daily for the presence of spirochetes beginning on day 2 postinfection and then for 7 to 10 days.

In vitro cultivation is an alternative to animal inoculation and may allow isolation of the organism from the blood or CSF. Kelly's medium and its most commonly used derivative, Barbour-Stoenner-Kelly (BSK) medium, support the growth of most but not all Borrelia spp. (16, 18, 19, 79, 80, 144, 214). A modification of BSK medium may be commercially available but has been formulated to optimize the growth of B. burgdorferi, not relapsing fever spirochetes. Better growth of relapsing fever species is achieved in some cases by increasing the amount of rabbit serum from 6 to 12% (vol/vol). The source of the bovine serum albumin for the BSK medium may sometimes be the determinant of whether the spirochetes can be cultivated in vitro or not. Supplementation of the medium with 5-fluorouracil, rifampin, phosphomycin, neomycin, and/or amphotericin B reduces the risk of contaminated cultures. Cultures are inoculated with several drops of blood or plasma and incubated at 34 to 36°C in tightly capped tubes for up to 2 weeks. Samples of the cultures are examined daily or every other day by dark-field or phase-contrast microscopy.

PCR may be performed on specimens of blood and joint tissues and has been used to study B. hermsii and B. turicatae infections of mice (177, 188). The technique is probably as sensitive as culture and has the advantage that the results can be obtained within a few hours. PCR was used to identify B. duttonii as the cause of human TBRF in southern Zaire (96). PCR may also be used for detecting and identifying Borrelia infections of ticks and mammalian hosts, especially in cases where the microorganism is uncultivable (28, 204).

No standardized, widely accepted serologic assay for relapsing fever infections presently exists. Elevated titers of antibodies that bind to the Proteus OX-K antigen in the Weil-Felix agglutination assay have been observed in both LBRF and TBRF (39, 103, 237). However, the basis of this reaction is not known, and this assay is not commonly available. Indirect immunofluorescence assays or enzyme-linked immunoassays for antibodies to whole cells of some TBRF species are currently available through some commercial and government reference laboratories, but these assays have not been comprehensively evaluated. The whole-cell assays include antigens common to other spirochetes and bacteria and consequently do not have high specificity. More promising is an immunoassay using the GlpQ protein, which is found in relapsing fever *Borrelia* spp. but not in the Lyme borreliosis *Borrelia* spp. An enzyme-linked immunosorbent assay based on recombinant GlpQ demonstrated higher specificity than whole-cell assays and was used in small studies of both TBRF and LBRF (183, 202).

TREATMENT

TBRF and LBRF *Borrelia* spp. are susceptible to penicillin and most other beta-lactam antibiotics, as well as to tetracyclines and to macrolides, such as erythromycin (21). The MICs of these antibiotics for *Borrelia* spp. are generally less than 0.1 µg/ml. The effectiveness of antibiotic treatment can be assessed by observing the clearance of spirochetes from the blood. Within 4 to 8 h of receiving the first dose of an effective antibiotic, patients should no longer have detectable spirochetes in the blood. Relapsing fever *Borrelia* spp. are also susceptible in vitro to chloramphenicol, vancomycin, and some fluoroquinolones, but there is less clinical experience with these antibiotics. Although parenteral vancomycin was effective in clearing *B. turicatae* from the blood of experimentally infected mice, active infection persisted in the brain (143). *Borrelia* spp. spirochetes are relatively resistant to rifampin, sulfonamides, and aminoglycosides.

Single oral doses of 100 mg of doxycycline, 500 mg of tetracycline, or 500 mg of erythromycin stearate or ethyl succinate have been shown to be effective in the treatment of adults with LBRF (56, 180, 181, 206). For children more than 8 years old, one of the following antibiotics is used in a single oral dose: doxycycline at 2 mg/kg of body weight, up to 100 mg; tetracycline at 12.5 mg/kg, up to 500 mg; or erythromycin at 12.5 mg/kg, up to 500 mg. For children 8 years old or less, the recommended treatment is a single oral dose of erythromycin at 12.5 mg/kg, up to 500 mg. An alternative single-dose oral treatment is chloramphenicol at 500 mg for adults and 12.5 to 25 mg/kg, up to 500 mg, for children (234). The overall recurrence rate after appropriate antibiotic treatment is less than 5%. Tetracyclines appear to be superior to erythromycins in efficacy and are preferred except for pregnant and nursing women and for children less than 9 years old. When the patient cannot take tetracycline orally, the intravenous dose is 250 or 500 mg for adults or 100 mg for doxycycline. Parenteral treatment with intramuscular penicillin G procaine is 600,000 to 800,000 U for adults and 400,000 U for children. If louse-borne typhus is suspected, the recommended antibiotics are doxycycline or chloramphenicol, but single doses will not be sufficient.

In comparison to LBRF, clinical evidence about management of TBRF is more anecdotal, but experience to date indicates that after single-dose treatments of TBRF the failure rate is 20% or higher (68, 136, 213). Recurrence of TBRF after single-dose treatments is likely the result of reinvasion of the blood by spirochetes from the brain once antibiotic levels decline below MICs in the blood (143, 197). The preferred oral treatment for adults with TBRF is 500 mg of tetracycline or 12.5 mg per kg every 6 h for 10 days or 100 mg of doxycycline twice daily for 10 days. When tetracyclines are contraindicated, the alternative is 500 mg of erythromycin or 12.5 mg per kg orally every 6 h for 10 days. As an alternative treatment for TBRF, beta-lactam antibiotics should be administered intravenously rather than orally, especially if central nervous system involvement is suspected or confirmed. For adults, either penicillin G (3 million U) intravenously every 4 h or ceftriaxone (2 g) intravenously once a day or in two divided doses, for a duration of 10 to 14 days, is effective intravenous treatment for Lyme borreliosis and would likely also be effective for relapsing fever with neurologic involvement.

Treatment of both LBRF and TBRF with antibiotics commonly results in the Jarisch-Herxheimer reaction (J-HR) soon after initiation of therapy (46, 48, 229, 230). Relapsing fever is one of the few infections for which antibiotic treatment itself can be expected to pose a significant risk of death or further morbidity. J-HR is effectively the same as the crisis that follows the appearance of neutralizing antibodies in the blood. In these situations, spirochetes are lysed by antibodies during the crisis and by antibiotics during J-HR, and spirochetal components are released into the circulation. Within 1 to 2 h of the start of treatment, the patient experiences intense rigors and becomes restless and apprehensive. This is accompanied by an elevation of temperature by 1 to 2°C, tachycardia, and a rise in blood pressure over 1 to 2 h. This phase is followed over the next few hours by diaphoresis, exhaustion, a decline in temperature, hypotension, and leukopenia. The shock-like state, in which there is dilated vasculature and the increased oxygen demands associated with fever (229), may be exacerbated by myocardial dysfunction if there is invasion of the heart.

At one time, J-HR was thought to be the consequence of endotoxin or antigen-antibody complexes (48, 116), but spirochetes do not have an endotoxin-like lipopolysaccharide, and changes in complement levels were not detected in patients with LBRF (229). A more likely mechanism for J-HR is the action of the abundant lipoproteins of spirochetes on the toll-like receptors 2 of macrophages and other cells (205, 227). This ligand-receptor binding induces the release of inflammatory cytokines (131). Levels of TNF, interleukin-6 (IL-6), and IL-8 rose severalfold over pretreatment levels during J-HR in patients treated for louse-borne relapsing fever (165). Infusion of antibodies to human TNF prior to administration of the penicillin reduced the severity of J-HR in one clinical trial (104).

In one study, the incidence of J-HR during treatment of LBRF was lower after receiving penicillin than with tetracycline (206), but this may be at the cost of a delay in the response of the illness (206, 229). Administration of corticosteroids, pentoxifylline (187), antipyretics, or naloxone has been of limited or no benefit in reducing morbidity or mortality from J-HR. Before treatment commences, steps should be taken to anticipate J-HR. This means provision of monitoring or constant nursing attention and ready access to resuscitative measures, such as intravenous fluids for volume expansion and inotropic cardiac agents.

PREVENTION

LBRF can be prevented by avoiding infestation or contact with human body lice. Although humans are reservoirs of the infection, there is no direct human-to-human transmission, with the exception of transplacental or perinatal transmission or contact with infected blood. The body louse lives in clothing and only attaches to body hair when feeding. Reduction of crowding, improved personal hygiene, and better access to washing facilities greatly decrease the potential for louse-borne diseases. More specific and immediate measures for delousing patients and household or shelter contacts are bathing, shaving of the scalp, and application of one of the following: 1% lindane shampoo (Kwell) or powder; 0.5% permethrin powder; 1% permethrin soap, lotion, or shampoo; 10% DDT (dichloro-diphenyl-trichloroethane) powder; 5% carbaryl powder; or 1% malathion powder (119, 213). The insecticides can be mixed with talcum powder. Infested clothes and bedding materials should be washed at a water temperature of at least 60°C and with either soap or 7% (wt/vol) DDT. Washed clothing and bedding should then be ironed if possible.

Log cabins and similar wood structures in forested areas pose a particular risk of TBRF when rodents nest in roofs, walls, and woodpiles; under eaves and porches; and in burrows under the house. In other natural environments, ticks may be in caves or shelters where animals sleep and nest. In villages or other inhabited areas, the ticks may be present in thatched roofs, mud walls, and crawl spaces under houses. In more agrarian environments, domestic animals such as pigs, goats, and sheep may be reservoirs for infection of humans if the livestock are adjacent to the living quarters and if the ticks have access to the human household. Sleeping on floors in buildings suspected of infestation should be avoided. Beds should preferably be of metal and should be moved away from walls. Insecticide-impregnated mosquito nets around the bed may be useful. For entry into infested caves, DEET (N,N-diethyl-m-toluamide) can be applied to the exposed skin, and permethrin can be sprayed on clothing.

The incidence of tick-borne relapsing fever can be reduced by construction of houses with sealed plank floors, concrete, or metal floors and walls (170). Efforts should be made to make the structure rodent proof (39, 174). Interiors of buildings infested with *Ornithodoros* ticks can be sprayed or fumigated with 0.5% diazinon, 0.5% malathion, or 0.5% lindane.

When *Ornithodoros* bites do occur on an occasional basis, such as during exploration of a cave in an area where relapsing fever is endemic, empiric evidence suggests that prophylactic tetracycline (500 mg orally four times daily) or doxycycline (100 mg orally once daily) for 2 to 3 days may reduce the risk of infection for individuals 8 years of age or older if taken within 2 days of the exposure. This regimen can also be used after accidental inoculation with infectious material in the laboratory or clinic. Oral erythromycin has been used as a prophylactic measure in conjunction with delousing measures in communities or camps in which there is an outbreak of LBRF.

At present there is no commercial or investigational vaccine for either LBRF or TBRF. Of the two diseases, the higher priority on a public health basis would be for a vaccine against LBRF. A relapsing fever vaccine based on the variable major proteins could be efficacious, but a successful subunit formulation would likely require inclusion of all or most variant antigens for a given species. Alternatively, a single subunit vaccine could be directed at the Vtp protein, which is expressed by the spirochetes at the time the ticks or lice begin to feed (200). Antibodies to Vtp might prevent acquisition at the point of tick feeding and before spirochetemia was underway.

Acknowledgments. I thank Willy Burgdorfer, Edward Korenberg, Victor Kryuchechnikov, and Tom Schwan for their comments and review of the manuscript.

My laboratory's research on relapsing fever and the *Borrelia* species that cause it has been supported by NIH grant AI 24424.

REFERENCES

1. Adler, S., O. Theodor, and H. Schieber. 1937. Observations on tick-transmitted human spirochaetosis in Palestine. *Ann. Trop. Med. Parasitol.* 31:25–35.
2. Ahmed, M., S. Abdel Wahab, M. Abdel Malik, A. Abdel Gadir, S. Salih, A. Omer, and A. Al Hassan. 1980. Louse-borne relapsing fever in the Sudan. A historical review and a clinico-pathological study. *Trop. Geogr. Med.* 32:106–111.

3. Alugupalli, K. R., R. M. Gerstein, J. Chen, E. Szomolanyi-Tsuda, R. T. Woodland, and J. M. Leong. 2003. The resolution of relapsing fever borreliosis requires IgM and is concurrent with expansion of B1b lymphocytes. *J. Immunol.* 170:3819–3827.

4. Alugupalli, K. R., A. D. Michelson, M. R. Barnard, D. Robbins, J. Coburn, E. K. Baker, M. H. Ginsberg, T. G. Schwan, and J. M. Leong. 2001. Platelet activation by a relapsing fever spirochaete results in enhanced bacterium-platelet interaction via integrin αIIbβ3 activation. *Mol. Microbiol.* 39:330–340.

5. Alugupalli, K. R., A. D. Michelson, I. Joris, T. G. Schwan, K. Hodivala-Dilke, R. O. Hynes, and J. M. Leong. 2003. Spirochete-platelet attachment and thrombocytopenia in murine relapsing fever borreliosis. *Blood* 102:2843–2850.

6. Anda, P., W. Sanchez-Yebra, M. del Mar Vitutia, E. Perez Pastrana, I. Rodriguez, N. S. Miller, P. B. Backenson, and J. L. Benach. 1996. A new Borrelia species isolated from patients with relapsing fever in Spain. *Lancet* 348:162–165.

7. Anderson, T. R., and L. E. Zimmerman. 1955. Relapsing fever in Korea. A clinicopathologic study of eleven fatal cases with special attention to association with salmonella infections. *Am. J. Pathol.* 31:1083–1109.

8. Arimitsu, Y., and K. Akama. 1973. Characterization of protective antibodies produced in mice infected with Borrelia duttonii. *Jpn. J. Med. Sci. Biol.* 26:229–237.

9. Babes, V. 1916. Hemorragies meningees et autres manifestations hemorragiques dans la fievre recurrente. *C. R. Seances Soc. Biol. (Paris)* 79:855–857.

10. Baltazard, M., M. Bahmanyar, and M. Chamsa. 1954. Sur l'usage du cobaye pour la differenciation des spirochetes recurrents. *Bull. Soc. Pathol. Exot.* 47:864–877.

11. Baltazard, M., C. Mofidi, and M. Bahmanyar. 1947. Solution aux difficulties de l'experimentation avec le spirochete d'Obermeier, S. recurrentis, agent de la fievre recurrente a poux. *C. R. Acad. Sci.* 224:1858–1860.

12. Barbour, A. G. 2003. Antigenic variation in Borrelia: relapsing fever and Lyme borreliosis, p. 319–356. *In* A. Craig and A. Scherf (ed.), *Antigenic Variation*. Academic Press, London, England.

13. Barbour, A. G. 2002. Antigenic variation by relapsing fever Borrelia species and other bacterial pathogens, p. 972–996. *In* N. L. Craig, R. Craigie, M. Gellert, and A. M. Lambowitz (ed.), *Mobile DNA II*. American Society for Microbiology, Washington, D.C.

14. Barbour, A. G. 2000. Borrelia infections: relapsing fever and Lyme disease, p. 57–70. *In* M. W. Cunningham and R. S. Fujinami (ed.), *Effects of Microbes on the Immune System*. Lippincott, Williams and Wilkins, Philadelphia, Pa.

15. Barbour, A. G. 2001. Borrelia: a diverse and ubiquitous genus of tick-borne pathogens, p. 153–174. *In* W. M. Scheld, W. A. Craig, and J. M. Hughes (ed.), *Emerging Infections 5*. ASM Press, Washington, D.C.

16. Barbour, A. G. 1986. Cultivation of Borrelia: a historical overview. *Zentralbl. Bakteriol. Mikrobiol. Hyg. A* 263:11–14.

17. Barbour, A. G. 1987. Immunobiology of relapsing fever. *Contrib. Microbiol. Immunol.* 8:125–137.

18. Barbour, A. G. 1984. Isolation and cultivation of Lyme disease spirochetes. *Yale J. Biol. Med.* 57:521–525.

19. Barbour, A. G. 1988. Laboratory aspects of Lyme borreliosis. *Clin. Microbiol. Rev.* 1:399–414.

20. Barbour, A. G. 1993. Linear DNA of Borrelia species and antigenic variation. *Trends Microbiol.* 1:236–239.

21. Barbour, A. G. 1999. Relapsing fever and other Borrelia infections, p. 535–546. *In* R. L. Guerrant, D. H. Walker, and P. F. Weller (ed.), *Tropical Infectious Diseases. Prin-ciples, Pathogens and Practice*. Churchill Livingston, Philadelphia, Pa.

22. Barbour, A. G. 2004. Specificity of Borrelia-tick vector relationships, p. 75–90. *In* S. H. Gillespie, G. L. Smith, and A. Osbourn (ed.), *SGM Symposium 63: Microbe-Vector Interactions in Vector-Borne Disease*. Cambridge University Press, Cambridge, England.

23. Barbour, A. G., O. Barrera, and R. C. Judd. 1983. Structural analysis of the variable major proteins of Borrelia hermsii. *J. Exp. Med.* 158:2127–2140.

24. Barbour, A. G., and V. Bundoc. 2001. In vitro and in vivo neutralization of the relapsing fever agent Borrelia hermsii with serotype-specific immunoglobulin M antibodies. *Infect. Immun.* 69:1009–1015.

25. Barbour, A. G., N. Burman, C. J. Carter, T. Kitten, and S. Bergstrom. 1991. Variable antigen genes of the relapsing fever agent Borrelia hermsii are activated by promoter addition. *Mol. Microbiol.* 5:489–493.

26. Barbour, A. G., C. J. Carter, and C. D. Sohaskey. 2000. Surface protein variation by expression site switching in the relapsing fever agent Borrelia hermsii. *Infect. Immun.* 78:7114–7121.

27. Barbour, A. G., and S. F. Hayes. 1986. Biology of Borrelia species. *Microbiol. Rev.* 50:381–400.

28. Barbour, A. G., G. O. Maupin, G. J. Teltow, C. J. Carter, and J. Piesman. 1996. Identification of an uncultivable Borrelia species in the hard tick Amblyomma americanum: possible agent of a Lyme disease-like illness. *J. Infect. Dis.* 173:403–409.

29. Barbour, A. G., and B. I. Restrepo. 2000. Antigenic variation in vector-borne pathogens. *Emerg. Infect. Dis.* 6:449–457.

30. Barbour, A. G., and H. G. Stoenner. 1985. Antigenic variation of Borrelia hermsii, p. 123–135. *In* M. I. Simon and I. Herskowitz (ed.), *Genome Rearrangement*. Alan R. Liss, Inc., New York, N.Y.

31. Barbour, A. G., S. L. Tessier, and H. G. Stoenner. 1982. Variable major proteins of Borrelia hermsii. *J. Exp. Med.* 156:1312–1324.

32. Barclay, A. J., and J. B. Coulter. 1990. Tick-borne relapsing fever in central Tanzania. *Trans. R. Soc. Trop. Med. Hyg.* 84:852–856.

33. Barstad, P. A., J. E. Coligan, M. G. Raum, and A. G. Barbour. 1985. Variable major proteins of Borrelia hermsii. Epitope mapping and partial sequence analysis of CNBr peptides. *J. Exp. Med.* 161:1302–1314.

34. Beck, M. 1937. California field and laboratory studies on relapsing fever. *J. Infect. Dis.* 60:64–80.

35. Beunders, B., and P. Van Thiel. 1932. Untersuchungen ueber die persistenz von Spirochaeta duttoni in mausegehirnen bei experimenteller febris recurrens. *Z. Hyg. Infektionskr.* 114:568–583.

36. Bodman, R. I., and I. S. Stewart. 1948. Louse-borne relapsing fever in Persia. *Br. Med. J.* 1948:291–292.

37. Bohls, S. W., and V. T. Schuhardt. 1933. Relapsing fever in Texas and the laboratory method of diagnosis. *Texas State J. Med.* 13:425–427.

38. Borgnolo, G., B. Hailu, A. Ciancarelli, M. Alaviva, and T. Woldemariam. 1993. Louse-borne relapsing fever. A clinical and an epidemiological study of 389 patients in Asella Hospital, Ethiopia. *Trop. Geograph. Med.* 45:66–69.

39. Boyer, K. M., R. S. Munford, G. O. Maupin, C. P. Pattison, M. D. Fox, A. M. Barnes, W. L. Jones, and J. E. Maynard. 1977. Tick-borne relapsing fever: an interstate outbreak originating at Grand Canyon National Park. *Am. J. Epidemiol.* 105:469–479.

40. Breitschwerdt, E. B., F. J. Geoly, D. J. Meuten, J. F. Levine, P. Howard, B. C. Hegarty, and L. C. Stafford. 1996. Myocarditis in mice and guinea pigs experimentally infected with a canine-origin Borrelia isolate from Florida. *Am. J. Vet. Res.* **57**:505–511.

41. Breitschwerdt, E. B., W. L. Nicholson, A. R. Kiehl, C. Steers, D. J. Meuten, and J. F. Levine. 1994. Natural infections with *Borrelia spirochetes* in two dogs from Florida. *J. Clin. Microbiol.* **32**:352–357.

42. Briggs, L. H. 1935. Relapsing fever. *Calif. West. Med.* **42**:1–13.

43. Briggs, L. H. 1922. Relapsing fever in California. *JAMA* **79**:941–944.

44. Brocklesby, D. W., G. R. Scott, and C. S. Rampton. 1963. Borrelia theileri and transient fevers in cattle. *Vet. Rec.* **75**:103–104.

45. Brown, V., B. Larouze, G. Desve, J. J. Rousset, M. Thibon, A. Fourrier, and V. Schwoebel. 1988. Clinical presentation of louse-borne relapsing fever among Ethiopian refugees in northern Somalia. *Ann. Trop. Med. Parasitol.* **82**:499–502.

46. Bryceson, A. 1976. Clinical pathology of the Jarisch-Herxheimer reaction. *J. Infect. Dis.* **133**:696–704.

47. Bryceson, A., E. Parry, P. Perine, D. Warrel, D. Vukotich, and C. Leithead. 1970. Louse-borne relapsing fever: a clinical and laboratory study of 62 cases in Ethiopia and a reconsideration of the literature. *Q. J. Med.* **153**:129–170.

48. Bryceson, A. D., K. E. Cooper, D. A. Warrell, P. L. Perine, and E. H. Parry. 1972. Studies of the mechanism of the Jarisch-Herxheimer reaction in louse-borne relapsing fever: evidence for the presence of circulating Borrelia endotoxin. *Clin. Sci.* **43**:343–354.

49. Bunikis, J., U. Garpmo, J. Tsao, J. Berglund, D. Fish, and A. G. Barbour. 2004. Sequence typing reveals extensive strain diversity of the Lyme borreliosis agents *Borrelia burgdorferi* in North America and *Borrelia afzelii* in Europe. *Microbiology* **150**:1741–1755.

50. Bunikis, J., U. Garpmo, J. Tsao, J. Berglund, D. Fish, and A. G. Barbour. 2004. Strain typing of relapsing fever *Borrelia* spp., including newly discovered species in hard ticks. *Emerg. Infect. Dis.* **10**:1661–1664.

51. Burgdorfer, W. 1951. Analyse des Infektionsverlaufes bei Ornithodorus moubata und der natürlichen Uebertragung von Spirochaeta duttoni. *Acta Trop.* **8**:196–262.

52. Burgdorfer, W., and M. G. Varma. 1967. Transstadial and transovarial development of disease agents in arthropods. *Annu. Rev. Entomol.* **12**:347–376.

53. Burman, N., S. Bergstrom, B. I. Restrepo, and A. G. Barbour. 1990. The variable antigens Vmp7 and Vmp21 of the relapsing fever bacterium Borrelia hermsii are structurally analogous to the VSG proteins of the African trypanosome. *Mol. Microbiol.* **4**:1715–1726.

54. Burman, N., A. Shamaei-Tousi, and S. Bergstrom. 1998. The spirochete *Borrelia crocidurae* causes erythrocyte rosetting during relapsing fever. *Infect. Immun.* **66**:815–819.

55. Butler, T., P. Hazen, C. K. Wallace, S. Awoke, and A. Habte-Michael. 1979. Infection with Borrelia recurrentis: pathogenesis of fever and petechiae. *J. Infect. Dis.* **140**:665–675.

56. Butler, T., P. K. Jones, and C. K. Wallace. 1978. Borrelia recurrentis infection: single-dose antibiotic regimens and management of the Jarisch-Herxheimer reaction. *J. Infect. Dis.* **137**:573–577.

57. Cadavid, D., and A. G. Barbour. 1998. Neuroborreliosis during relapsing fever: review of the clinical manifestations, pathology, and treatment of infections in humans and experimental animals. *Clin. Infect. Dis.* **26**:151–164.

58. Cadavid, D., V. Bundoc, and A. G. Barbour. 1993. Experimental infection of the mouse brain by a relapsing fever Borrelia species: a molecular analysis. *J. Infect. Dis.* **168**:143–151.

59. Cadavid, D., A. R. Pachner, L. Estanislao, R. Patalapati, and A. G. Barbour. 2001. Isogenic serotypes of Borrelia turicatae show different localization in the brain and skin of mice. *Infect. Immun.* **69**:3389–3397.

60. Cadavid, D., P. M. Pennington, T. A. Kerentseva, S. Bergstrom, and A. G. Barbour. 1997. Immunologic and genetic analyses of VmpA of a neurotropic strain of *Borrelia turicatae.* *Infect. Immun.* **65**:3352–3360.

61. Cadavid, D., D. D. Thomas, R. Crawley, and A. G. Barbour. 1994. Variability of a bacterial surface protein and disease expression in a possible mouse model of systemic Lyme borreliosis. *J. Exp. Med.* **179**:631–642.

62. Calero, C. 1946. Relapsing fever on the isthmus of Panama. Report of 106 cases. *Am. J. Trop. Med.* **26**:761–769.

63. Campbell, G. L., W. S. Paul, M. E. Schriefer, R. B. Craven, K. E. Robbins, and D. T. Dennis. 1995. Epidemiologic and diagnostic studies of patients with suspected early Lyme disease, Missouri, 1990–1993. *J. Infect. Dis.* **172**:470–480.

64. Carley, J. G., and J. H. Pope. 1962. A new species of Borrelia (*B. queenslandia*) from *Rattus villosissimus* in Queensland. *Aust. J. Exp. Biol. Med. Sci.* **40**:255–262.

65. Carter, C. J., S. Bergstrom, S. J. Norris, and A. G. Barbour. 1994. A family of surface-exposed proteins of 20 kilodaltons in the genus *Borrelia*. *Infect. Immun.* **62**:2792–2799.

66. Casjens, S., N. Palmer, R. van Vugt, W. M. Huang, B. Stevenson, P. Rosa, R. Lathigra, G. Sutton, J. Peterson, R. J. Dodson, D. Haft, E. Hickey, M. Gwinn, O. White, and C. M. Fraser. 2000. A bacterial genome in flux: the twelve linear and nine circular extrachromosomal DNAs in an infectious isolate of the Lyme disease spirochete Borrelia burgdorferi. *Mol. Microbiol.* **35**:490–516.

67. Charters, A. 1942. Relapsing fever in Abyssinia. *Trans. R. Soc. Trop. Med. Hyg.* **35**:271–279.

68. Cherry, J. 1955. The prevention and treatment of tick-borne relapsing fever with special reference to aureomycin and terramycin. *Trans. R. Soc. Trop. Med. Hyg.* **49**:563–573.

69. Chohan, I. S. 1967. Tick-borne relapsing fever in Kashmir: mice inoculation—a diagnostic method of choice. *Ind. J. Pathol. Bacteriol.* **10**:289–294.

70. Chorine, V., and O. Crouge. 1942. Virulence du sang du cobaye infecte avec le *Spirochaeta hispanica*. *Ann. Inst. Pasteur* **68**:518–523.

71. Clark, H. C., L. H. Dunn, and J. Benavides. 1931. Experimental transmission to man of a relapsing fever spirochete in a wild monkey of Panama, Leontocebus geoffroyi. *Am. J. Trop. Med.* **11**:243–257.

72. Clastrier, J. 1941. Etude experimentale de deux souches de Spirochaeta hispanicum isolees en Algerie. *Arch. Inst. Pasteur Alger.* **19**:228–239.

73. Cobey, F. C., S. H. Goldbarg, R. A. Levine, and C. L. Patton. 2001. Short report: Detection of borrelia (relapsing fever) in rural Ethiopia by means of the quantitative buffy coat technique. *Am. J. Trop. Med. Hyg.* **65**:164–165.

74. Coffey, E. M., and W. C. Eveland. 1967. Experimental relapsing fever initiated by Borrelia hermsi. II. Sequential appearance of major serotypes in the rat. *J. Infect. Dis.* **117**:29–34.

75. Coghill, N. 1949. Clinical manifestations of tick-borne relapsing fever with special reference to the disease in Cyprus. *J. R. Army Med. Corps* **92**:2–33.

76. Connolly, S. E., and J. L. Benach. 2001. Cutting edge: the spirochetemia of murine relapsing fever is cleared by complement-independent bactericidal antibodies. *J. Immunol.* **167**:3029–3032.

77. Cooley, R. A., and G. M. Kohls. 1944. *The Argasidae of North America, Central America, and Cuba.* Notre Dame University Press, South Bend, Ind.

78. Cunningham, J., and A. G. L. Fraser. 1937. Further observations on Indian relapsing fever. III. Persistence of spirochaetes in the blood and organs of infected animals. *Indian J. Med. Res.* 24:581–592.

79. Cutler, S. J., C. O. Akintunde, J. Moss, M. Fukunaga, K. Kurtenbach, A. Talbert, H. Zhang, D. J. Wright, and D. A. Warrell. 1999. Successful in vitro cultivation of *Borrelia duttonii* and its comparison with *Borrelia recurrentis. Int. J. Syst. Bacteriol.* 49:1793–1799.

80. Cutler, S. J., D. Fekade, K. Hussein, K. A. Knox, A. Melka, K. Cann, A. R. Emilianus, D. A. Warrell, and D. J. Wright. 1994. Successful in-vitro cultivation of Borrelia recurrentis. *Lancet* 343:242.

81. DaMassa, A. J., and H. E. Adler. 1979. Avian spirochetosis: natural transmission by Argas (Persicargas) sanchezi (Ixodoidea: argasidae) and existence of different serologic and immunologic types of Borrelia anserina in the United States. *Am. J. Vet. Res.* 40:154–157.

82. Davis, G. E. 1952. Biology as an aid to the identification of two closely related species of ticks of the genus Ornithodoros. *J. Parasitol.* 38:477–480.

83. Davis, G. E. 1952. Observations on the biology of the argasid tick, Ornithodoros brasiliensis Aragao, 1923; with the recovery of a spirochete, Borrelia brasiliensis, n. sp. *J. Parasitol.* 38:473–476.

84. Davis, G. E. 1956. A relapsing fever spirochete, Borrelia mazzottii (sp. nov.) from Ornithodoros talaje from Mexico. *Am. J. Hyg.* 63:13–17.

85. Davis, G. E. 1943. Relapsing fever: the tick *Ornithodoros turicata* as a spirochetal reservoir. *Public Health Rep.* 58:839–842.

86. Davis, G. E. 1952. The relapsing fevers: tick-spirochete specificity studies. *Exp. Parasitol.* 1:406–410.

87. Davis, G. E. 1940. Ticks and relapsing fever in the United States. *Public Health Rep.* 55:2347–2351.

88. Davis, G. E., H. L. Wynns, and M. D. Beck. 1941. Relapsing fever: Ornithodoros parkeri, a vector in California. *Public Health Rep.* 56:2426–2428.

89. Davis, H., J. M. Vincent, and J. Lynch. 2002. Tick-borne relapsing fever caused by *Borrelia turicatae. Pediatr. Infect. Dis. J.* 21:703–705.

90. Dennis, D., S. Awoke, E. Doberstein, and J. Fresh. 1976. Bleeding in louse-borne relapsing fever in Ethiopia. *East Afr. Med. J.* 53:220–225.

91. Dewar, H., and R. Walmsley. 1945. Relapsing fever with nephritis and subarachnoid haemorrhage. *Lancet* i:630–631.

92. Diab, F. M., and Z. R. Soliman. 1977. An experimental study of Borrelia anserina in four species of Argas ticks. 1. Spirochete localization and densities. *Z. Parasitenkd.* 53:201–212.

93. Donelson, J. E. 1995. Mechanisms of antigenic variation in Borrelia hermsii and African trypanosomes. *J. Biol. Chem.* 270:7783–7786.

94. Dunn, L. H. 1933. Notes on relapsing fever in Panama with special reference to animal hosts. *Am. J. Trop. Med.* 13:201–209.

95. Dunn, L. H. 1927. Studies on the South American tick Ornithodoros venezuelensis Brumpt in Colombia. *J. Parasitol.* 13:249–255.

96. Dupont, H. T., B. La Scola, R. Williams, and D. Raoult. 1997. A focus of tick-borne relapsing fever in southern Zaire. *Clin. Infect. Dis.* 25:139–144.

97. Duray, P. H. 1987. The surgical pathology of human Lyme disease: an enlarging picture. *Am. J. Surg. Pathol.* 11:47–60.

98. Dworkin, M. S., D. E. Anderson, Jr., T. G. Schwan, P. C. Shoemaker, S. N. Banerjee, B. O. Kassen, and W. Burgdorfer. 1998. Tick-borne relapsing fever in the northwestern United States and southwestern Canada. *Clin. Infect. Dis.* 26:122–131.

99. Dworkin, M. S., T. G. Schwan, and D. E. Anderson, Jr. 2002. Tick-borne relapsing fever in North America. *Med. Clin. North. Am.* 86:417–433.

100. Dworkin, M. S., P. C. Shoemaker, C. L. Fritz, M. E. Dowell, and D. E. Anderson, Jr. 2002. The epidemiology of tick-borne relapsing fever in the United States. *Am. J. Trop. Med. Hyg.* 66:753–758.

101. Dykhuizen, D. E., and G. Baranton. 2001. The implications of a low rate of horizontal transfer in Borrelia. *Trends Microbiol.* 9:344–350.

102. Eicken, C., V. Sharma, T. Klabunde, M. B. Lawrenz, J. M. Hardham, S. J. Norris, and J. C. Sacchettini. 2002. Crystal structure of Lyme disease variable surface antigen VlsE of Borrelia burgdorferi. *J. Biol. Chem.* 277:21691–21696.

103. Elsdon-Dew, R. 1943. Relapsing fever and B. proteus X Kingbury. *Nature* 152:565.

104. Fekade, D., K. Knox, K. Hussein, A. Melka, D. G. Lalloo, R. E. Coxon, and D. A. Warrell. 1996. Prevention of Jarisch-Herxheimer reactions by treatment with antibodies against tumor necrosis factor alpha. *N. Engl. J. Med.* 335:311–315.

105. Felsenfeld, O. 1965. Borrelia, human relapsing fever, and parasite-vector-host relationships. *Bacteriol. Rev.* 29:46–74.

106. Felsenfeld, O. 1971. *Borrelia: Strains, Vectors, Human and Animal Borreliosis.* Warren H. Greene, Inc., St. Louis, Mo.

107. Ferdows, M. S., P. Serwer, G. A. Griess, S. J. Norris, and A. G. Barbour. 1996. Conversion of a linear to a circular plasmid in the relapsing fever agent *Borrelia hermsii. J. Bacteriol.* 178:793–800.

108. Filippova, N. A. 1966. *Argasidae.* Nauka, Moscow, Russia.

109. Fraenkel, C. J., U. Garpmo, and J. Berglund. 2002. Determination of novel Borrelia genospecies in Swedish *Ixodes ricinus* ticks. *J. Clin. Microbiol.* 40:3308–3312.

110. Fraser, C. M., S. Casjens, W. M. Huang, G. G. Sutton, R. Clayton, R. Lathigra, O. White, K. A. Ketchum, R. Dodson, E. K. Hickey, M. Gwinn, B. Dougherty, J. F. Tomb, R. D. Fleischmann, D. Richardson, J. Peterson, A. R. Kerlavage, J. Quackenbush, S. Salzberg, M. Hanson, R. van Vugt, N. Palmer, M. D. Adams, J. Gocayne, J. C. Venter, et al. 1997. Genomic sequence of a Lyme disease spirochaete, Borrelia burgdorferi. *Nature* 390:580–586.

111. Fuchs, P. C., and A. A. Oyama. 1969. Neonatal relapsing fever due to transplacental transmission of Borrelia. *JAMA* 208:690–692.

112. Fukunaga, M., and Y. Koreki. 1995. The flagellin gene of Borrelia miyamotoi sp. nov. and its phylogenetic relationship among Borrelia species. *FEMS Microbiol. Lett.* 134:255–258.

113. Fukunaga, M., K. Okada, M. Nakao, T. Konishi, and Y. Sato. 1996. Phylogenetic analysis of *Borrelia* species based on flagellin gene sequences and its application for molecular typing of Lyme disease borreliae. *Int. J. Syst. Bacteriol.* 46:898–905.

114. Fukunaga, M., Y. Takahashi, Y. Tsuruta, O. Matsushita, D. Ralph, M. McClelland, and M. Nakao. 1995. Genetic and phenotypic analysis of *Borrelia miyamotoi* sp. nov., isolated from the ixodid tick *Ixodes persulcatus*, the vector for Lyme disease in Japan. *Int. J. Syst. Bacteriol.* 45:804–810.

115. Fukunaga, M., Y. Ushijima, L. Y. Aoki, and A. Talbert. 2001. Detection of Borrelia duttonii, a tick-borne relapsing

fever agent in central Tanzania, within ticks by flagellin gene-based nested polymerase chain reaction. *Vector Borne Zoonotic Dis.* 1:331–338.

116. **Galloway, R. E., J. Levin, T. Butler, G. B. Naff, G. H. Goldsmith, H. Saito, S. Awoke, and C. K. Wallace.** 1977. Activation of protein mediators of inflammation and evidence for endotoxemia in Borrelia recurrentis infection. *Am. J. Med.* 63:933–938.

117. **Gambles, R. M., and N. F. Coghill.** 1948. Relapsing fever in Cyprus. *Ann. Trop. Med. Parasitol.* 42:288–303.

118. **Garcia-Monco, J. C., N. S. Miller, P. B. Backenson, P. Anda, and J. L. Benach.** 1997. A mouse model of Borrelia meningitis after intradermal injection. *J. Infect. Dis.* 175:1243–1245.

119. **Garnham, P., C. Davis, R. Heisch, and G. Timms.** 1947. An epidemic of louse-borne relapsing fever in Kenya. *Trans. R. Soc. Trop. Med. Hyg.* 41:141–170.

120. **Geigy, R., and G. Sarasin.** 1958. Isolatstamme von *Borrelia duttoni* und immunisierungsverhalten gegenuber der weissen maus. *Acta Trop.* 15:254–258.

121. **Godeluck, B., J. M. Duplantier, K. Ba, and J. F. Trape.** 1994. A longitudinal survey of Borrelia crocidurae prevalence in rodents and insectivores in Senegal. *Am. J. Trop. Med. Hyg.* 50:165–168.

122. **Gylfe, A., S. Bergstrom, J. Lundstrom, and B. Olsen.** 2000. Reactivation of Borrelia infection in birds. *Nature* 403:724–725.

123. **Hamase, A., Y. Takahashi, K. Nohgi, and M. Fukunaga.** 1996. Homology of variable major protein genes between *Borrelia hermsii* and *Borrelia miyamotoi. FEMS Microbiol. Lett.* 140:131–137.

124. **Hamilton, J. B.** 1943. Ocular complications in relapsing fever. *Br. J. Ophthalmol.* 27:68–80.

125. **Hardy, P. H., Jr., and J. Levin.** 1983. Lack of endotoxin in Borrelia hispanica and Treponema pallidum. *Proc. Soc. Exp. Biol. Med.* 174:47–52.

126. **Hayes, L. J., D. J. Wright, and L. C. Archard.** 1988. Segmented arrangement of Borrelia duttonii DNA and location of variant surface antigen genes. *J. Gen. Microbiol.* 134:1785–1793.

127. **Hendson, M., and R. S. Lane.** 2000. Genetic characteristics of *Borrelia coriaceae* isolates from the soft tick *Ornithodoros coriaceus* (Acari: Argasidae). *J. Clin. Microbiol.* 38:2678–2682.

128. **Herms, W. B., and C. M. Wheeler.** 1935. Tick transmission of California relapsing fever. *J. Econ. Entomol.* 28:846–855.

129. **Hinnebusch, B. J., A. G. Barbour, B. I. Restrepo, and T. G. Schwan.** 1998. Population structure of the relapsing fever spirochete *Borrelia hermsii* as indicated by polymorphism of two multigene families that encode immunogenic outer surface lipoproteins. *Infect. Immun.* 66:432–440.

130. **Hinnebusch, J., and K. Tilly.** 1993. Linear plasmids and chromosomes in bacteria. *Mol. Microbiol.* 10:917–922.

131. **Hirschfeld, M., C. J. Kirschning, R. Schwandner, H. Wesche, J. H. Weis, R. M. Wooten, and J. J. Weis.** 1999. Cutting edge: inflammatory signaling by Borrelia burgdorferi lipoproteins is mediated by toll-like receptor 2. *J. Immunol.* 163:2382–2386.

132. **Holt, S. C.** 1978. Anatomy and chemistry of spirochetes. *Microbiol. Rev.* 38:114–160.

133. **Hoogstraal, H.** 1985. Argasid and nuttalliellid ticks as parasites and vectors. *Adv. Parasitol.* 24:135–238.

134. **Hoogstraal, H.** 1979. Ticks and spirochetes. *Acta Trop.* 36:133–136.

135. **Horrenberger, R.** 1954. Spirochaeta hispanica chez les rats d'Alger (nouvelle enquete). *Arch. l'Inst. Pasteur Alger.* 32:18–22.

136. **Horton, J., and M. Blaser.** 1985. The spectrum of relapsing fever in the Rocky Mountains. *Arch. Intern. Med.* 145:871–875.

137. **Hovind-Hougen, K.** 1976. Treponema and Borrelia morphology, p. 7–18. *In* R. C. Johnson (ed.), *The Biology of Parasitic Spirochetes*. Academic Press, New York, N.Y.

138. **James, A. M., D. Liveris, G. P. Wormser, I. Schwartz, M. A. Montecalvo, and B. J. Johnson.** 2001. Borrelia lonestari infection after a bite by an Amblyomma americanum tick. *J. Infect. Dis.* 183:1810–1814.

139. **Johnson, R. C.** 1976. Comparative spirochete physiology and cellular composition, p. 39–48. *In* R. C. Johnson (ed.), *The Biology of Parasitic Spirochetes*. Academic Press, New York, N.Y.

140. **Jongen, V. H., J. van Roosmalen, J. Tiems, J. Van Holten, and J. C. Wetsteyn.** 1997. Tick-borne relapsing fever and pregnancy outcome in rural Tanzania. *Acta Obstet. Gynecol. Scand.* 76:834–838.

141. **Judge, D., I. Samuel, P. Perine, and D. Vukotic.** 1974. Louse-borne relapsing fever in man. *Arch. Pathol.* 97:136–140.

142. **Judge, D. M., J. T. La Croix, and P. L. Perine.** 1974. Experimental louse-borne relapsing fever in the grivet monkey, Cercopithecus aethiops. II. Pathology. *Am. J. Trop. Med. Hyg.* 23:962–968.

143. **Kazragis, R. J., L. L. Dever, J. H. Jorgensen, and A. G. Barbour.** 1996. In vivo activities of ceftriaxone and vancomycin against *Borrelia* spp. in the mouse brain and other sites. *Antimicrob. Agents Chemother.* 40:2632–2636.

144. **Kelly, R.** 1971. Cultivation of Borrelia hermsi. *Science* 173:443–444.

145. **Kemp, H. A., W. H. Moursund, and H. E. Wright.** 1935. Relapsing fever in Texas. V. A survey of the epidemiology and clinical manifestations of the disease as it occurs in Texas. *Am. J. Trop. Med.* 15:495–506.

146. **Kisinza, W. N., P. J. McCall, H. Mitani, A. Talbert, and M. Fukunaga.** 2003. A newly identified tick-borne Borrelia species and relapsing fever in Tanzania. *Lancet* 362:1283–1284.

147. **Kitten, T., and A. G. Barbour.** 1990. Juxtaposition of expressed variable antigen genes with a conserved telomere in the bacterium Borrelia hermsii. *Proc. Natl. Acad. Sci. USA* 87:6077–6081.

148. **Kitten, T., and A. G. Barbour.** 1992. The relapsing fever agent Borrelia hermsii has multiple copies of its chromosome and linear plasmids. *Genetics* 132:311–324.

149. **Kitten, T., A. V. Barrera, and A. G. Barbour.** 1993. Intragenic recombination and a chimeric outer membrane protein in the relapsing fever agent *Borrelia hermsii. J. Bacteriol.* 175:2516–2522.

150. **Konishi, H., M. G. Morshed, H. Akitomi, and T. Nakazawa.** 1993. In vitro cultivation of Borrelia duttonii on cultures of SflEp cells. *Microbiol. Immunol.* 37:229–232.

151. **Korenberg, E. I.** 1993. Borrelioses, p. 382–391. *In* V. I. Pokrovsky (ed.), *Epidemiology of Infectious Diseases: A Manual.* Meditsina, Moscow, Russia. (In Russian.)

152. **Krakowski, J., and E. Edelstein.** 1949. A survey of 25 cases of tick-borne relapsing fever observed at number 9 army hospital. *Harefuah* (Tel-Aviv foreign ed.) 5/6:23–24.

153. **Kurtti, T. J., U. G. Munderloh, G. G. Ahlstrand, and R. C. Johnson.** 1988. Borrelia burgdorferi in tick cell culture: growth and cellular adherence. *J. Med. Entomol.* 25:256–261.

154. **Lane, R. S., W. Burgdorfer, S. F. Hayes, and A. G. Barbour.** 1985. Isolation of a spirochete from the soft tick, Ornithodoros coriaceus: a possible agent of epizootic bovine abortion. *Science* 230:85–87.

155. **Lane, R. S., and S. A. Manweiler.** 1988. Borrelia coriaceae in its tick vector, Ornithodoros coriaceus (Acari: Argasidae),

with emphasis on transstadial and transovarial infection. *J. Med. Entomol.* **25:**172–177.

156. **Longanecker, D. S.** 1951. Laboratory and field studies on the biology of the relapsing fever tick vector (Ornithodoros hermsi) in the high mountains of California. *Am. J. Trop. Med.* **31:**373–380.

157. **Magoun, L., W. R. Zuckert, D. Robbins, N. Parveen, K. R. Alugupalli, T. G. Schwan, A. G. Barbour, and J. M. Leong.** 2000. Variable small protein (Vsp)-dependent and vsp-independent pathways for glycosaminoglycan recognition by relapsing fever spirochaetes. *Mol. Microbiol.* **36:**886–897.

158. **Matton, P., and H. Van Melckebeke.** 1990. Bovine borreliosis: comparison of simple methods for detection of the spirochaete in the blood. *Trop. Anim. Health Prod.* **22:**147–152.

159. **Mazzotti, L.** 1943. Transmission experiments with *Spirochaeta turicatae* and *S. venezuelensis* with four species of Ornithodoros. *Am. J. Hyg.* **38:**203–206.

160. **McDowell, J. V., E. Tran, D. Hamilton, J. Wolfgang, K. Miller, and R. T. Marconi.** 2003. Analysis of the ability of spirochete species associated with relapsing fever, avian borreliosis, and epizootic bovine abortion to bind factor H and cleave c3b. *J. Clin. Microbiol.* **41:**3905–3910.

161. **Meier, J. T., M. I. Simon, and A. G. Barbour.** 1985. Antigenic variation is associated with DNA rearrangements in a relapsing fever Borrelia. *Cell* **41:**403–409.

162. **Meleney, H. E.** 1928. Relapse phenomena of Spironema recurrentis. *J. Exp. Med.* **48:**65–82.

163. **Melkert, P. W.** 1988. Relapsing fever in pregnancy: analysis of high-risk factors. *Br. J. Obstet. Gynaecol.* **95:**1070–1072.

164. **Mitiku, K., and G. Mengistu.** 2002. Relapsing fever in Gondar, Ethiopia. *East Afr. Med. J.* **79:**85–87.

165. **Negussie, Y., D. G. Remick, L. E. DeForge, S. L. Kunkel, A. Eynon, and G. E. Griffin.** 1992. Detection of plasma tumor necrosis factor, interleukins 6, and 8 during the Jarisch-Herxheimer reaction of relapsing fever. *J. Exp. Med.* **175:**1207–1212.

166. **Newman, K., Jr., and R. C. Johnson.** 1981. In vivo evidence that an intact lytic complement pathway is not essential for successful removal of circulating *Borrelia turicatae* from mouse blood. *Infect. Immun.* **31:**465–469.

167. **Newman, K., Jr., and R. C. Johnson.** 1984. T-cell-independent elimination of *Borrelia turicatae*. *Infect. Immun.* **45:**572–576.

168. **Nicolle, C., and C. Anderson.** 1927. Etude comparative de quelques viru recurrents, pathogenes pour l'homme. *Arch. Inst. Pasteur Tunis* **16:**123–206.

169. **Nordstrand, A., A. Shamaei-Tousi, A. Ny, and S. Bergstrom.** 2001. Delayed invasion of the kidney and brain by *Borrelia crocidurae* in plasminogen-deficient mice. *Infect. Immun.* **69:**5832–5839.

170. **Ordman, D.** 1943. Epidemiological observations on an outbreak of tick relapsing fever in Northern Transvaal. *S. Afr. Med. J.* **1943**(June 12):180–182.

171. **Ordman, D., and F. Jones.** 1940. Some clinical aspects of tick relapsing fever in natives in South Africa. *S. Afr. Med. J.* **14:**81–83.

172. **Parsons, L.** 1947. Relapsing fever at Lake Tahoe, California-Nevada. *Am. J. Clin. Pathol.* **17:**388–392.

173. **Paster, B. J., and F. E. Dewhirst.** 2000. Phylogenetic foundation of spirochetes. *J. Mol. Microbiol. Biotechnol.* **2:**341–344.

174. **Paul, W. S., G. Maupin, A. O. Scott-Wright, R. B. Craven, and D. T. Dennis.** 2002. Outbreak of tick-borne relapsing fever at the north rim of the Grand Canyon: evidence for effectiveness of preventive measures. *Am. J. Trop. Med. Hyg.* **66:**71–75.

175. **Pavlovsky, Y. N.** 1963. Tick-borne relapsing fever, p. 138–184. *In* Y. N. Pavlovsky (ed.), *Human Disease with Natural Foci.* Foreign Languages Publishing House, Moscow, Russia.

176. **Penningon, P. M., D. Cadavid, J. Bunikis, S. J. Norris, and A. G. Barbour.** 1999. Extensive interplasmidic duplications change the virulence phenotype of the relapsing fever agent borrelia turicatae. *Mol. Microbiol.* **34:**1120–1132.

177. **Pennington, P. M., C. D. Allred, C. S. West, R. Alvarez, and A. G. Barbour.** 1997. Arthritis severity and spirochete burden are determined by serotype in the *Borrelia turicatae*-mouse model of Lyme disease. *Infect. Immun.* **65:**285–292.

178. **Pennington, P. M., D. Cadavid, and A. G. Barbour.** 1999. Characterization of VspB of *Borrelia turicatae*, a major outer membrane protein expressed in blood and tissues of mice. *Infect. Immun.* **67:**4637–4645.

179. **Perine, P., E. Parry, D. Vukotich, D. A. Warrell, and A. D. Bryceson.** 1971. Bleeding in louse-borne relapsing fever. I. Clinical studies in 37 patients. *Trans. R. Soc. Trop. Med. Hyg.* **65:**776–781.

180. **Perine, P. L., D. W. Krause, S. Awoke, and J. E. McDade.** 1974. Single-dose doxycycline treatment of louse-borne relapsing fever and epidemic typhus. *Lancet* **ii:**742–744.

181. **Perine, P. L., and B. Teklu.** 1983. Antibiotic treatment of louse-borne relapsing fever in Ethiopia: a report of 377 cases. *Am. J. Trop. Med. Hyg.* **32:**1096–1100.

182. **Plasterk, R. H., M. I. Simon, and A. G. Barbour.** 1985. Transposition of structural genes to an expression sequence on a linear plasmid causes antigenic variation in the bacterium *Borrelia hermsii*. *Nature* **318:**257–263.

183. **Porcella, S. F., S. J. Raffel, M. E. Schrumpf, M. E. Schriefer, D. T. Dennis, and T. G. Schwan.** 2000. Serodiagnosis of louse-borne relapsing fever with glycerophosphodiester phosphodiesterase (GlpQ) from *Borrelia recurrentis*. *J. Clin. Microbiol.* **38:**3561–3571.

184. **Quin, C., and E. Perkins.** 1946. Tick-borne relapsing fever in East Africa. *Trop. Med. Hyg.* **49:**30–32.

185. **Ras, N. M., B. Lascola, D. Postic, S. J. Cutler, F. Rodhain, G. Baranton, and D. Raoult.** 1996. Phylogenesis of relapsing fever *Borrelia* spp. *Int. J. Syst. Bacteriol.* **46:**859–865.

186. **Rawlings, J. A.** 1995. An overview of tick-borne relapsing fever with emphasis on outbreaks in Texas. *Tex. Med.* **91:**56–59.

187. **Remick, D. G., Y. Negussie, D. Fekade, and G. Griffin.** 1996. Pentoxifylline fails to prevent the Jarisch-Herxheimer reaction or associated cytokine release. *J. Infect. Dis.* **174:**627–630.

188. **Restrepo, B. I., and A. G. Barbour.** 1994. Antigen diversity in the bacterium B. hermsii through "somatic" mutations in rearranged vmp genes. *Cell* **78:**867–876.

189. **Restrepo, B. I., C. J. Carter, and A. G. Barbour.** 1994. Activation of a vmp pseudogene in Borrelia hermsii: an alternate mechanism of antigenic variation during relapsing fever. *Mol. Microbiol.* **13:**287–299.

190. **Restrepo, B. I., T. Kitten, C. J. Carter, D. Infante, and A. G. Barbour.** 1992. Subtelomeric expression regions of Borrelia hermsii linear plasmids are highly polymorphic. *Mol. Microbiol.* **6:**3299–3311.

191. **Rich, S. M., P. M. Armstrong, R. D. Smith, and S. R. Telford III.** 2001. Lone star tick-infecting borreliae are most closely related to the agent of bovine borreliosis. *J. Clin. Microbiol.* **39:**494–497.

192. **Rich, S. M., S. A. Sawyer, and A. G. Barbour.** 2001. Antigen polymorphism in Borrelia hermsii, a clonal pathogenic bacterium. *Proc. Natl. Acad. Sci. USA* **98:**15038–15043.

193. **Russell, H.** 1936. Observations on immunity in relapsing fever and trypanosomiasis. *Trans. R. Soc. Trop. Med. Hyg.* **30:**179–190.

194. Sadziene, A., M. Jonsson, S. Bergstrom, R. K. Bright, R. C. Kennedy, and A. G. Barbour. 1994. A bactericidal antibody to *Borrelia burgdorferi* is directed against a variable region of the OspB protein. *Infect. Immun.* **62:**2037–2045.

195. Salih, S., D. Mustafa, S. Abdel-Wahab, M. Ahmed, and A. Omer. 1977. Louse-borne relapsing fever. I. A clinical and laboratory study of 363 cases in the Sudan. *Trans. R. Soc. Trop. Med. Hyg.* **71:**43–48.

196. Schmidtmann, E. T., R. B. Bushnell, E. C. Loomis, M. N. Oliver, and J. H. Theis. 1976. Experimental and epizootiologic evidence associating Ornithodoros coriaceus (Acari: Agrasidae) with the exposure of cattle to epizootic bovine abortion in California. *J. Med. Entomol.* **13:**292–299.

197. Schuhardt, V., and E. Hemphill. 1946. Brain involvement as a possible cause of relapse after treatment in spirochaetal relapsing fever. *Science* **103:**422–423.

198. Schuhardt, V. T., and M. Wilkerson. 1951. Relapse phenomena in rats infected with single spirochetes (*Borrelia recurrenis* var. *turicatae*). *J. Bacteriol.* **62:**215–219.

199. Schwan, T. G., J. M. Battisti, S. F. Porcella, S. J. Raffel, M. E. Schrumpf, E. R. Fischer, J. A. Carroll, P. E. Stewart, P. Rosa, and G. A. Somerville. 2003. Glycerol-3-phosphate acquisition in spirochetes: distribution and biological activity of glycerophosphodiester phosphodiesterase (GlpQ) among *Borrelia* species. *J. Bacteriol.* **185:**1346–1356.

200. Schwan, T. G., and B. J. Hinnebusch. 1998. Bloodstream-versus tick-associated variants of a relapsing fever bacterium. *Science* **280:**1938–1940.

201. Schwan, T. G., P. F. Policastro, Z. Miller, R. L. Thompson, T. Damrow, and J. E. Keirans. 2003. Tick-borne relapsing fever caused by Borrelia hermsii, Montana. *Emerg. Infect. Dis.* **9:**1151–1154.

202. Schwan, T. G., M. E. Schrumpf, B. J. Hinnebusch, D. E. Anderson, Jr., and M. E. Konkel. 1996. GlpQ: an antigen for serological discrimination between relapsing fever and Lyme borreliosis. *J. Clin. Microbiol.* **34:**2483–2492.

203. Sciotto, C. G., B. A. Lauer, W. L. White, and G. R. Istre. 1983. Detection of Borrelia in acridine orange-stained blood smears by fluorescence microscopy. *Arch. Pathol. Lab. Med.* **107:**384–386.

204. Scoles, G. A., M. Papero, L. Beati, and D. Fish. 2001. A relapsing fever group spirochete transmitted by Ixodes scapularis ticks. *Vector Borne Zoonotic Dis.* **1:**21–34.

205. Scragg, I. G., D. Kwiatkowski, V. Vidal, A. Reason, T. Paxton, M. Panico, A. Dell, and H. Morris. 2000. Structural characterization of the inflammatory moiety of a variable major lipoprotein of Borrelia recurrentis. *J. Biol. Chem.* **275:**937–941.

206. Seboxa, T., and S. I. Rahlenbeck. 1995. Treatment of louse-borne relapsing fever with low dose penicillin or tetracycline: a clinical trial. *Scand. J. Infect. Dis.* **27:**29–31.

207. Shamaei-Tousi, A., M. J. Burns, J. L. Benach, M. B. Furie, E. I. Gergel, and S. Bergstrom. 2000. The relapsing fever spirochaete, Borrelia crocidurae, activates human endothelial cells and promotes the transendothelial migration of neutrophils. *Cell. Microbiol.* **2:**591–599.

208. Shamaei-Tousi, A., O. Collin, A. Bergh, and S. Bergstrom. 2001. Testicular damage by microcirculatory disruption and colonization of an immune-privileged site during *Borrelia crocidurae* infection. *J. Exp. Med.* **193:**995–1004.

209. Shamaei-Tousi, A., P. Martin, A. Bergh, N. Burman, T. Brännström, and S. Bergström. 1999. Erythrocyte-aggregating relapsing fever spirochete Borrelia crocidurae induces formation of microemboli. *J. Infect. Dis.* **180:**1929–1938.

210. Shanbaky, N. M., and N. Helmy. 2000. First record of natural infection with Borrelia in Ornithodoros (Ornithodoros)

savignyi. Reservoir potential and specificity of the tick to Borrelia. *J. Egypt Soc. Parasitol.* **30:**765–780.

211. Sharma, S. P., W. Amanfu, and T. C. Losho. 2000. Bovine borreliosis in Botswana. *Onderstepoort J. Vet. Res.* **67:**221–223.

212. Smith, R. D., J. Brener, M. Osorno, and M. Ristic. 1978. Pathobiology of Borrelia theileri in the tropical cattle tick, Boophilus microplus. *J. Invertebr. Pathol.* **32:**182–190.

213. Southern, P., and J. Sanford. 1969. Relapsing fever. A clinical and microbiological review. *Medicine* **48:**129–149.

214. Stoenner, H. G. 1974. Biology of Borrelia hermsii in Kelly medium. *Appl. Microbiol.* **28:**540–543.

215. Stoenner, H. G., T. Dodd, and C. Larsen. 1982. Antigenic variation of Borrelia hermsii. *J. Exp. Med.* **156:**1297–1311.

216. Sundnes, K., and A. Haimanot. 1993. Epidemic of louse-borne relapsing fever in Ethiopia. *Lancet* **342:**1213.

217. Tabuchi, N., H. Mitani, S. Seino, and M. Fukunaga. 2002. The 44-kb linear plasmid molecule in the relapsing fever agent Borrelia duttonii strain Ly serve as a preservation of vmp genes. *Microbiol. Immunol.* **46:**159–165.

218. Takahashi, Y., S. J. Cutler, and M. Fukunaga. 2000. Size conversion of a linear plasmid in the relapsing fever agent Borrelia duttonii. *Microbiol. Immunol.* **44:**1071–1074.

219. Takayama, K., R. J. Rothenberg, and A. G. Barbour. 1987. Absence of lipopolysaccharide in the Lyme disease spirochete, Borrelia burgdorferi. *Infect. Immun.* **55:**2311–2313.

220. Thomas, N. J., J. Bunikis, A. G. Barbour, and M. J. Wolcott. 2002. Fatal spirochetosis due to a relapsing fever-like Borrelia sp. in a northern spotted owl. *J. Wildl. Dis.* **38:**187–193.

221. Thompson, R. S., W. Burgdorfer, R. Russell, and B. J. Francis. 1969. Outbreak of tick-borne relapsing fever in Spokane County, Washington. *JAMA* **210:**1045–1050.

222. Trape, J. F., J. M. Duplantier, H. Bouganali, B. Godeluck, F. Legros, J. P. Cornet, and J. L. Camicas. 1991. Tick-borne borreliosis in west Africa. *Lancet* **337:**473–475.

223. Trape, J. F., B. Godeluck, G. Diatta, C. Rogier, F. Legros, J. Albergel, Y. Pepin, and J. M. Duplantier. 1996. The spread of tick-borne borreliosis in West Africa and its relationship to sub-Saharan drought. *Am. J. Trop. Med. Hyg.* **54:**289–293.

224. van Holten, J., J. Tiems, and V. H. Jongen. 1997. Neonatal Borrelia duttoni infection: a report of three cases. *Trop. Doct.* **27:**115–116.

225. Varma, M. G. R. 1956. Infections of *Ornithodoros* ticks with relapsing fever spirochaetes, and the mechanisms of their transmission. *Ann. Trop. Med. Parasitol.* **50:**18–31.

226. Vidal, V., S. Cutler, I. G. Scragg, D. J. Wright, and D. Kwiatkowski. 2002. Characterisation of silent and active genes for a variable large protein of Borrelia recurrentis. *BMC Infect. Dis.* **2:**25.

227. Vidal, V., I. G. Scragg, S. J. Cutler, K. A. Rockett, D. Fekade, D. A. Warrell, D. J. Wright, and D. Kwiatkowski. 1998. Variable major lipoprotein is a principal TNF-inducing factor of louse-borne relapsing fever. *Nat. Med.* **4:**1416–1420.

228. Walker, T., M. G. Luna, J. Bunikis, and A. G. Barbour. Tick-borne relapsing fever in the eastern Sierra mountains. Submitted for publication.

229. Warrell, D. A., P. L. Perine, D. W. Krause, D. H. Bing, and S. J. MacDougal. 1983. Pathophysiology and immunology of the Jarisch-Herxheimer-like reaction in louse-borne relapsing fever: comparison of tetracycline and slow- release penicillin. *J. Infect. Dis.* **147:**898–909.

230. Webster, G., J. D. Schiffman, A. S. Dosanjh, M. R. Amieva, H. A. Gans, and T. C. Sectish. 2002. Jarisch-Herxheimer reaction associated with ciprofloxacin administration for tick-borne relapsing fever. *Pediatr. Infect. Dis. J.* **21:**571–573.

231. Wengrower, D., H. Knobler, S. Gillis, and T. Chajek-Shaul. 1984. Myocarditis in tick-borne relapsing fever. *J. Infect. Dis.* **149:**1033.

232. Wheeler, C., W. Herms, and K. Meyer. 1935. A new tick vector of relapsing fever in California. *Proc. Soc. Exp. Biol. Med.* **32:**1290–1292.

233. Wood, R. C., and K. C. Dixon. 1945. Tick-borne relapsing fever in Cyprus. *Br. Med. J.* **2:**526–528.

234. World Health Organization. 2001. *WHO Model Prescribing Information. Drugs Used in Bacterial Infections.* World Health Organization, Geneva, Switzerland.

235. Yagupsky, P., and S. Moses. 1985. Neonatal Borrelia species infection (relapsing fever). *Am. J. Dis. Child.* **139:**74–76.

236. Zaher, M. A., Z. R. Soliman, and F. M. Diab. 1977. An experimental study of Borrelia anserina in four species of Argas ticks. 2. Transstadial survival and transovarial transmission. *Z. Parasitenkd.* **53:**213–223.

237. Zarafonetis, C. J. D., H. S. Ingraham, and J. F. Berrry. 1946. Weil-Felix and typhus complementation fixation tests, with special reference to *B. proteus* OX-K agglutination. *J. Immunol.* **52:**189–199.

238. Zhang, J. R., J. M. Hardham, A. G. Barbour, and S. J. Norris. 1997. Antigenic variation in Lyme disease borreliae by promiscuous recombination of VMP-like sequence cassettes. *Cell* **89:**275–285.

239. Zhong, J., and A. G. Barbour. 2004. Cross-species hybridization of a Borrelia burgdorferi DNA array reveals infection- and culture associated genes of the unsequenced genome of the relapsing fever agent Borrelia hermsii. *Mol. Microbiol.* **51:**729–748.

240. Zückert, W. R., T. A. Kerentseva, C. L. Lawson, and A. G. Barbour. 2001. Structural conservation of neurotropism-associated VspA within the variable Borrelia Vsp-OspC lipoprotein family. *J. Biol. Chem.* **276:**457–463.

241. Zückert, W. R., J. E. Lloyd, P. E. Stewart, P. A. Rosa, and A. G. Barbour. 2004. Cross-species surface display of functional spirochetal lipoproteins by recombinant *Borrelia burgdorferi. Infect. Immun.* **72:**1463–1469.

Chapter 17

Rocky Mountain Spotted Fever and Other Spotted Fever Group Rickettsioses

KEVIN R. MACALUSO AND ABDU F. AZAD

INTRODUCTION

Rickettsioses, caused by members of the typhus group and spotted fever group (SFG) rickettsiae, are significant, underrecognized diseases found worldwide. Currently, nine different SFG rickettsiae are recognized in the Western hemisphere. However, only four species, *Rickettsia akari*, *Rickettsia parkeri*, *Rickettsia rickettsii*, and *Rickettsia felis*, are known to cause human disease. While the last of these four is the causative agent of a flea-borne typhus-like rickettsiosis (22) that has only recently been described (7), *R. akari*, *R. parkeri*, and *R. rickettsii* are transmitted by arachnids (mites and ticks).

Rickettsialpox, the disease in humans associated with *R. akari* infection, was first described in New York City in 1946 (47). Since its original description, the distribution of rickettsialpox has been broadened to a number of cities in the northeastern United States, including Boston, Cleveland, Philadelphia, Pittsburgh, and West Hartford, and more recently the southeastern United States (28). The clinical and epidemiological characteristics of rickettsialpox, including the enzootic cycle of *R. akari* between the reservoir house mouse (*Mus musculus*) and the vector house mouse mite (*Liponyssoides sanguineus*), were described within months of the discovery (39).

Although human rickettsiosis associated with *R. parkeri* has only recently been described in the literature (39a), this rickettsia was recognized to cause a mild febrile illness in guinea pigs at the time of its discovery in 1939 (39b). *R. parkeri*, like *R. rickettsii*, is a New World, tick-borne member of the SFG; however, based on preliminary information, the disease that it causes in humans (Color Plate 14D to F) appears more similar to infections caused by eschar-associated, Old World rickettsiae, including *Rickettsia conorii* and *Rickettsia africae*. To date, *R. parkeri* has been detected in *Amblyomma* ticks from Alabama, Georgia, Kentucky, Mississippi, and Texas. *R. parkeri* was first isolated from *Amblyomma maculatum*, but recently *Amblyomma americanum* ticks have also been shown to be a competent vector of this rickettsia in laboratory studies (16a). The parameters of *R. parkeri* maintenance and transmission in nature are yet to be clearly defined.

While the history of *R. akari* and *R. parkeri* infection in the United States is relatively recent, *R. rickettsii*, the etiological agent of Rocky Mountain spotted fever (RMSF), has a long and very interesting history in the United States. The identification of *R. rickettsii* and demonstration of its relationship with ixodid ticks have fascinated researchers worldwide and have led to the identification of other tick-borne rickettsiae. Consequently, there are several other, more-prevalent, species of SFG rickettsiae in North America in a variety of tick vectors that are not associated with human disease (Table 1). With the ongoing characterization of the relationship between rickettsiae and the tick vector, the effect of the presence of these nonpathogenic rickettsiae on the ecology and distribution of *R. rickettsii* is the focus of research in a number of laboratories.

RMSF was first described in the 1890s, and researchers have worked to characterize its manifestations, develop effective therapeutics, examine the biological aspects of the agent, and in particular to understand its survival and multiplication within its arthropod host. A historical account of the disease, including the stories of the principal investigators who pioneered the field of rickettsiology, has recently been published in an excellent book by Robert Philip (40). Because this chapter deals primarily with human health and tick-borne SFG rickettsiae described in North, Central, and South America, the majority of the content will be in reference to *R. rickettsii*. Information concerning the other SFG rickettsiae that are

Kevin R. Macaluso • Department of Pathobiological Sciences, School of Veterinary Medicine, Louisiana State University, Baton Rouge, LA 70803. **Abdu F. Azad** • Department of Microbiology and Immunology, School of Medicine, University of Maryland, Baltimore, MD 21201.

Table 1. Spotted fever group *Rickettsia* species, arthropod vector, and distribution described in the United States

Species	Vector	Distribution in United States
R. rickettsii	*D. andersoni, D. variabilis*	Widespread
R. montanensis	*D. andersoni*	Montana, Virginia, Ohio
	D. variabilis	Massachusetts, Connecticut, North Carolina, South Carolina, New York
R. parkeri	*A. americanum, Amblyomma maculatum*	Alabama, Texas, Georgia, Mississippi, Kentucky
R. peacockii	*D. andersoni*	Montana, Colorado
R. rhipicephali	*R. sanguineus, D. andersoni, D. variabilis, D. occidentalis*	Mississippi, Texas, North Carolina, South Carolina, Montana, California
R. bellii	*D. variabilis*	Widespread
R. canadensis	*H. leporispalustris*	Montana
R. akari	*L. sanguineus*	New York and other large metropolitan centers
R. felis[a]	*Ctenocephalides felis*	Texas, California

[a] *R. felis* is a flea-borne *Rickettsia* member of the SFG (7, 22).

known or suspected to cause human disease in other regions of the world will be addressed in a separate chapter. Furthermore, because a number of excellent reviews have been published regarding the biology of *Rickettsia* (18, 32), the various aspects of RMSF, including issues of ecology (45, 49) and clinical characteristics (52), this chapter aims to expand on that base of knowledge and update the reader on the current trends of research on tick-borne rickettsioses.

ETIOLOGICAL AGENT AND DEVELOPMENT WITHIN THE TICK HOST

While this chapter focuses on tick transmission of *R. rickettsii*, a brief overview of rickettsiae should be included. Rickettsiae are gram-negative obligate intracellular microorganisms that belong to the α-subdivision of the *Proteobacteria*. Several other medically important genera are included in this subdivision, including *Orientia, Anaplasma,* and *Ehrlichia* (13). Structurally, rickettsiae are coccobacilli, (rod-shaped) bacteria that average 0.7 to 2.0 μm by 0.3 to 0.5 μm in size (Fig. 1). The trilaminar cell wall of rickettsiae is surrounded by a translucent zone that has been termed the slime layer. Although the specific function of this layer is not known, physical changes have been observed during tick feeding, linking it to a role in transmission. Furthermore, tick feeding results in growth of the slime layer, which has been attributed to virulence. The morphological changes that take place are considered to be induced during tick feeding and are called reactivation (19). Due to their obligate intracellular lifestyle, rickettsiae invade a number of cell types. However, the cells that are targeted for infection depend on both the host and the rickettsiae. In humans, the organisms preferentially infect endothe-

lial cells. By a mechanism yet unknown, SFG rickettsiae enter host cells via receptor-mediated endocytosis and escape from the endosome prior to the formation of an endolysosome (34). Although documented to invade the nucleus, they primarily reside and replicate freely in the cytoplasm of the host cell. Utilizing host-derived molecules, rickettsiae synthesize actin tails (Color Plate 12) to facilitate movement and propel themselves from one cell to the next (21). Recently, genomes for both typhus and SFG rickettsiae have been sequenced (1, 37). While an efficient system of genetic manipulation is lacking for rickettsiae (53), complementation studies have been used to assign function to a number of rickettsial genes including *groESL* (41), *invA* (16), and *lepB* (42). The identification and characterization of virulence factors will aid in our understanding of the disease associated with rickettsial infection.

With the exception of *R. felis*, SFG rickettsiae are associated with mites and ticks, which serve as the vectors and reservoirs for the agent (2). Within the tick, *R. rickettsii* systematically infects all organs including the salivary glands, midgut, and ovary tissues (34). The infection of the ovaries is critical because it allows the rickettsiae to invade developing tick oocytes and thus be maintained in the developing egg. This process of passing an infectious agent from adult to the progeny is termed transovarial transmission. Rickettsiae are then found to infect each subsequent life stage: larval, nymphal, and adult, via transstadial transmission (32). This intimate relationship between the bacteria and vector has evolved into a mechanism of maintenance that ensures rickettsial survival, even in the absence of a vertebrate host.

In the United States, most genera of ixodid ticks have been associated with rickettsial infection. While *A. americanum, Haemaphysalis leporispalustris,* and

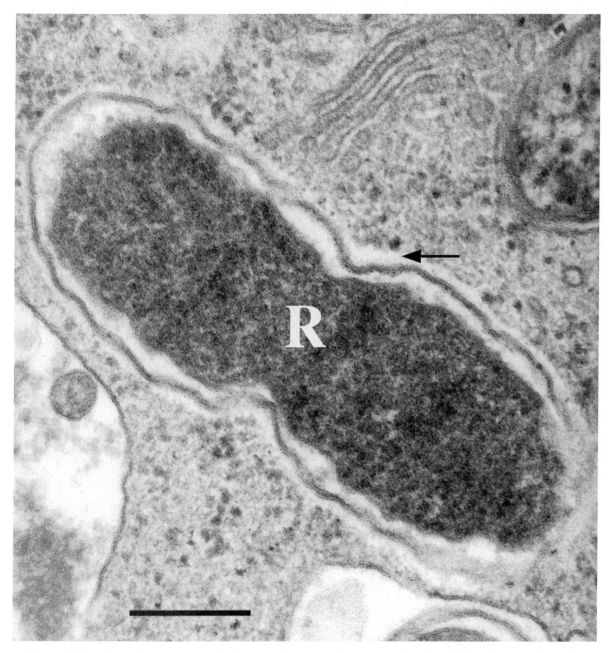

Figure 1. Transmission electron micrograph of *R. peacockii* strain DaE100R (R) within the cytoplasm of DAE100 (*D. andersoni* embryonic cell line) host cell. The arrow identifies the translucent zone that has been termed the slime layer. Bar, 0.2 μm. Image courtesy of A. T. Palmer and T. J. Kurtti.

Dermacentor parumapertus have been implicated as vectors of *R. rickettsii*, only two ticks, *Dermacentor andersoni* and *Dermacentor variabilis* (Color Plate 1B), are considered the primary vectors of *R. rickettsii*. The other SFG rickettsiae have also been documented in these two species of *Dermacentor* (4), as well as *Dermacentor occidentalis*, *Ixodes pacificus*, *Ixodes brunneus*, *Ixodes cookei*, *Ixodes dentatus*, *Ixodes scapularis*, *Ixodes texanus*, and *Rhipicephalus sanguineus* (reviewed in reference 45).

The interaction of SFG rickettsiae with their tick host, resulting in successful propagation of the rickettsiae, continues to be the focus of research interests. Initial studies identified an increased incidence of RMSF in the western portion of the Bitter Root Valley, Montana, compared to the eastern half of the valley. Examination of the rickettsiae present in ticks on both sides of the valley revealed a similar but antigenically different rickettsial organism on the eastern side, compared to the *R. rickettsii* identified on the western side of the valley (10). The lower level of occurrence of RMSF was correlated with the presence of the different rickettsiae, which were then grouped under the term east side agent. These studies characterized the organism as a nonpathogenic rickettsia whose growth is restricted to the ovaries of the tick *D. andersoni* (10). Furthermore, it was shown that ticks infected with this nonpathogenic organism were able to acquire *R. rickettsii* from a rickettsemic animal and maintain the infection transstadially but not transovarially. It was also demonstrated that the *D. andersoni* originally infected with *R. rickettsii* and subsequently exposed to the east side agent favored transovarial transmission of the nonpathogenic east side agent. These studies aided in explaining the distribution of RMSF in the valley, as well as offering a feasible explanation for the current relatively low prevalence of RMSF in the Rocky Mountain area, which corresponds to the distribution of *D. andersoni*. Molecular characterization of the rickettsia in ticks (35) and successful identification of the east side agent resulted in the description of a novel species now called *R. peacockii* (48).

The ability of the nonpathogenic *R. peacockii* to inhibit transmission of the pathogenic *R. rickettsii* has been termed transovarial transmission interference. In the same studies, it was reported that two other nonpathogenic rickettsiae, *Rickettsia montanensis* and *Rickettsia rhipicephali*, were also able to prevent transmission of pathogenic *R. rickettsii* via transovarial transmission (8). While this interference was suspected to be related to the pathogenic and nonpathogenic nature of the rickettsiae, recent studies have illustrated that this interference will occur independently of the pathogenicity of the rickettsiae. It has been demonstrated that *R. montanensis* and *R. rhipicephali* were able to block the transovarial transmission of each other in a tick reciprocal challenge model (30). The mechanism(s) that facilitates the inhibition of dual infection remains unknown but is the focus of intense research (31, 33). It is hypothesized that regulation of the molecules utilized by rickettsiae for attachment, invasion, and/or survival in the ovaries during the primary infection render the ovaries unavailable for the secondary infection. Similar interference actions between closely related organisms have been reported for other bacteria in the arthropod (12).

While it does appear that a number of species of rickettsia are capable of infecting one species of tick, the relationship between the tick and rickettsiae is also not as indiscriminant as field infection surveys might imply. Whether this is a stable (transovarially maintained) infection or more of a transient one is not clear. Furthermore, there is evidence of rickettsia-tick primary host relationships. Laboratory studies have explored the fitness cost to ticks that maintain rick-

ettsiae. Initial studies utilizing *R. rickettsii* (Sawtooth strain) reported that ticks were capable of maintaining the rickettsiae through 12 generations via transovarial transmission alone (9). However, in this study it was also noticed that the viability of feeding ticks and eventual reproductive success appeared to diminish by the fifth filarial generation. Subsequent studies using highly pathogenic strains of *R. rickettsii* (e.g., Sawtooth and Como-96) clearly illustrated an adverse effect on *D. andersoni* when maintained transovarially (36). Similarly, *D. andersoni* naturally infected with either *R. montanensis* (M/5-6) or *R. rhipicephali* also had decreased fecundity and were unable to pass either rickettsiae to their progeny. However, when *D. variabilis* were exposed to either of these two rickettsiae in a laboratory setting, no differences in engorgement weight, time to onset of oviposition, or egg clutch size were observed during the first or second generation of infected ticks (29). The differences in the observations could be due to strain variations in each rickettsial species. Although unexamined, strain variation is likely the direct result of the culture or passage history of each laboratory strain used, as seen with other tick-borne bacteria (i.e., *Borrelia*). Interestingly, *D. variabilis*, ticks most commonly associated with *R. montanensis*, were unable to maintain an infection with *R. rhipicephali* through two generations (30).

ECOLOGY

Although humans serve only as an accidental host, the role of small mammals in the maintenance cycle of SFG rickettsiae must not be overlooked (reviewed in reference 49). Both lagomorphs and rodents are suspected of serving as potential reservoirs of *R. rickettsii*. However, only a few mammals, including golden-mantled ground squirrels (*Spermophilus lateralis*), meadow voles (*Microtus pennsylvanicus*), chipmunks (e.g., *Eutamias amoenus*), and snowshoe hares (*Lepus americanus*), from which *R. rickettsii* has been isolated are capable of maintaining rickettsemias at levels high enough to infect ticks under laboratory conditions (reviewed in reference 45). While the tick is capable of maintaining the rickettsial infection via transovarial transmission, a mammalian host is the sole means for the transmission of rickettsiae from one tick to another. *Rickettsia*-infected immature ticks that feed on small mammals create a pool of infected mammalian hosts that serve as reservoirs for uninfected ticks to feed upon (20). Although it appears that the rickettsial infection in these small mammals is fleeting (<8 days), the combination of rickettsial infection, heavy tick burden, and relatively small home range of most small mammals allows for the development of a focus of hyperinfection in a tick population. Thus, these small mammals serve as the amplifying hosts, spreading infection within the tick population, while the tick serves as the long-term reservoir host. Additionally, the newly infected nymphal ticks maintain the infection after their molt. The increase in adult *Rickettsia*-infected ticks that feed on large mammals, including humans, also facilitates the development of foci of infection and the spread of RMSF.

While some species of rickettsia, e.g., *Rickettsia prowazekii*, the etiological agent of louse-borne typhus, is spread to a host when a rickettsia-infected blood meal is passed through in the form of fecal material and subsequently rubbed into abrasions in the host skin, it is generally thought that ticks transmit rickettsia to humans via feeding. Ticks transmit rickettsiae in the saliva, which is deposited through the mouthparts into the host during tick feeding. *Rickettsia*, like many other arthropod-borne disease agents, is believed to take advantage of the tick's ability to modulate the host's immune response at the tick feeding site. Although not specifically examined in rickettsiae, transmission during the relatively long feeding period of ticks likely facilitates rickettsial establishment in the host at an immunologically privileged site (55).

EPIDEMIOLOGY

Due to the intimate relationship between rickettsiae and their tick hosts, the distribution of rickettsiae is limited solely to the geographic distribution of these arthropod hosts. While the various members of the SFG are present throughout the United States, for epidemiological purposes only *R. rickettsii* will be discussed. Indeed, the incidence of RMSF reported has varied over the last 60 years (Fig. 2). Within the second half of this period, the incidence rate has increased much more rapidly and has been steadily higher than during the first half. However, fluctuations in prevalence are still observed. A sharp increase

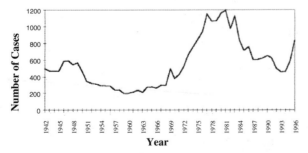

Figure 2. RMSF cases reported to the CDC from 1942 to 1996. (Image from http://www.cdc.gov/ncidod/dvrd/rmsf/Epidemiology.htm.)

in the 1970s was sustained for nearly 2 decades before the number of reported cases began to decline in the late 1980s. Since the early 1990s, an increase in incidence has again been observed. While the increase could be attributed to better and/or more vigilant reporting of disease to the Centers for Disease Control and Prevention (CDC), an increase in cases may also likely be due to the increased establishment of humans in suburban areas that are endemic foci for zoonotic diseases (17).

RMSF was originally described in the western United States, with the focus of the seminal research in Montana. However, in the last 100 years there has been a clearly evident shift in the distribution of cases from the western to the eastern portion of the United States (2), with the occurrence of RMSF currently highest in the south-Atlantic region (Fig. 3). In fact, according to CDC reports, approximately 77% of the reported cases between 1994 and 1998 were observed in the southern and southeastern regions of the United States (www.cdc.gov). In these regions, the states North Carolina, Tennessee, Georgia, and South Carolina account for some 42% of the cases of RMSF in the entire United States. Outside these regions, Oklahoma has the second-highest number of reported cases, accounting for approximately 8% of the national total.

Aside from the geographical distribution of RMSF in the United States, which results in an increased risk of infection based on location, other factors have been associated with infection. A higher incidence of infection is observed in males, Caucasians, and children (51). In the United States, the spring and summer seasons (April through September) are the primary months in which there is an increased incidence of RMSF (Fig. 4). Although not shown in Fig. 4, there is evidence that infection peaks earlier (May to June) in northern areas, but somewhat later (June to July) in the southern areas. The differences in peak incidence of RMSF correlated with the cooler and warmer temperatures associated with the northern and southern regions, respectively (25). The seasonal pattern of RMSF cases is correlated to the seasonal activity of the adult *Dermacentor* tick, which is the only life stage that feeds on humans and appears to be correlated with the tick's response to changing day length (diapause). In the northernmost part of its geographic range, the immature tick feeds in late spring or early summer. Consequently, adult ticks emerging following the nymphal blood meal diapause over fall and winter in response to declining photoperiod and air temperature. They reemerge the following spring to seek hosts and transmit infection. In the southern parts of the tick's range, immature ticks feed and molt in early spring. In this region, adult ticks emerge in late spring

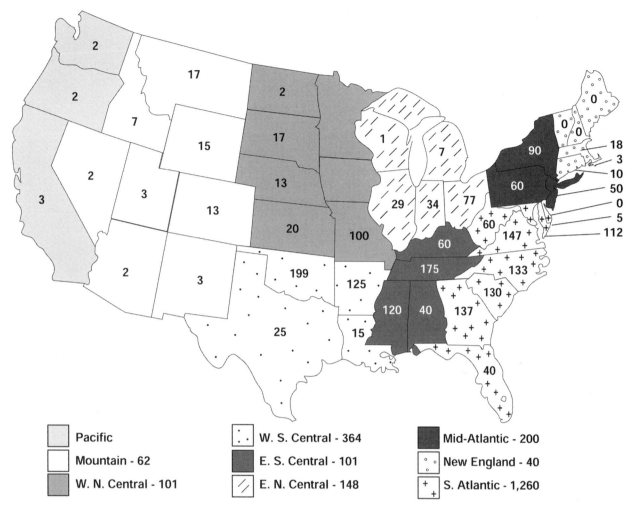

Figure 3. Regional distribution of reported RMSF as determined by cases reported to the CDC by individual states from 1994 to 1998. (Image redrawn from http://www.cdc.gov/ncidod/dvrd/rmsf/Epidemiology.htm.)

and commence host-seeking activity in response to longer day length and increasing photoperiod, delaying disease transmission to early summer or midsummer. Transmission of *R. rickettsii* to humans is almost

solely due to the bite of an infected tick. However, direct contact with infected blood (54) and aerosol inoculation (3) are also potential means of infection.

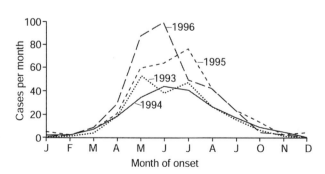

Figure 4. Seasonal distribution of RMSF cases reported to the CDC during each month for the years 1993 to 1996. (Image redrawn from http://www.cdc.gov/ncidod/dvrd/rmsf/Epidemiology. htm.)

CLINICAL FEATURES OF RMSF

In mammals, *R. rickettsii* infection results in fever, typically associated with a rash, which has been designated by many different names, depending on the locale. For example, disease associated with *R. rickettsii* infection is called Brazilian spotted fever or fiebre maculosa in Brazil, fiebre manchada in Mexico, and Tobia fever in Colombia (reviewed in reference 15). While there are many names for the disease associated with *R. rickettsii* infection, it is only this species that has been associated with spotted fever in the Western hemisphere. Human infection with *R. akari* has also been documented in the United States, primarily in the northeast; however, this is a self-limited illness that has manifestations more characteristic of a viral infection than of RMSF.

While the classical triad of findings for RMSF include fever, rash, and a history of tick bite, one or more of these may not be evident when a patient initially seeks medical attention. Rather, early presentation is nonspecific and may resemble a viral infection (26). Human infection with *R. rickettsii* initially results in fever and sometimes chills, headache, and myalgia. Also, gastrointestinal symptoms including nausea, vomiting, abdominal pain, and lack of appetite may develop early in some patients, especially children. The majority (~90%) of patients will develop a skin rash during infection (Color Plate 11A and C). The rash will begin as a macropapular eruption on the ankles and wrists, which spreads to cover the entire body. However, the rash is not always evident until later in the course of the illness. For a thorough description of the classical manifestations of RMSF, as well as some of the abnormal manifestations observed during infection, the reader is referred to Walker and Lane (52).

In addition to the flu-like symptoms described above, a person infected with *R. rickettsii* may also develop neurological problems, as well as muscle (skeletal and heart) and organ (kidney, gastrointestinal, lung, and liver) injury (52). Severe cases of advanced rickettsial infections can also result in acute renal failure (11), pulmonary infiltrates and edema (Color Plate 11B and F), and gangrene (27). Loss of fingers or toes due to injury to the peripheral circulatory system has been reported among some survivors of severe RMSF in which irreversible skin and tissue damage had occurred (27). A major complication in some cases is DIC (disseminated intravascular coagulopathy), which can lead to cardiac arrest or stroke, in addition to the other complications noted above. Finally, rickettsial meningoencephalitis (23) and neurological damage (Color Plate 11G to I) have been identified in infected patients, resulting in long-term impairment (6).

PATHOLOGY

Although the mechanisms are not well defined, rickettsia-induced vascular injury occurs after *R. rickettsii* invades endothelial cells within the human host. The vasculitis (Color Plate 11C, E, G, and H) results in increased vascular permeability with movement of fluid to the interstitium and a secondary host cellular response (Color Plate 11D) (46). Subsequently, a generalized lymphohistiocytic vasculitis will occur involving most organs of the body. Within the skin, lymphohistiocytic small-vessel vasculitis progresses to leukocytoclastic vasculitis and is considered a form of septic vasculitis (24).

DIAGNOSIS

Because rickettsial infections are similar to nonspecific viral infections, they are often overlooked or misdiagnosed. Due to this nature of the disease, antibiotic treatment should start prior to a definitive diagnosis (see Chapter 5). Laboratory diagnosis of rickettsial infection has progressed dramatically in the last 10 years. It is now standard practice to use molecular techniques to characterize the rickettsial infection in the patient, as well as in the tick vector. In addition to PCR-based analysis, several antigen-based detection systems have been developed for efficient, cost-effective rickettsial diagnosis (reviewed in reference 26). Depending on the rationale for rickettsial identification (disease confirmation or field infection surveys), different applications can be utilized.

If the objective is primarily to confirm or identify *R. rickettsii* infection in a patient, serological assays are typically preferred. The most commonly used assay is the indirect immunofluorescence assay (IFA). Rickettsial antigen slides are prepared and used as a target for screening host serum for antibodies specific for rickettsiae. It is preferable that both acute and convalescent serum samples be taken from the patient, as a rise in antibody titer, specific for rickettsiae, is correlated with recent rickettsial infection (51). Antigen slides are typically prepared in diagnostic laboratories, and variations using several species-specific antigens on one slide are commercially available. Limitations to the IFA assay include the fact that patients who present early in the infectious process (e.g., within 2 weeks of onset) have not produced detectable levels of antibodies at the time of the first visit. In addition, because antibody production to rickettsiae may persist long after an initial infection, positive IFA results may provide a false-positive result for a current presentation (26).

Another technique used to diagnose rickettsial infection is immunostaining. Immunohistochemical localization of SFG rickettsial antigens in various tissues can be visualized by an immunoalkaline phosphatase stain with naphthol phosphate-fast red substrate and hematoxylin counterstaining. This technique can be used with skin biopsies of the patient's rash prior to antibiotic treatment, as well as on tissue sections obtained postmortem. While this method can detect infection earlier than serologic assays, limitations to this assay include its sensitivity and specificity (38).

If the objective is to characterize the organism, then culture is the best, most-thorough technique for definitive identification. Several techniques for the isolation of rickettsiae in chicken egg yolk sac and mammalian and tick cell lines have been well described previously (32). While culture allows isolation of the disease-causing agent, additional serologic and molecular assays must be carried out to actually identify the specific *Rickettsia*. Because culturing is a two-step process and very time-consuming, it is not a practical diagnostic method. Great caution must also be used when handling all rickettsiae, due to their ability to be aerosolized.

PCR-based techniques have greatly facilitated the diagnosis of human infections, the assessment of the prevalence of the pathogen in ticks, and, as a result, our understanding of the distribution and variation of different rickettsiae in the United States (14) and abroad. The standard protocol for identification with the PCR-based technique is to amplify a hypervariable portion of the gene that encodes the SFG-specific outer membrane protein A (43). By use of a combination of PCR and restriction fragment length polymorphism analysis, all but two species of rickettsiae can be differentiated (44). Unique banding patterns are a result of enzymatic digestion of the PCR amplicon, which allows for rapid and accurate identification of the infecting species. Additionally, most described species have this portion of their gene on the database, and so further sequence analysis and comparison allow for definitive identification. Several templates have proven successful with these techniques, including tick (all life stages), animal tissue, and animal sera. Interestingly, a multiplex real-time PCR field application is currently being developed that will allow for specific rickettsial identification in the field without the requirement of RFLP or sequencing (26).

TREATMENT AND PREVENTION

As described above, serologic diagnosis is unreliable early in infection, when most patients present clinically. In addition, although immunohistochemical or PCR studies of skin biopsies (and, in the case of PCR, possibly blood) may be more sensitive early in infection, they may not be readily available, the results may take time to obtain, and the methods are not sufficiently sensitive to rule out the diagnosis. Patients treated early in the course of the disease (e.g., within 4 days of disease onset) generally do well, with mortality rates of <5%. In contrast, patients for whom the diagnosis is not suspected and in whom treatment is delayed frequently have or develop organ impairment and tend to experience much greater morbidity and mortality. For these reasons, RMSF must be considered in patients with an otherwise unexplained illness that is clinically consistent (e.g., acute-onset fever and disseminated rash, usually with headache) and who may have been exposed to infected ticks (whether through travel or residence). In such individuals, the

prompt initiation of appropriate therapy may be lifesaving and is usually indicated while awaiting the results of diagnostic tests (see Chapter 5). Documented effective treatment of *R. rickettsii* infection has been limited to tetracycline compounds (e.g., particularly doxycycline [46] and chloramphenicol). Newer fluoroquinolones are active in vitro but have been unproven in patients. The long plasma half-life, favorable safety profile, and well-documented and consistent efficacy of doxycycline make it the treatment of choice. Doxycycline is typically administered as 100 mg every 12 h for adults (which may be given intravenously in critically ill patients or if oral therapy cannot be tolerated) or 4 mg/kg of body weight per day in two equal doses for children under 45 kg (100 lbs). The use of tetracyclines (including doxycycline) has often been considered to be relatively contraindicated in children under 8 years old and in pregnant women due to potential effects on dental enamel and, in the case of pregnancy, fetal bone formation; chloramphenicol may be a potential alternative in such settings. However, it is important to note that retrospective studies suggest that it may not be as effective as doxycycline for treating RMSF. Thus, doxycycline is still considered to be the preferred treatment for RMSF, particularly in seriously ill patients. An infectious disease specialist or the CDC should be consulted when such questions arise. Treatment should persist for a minimum of three days after the fever subsides and there is definitive sign of clinical improvement. Typical duration of antibiotic treatment is 5 to 10 days. It should also be mentioned that there are anecdotal reports and some laboratory studies which suggest that sulfa-containing antimicrobial agents may exacerbate the clinical severity of rickettsial infections (5, 50).

While a number of potentially promising anti-tick and transmission blocking vaccine candidates are currently being pursued, no viable vaccine has been marketed. Likewise, attenuated vaccines for the prevention of RMSF in humans have also proved to be unreliable. Therefore, the best prevention of RMSF and all tickborne diseases is still mechanical prevention of tick attachment to the host. Measures to prevent tick exposure include tucking the pants into the socks and tucking the shirt into the pants. The use of chemical repellents (e.g., DEET) on the clothing may also aid in prevention of tick attachment. When recreating or working in areas in which RMSF is endemic, a thorough inspection of the body should follow. Early removal of attached ticks is essential, since microbial transmission can occur within 12 to 24 h due to reactivation of rickettsiae in the tick's body tissues. Attached ticks should be carefully removed with forceps. The tick should then be saved in alcohol for future reference.

Acknowledgments. We thank D. E. Sonenshine for reading and critical comments concerning this chapter. We thank T. J. Kurtti and A. T. Palmer (University of Minnesota) and J. A. Simser (University of Maryland, Baltimore) for providing images of rickettsiae.

This work is supported in part by grants AI43006 (A.F.A.) and AI051857 (K.R.M.) from the National Institutes of Health.

REFERENCES

1. **Andersson, S. G., A. Zomorodipour, J. O. Andersson, T. Sicheritz-Ponten, U. C. Alsmark, R. M. Podowski, A. K. Naslund, A. S. Eriksson, H. H. Winkler, and C. G. Kurland.** 1998. The genome sequence of *Rickettsia prowazekii* and the origin of mitochondria. *Nature* **396:**133–140.

2. **Azad, A. F., and C. B. Beard.** 1998. Rickettsial pathogens and their arthropod vectors. *Emerg. Infect. Dis.* **4:**179–186.

3. **Azad, A. F., and S. Radulovic.** 2003. Pathogenic rickettsiae as bioterrorism agents. *Ann. N. Y. Acad. Sci.* **990:**734–748.

4. **Bell, E. J., G. M. Kohls, H. G. Steonner, and D. B. Lackman.** 1963. Non-pathogenic rickettsias related to the spotted fever group isolated from ticks, *Dermacentor variabilis* and *Dermacentor andersoni* from eastern Montana. *J. Immunol.* **90:**770–781.

5. **Beltrán, R. R., and J. I. Herrero Herrero.** 1992. Deleterious effect of trimethoprim-sulfamethoxazole in Mediterranean spotted fever. *Antimicrob. Agents Chemother.* **36:**1342–1343.

6. **Bergeron, J. W., R. L. Braddom, and D. L. Kaelin.** 1997. Persisting impairment following Rocky Mountain spotted fever: a case report. *Arch. Phys. Med. Rehabil.* **78:**1277–1280.

7. **Bouyer, D. H., J. Stenos, P. Crocquet-Valdes, C. G. Moron, V. L. Popov, J. E. Zavala-Velazquez, L. D. Foil, D. R. Stothard, A. F. Azad, and D. H. Walker.** 2001. *Rickettsia felis*: molecular characterization of a new member of the spotted fever group. *Int. J. Syst. Evol. Microbiol.* **51:**339–347.

8. **Burgdorfer, W.** 1988. Ecological and epidemiological considerations of Rocky Mountain spotted fever and scrub typhus, p. 33–50. *In* D. H. Walker (ed.), *Biology of Rickettsial Diseases*, vol. 1. CRC Press, Inc., Boca Raton, Fla.

9. **Burgdorfer, W., and L. P. Brinton.** 1975. Mechanisms of transovarial infection of spotted fever rickettsiae in ticks. *Ann. N. Y. Acad. Sci.* **266:**61–72.

10. **Burgdorfer, W., S. F. Hayes, and A. J. Mavros.** 1981. Nonpathogenic rickettsiae in *Dermacentor andersoni*: a limiting factor for the distribution of *Rickettsia rickettsii*. p. 585–594. *In* W. Burgdorfer and R. L. Anacker (ed.), *Rickettsiae and Rickettsial Diseases*. Academic Press, Inc., New York, N.Y.

11. **Conlon, P. J., G. W. Procop, V. Fowler, M. A. Eloubeidi, S. R. Smith, and D. J. Sexton.** 1996. Predictors of prognosis and risk of acute renal failure in patients with Rocky Mountain spotted fever. *Am. J. Med.* **101:**621–626.

12. **de La Fuente, J., E. F. Blouin, and K. M. Kocan.** 2003. Infection exclusion of the rickettsial pathogen *Anaplasma marginale* in the tick vector *Dermacentor variabilis*. *Clin. Diagn. Lab. Immunol.* **10:**182–184.

13. **Dumler, J. S., A. F. Barbet, C. P. Bekker, G. A. Dasch, G. H. Palmer, S. C. Ray, Y. Rikihisa, and F. R. Rurangirwa.** 2001. Reorganization of genera in the families Rickettsiaceae and Anaplasmataceae in the order Rickettsiales: unification of some species of *Ehrlichia* with *Anaplasma*, *Cowdria* with *Ehrlichia* and *Ehrlichia* with *Neorickettsia*, descriptions of six new species combinations and designation of *Ehrlichia equi* and 'HGE agent' as subjective synonyms of *Ehrlichia phagocytophila*. *Int. J. Syst. Evol. Microbiol.* **51:**2145–2165.

14. **Gage, K. L., M. E. Schrumpf, R. H. Karstens, W. Burgdorfer, and T. G. Schwan.** 1994. DNA typing of rickettsiae in naturally infected ticks using a polymerase chain reaction/restriction fragment length polymorphism system. *Am. J. Trop. Med. Hyg.* **50:**247–260.

15. **Galvao, M. A., C. L. Mafra, C. Moron, E. Anaya, and D. H. Walker.** 2003. Rickettsiosis of the genus *Rickettsia* in South America. *Ann. N. Y. Acad. Sci.* **990:**57–61.

16. **Gaywee, J., W. Xu, S. Radulovic, M. J. Bessman, and A. F. Azad.** 2002. The *Rickettsia prowazekii* invasion gene homolog (*invA*) encodes a Nudix hydrolase active on adenosine (5')-pentaphospho-(5')-adenosine. *Mol. Cell. Proteomics* **1:**179–185.

16a. **Goddard, J.** 2003. Experimental infection of lone star ticks, *Amblyomma americanum* (L.), with *Rickettsia parkeri* and exposure of guinea pigs to the agent. *J. Med. Entomol.* **40:**686–689.

17. **Gubler, D. J.** 1998. Resurgent vector-borne diseases as a global health problem. *Emerg. Infect. Dis.* **4:**442–450.

18. **Hadstack, T.** 1996. The biology of rickettsiae. *Infect. Agents Dis.* **5:**127–143.

19. **Hayes, S. F., and W. Burgdorfer.** 1982. Reactivation of *Rickettsia rickettsii* in *Dermacentor andersoni* ticks: an ultrastructural analysis. *Infect. Immun.* **37:**779–785.

20. **Hayes, S. F., and W. Burgdorfer.** 1989. Interactions between rickettsial endocytobionts and their tick hosts, p. 235–251. *In* W. Schwemmler and G. Gassner (ed.), *Insect Endocyobiosis: Morphology, Physiology, Genetics, Evolution*. CRC Press, Inc., Boca Raton, Fla.

21. **Heinzen, R. A., S. S. Grieshaber, L. S. Van Kirk, and C. J. Devin.** 1999. Dynamics of actin-based movement by *Rickettsia rickettsii* in Vero cells. *Infect. Immun.* **67:**4201–4207.

22. **Higgins, J. A., S. Radulovic, M. E. Schriefer, and A. F. Azad.** 1996. *Rickettsia felis*: a new species of pathogenic rickettsia isolated from cat fleas. *J. Clin. Microbiol.* **34:**671–674.

23. **Horney, L. F., and D. H. Walker.** 1988. Meningoencephalitis as a major manifestation of Rocky Mountain spotted fever. *South. Med. J.* **81:**915–918.

24. **Kao, G. F., C. D. Evancho, O. Ioffe, M. H. Lowitt, and J. S. Dumler.** 1997. Cutaneous histopathology of Rocky Mountain spotted fever. *J. Cutan. Pathol.* **24:**604–610.

25. **Kaplan, J. E., and V. F. Newhouse.** 1984. Occurrence of Rocky Mountain spotted fever in relation to climatic, geophysical, and ecologic variables. *Am. J. Trop. Med. Hyg.* **33:**1281–1282.

26. **Kelly, D. J., A. L. Richards, J. Temenak, D. Strickman, and G. A. Dasch.** 2002. The past and present threat of rickettsial diseases to military medicine and international public health. *Clin. Infect. Dis.* **34:**S145–S169.

27. **Kirkland, K. B., P. K. Marcom, D. J. Sexton, J. S. Dumler, and D. H. Walker.** 1993. Rocky Mountain spotted fever complicated by gangrene: report of six cases and review. *Clin. Infect. Dis.* **16:**629–634.

28. **Krusell, A., J. A. Comer, and D. J. Sexton.** 2002. Rickettsialpox in North Carolina: a case report. *Emerg. Infect. Dis.* **8:**727–728.

29. **Macaluso, K. R., D. E. Sonenshine, S. M. Ceraul, and A. F. Azad.** 2001. Infection and transovarial transmission of rickettsiae in *Dermacentor variabilis* ticks acquired by artificial feeding. *Vector Borne Zoonotic Dis.* **1:**45–53.

30. **Macaluso, K. R., D. E. Sonenshine, S. M. Ceraul, and A. F. Azad.** 2002. Rickettsial infection in *Dermacentor variabilis* (Acari: Ixodidae) inhibits transovarial transmission of a second *Rickettsia*. *J. Med. Entomol.* **39:**809–813.

31. **Macaluso, K. R., A. Mulenga, J. A. Simser, and A. F. Azad.** 2003. Differential expression of genes in uninfected and

Rickettsia-infected *Dermacentor variabilis* as assessed by differential display PCR. *Infect. Immun.* **71**:6165–6170.

32. **McDade, J. E., and V. F. Newhouse.** 1986. Natural history of *Rickettsia rickettsii. Annu. Rev. Microbiol.* **40**:287–309.

33. **Mulenga, A., K. R. Macaluso, J. A. Simser, and A. F. Azad.** 2003. Dynamics of *Rickettsia*-tick interactions: identification and characterization of differentially expressed mRNAs in uninfected and infected *Dermacentor variabilis. Insect Mol. Biol.* **12**:185–193.

34. **Munderloh, U. G., and T. J. Kurtti.** 1995. Cellular and molecular interrelationships between ticks and prokaryotic tick-borne pathogens. *Annu. Rev. Entomol.* **40**:221–243.

35. **Niebylski, M. L., M. E. Schrumpf, W. Burgdorfer, E. R. Fischer, K. L. Gage, and T.G. Schwan.** 1997. *Rickettsia peacockii* sp. nov., a new species infecting wood ticks, *Dermacentor andersoni*, in western Montana. *Int. J. Sys. Bacteriol.* **47**:446–452.

36. **Niebylski, M. L., M. G. Peacock, and T. G. Schwan.** 1999. Lethal effect of *Rickettsia rickettsii* on its tick vector (*Dermacentor andersoni*). *Appl. Environ. Microbiol.* **65**:773–778.

37. **Ogata, H., S. Audic, P. Renesto-Audiffren, P. E. Fournier, V. Barbe, D. Samson, V. Roux, P. Cossart, J. Weissenbach, J. M. Claverie, and D. Raoult.** 2001. Mechanisms of evolution in *Rickettsia conorii* and *R. prowazekii. Science* **293**:2093–2098.

38. **Paddock, C. D., P. W. Greer, T. L. Ferebee, J. Singleton, Jr., D. B. McKechnie, T. A. Treadwell, J. W. Krebs, M. J. Clarke, R. C. Holman, J. G. Olson, J. E. Childs, and S. R. Zaki.** 1999. Hidden mortality attributable to Rocky Mountain spotted fever: immunohistochemical detection of fatal, serologically unconfirmed disease. *J. Infect. Dis.* **179**:1469–1476.

39. **Paddock, C. D., S. R. Zaki, T. Koss, J. Singleton, Jr, J. W. Sumner, J. A. Comer, M. E. Eremeeva, G. A. Dasch, B. Cherry, and J. E. Childs.** 2003. Rickettsialpox in New York City: a persistent urban zoonosis. *Ann. N. Y. Acad. Sci.* **990**:36–44.

39a. **Paddock, C. D., J. W. Sumner, J. A. Comer, S. R. Zaki, C. S. Goldsmith, J. Goddard, S. L. F. McLellan, C. T. Tamminga, and C. A. Ohl.** 2004. *Rickettsia parkeri*: a newly recognized cause of spotted fever rickettsiosis in the United States. *Clin. Infect. Dis.* **38**:805–811.

39b. **Parker, R. R., G. M. Kohls, G. W. Cox, and G. E. Davis.** 1939. Observations on an infectious agent from *Amblyomma maculatum. Public Health Rep.* **54**:1482–1484.

40. **Philip, R. N.** 2000. *Rocky Mountain Spotted Fever in Western Montana: Anatomy of a Pestilence.* Bitter Root Valley Historical Society, Hamilton, Mont.

41. **Radulovic, S., M. S. Rahman, M. S. Beier, and A. F. Azad.** 2002. Molecular and functional analysis of the *Rickettsia typhi* groESL operon. *Gene* **298**:41–48.

42. **Rahman, M. S., J. A. Simser, K. R. Macaluso, and A. F. Azad.** 2003. Molecular and functional analysis of the *lepB* gene, encoding a type I signal peptidase from *Rickettsia rickettsii* and *Rickettsia typhi. J. Bacteriol.* **185**:4578–4584.

43. **Regnery, R. L., C. L. Spruill, and B. D. Plikaytis.** 1991. Genotypic identification of rickettsiae and estimation of intraspecies sequence divergence for portions of two rickettsial genes. *J. Bacteriol.* **173**:1576–1589.

44. **Roux, V., P. Fournier, and D. Raoult.** 1996. Differentiation of spotted fever group rickettsiae by sequencing and analysis of restriction fragment length polymorphism of PCR-amplified DNA of the gene encoding the protein rOmpA. *J. Clin. Microbiol.* **34**:2058–2065.

45. **Schreifer, M. E., and A. Azad.** 1994. Changing ecology of Rocky Mountain spotted fever, p. 314–326. *In* D. E. Sonenshine and T. N. Mather (ed.), *Ecological Dynamics of Tick-Borne Zoonoses.* Oxford University Press, New York, N.Y.

46. **Sexton, D. J.** 2000. Rocky Mountain spotted fever, p. 435–438. *In* G. Thomas Strickland (ed.), *Hunter's Tropical Medicine and Emerging Infectious Diseases*, 8th edition. W. B. Saunders Co., Philadelphia, Pa.

47. **Shankman, B.** 1946. Report of an outbreak of endemic febrile illness, not yet identified, occurring in New York City. *N.Y. State J. Med.* **46**:2156–2159.

48. **Simser, J. A., A. T. Palmer, U. G. Munderloh, and T. J. Kurtti.** 2001. Isolation of a spotted fever group *Rickettsia, Rickettsia peacockii*, in a Rocky Mountain wood tick, *Dermacentor andersoni*, cell line. *Appl. Environ. Microbiol.* **67**:546–552.

49. **Sonenshine, D. E.** 1993. *Biology of Ticks*, vol. 2. Oxford University Press, New York, N.Y.

50. **Topping, N. H.** 1939. Experimental Rocky Mountain spotted fever and epidemic typhus treated with prontosil or sulfapyridine. *Public Health Rep.* **54**:1143–1147.

51. **Treadwell, T. A., R. C. Holman, M. J. Clarke, J. W. Krebs, C. D. Paddock, and J. E. Childs.** 2000. Rocky Mountain spotted fever in the United States, 1993–1996. *Am. J. Trop. Med. Hyg.* **63**:21–26.

52. **Walker, D. H., and T. W. Lane.** 1988. Rocky Mountain spotted fever: clinical signs, symptoms, and pathophysiology, p. 63–78. *In* D. H. Walker (ed.), *Biology of Rickettsial Diseases*, vol. 1. CRC Press, Inc., Boca Raton, Fla.

53. **Wood, D. O., and A. F. Azad.** 2000. Genetic manipulation of rickettsiae: a preview. *Infect. Immun.* **68**:6091–6093.

54. **Wells, G. M., T. E. Woodward, P. Fiset, and R. B. Hornick.** 1978. Rocky Mountain spotted fever caused by blood transfusion. *JAMA* **239**:2763–2765.

55. **Wikel, S. K.** 1996. Host immunity to ticks. *Annu. Rev. Entomol.* **41**:1–22.

Tick-Borne Diseases of Humans
Edited by Jesse L. Goodman et al.
© 2005 ASM Press, Washington, D.C.

Chapter 18

Mediterranean Spotted Fever and Other Tick-Borne Rickettsioses

PIERRE-EDOUARD FOURNIER AND DIDIER RAOULT

INTRODUCTION

Rickettsioses are arthropod-borne infections caused by bacteria belonging to the genus *Rickettsia* within the family *Rickettsiaceae* in the order *Rickettsiales*. Most of these zoonoses are transmitted by ticks, but some are vectored by lice, fleas, or mites. Tick-borne rickettsioses have specific geographic distributions, directly dependent on the distribution of their vectors. These rickettsioses are among the oldest known arthropod-borne diseases (186). Rocky Mountain spotted fever (RMSF) was first reported in 1899 by Maxcey; its vector, *Dermacentor andersoni*, was described in 1909 (198, 262). One year later, Conor and Bruch described Mediterranean spotted fever (MSF) in Tunisia (43). Until 1984, only three additional tick-transmitted rickettsioses were reported, including Siberian tick typhus, Israeli spotted fever, and Queensland tick typhus. Over the last 12 years, another 10 of these infections have been characterized, including Astrakhan fever, Flinders Island spotted fever (FISF), African tick-bite fever (ATBF), Japanese spotted fever (JSF), tick-borne lymphadenitis (TIBOLA), lymphangitis-associated rickettsiosis (LAR) due to *Rickettsia sibirica mongolotimonae*, and unnamed infections caused by *Rickettsia helvetica*, *Rickettsia aeschlimannii*, *Rickettsia parkeri*, and "*Rickettsia heilongjiangensis*." Thus, many of the tick-borne rickettsioses are considered to be emerging infections. Several rickettsiae have only been isolated from ticks and thus have been considered likely to be nonpathogenic. A priori, it is difficult to predict which rickettsiae are potential human pathogens. Furthermore, different isolates of the same species vary in virulence for the same host (136). For many years, the sole method for isolating rickettsiae was to inoculate animals, with guinea pigs being the favored system. This practice resulted in the selection of strains that were pathogenic for their experimental host. Only later did alternative isolation methods involving chicken embryos or cell culture become available to permit the characterization of new isolates. It is potentially misleading to rely on the results of studies of strains obtained from a specific animal model in making unbiased deductions regarding human pathogenicity. Pathogenicity may, in fact, be linked to the ability of the host arthropod to bite humans; for example, new rickettsiae found in the ladybird beetle (AB bacterium) and in the pea aphid (pea aphid rickettsia) (12, 40, 257) have not been implicated in human disease, probably because their hosts do not bite humans. When a rickettsia is found in an arthropod capable of biting humans, it should be considered a potential human pathogen.

Various circumstances have played a role in the recent description of new rickettsioses, including (i) the curiosity of clinicians which was highlighted in the case of the description of JSF by Mahara et al. (131) or the description of FISF by R. S. Stewart (228); (ii) the modification of human behavior, as seen in ATBF with the development of tourism to sub-Saharan Africa (68); and (iii) the development of new diagnostic tools, including new cell culture systems (134) or new serology and molecular methods (119).

In this chapter, we will consider various aspects of tick-borne rickettsioses, including the description of rickettsiae, their vectors and the relationships between rickettsiae and ticks, an overview of the various diseases recognized to date (excluding RMSF, which is the subject of Chapter 17), a description of rickettsiae of unknown pathogenicity, and a report on modern diagnostic tools and treatments used for tick-transmitted rickettsioses.

BACTERIA

Bacteria within the genus *Rickettsia* are small bacilli belonging to the order *Rickettsiales*. These bac-

Pierre-Edouard Fournier and Didier Raoult • Unité des Rickettsies, CNRS UMR 6020, Faculté de Médecine, Université de la Méditerranée, Marseille, France.

teria are strictly associated with eukaryotic cells and associated with arthropods, which serve as vectors or even reservoirs.

Taxonomy and Phylogeny

Bacteria within the order *Rickettsiales* were initially described as short gram-negative bacilli retaining basic fuchsin dye when stained by the Gimenez method (81) and growing in strict association with eukaryotic cells. The order *Rickettsiales* was historically divided into the families *Rickettsiaceae, Bartonellaceae,* and *Anaplasmataceae.* Within the family *Rickettsiaceae,* the tribe *Rickettsiae* was composed of the genera *Rickettsia, Coxiella,* and *Rochalimaea* (255). The development of PCR and nucleotide sequencing, particularly the study of 16S rRNA or rDNA (261), has considerably modified the taxonomic classification of bacteria, in particular intracellular bacteria that express few phenotypic criteria commonly used for identification and classification. 16S rRNA analysis has led to the reclassification of several species: *Coxiella burnetii* was removed from the order *Rickettsiales* and reclassified in the gamma subgroup of *Proteobacteria* (253). The genera *Rochalimaea, Grahamella,* and *Bartonella* were unified but retained in the alpha subgroup of *Proteobacteria.*

The genus *Rickettsia* remains the only genus within the tribe *Rickettsiae.* It was initially divided into the typhus group (TG), the spotted fever group (SFG), and the scrub typhus group (STG) (255). The differentiation of these three groups was historically based on several factors (255), including (i) the intracellular location of each species, which is related to the ability of a specific rickettsia to polymerize actin in the cytoplasm, allowing intracellular mobility (97, 237) in the nucleus and the cytoplasm for the SFG rickettsiae and *Rickettsia canadensis* and only in the cytoplasm for the others; (ii) an optimal growth temperature of 32°C for the SFG rickettsiae and 35°C for the TG and *Orientia tsutsugamushi*; and (iii) the cross-reaction of sera from a patient with rickettsial infection to the somatic antigens of three *Proteus* strains, including OX19 (TG and *Rickettsia rickettsii*), OX2 (SFG), and OXK (*O. tsutsugamushi*) (273). This classification underwent many modifications on the basis of 16S rRNA sequence comparison. The position of *Rickettsia tsutsugamushi,* the only member of the STG, is distinct enough to warrant transfer into a new genus, *Orientia,* as *O. tsutsugamushi* (232). In addition, Stothard et al. proposed that a new group named the ancestral group be created inside the genus *Rickettsia,* including *R. canadensis, Rickettsia bellii* and the AB bacterium (230). Currently, the genus *Rickettsia* is composed of the ancestral group, the TG composed of *Rickettsia prowazekii* and

Rickettsia typhi, and the SFG composed of 18 recognized species. However, the taxonomic definition of a rickettsial species remains controversial. The traditional identification methods used in bacteriology cannot be applied to rickettsiae because of their strictly intracellular nature. Thus, if one applies the same DNA-DNA relatedness cutoff used for other bacterial genera (251) to the rickettsial species *R. rickettsii, Rickettsia conorii, Rickettsia montanensis,* and *Rickettsia sibirica,* which are distinguished by their association with different vectors and differences in their epidemiological and pathogenic characteristics, they would all belong to the same species (140, 246). In the first half of the 20th century the distinctive immunogenic properties of rickettsial antigens were used to distinguish between rickettsiae. Cross-immunity and vaccine protection tests (167) in guinea pigs and complement fixation (169) or toxin neutralization (21) tests were successfully applied to the differentiation of *R. rickettsii, R. sibirica,* and *R. conorii.* In 1978, R. N. Philip et al. developed the indirect microimmunofluorescence (MIF) serologic typing test with mouse sera, which is currently the reference method for the identification of new SFG rickettsiae (165). Based on this method, a recognized SFG rickettsial species is in fact a serotype. The advent of purification methods (254) enabling the separation of rickettsiae from host cell components has allowed the study of rickettsial proteins and the understanding of the mechanisms on which these serological identification techniques have been based. The antigenic determinants for the serotyping scheme are the high-molecular-weight outer membrane proteins rOmpA and rOmpB and the cytoplasmic protein PS120. With the development of a new cell culture isolation technique (e.g., the shell vial technique) (134), more strains have been isolated over the past few years. These strains have been characterized by a polyphasic approach involving phenotypic criteria: pathogenic and ecological characteristics, serotyping, protein analysis by sodium dodecyl sulfate-polyacrylamide gel electrophoresis (SDS-PAGE) (2, 145), and genotypic criteria (restriction fragment length polymorphism (RFLP) analysis of PCR amplification products (58, 194), macrorestriction analysis by pulsed-field gel electrophoresis (205), and use of monoclonal antibodies (267). From these analyses, it appeared that no consensus criteria for the definition of rickettsial species exist. With the development of molecular approaches, the use of MIF serotyping as a reference method should be questioned. Recently, Maiden et al. (132) and the ad hoc committee for the reevaluation of the species definition in bacteriology (225) have demonstrated the usefulness of multiple gene sequencing for taxonomy. For rickettsiae, comparison of sequences from different genes allowed significant phylogenetic inferences to be made at different taxonomic levels, ranging from those between closely related species to those between more distantly related organisms. Several phylogenetic analyses of the rickettsiae, based on 16S rRNA gene sequence comparison, have been carried out (206, 230). These studies have confirmed the evolutionary unity of the genus (Fig. 1), but since the sequences were almost identical, significant inferences about intragenus phylogeny were not possible. Four divergent genes that encode the enzyme citrate synthase (224), the outer membrane proteins rOmpA (69) and rOmpB (207), and the cytoplasmic protein PS120 (215) have been sequenced to find more sensitive and significant phylogenetic relationships among rickettsiae. The results of the comparison of these sequences demonstrated the following. (i) *R. canadensis*, *R. bellii*, and the AB bacterium lie outside both the TG and the SFG on an evolutionary lineage, which diverged before the separation of these two groups, thus confirming the hypothesis of Stothard et al. (230). (ii) The TG comprised *R. prowazekii* and *R. typhi* only. (iii) The tick-borne *R. helvetica* and *Rickettsia australis* and the mite-borne *Rickettsia akari* were associated with the SFG cluster. (iv) The SFG rickettsiae can be subdivided into four groups, the *R. rickettsii* group, the *Rickettsia massiliae* group, the *R. akari* group, and the *R. helvetica* group (Tables 1 and 2). Comparison of phylogenetic inferences derived from any of these four gene sequences indicated similar evolutionary models (Fig. 1), but it is best if more than one gene is analyzed during the characterization of putative new species, since phylogenetic analysis must stem from identical results obtained from different genes and analysis methods.

We have recently proposed gene sequence-based criteria for the classification of rickettsial isolates at the genus, group, and species levels, using sequences from the 16S rDNA, *gltA*, *ompA*, *ompB*, and *sca4* (gene D) genes (63a).

The 18 currently validated SFG species include 13 species pathogenic for humans: *R. rickettsii*, the agent of RMSF (26); *R. conorii*, which causes MSF (27), Israeli spotted fever (83), and Astrakhan fever (232); *R. akari*, responsible for rickettsialpox (103); *R. sibirica*, the agent of Siberian tick typhus (STT) (271) and LAR (65a); *R. australis*, which causes Queensland tick typhus (QTT) (160); *Rickettsia japonica*, responsible for Japanese spotted fever (JSF) (242), *Rickettsia slovaca*, the agent of TIBOLA (216); *Rickettsia africae*, which causes African tick-bite fever (ATBF) (109); *Rickettsia honei*, responsible for FISF (227); *Rickettsia felis*, the agent of flea typhus (23); and *R. helvetica* (17), *R. parkeri* (115), and *R. aeschlimannii* (16), which are agents of unnamed infections (Table 1). Five species of as-yet-unreported pathogenicity also belong to the SFG: *R. bellii* (164),

R. massiliae (18), *Rickettsia rhipicephali* (32), *R. montanensis* (255), and *Rickettsia peacockii* (141). In addition to these 18 recognized species, more than 20 rickettsial strains whose taxonomic classification is not yet established have been described. Among them, "*R. heilongjiangensis*" is the agent of an unnamed disease.

Genomics

Until 2001, the genome size of rickettsiae was estimated by pulsed-field gel electrophoresis and ranged from 1.1 to 1.6 Mb. In 2001, the first genome of a tick-transmitted rickettsia (e.g., *R. conorii* strain Seven) was fully sequenced (148). The analysis of the sequences obtained has highlighted unique characteristics among bacterial genomes. Its size is 1,268,755 nucleotides and comprises 1,374 open reading frames (ORFs). Intriguingly, 656 95- to 150-nucleotide-long palindromic repeat fragments have been discovered (146, 147). Their distribution throughout the genome is irregular, with some inserted into protein-encoding genes but compatible with the encoded protein's three-dimensional fold and functions. Their role is currently unknown, but they may serve as mobile elements regulating protein expression. Further comparison of the *R. conorii* genome with that of *R. prowazekii* provided additional data on the evolution of rickettsial genomes (148). Only 804 of the 1,374 ORFs of *R. conorii* are present in the *R. prowazekii* genome, which contains only 834 ORFs. The two genomes exhibit a nearly identical gene localization. This provided clues to the degradation of rickettsial genomes, from complete transcribed genes to split transcribed genes and then to split untranscribed genes (148).

Pathophysiology

Rickettsiae are strictly associated with eukaryotic cells and cannot multiply extracellularly. Following the tick bite and a prolonged attachment of the tick to its host, the rickettsiae invade their target endothelial cells. Evidence for the role of the 52-kDa beta-peptide in attachment to cells has been described (78). This beta-peptide is a product of the maturation of the rOmpB protein (78). Gilmore et al. have observed that the Iowa strain of *R. rickettsii*, which does not possess the beta-peptide, is avirulent, thus demonstrating its role in cell attachment (78). Phospholipase activity has been linked to the infection stage (122, 260). A very active rickettsial multiplication occurs at the site of the bite, which results in ischemia and formation of the inoculation eschar. Inside the cells, rickettsiae escape from the phagosome vacuole and live free in the cytosol (97, 236, 237). Several copies of the ATP/ADP

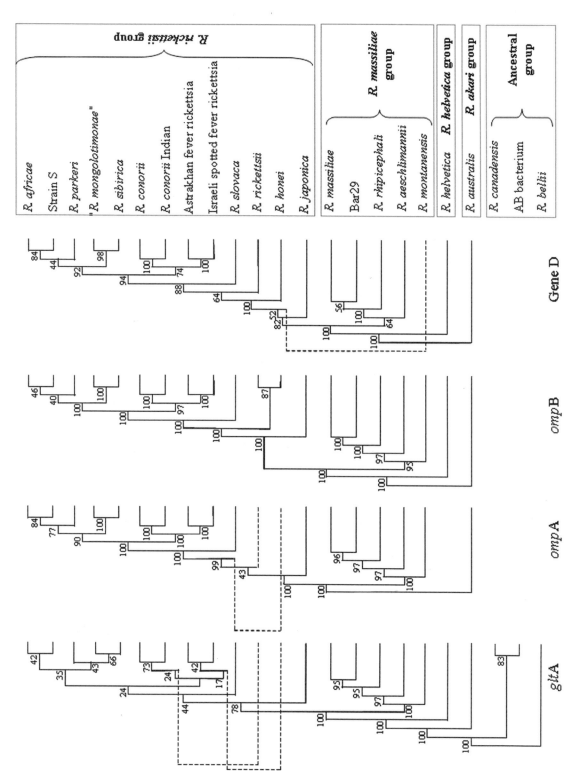

Figure 1. Phylogenetic organization of tick-transmitted rickettsiae based on the comparison of *gltA*, *ompA*, *ompB*, and *sca4* (gene D) gene sequences by the parsimony method.

Table 1. Pathogenic tick-transmitted rickettsiae

Species (reference)	Disease (reference)	Vector(s)	Geographic distribution
R. rickettsii group			
R. rickettsii[a] (260)	RMSF (196)	*D. andersoni, D. variabilis,* *A. americanum,* *Amblyomma cajennense,* *R. sanguineus*	North, Central, and South America
R. conorii conorii[a] (27)	MSF (43)	*R. sanguineus*	Mediterranean region, Black Sea, sub-Saharan Africa, India
R. conorii israelensis (85)	Israeli spotted fever (83)	*R. sanguineus*	Israel, Portugal
R. conorii caspia (47)	Astrakhan fever (232)	*R. pumilio, R. sanguineus*	Astrakhan, Russia, Kosovo, Chad
R. sibirica sensu stricto[a] (269)	STT (125)	*Dermacentor nuttali,* *D. marginatus,* *Dermacentor pictus,* *D. silvarum, H. concinna,* *Haemaphysalis punctata,* *R. sanguineus*	Siberia, Pakistan, Northern China, Mongolia
R. honei[a] (225)	FISF (226)	*Ixodes* spp., *Rhipicephalus* spp.	Flinders Island (Australia), Thailand
R. japonica[a] (242)	JSF (127)	*H. longicornis, H. flava,* *Haemaphysalis formosensis,* *Haemaphysalis hystricis,* *D. taiwanensis, I. ovatus*	Japan, China
R. sibirica mongolotimonae (26)	Lymphangitis-associated rickettsiosis (176)	*H. asiaticum*	Mongolia, China, France, Algeria, sub-Saharan Africa
"*R. heilongjiangensis*" (61)	Unnamed spotted fever (61)	*D. silvarum*	China
R. africae[a] (111)	ATBF (110)	*A. variegatum, A. hebraeum*	Sub-Saharan Africa, French West Indies
R. slovaca[a] (193)	TIBOLA (148)	*D. reticulatus, D. marginatus*	France, Spain, Switzerland, Hungary, Slovakia, Russia
R. parkeri (115)	Unnamed spotted fever (150a)	*A. maculatum*	United States
R. massiliae group			
R. aeschlimannii[a] (16)	Unnamed spotted fever (179)	*H. marginatus*	Morocco
R. helvetica group			
R. helvetica[a] (29)	Unnamed spotless fever (66)	*Ixodes* spp.	Eurasia
R. akari group			
R. australis[a] (158)	Queensland tick typhus (168)	*I. holocyclus*	Australia

[a] Currently validated species.

translocase gene are present in the *R. conorii* genome (148). It is likely that rickettsiae use ATP produced by the host cells as a source of energy (259). In contrast to TG rickettsiae, those transmitted by ticks are able to penetrate and multiply inside the nucleus. This mobility is attributed to actin polymerization (30, 97, 237). Rickettsiae multiply by scissiparity (reproduction by fission) and are released into the bloodstream by cell projections or by the detachment of infected cells. Subsequent to this rickettsiemia, new endothelial cells are infected. This proliferation of rickettsiae in the vascular endothelium results in vasculitis, which is the basis of the main clinical symptoms: fever, headache, and cutaneous eruption. Furthermore, von Willebrand factor and thrombomodulin are released into the bloodstream. In addition, the antithrombotic proper-

ties of the endothelium are diminished, which results in risks of thrombosis, especially in malignant forms.

RELATIONSHIPS BETWEEN TICKS AND RICKETTSIAE

Ticks are the main vectors and reservoirs of SFG rickettsiae (Tables 1 and 2). Rickettsiae infect and multiply in almost all organs of their invertebrate hosts. When the ovaries and oocytes of an adult female tick are infected, rickettsiae may be transmitted transovarially to at least some of the offspring. The percentage of infected eggs obtained from females of the same tick species infected with the same rickettsial strain may vary for as-yet-unknown reasons (31, 35).

Table 2. Rickettsiae of unknown pathogenicity

Species (reference)[a]	Vector(s)	Geographic distribution
R. rickettsii group		
Souche S (54)	*R. sanguineus*	Armenia
"*R. hulinii*" (270)	*H. concinna*	China
R. peacockii[b] (150)	*D. andersoni*	United States
JC880 (197)	*R. sanguineus*	Pakistan
Rav1 (153)	*A. variegatum*	Sub-Saharan Africa
Rav3 (153)	*A. variegatum*	Sub-Saharan Africa
Rav9 (153)	*A. variegatum*	Sub-Saharan Africa
R. massiliae group		
R. massiliae[b] (18)	*R. turanicus, R. sanguineus, Rhipicephalus* spp.	France, Greece, Spain, Portugal, sub-Saharan Africa
R. rhipicephali[b] (34)	*R. sanguineus, D. andersoni, D. variabilis, D. occidentalis*	United States, France, Portugal, Central Africa
R. montanensis[b] (115)	*D. variabilis, D. andersoni*	United States
Bar 29 (19)	*R. sanguineus*	Spain
"*R. amblyommii*" (171)	*A. americanum*	United States
DnS14 (220)	*D. silvarum, D. niveus*	Siberia, Kazakhstan
RpA4 (220)	*D. reticulatus, D. niveus*	Russia, Kazakhstan
R. helvetica group		
AT1 (65)	*A. testudinarium*	Japan
"*R. monacensis*" (221)	*I. ricinus*	Slovakia, Germany
IRS3 (212)	*I. ricinus*	Slovakia
IRS4 (212)	*I. ricinus*	Slovakia
Ancestral group		
R. canadensis[b] (136)	*H. leporispalustris*	Canada
R. bellii[b] (162)	*D. andersoni, D. occidentalis, D. albipictus, D. variabilis, O. concanensis, A. cooleyi, H. leporispalustris*	United States
"*Candidatus* R. tarasevichiae" (219)	*I. persulcatus*	Russia

[a] Only rickettsiae for which DNA sequences permitted their phylogenetic classification are included.
[b] Currently validated species.

Once an egg is infected, all subsequent life stages of the tick will be infected (the rate of transstadial transmission is therefore 100%). Ixodid ticks are blood-sucking arthropods throughout all developmental stages, apart from some of the adult male ticks in some *Ixodes* species. Rickettsiae infecting the ticks' salivary glands can be transmitted to vertebrate hosts during feeding. Therefore, since larvae, nymphs, and adults may all be infective for susceptible vertebrate hosts, the ticks must be regarded as the main reservoir host of rickettsiae. Sexual transmission from male to female ticks in *Ixodes ricinus* and *D. andersoni* ticks has been described (92, 163). Uninfected, immature *D. andersoni* ticks were allowed to feed simultaneously with adults infected with *R. rickettsii* on the same uninfected guinea pigs. The rickettsiae were transmitted both to the guinea pigs and to the uninfected immature ticks, showing that a rickettsemic blood meal is a mode of uptake (161). Long-term starvation of a tick does not kill its infecting rickettsiae, although it may alter some of their properties. For example,

R. rickettsii in *D. andersoni* ticks loses its virulence for guinea pigs when the ticks are subjected to physiological stress, such as long periods of starvation. However, subsequent exposure of these ticks to a temperature of 37°C for 24 to 48 h or refeeding them on laboratory animals restores the original virulence of the bacteria. This long-recognized phenomenon is known as reactivation (224). While there is wide consensus about this part of the rickettsial cycle, the role of vertebrate reservoirs in maintaining zoonotic foci has yet to be agreed upon. For vertebrates to be efficient reservoirs of rickettsiae, they need to be normal hosts of the vector, and to be susceptible to the rickettsiae, and they should develop a relatively long duration of rickettsiemia. If they did not fulfill these criteria, ticks would not be able to acquire rickettsiae from the bloodstream of their hosts. Humans are not good reservoirs for rickettsiae, since they are seldom infested with large numbers of ticks for a long period and rickettsemia is usually of only short duration, especially with antibiotic intervention.

Although yet to be demonstrated, there is potentially another method by which rickettsiae may be transmitted between ticks. The social behavior of ticks is determined mainly by the effects of different pheromones (90, 157). Some pheromones are responsible for the aggregation of ticks on the host, enhancing the chance for meeting and copulation. Under such circumstances, ticks would also feed, and thus the mouthparts of several different ticks would be in the skin of the host in close proximity. Under such feeding conditions, the direct spread of rickettsiae to uninfected ticks might be possible without causing infection of the animal being fed upon. Little is known about the effects of rickettsial infection on ticks, although Burgdorfer and colleagues reported that rickettsial infection lowered tick fertility (31, 35). Ixodid ticks are highly adapted to maintaining a favorable water balance in arid environments, often feeding on a specific host only seasonally and surviving for months or years when these hosts are absent (101). They are slow-feeding ticks, taking days to engorge. It is difficult to determine the association between rickettsial and tick species because specific characterization of species and subspecies in both phyla lacks sensitivity. Consequently, it is difficult to determine how long a tick species has been associated with a rickettsial species and therefore if coevolution has occurred. The range of host specificity of a tick varies greatly from one species to another, although larval and nymph stages are usually less specific in their choice of host and bite humans more often than adult ticks. Some species, such as the brown dog tick *Rhipicephalus sanguineus*, are very host specific and rarely bite humans (79), whereas others, such as *I. ricinus* in Europe or *Amblyomma* species in Africa, will bite any mammal. This explains the multiple eschars observed with ATBF. Indeed, tick ecology determines all the epidemiological aspects of tick bite fevers.

The geographical distribution of *Rickettsia* spp. is determined by the incidence of their tick hosts, and the seasonal incidence of disease parallels tick activity. It should be noted that immature stages of ticks can be involved in disease transmission and that their incidence differs from that of the adult population. For example, MSF, caused by *R. conorii*, is transmitted by *R. sanguineus*, whose adult populations peak in May. Most MSF cases, however, occur in August, 3 months later (189), suggesting that larvae or nymphs are responsible, particularly since the immature stages of numerous tick species bite humans (79) and their highest incidence occurs in August. The infecting tick bite is painless, and the tick is not usually observed, especially when smaller larvae or nymphs are involved. When not engorged, these stages are about the size of a pinhead. A history of tick bite is an important finding but is often absent. In several cases of MSF, ticks have been found at the site of the bite on patients who have been febrile for several days. The patients had simply not noticed the presence of the ticks, which must have been attached for more than 10 days, since the incubation period for the disease is usually 7 days. In areas of the United States or Africa where huge numbers of ticks are found, patients with rickettsiosis can easily identify attached ticks.

The risk of ticks transmitting rickettsiae and consequently the prevalence of a specific disease are dependent on several parameters. (i) The prevalence of rickettsia-infected ticks, which can vary greatly, is obviously important. For example, up to 12% of *R. sanguineus* ticks are infected with *R. conorii* in southern France (159), whereas only 0.5% of *Dermacentor variabilis* ticks in North Carolina are infected by *R. rickettsii* (248). (ii) The affinity of a specific tick for human beings also varies. For example, in Mediterranean countries, although nearly everybody is in contact with the dog tick *R. sanguineus*, the prevalence of MSF is only 50 per 100,000 inhabitants. The reason is the low affinity of this tick for alternate hosts. (iii) The abundance of the tick itself is important and is influenced by many factors, including climatic and ecological conditions (91, 133).

DISEASES

The following is a brief description of the currently described rickettsial diseases, excluding RMSF. The signs and symptoms of rickettsioses are compared in Table 3.

Mediterranean Spotted Fever

MSF was first described in Tunisia in 1910 by Conor and Bruch (43). As characteristic skin eruptions were papular rather than macular, the disease was referred to as boutonneuse fever. The eschar at the site of the tick bite (Color Plate 13A to C) was described in Marseille in 1925 by Olmer (149). The disease is encountered throughout the Mediterranean region, in sub-Saharan Africa (238), India, and around the Black Sea (Color Map 9) (55). An MSF-like disease was described in Vladivostock in the eastern part of Russia near Japan, but no direct evidence of *R. conorii* infection was reported. An increase in the number of MSF cases in France, Italy, Spain, and Portugal paralleled that of RMSF in the United States during the 1970s (133). This increase in incidence was correlated with higher temperatures and lower rainfall in Spain and with a decrease in the number of days of frost during the preceding year in France (188). Although *R. conorii* is considered to cause a less severe disease than *R. rickettsii*, severe forms of MSF, named

Table 3. Compared symptoms of tick-transmitted rickettsioses (184)[a]

Disease	Cutaneous rash (%)	Inoculation eschar (%)	Multiple eschars (%)	Headache (%)	Enlarged lymph nodes (%)
RMSF	88	Rare*	0	80	0
MSF	97	72	0	56	Rare*
Israeli spotted fever	100	0	0	NA	0
Astrakhan fever	100	23	0	92	0
STT	100	77	0	100	Yes*
QTT	100	65	NA	0	Yes*
JSF	100	48	0	22	0
ATBF	46	95	54	5	43
FISF	85	25	0	73	Yes*
TIBOLA	6	100	0	20	100
Lymphangitis-associated rickettsiosis	78	89	22	55	55
R. helvetica infection	0	Yes*	0	Yes*	0
"R. heilongjiangensis" infection	92	92	0	100	77
R. parkeri	Yes*	Yes*	Yes*	Yes*	Yes*

[a] *, no numerical data were available for these variables. NA, not applicable.

malignant MSF, have been reported in 6% of patients and the mortality rate may reach 2.5% (190). Therefore, MSF should not be considered a mild spotted fever. As MSF is not a reportable disease except in Italy, its exact incidence is unknown. The Reference Center for the Diagnosis and Study of Rickettsioses, located in Marseille, France, estimates the incidence to be around 50 cases per year per 100,000 inhabitants in the Marseille area. As the disease is transmitted by *R. sanguineus*, which infects dogs, it is also encountered in urban areas. Because of a frequent lack of several classical clinical features, a diagnosis score has been proposed to facilitate the diagnosis of this disease (Table 4) (189). In France, MSF occurs between May and October, with most cases being diagnosed in July and August. It involves mostly men and boys under 10 years of age or older than 50 years. The tick bite, mostly from immature stages, is often unreported by patients. The tick needs to remain attached to the patient for at least 20 h to transmit *R. conorii*. After an asymptomatic incubation of 6 days, the onset of signs is generally sudden and marked by elevated fever (>39°C), headache, arthralgia, and myalgia. At this stage, the presence of the eschar (50% of cases), usually found on the limbs, helps to establish the diagnosis (Color Plate 13A to C). In a few cases, the inoculation occurred through conjunctivae and patients presented with conjunctivitis. One to 7 days (median, 4 days) following the onset of fever, a generalized maculopapular rash, involving the palms and soles but sparing the face, develops (Color Plate 13E). Usually, patients will recover within 10 days without any sequellae. Six percent of patients will develop malignant forms of the disease. Risk factors for severe forms include age of >60 years, diabetes mellitus, chronic alcoholism, glucose-6-phosphate dehydrogenase deficiency (168), cardiac insufficiency, and im-

munosuppression. These forms are characterized by a purpuric rash and neurological, renal, hepatic, cerebral, myocardial, or cardiac problems which may result in multiple-organ dysfunction syndrome, especially in elderly people (192). Thrombosis of the deep venous vessels and acute pericarditis have also been described as complications of boutonneuse fever (48,

Table 4. Score for diagnosis of MSF[a]

Criteria	No. of points
Epidemiological criteria	
Life or travel in areas of endemicity	2
Onset of symptoms between May . . . . and September	2
Reported contact with dog ticks	2
Clinical criteria	
Fever greater than 39°C (102°F)	5
Inoculation eschar	5
Maculo papular or purpuric cutaneous rash	5
Two of three clinical criteria	3
All three clinical criteria	5
Aspecific biological criteria	
Thrombocyte count, <150 g/liter	1
SGOT and/or SGPT >50 UI/liter	1
Bacteriological criteria	
Isolation of *R. conorii* from clinical specimens	25
Detection of *R. conorii* from skin biopsy	25
by immunofluorescence	
Serological criteria	
Unique serum with total Ig of ≥1:128	5
Unique serum with IgG of ≥1:128	10
and IgM of ≥1:64	
Fourfold increase in Ig titers between two	20
sera sampled 2 weeks apart	

[a] When the score is greater than 25 for a patient, the diagnosis of MSF is likely.

117). Variations in the severity of MSF have been encountered in different countries and even in different areas of the same country. For example, in the northeastern part of Catalonia in Spain, the disease is milder than elsewhere in Spain (56, 63, 209). Rare forms of MSF such as those associated with facial nerve palsy (22) or Guillain-Barré syndrome (46, 171) have been reported.

In India, a specific *R. conorii* strain, termed *R. conorii indica*, is responsible for typical forms of MSF. Parola et al. reported an imported case of MSF caused by *R. conorii indica* in France (154).

Siberian Tick Typhus

STT was first described in Primorye in the spring-summer season of 1934 to 1935. It is well described in the former USSR, where literature relating to SFG and TG rickettsioses is abundant (55, 125, 196). The disease is also prevalent in Pakistan (200) and has recently been documented in northern China (60, 270). It is prevalent in many tick species, including *Dermacentor*, *Haemaphysalis*, and *Rhipicephalus* spp., and has been identified in rodents, including mice, rats, and hedgehogs (41, 210). The incubation period is usually 4 to 7 days following a tick bite. Thereafter, an ulcerated necrotic lesion appears at the inoculation site, often accompanied by regional lymphadenopathy (Color Plate 13G). Fever (38 to 39°C), headache, myalgia, and digestive disturbances are concomitant symptoms and can last for 6 to 10 days without treatment. The rash, which may be purpuric, usually occurs 2 to 4 days after the onset of clinical symptoms. The central nervous system is often affected during infection. This disease is considered to be a mild spotted fever and is seldom associated with severe complications (196).

Israeli Spotted Fever

The first cases of rickettsial spotted fever were reported in the late 1940s in Israel and were diagnosed as RMSF (83). The number of cases increased following the development of new settlements in the rural areas of Israel. Although the disease presents with clinical features similar to those of MSF, the typical eschar at the inoculation site is usually absent. In 1974, Goldwasser et al. (85) isolated and characterized the rickettsial agent of the disease, finding it to be closely related to but slightly different from *R. conorii*. It is transmitted to humans by *R. sanguineus*. Antigenically, the causative organism, *R. conorii israelensis*, is distinguishable from *R. conorii conorii*, and comparison of rOmpA, rOmpB, and PS120 gene sequences has also demonstrated it to be distinct (84, 204, 207, 215). Several fatal cases and severe forms have been described, especially in children and in patients with glucose-6-phosphate dehydroge-

nase deficiency, and the prevalence of the disease seems to be increasing (83, 85, 86, 193, 268). The incubation period ranges from 7 to 8 days after the tick bite, and the symptoms observed in all the patients are fever and a rash which usually starts on the hands and feet and extends to the rest of the skin. The prevalence of arthralgia, headache, vomiting, and myalgia varies from 13 to 33%. A primary lesion, resembling a small pinkish papule rather than a real eschar, is found less often (7%) than spleno- or hepatomegaly (30 to 35%) (86). Asymptomatic infections have been described and authenticated by seroconversion (211). However, the test used was not specific enough to ensure that *R. conorii israelensis* was definitely the agent provoking seroconversion. In 1999, Israeli spotted fever was identified in Sicily and Portugal (8).

Astrakhan Fever

Around the Caspian Sea, an eruptive febrile summer disease has been observed since 1983. It was apparently unknown before this time and was sufficient to be considered a new disease, named Astrakhan fever (234). The presence of a tache noire was reported in only 20% of patients. The Gamaleya Institute for Epidemiology and Microbiology in Moscow, Russia, tested sera from patients with Astrakhan fever by using the complement fixation test and observed the presence of antibodies in 50 to 70% of patient specimens (13, 233–235) when *R. conorii conorii* was used as the antigen. The clinical and epidemiological aspects have been described to include *R. sanguineus* and *Rhipicephalus pumilio* ticks as vectors (56, 234). The causative agent of the disease, named *R. conorii caspia*, isolated from both patients (47) and ticks (57), is closely related to but distinct from *R. conorii conorii*.

R. conorii caspia has recently been isolated from French military personnel in Chad (71) and from ticks in Kosovo, Serbia (64).

Queensland Tick Typhus

QTT has been recognized as a disease since 1946, when the first cases were observed among troops training in the bush of northern Queensland, Australia (170). This rickettsiosis is distributed all along the eastern coast of Australia (53, 218, 219). More than one causative agent of rickettsiosis is found in Australia. *R. australis*, the etiologic agent of QTT, is prevalent in the northeastern part of the country, while *R. honei* (227) has been isolated from patients with rickettsiosis on Flinders Island, which lies close to Tasmania in the far south. This latter new disease will be discussed below. The areas of endemic infection by the two organisms have yet to be established. Although *R. australis* and *R. honei* show clear biological and genotypic differences (10), the clinical features of the diseases they cause are quite similar. After a sudden onset of illness characterized by fever, headache, and myalgia, patients usually develop a rash (maculopapular or vesicular) within the first 10 days. An eschar seems to be more prevalent in cases from northern Australia (65%). Bites clearly associated with ticks are reported more often in northern Australia, where lesions attributed to insect bites are frequently mentioned. Lymphadenopathy is also a common feature. Only a single fatal case of QTT has been reported to date (220). The common tick species biting humans in Queensland is *Ixodes holocyclus*. This and *Ixodes tasmani* have been confirmed in a study from Queensland to harbor *R. australis* (38). The latter tick seems to play a role in the maintenance of this rickettsia in small animals (38). Moreover, Cook and Campbell (44) detected antibodies in 54 of 307 bandicoots and rodents trapped in northern Queensland.

Japanese or Oriental Spotted Fever

JSF was first described by Mahara, a Japanese physician, and colleagues in 1985 (128, 129, 131). Mahara was alerted by two cases of highly febrile exanthema within 3 months of each other during the summer of 1984. Both patients lived in the countryside, one had a black eschar, and both had collected bamboo shoots on the same mountain. The patients' sera tested positive by the Weil-Felix test (128) and then by MIF with *R. montanensis* as antigen (241). Since that date, the causative organism, *R. japonica*, has been isolated from patients (244) and characterized as a new SFG rickettsia. The disease is now known to be endemic in the southwestern part of Japan, where more than 100 cases have been described. The agent, *R. japonica* (269), and its tick vectors, *Haemaphysalis longicornis* (243) and *Dermacentor taiwanensis* (231), have now been characterized. The ticks *Ixodes ovatus*, *Ixodes persulcatus*, *I. monospinosus*, and *Haemaphysalis flava* have also been incriminated as vectors of this rickettsia (65, 106). It is interesting that this disease is a typical spotted fever, as described in 1899 for RMSF and in 1909 for MSF. That it was not identified until 1986 in Japan, a country with an excellent medical infrastructure, is very surprising. The first diagnosis was made by the Weil-Felix test, which is also used to diagnose scrub typhus, a disease endemic in parts of Japan although not in the area where Mahara observed his cases. This test was chosen because of suspicion of an atypical scrub typhus with a novel clinical presentation and epidemiology. JSF occurs from April to October and is accompanied by fever, headache, an inoculation eschar, and a maculopapular rash. Cases of encephalitis caused by *R. japonica* have also been reported (6, 130).

Flinders Island Spotted Fever and Thai Tick Typhus

FISF was described in 1991 by Stewart, the only medical doctor on Flinders Island in Tasmania, south of Australia. He described 26 cases, observed over 12 years, of a summer febrile illness associated with a rash that was erythematous in the majority of patients and purpuric in two patients with severe cases associated with thrombocytopenia (228). The patients presented with a local lesion (eschar) in 25% of cases and enlarged local nodes in 55% of cases. The patients' sera were initially assayed serologically by the Weil-Felix test and subsequently by MIF, and the results confirmed that the agent was an SFG rickettsia. At the time of Stewart's observations, three rickettsial diseases were known in Australia: murine typhus, scrub typhus, and QTT, as described above. The main clinical differences between QTT and FISF are the occurrence of a vesicular rash and local lymph node enlargement in QTT. The fact that the disease was observed far from its described area of endemicity led to the suggestion that it was a distinct rickettsial infection. This suggestion was confirmed in 1992 (10), when a new isolate was obtained from patients. The isolate was characterized by sequencing of the 17-kDa antigen gene and proposed as a new species, *R. honei* (11, 227).

In Thailand, a rickettsia isolated from pooled ticks and initially named Thai tick typhus rickettsia (200) has been shown to be identical to *R. honei* (227).

African Tick Bite Fever

The history of ATBF takes place in two periods. During the 1930s, Pijper described a very mild disease that was transmitted by tick bite in South Africa and whose epidemiological and clinical features were different from those of MSF, the only known tick-borne rickettsiosis at that time. This disease often occurred without a rash in people infected in the bush by the bite of ticks of the *Amblyomma* complex. Pijper isolated the causative agent and determined that it was different from *R. conorii* by cross-protection studies with guinea pigs. Unfortunately, the isolate was lost and Pijper's data (166, 167) were forgotten. Pijper's successor, Gear (74, 75), isolated *R. conorii* from a *Rhipicephalus* tick in South Africa, and therefore ATBF was considered to be a variant of MSF. However, in 1990, Kelly and Mason (111) isolated rickettsial strains from *Amblyomma hebraeum* ticks in Zimbabwe. They demonstrated that the strains were distinct from *R. conorii* and were indistinguishable from isolates obtained from *Amblyomma variegatum*, *Amblyomma gemma*, and *Amblyomma cohaerens* ticks collected in Ethiopia (33). This rickettsia was shown to be much more prevalent in ticks in Zimbabwe than was *R. conorii* and to infect *Ambly-*

omma ticks, which bite a wide range of animals including humans, as opposed to *R. sanguineus* complex ticks, which rarely bite humans (80). A high seroprevalence of antibodies against this new isolate was also demonstrated in the population, with infection frequencies reaching 80% in some areas of endemicity (112). In 1994, the same rickettsia was isolated from a patient's blood and named *R. africae* (109, 110). This finding confirmed Pijper's work and the presence of a second tick-transmitted rickettsiosis in Africa (109, 110, 113). Several cases have subsequently been reported among travellers returning from either Zimbabwe or South Africa. An unusual feature for a rickettsiosis is that ATBF often occurs as clustered cases (68, 182). The epidemiological and clinical features of ATBF have recently been detailed among patients suffering from symptoms reminiscent of tick-borne rickettsiosis (182). ATBF occurs in travelers to rural areas of sub-Saharan Africa in contact with *Amblyomma* ticks. It is generally milder than MSF (25, 182). The incubation period ranges from 6 to 7 days. A maculopapular or vesicular rash is present in 46% of patients. The inoculation eschar is present in 95% of cases, and there are multiple eschars in 54% (see Color Plate 14A to C). The latter characteristic is very unusual among other rickettsioses and rules out MSF. A lymph node in the draining area of the eschar(s) is found in 43% of cases. As a rule, the illness is uncomplicated. The prevalence of ATBF is high. The attack rate has been reported to be 14% in United States military citizens in Botswana (108) and from 3.9 to 8.6% among travellers to sub-Saharan Africa (107, 182). A prospective study by Jensenius et al. of a cohort of 940 Norwegian travelers to sub-Saharan Africa showed that the disease was even milder than previously expected (106a). In 1998, Parola et al. reported cases of ATBF from Guadeloupe, in the French West Indies (156). It was hypothesized that infected *Amblyomma* ticks had been brought from Africa to the West Indies on cattle at the time of the colonization of these islands by Europeans. This phenomenon has been highlighted recently with the discovery of infected live *Amblyomma* ticks from South Africa transported to Great Britain (182) and Florida (36). It should be noted that ATBF is characterized by a delayed seroconversion when compared to MSF (67). Therefore, a late-phase serum should be obtained more than 4 weeks after the onset of symptoms for accurate serological diagnosis of this rickettsiosis.

Tick-Borne Lymphadenitis (TIBOLA) or *Dermacentor*-Borne-Necrosis- Erythemalymphadenopathy (DEBONEL)

R. slovaca was first isolated in 1968 from a *Dermacentor marginatus* tick in Slovakia (195), but it was not until 1997 that the first documented case of *R. slovaca* was reported in a patient bitten by *D. marginatus* in France (177). The woman had presented with fever and an eschar at the site of the tick bite to the scalp which was surrounded by an inflammatory erythema. She also suffered from painful cervical lymph nodes and fatigue. Similar undocumented cases had previously been reported in France, Spain, Slovakia, and Hungary, where this disease was named wood scar, DEBONEL, or TIBOLA (116, 150). *R. slovaca* was found in all European countries where *D. marginatus* ticks were screened for rickettsial infections, including France, Portugal, Switzerland, Yugoslavia, Slovakia, Ukraine, Armenia, and Siberia (216, 222). In 2002, a series of 17 culture- and/or PCR-proven cases of *R. slovaca* infection from France or Hungary were reported (184). Patients presented with a single inoculation eschar to the scalp (Color Plate 15A) and enlarged cervical lymph nodes (Color Plate 15B) following a *Dermacentor* bite to the scalp. The median duration of incubation was 7 days. Fifteen patients were diagnosed between October and May. Lymph nodes were painful in 10 patients. Only two patients presented with fever, and only one developed a cutaneous rash. No complications were observed, but four patients developed a localized alopecia at the site of the bite and three suffered from persistent asthenia. Only 50% of patients developed detectable antibodies, which may reflect the fact that this disease is a localized infection.

Lymphangitis-Associated Rickettsiosis

R. sibirica mongolotimonae was first isolated in 1991 from *Hyalomma asiaticum*, collected in Inner Mongolia, and named isolate HA-91 (270). It was antigenically and genotypically unique among SFG rickettsiae. In 1996, an indistinguishable isolate was obtained from the blood and the skin of a 63-year-old patient in southern France (178). The patient was hospitalized in March (an atypical month for MSF) with a mild disease characterized only by a discrete rash and an inoculation eschar in the left groin. This patient was a resident of Marseille, France, with no prior travel history. The only possibly relevant history was that the patient had collected compost from a garden where migratory birds were resting (178). Birds carry ticks, and *Hyalomma* species can parasitize birds. A second human case was diagnosed in May 1998 in a human immunodeficiency virus-positive patient who had been gardening in a rural area of Marseille (70). The patient presented with fever, headache, an eschar, lymphangitis, and painful satellite lymphadenopathy. In 2001, *R. sibirica mongolotimonae* was detected in *Hyalomma truncatum* ticks collected in sub-Saharan

Africa (155). This finding has highlighted the risk of *R. sibirica mongolotimonae* infections in Africa and also the role of *Hyalomma* ticks as vectors of this rickettsia. In southern France, the vector has yet to be described, but it is hypothesized that the patients were bitten by migratory bird ticks. Recent studies from France (65a) and South Africa (172a) have shown that lymphangitis-associated rickettsiosis is also present in Algeria and South Africa. The disease is characterized by a febrile maculopapular rash. The inoculation eschar may be multiple in 22% of cases, 55% of patients may present with enlarged lymph nodes, and 44% may present with a lymphangitis expanding from the inoculation eschar to a draining node.

Infection Due to *R. helvetica*

R. helvetica was first isolated from *I. ricinus* in Switzerland in 1979 (29). This rickettsia has also been found in *Ixodes* ticks from France, Italy, Sweden, and Japan (65, 106, 142, 153). In 2000, a French patient was reported to have specifically seroconverted to *R. helvetica* in the course of an unexplained febrile illness (66). In the same study, the authors reported a seroprevalence of 9.2% against *R. helvetica* among forest workers from eastern France, the area where the patient lived. Involvement of this species in human infection was also reported in 1999 in young Swedish patients who died from acute perimyocarditis (143). *R. helvetica* was detected in various tissue specimens from both patients, and their sera reacted with SFG rickettsia antigens. In 2002, an association of *R. helvetica* with sarcoidosis has been proposed (144). However, as the data are mainly based on PCR analyses, these findings need to be confirmed.

Infection Due to *R. aeschlimannii*

R. aeschlimannii was first obtained from *Hyalomma marginatum* ticks in Morocco in 1997 (16) and then isolated from *H. marginatum* ticks from sub-Saharan Africa (155). In August 2000, a first case of *R. aeschlimannii* infection was diagnosed in a 36-year-old patient who had travelled to Morocco (181). This patient presented with an inoculation eschar to the ankle, a fever of 39.5°C, and a generalized maculopapular rash. The diagnosis was obtained by PCR amplification and sequencing of a fragment of the *ompA* gene of *R. aeschlimannii*. A second case was reported in a South African patient who removed a *Rhipicephalus appendiculatus* tick from his right thigh after a hunting trip (172). Early doxycycline therapy prevented the development of symptoms, but *R. aeschlimannii* was detected by PCR from a biopsy of the bite site.

Infection Due to "*R. heilongjiangensis*"

"*R. heilongjiangensis*" was first isolated in 1982 from *Dermacentor silvarum* ticks collected in the Heilongjiang province of China (61). Between May and July 1992, 12 patients presenting with fever, headache, rash, eschar, regional lympadenopathy, and conjunctivitis following a tick bite in the province were reported to be infected by this strain on the basis of serological results (124). Between May and June 1996, rickettsial isolates identical to "*R. heilongjiangensis*" were obtained from seven patients with clinical manifestations of SFG rickettsiosis, thus confirming the pathogenic role of this rickettsia (264). A recent series of "*R. heilongjiangensis*" infections demonstrated that the disease presented as a mild febrile rash in summer, with a single inoculation eschar in 92% of patients, enlarged lymph nodes in 77% of patients, and a lymphangitis expanding from the eschar to a draining node in 15% of patients (138a).

Infection Due to *R. parkeri*

R. parkeri was isolated in 1937 (151) from *Amblyomma maculatum* collected from Texan cows. It has never been recovered outside the United States. It has been shown to share a close genotypic relationship with *R. africae*, which also parasitizes *Amblyomma* species in sub-Saharan Africa. The first case of proven *R. parkeri* infection has recently been reported in a 40-year-old man who developed a febrile maculopapular rash associated with multiple eschars on his lower extremities and an enlarged inguinal lymph node (150a). The patient lived in a suburban area of South Virginia, where he was frequently exposed to ticks. He fully recovered following a doxycycline therapy.

RICKETTSIAE OF UNKNOWN PATHOGENICITY

Rickettsiae of unknown pathogenicity constitute a reservoir of potential pathogens (Table 2). Therefore, they should be considered bacteria of unknown pathogenicity rather than nonpathogenic. Indeed, the most recently described pathogenic rickettsiae, including *R. africae*, *R. slovaca*, *R. helvetica*, *R. aeschlimannii*, *R. sibirica mongolotimonae*, and "*R. heilongjiangensis*" have been demonstrated to be pathogenic for humans, whereas they had been initially isolated from ticks only.

R. rhipicephali (32) was first reported from Mississippi in 1975 (34). It was isolated from *R. sanguineus* and has subsequently been detected in France (49) and Portugal (9) in the same tick species. It has been suspected as causing fever in a patient following a dog tick bite (32). In the United States, *R. rhipicephali* has been isolated frequently from *D. occidentalis* and *Dermacentor andersoni* and occasionally from *D. variabilis* (72).

An unnamed rickettsia, JC880, was reported in Pakistan (199, 200) in 1970 and 1973; five isolates were available and have now been shown to be distinct from *R. conorii*, *R. sibirica*, Thai tick typhus rickettsia, *R. parkeri*, *R. rickettsii*, *R. akari*, and *R. australis*.

R. massiliae (18) parasitizes *R. sanguineus* and *Rhipicephalus turanicus* in France (14), Portugal (9) and Greece (7) and *Rhipicephalus muhsamae* in Mali (155, 239). A closely related strain (Bar 29) has also been isolated in Barcelona from *R. sanguineus* (19). This bacterium is identical to an isolate that was previously described as MTU5 (14) and is slightly different from *R. massiliae* by antigenic and phenotypic criteria. The geographic distribution of this rickettsia and its predominance in *Rhipicephalus* species in certain areas such as Catalonia, Spain, make it a pathogen of potential importance. This bacterium exhibits a natural resistance to rifampin in cell cultures (19).

Strain S (54) has been isolated from *R. sanguineus* in Armenia. Spotted fever is endemic in that country, where *R. sibirica*, a known pathogen, has also been isolated. Consequently, the pathogenic role of strain S is unknown and requires investigation.

R. bellii (164) is the species most frequently isolated from ticks in the United States. It was first obtained from *D. variabilis* in 1966 by Bell and has subsequently been recovered from *D. andersoni*, *D. occidentalis*, and *D. albipictus* and from members of other tick genera such as *Ornithodoros concanensis*, *Argas cooleyi*, and *Haemophysalis leporispalustris* (164). The species is apparently confined to America, where its pathogenic role has yet to be discovered.

R. montanensis (20) was first isolated from *D. variabilis* and *D. andersoni* in Montana in 1953. It is not pathogenic for guinea pigs but has been isolated from rodents (genera *Microtus* and *Peromiscus*) (20).

Unnamed species were isolated from *D. occidentalis* in California and *Dermacentor parumapertus* in Nevada and Utah (162, 229).

R. peacockii, the eastside agent, is a rickettsia strictly located in *D. andersoni* ovarial tissue in Montana (152). It is not found in hemocytes but has recently been grown in a *D. andersoni* cell line (DAE 100). Sequencing of 16S rRNA- and rOmpA-encoding genes showed that it is close to but distinct from *R. rickettsii* (141).

The strain DnS14 has been detected in *D. silvarum* from eastern Siberia and from *Dermacentor niveus* from Kazakhstan (222). This strain belongs to the *R. massiliae* group.

The strain RpA4 has been detected in *Dermacentor reticulatus* from Russia and *D. niveus* from Kazakhstan (222). This strain belongs to the *R. massiliae* group.

A rickettsia isolated from blood and lymph nodes of patients and from *Amblyomma americanum* ticks collected in Texas has been described. This rickettsia, named *R. texiana*, was responsible for over 1,000 cases of Bullis fever among World War II troops in training at Camp Bullis (5).

An unnamed rickettsial species isolated from *A. americanum* in 1971 in Alabama by Burgdorfer was described in 1978 (165).

"*Rickettsia amblyommii*" (173) has recently been isolated from the lone star tick *A. americanum*. Little is known about its prevalence or its pathogenicity.

Three uncultivated rickettsiae, named Rav1, Rav3, and Rav9, were detected by PCR from *A. variegatum* ticks in Niger and Mali (155). Based on *ompA* and *gltA* analyses, they were found to be closely related to but different from *R. africae*.

R. canadensis was first isolated from *H. leporispalustris* ticks removed from rabbits in Ontario, Canada (138). It was first considered a member of the TG rickettsia, based on serologic cross-reactions (105). However, the genetic data obtained by the sequences of both the 16S rRNA and the citrate synthase gene showed that *R. canadensis* is outside the TG (206–208, 215). The role of *R. canadensis* as a human pathogen has not been established. Serological evidence of human infection has been reported (24) in four patients presenting with an RMSF-like disease in California and Texas. A role for *R. canadensis* in acute cerebral vasculitis is also suspected (94, 123, 256) but warrants further investigation.

An unnamed species has been obtained from *Ixodes pacificus* ticks in Oregon (104).

"*R. hulinii*" was isolated from *Haemaphysalis concinna* ticks in China (272, 273). This species is closely related to *R. japonica*.

The closely related strains IRS3 (for *I. ricinus* Slovakia 3) and IRS 4 have been detected by PCR from *I. ricinus* ticks in Slovakia (214). These rickettsiae are phylogenetically grouped with *R. helvetica*, the strain AT-1, and "*Rickettsia monacensis*." IRS4 has recently been successfully cultivated from ticks (217).

"*R. monacensis*" was isolated from *I. ricinus* ticks collected in a city park in Munich, Germany (223). It was cultivated in DAE100 cells, derived from *D. andersoni*, and in IRE11 cells, derived from *I. ricinus*. "*R. monacensis*" is closely related to the IRS3 and to four strains within the *R. helvetica* group.

The strain AT-1 has been isolated from *Amblyomma testudinarium* ticks from Japan. It is phylogenetically close to but different from the strains IRS3 and IRS4 detected in *I. ricinus* in Slovakia and also belongs to the *R. helvetica* group (65, 106).

"*Candidatus* Rickettsia tarasevichiae" was detected in *I. persulcatus* ticks from various areas of Russia (221). It is phylogenetically closely related to *R. canadensis*.

DIAGNOSIS OF TICK-TRANSMITTED RICKETTSIOSES

Clinical Presentation

Although the advent of novel diagnostic tools such as the shell vial assay (134) and DNA detection assays has dramatically improved the efficiency of diagnosing rickettsioses and identifying their agents, it is important to consider that diseases such as RMSF and MSF have been initially described solely on the basis of clinical evidence, thus emphasizing the importance of clinical features for diagnosis. Careful clinical examination and epidemiologic investigation of patients with potential rickettsioses is critical. Clinically, the mainstay of the diagnosis has always been the presence of a characteristic rash. The typical clinical picture during rickettsiosis is high fever (39.5 to 40°C), headache, and rash. The disease can be mild or severe but will usually last for 2 to 3 weeks. This very basic knowledge should always be considered. In 1910, Conor and Bruch characterized MSF from only two cases because it was different from viral eruptions, which are usually milder and of shorter duration (43). They concluded that the two cases were equivalent to RMSF. In Astrakhan, an exanthematic infection was mistakenly suspected of being due to an echovirus, enterovirus, or arbovirus infection when it was, in fact, a rickettsiosis. The physicians making the diagnosis were not aware that the clinical presentation that they were facing was pathognomonic of a rickettsial eruption. Another example is the multiplicity of inoculation eschars, which is very unusual among rickettsioses. This feature observed in patients in sub-Saharan Africa should orient the diagnosis towards *R. africae*, whereas in southern France, *R. sibirica mongolotimonae* should be suspected. A diagnosing physician must therefore have a high index of suspicious and good knowledge of the literature when diagnosing rickettsial diseases.

Nonspecific Laboratory Findings

Most of the knowledge on nonspecific biological variations in the course of rickettsioses has been collected from MSF and RMSF. In MSF, anemia may occur in 12% of patients (51). The leukocyte count is usually normal, but leukopenia is observed in 12 to 20% of cases and leukocytosis in 11 to 28% of cases.

Thrombocytopenia occurs in 12.5 to 30% of cases. Levels of inflammatory proteins from the acute phase response (e.g., C-reactive protein and fibrinogen) are often increased. There may be a striking elevation of transaminases, with serum glutamic oxaloacetic transaminase (SGOT) and serum glutamic pyruvate transaminase (SGPT) levels increased in 37 to 39% of patients with MSF (51, 87). Elevated levels of bilirubin, lactic dehydrogenase, and creatine phosphokinase may be observed in 9, 44, and 18% of cases, respectively (51). Hypoproteinemia is observed in up to 3% of cases in MSF versus 18% in RMSF (51, 98). Increased levels of blood urea nitrogen and creatinine occur in 25 and 17% of patients, respectively (51). In severe cases, coagulopathy marked by decreased clotting factors may cause bleeding or thrombosis, hypocalcemia is frequent, and hyponatremia caused by increased secretion of antidiuretic hormone is common (51, 191).

Serology

Serological assays are the simplest diagnostic tests to perform, since serum is the easiest human blood specimen to obtain and it can readily be sent to a reference laboratory. The Weil-Felix test was the first serological assay to be developed. It involves antigens from three *Proteus* strains: *Proteus vulgaris* OX2, *P. vulgaris* OX19, and *Proteus mirabilis* OXK. This test is used to diagnose rickettsiosis based on serological cross-reactions (180). Antibody reaction to strain OX19 identifies TG rickettsiae (louse-borne *R. prowazekii* and flea-borne *R. typhi*) and *R. rickettsii*, reaction to OX2 identifies SFG rickettsiae, and reaction to OXK identifies *O. tsutsugamushi* (252). Although this test lacks sensitivity and specificity, it has the advantage of detecting early rising antibodies and is simple to carry out. Therefore, it continues to be used in some localities in many countries as a first line test.

Techniques such as immunoperoxidase assay or complement fixation tests, which lack both sensitivity and specificity, are no longer recommended (119).

Currently, the most commonly used and the reference serological test is the indirect immunofluorescence assay (119). It has been improved as a micromethod (MIF) and can simultaneously detect antibodies to several antigens with the same drop of serum in a single well containing multiple dots. This limits the titer variations linked to reader subjectivity. MIF has also been demonstrated to be applicable to blood dried on blotting paper and thus to specimens collected in situations where adequate preservation of serum specimens is not possible (62). It allows determination of both immunoglobulin G (IgG) and IgM antibodies. The early phase serum (<15 days following onset of symptoms) is often negative. Therefore, a late or convalescence-phase serum (>15 days) is required. A seroconversion marked by a fourfold or greater increase in antibody titers has a great value for the diagnosis of a rickettsiosis. Cutoff values of 1:64 for total Igs and 1:32 for IgM are used for the diagnosis. For ATBF, it has been demonstrated that the seroconversion is delayed by comparison with other tick-transmitted rickettsioses; therefore, the convalescence-phase serum should be sampled a minimum of 4 weeks following the onset of symptoms (67). In *R. slovaca* infection, the serological response is weak, possibly because of the lack of generalized infection; thus, other diagnostic methods should be used, such as culture or PCR analysis of skin or lymph node biopsies (184). However, although MIF is highly sensitive, cross-reactions can occur between rickettsiae and with *Ehrlichia*, *Bartonella*, *Legionella*, and *Proteus* infections (95, 96, 180). These cross-reacting antibodies appear to be directed against the lipopolysaccharide. Additional false-positive IgM antibodies are observed with the rheumatoid factor and in viral and parasitic infections generating unspecific lymphocyte B proliferation (i.e., cytomegalovirus, Epstein-Barr virus, and malaria). To identify the infecting *Rickettsia* species by discriminating cross-reacting antibodies between two or more antigens, cross-adsorption has been developed and successfully applied to samples from patients with rickettsioses (68, 93). The test serum is first mixed separately with the bacteria involved in the cross-reaction and then tested against each of these antigens. Cross-adsorption results in the disappearance of both homologous and heterologous antibodies when adsorption is performed with the bacterium responsible for the disease, whereas only heterologous antibodies are removed when adsorption is performed with the bacterium responsible for the cross-reaction. Although this technique is accurate, it is limited because it is very expensive and time-consuming, since a large number of rickettsiae are required for each absorption step.

The enzyme-linked immunosorbent assay was first introduced for detection of antibodies against *R. typhi* and *R. prowazekii* (89). This technique is highly sensitive and reproducible, allowing differentiation of IgG and IgM antibodies. The method was later adapted to the diagnosis of RMSF (246).

The Western blot immunoassay (WB) (179), employing antigens that are analyzed by electroblotting and SDS-PAGE, allows differentiation among SFG rickettsiae, provided that acute-phase sera are used. This test is able to detect early antibodies when other tests are still negative. WB detects two types of antigens, lipopolysaccharide and high-molecular-weight proteins (rOmpA, rOmpB, and PS120). These pro-

teins are species specific (15, 180) and provide the basis for rickettsial serotyping (165). However, although inoculated mice produce a predominance of antibodies against these proteins, human beings do not, and cross-reactions between rickettsial proteins make it difficult to identify the infecting rickettsia to the species level (95, 96). If sera are collected very early in infection, strong homologous reactions are often observed, making a specific diagnosis possible. However, as this rarely occurs, more specific methods are needed. Moreover, WB is time-consuming, available only in specialized settings, and lacks reproducibility. WB may be completed by cross-absorption (25, 68).

It should be emphasized that serological testing is insensitive early in acute infection, can give nonspecific results, and, therefore, should be considered only the first step in diagnosing or recognizing a rickettsial disease. In general, direct evidence for the identity of a rickettsial pathogen is required before purported new syndromes, new manifestations, or new areas of endemic infection can be defined. This evidence should be based on a combination of culture, microscopic, or genetic detection techniques and not solely on serology. In fact, the literature is full of serologically based evidence for new diseases or new clinical forms of disease that must be viewed with some degree of skepticism. Multiple sclerosis, myocardial infarction, and schizophrenia have all been falsely reported to be related to rickettsioses on the basis of serological tests and have led to the prescription of incorrect therapeutic regimens (82, 120).

Isolation of Rickettsiae

Rickettsiae are characterized by Gimenez staining, although some other bacteria also retain the basic fuchsin stain and must be distinguished from rickettsiae on the basis of culture requirements. For example, coinfection of ticks by "*Wolbachia*"-like organisms is possible, and these organisms may appear as rickettsiae in nonspecific stains. Culture of rickettsiae should be reserved for specialized laboratories equipped with biohazard facilities; also, *R. rickettsii* has been recognized as a potential agent of bioterrorism. *Rickettsia* has been isolated by several different methods. Animal inoculation has been widely used, originally with guinea pigs and subsequently with rats and voles. Embryonated eggs have also been employed. However, cell culture is currently the most widely used system for primary isolation. The shell vial cell culture method, a microculture system derived from a commercially available method for cytomegalovirus culture and early antigen detection but without the addition of antibiotics except cotrimoxazole (114), has been shown to be highly efficient for obtaining rickettsial isolates from human specimens (9, 12, 57, 134, 245). This method comprises a centrifugation step, which increases the ratio and adherence of rickettsiae to cells. Another advancement for the successful isolation of rickettsiae has been the use of various cell lines such as tick or mammalian cells. One of the most useful cell lines for the isolation of tick-borne rickettsiae is the HEL (human embryonic lung fibroblast) cell line. The multiplication of cell lines allows a variety of culture conditions. Varying culture temperature is also useful. Heparinized blood (leukocytic buffy coat), skin and lymph node biopsies, cerebrospinal fluid taken before antibiotic therapy, and ticks may be used for cell culture (59).

The best human specimen is undoubtedly biopsy of skin from the inoculation site eschar. Each sample is assayed in triplicate. Rickettsiae are detected directly inside the shell vial by immunofluorescence staining and microscopic examination of coverslips. After fixation with acetone, the coverslips are incubated with the patient's serum and various monoclonal antibodies. The culture is kept for 2 weeks, with examination of one shell vial each week. After this time, if immunofluorescence is negative, the culture is considered negative. If immunofluorescence is positive, parallel shell vials are inoculated onto confluent monolayers of HEL cells in culture flasks in an attempt to obtain isolates of *Rickettsia* spp. Usually, culture of rickettsiae takes 3 to 7 days. Many rickettsiae, including *R. conorii*, *R. rickettsii*, *R. massiliae*, *R. aeschlimannii*, *R. slovaca*, *R. helvetica*, *R. sibirica mongolotimonae*, and *R. africae*, have been isolated by this method. Although this assay is useful, about one-third of the isolates are lost on passage for unknown reasons. The importance of culture cannot, however, be underestimated, since obtaining an isolate from a tick or a patient is the ultimate goal in rickettsial disease description (102).

Immunological Detection of Rickettsiae

Skin biopsy specimens have been used in the diagnosis of both RMSF and MSF since the early work of Walker et al. (247). Samples can be tested fresh, frozen, or after fixation and paraffin embedding. The inoculation eschar, when present, should definitely be biopsied, because it contains large numbers of rickettsiae (139). The detection of rickettsiae in skin biopsy specimens by utilizing coated magnetic beads has also proven to be useful (247, 249). Prior to detection, biopsy samples are cut into small pieces and subjected to collagenase treatment. Endothelial cells are then recovered from these digestion mixtures with immunomagnetic beads. This technique allows rickettsiae to be recovered with relative ease, even from samples

from patients receiving antibiotic therapy. Other clinical samples obtained at autopsy can be tested in the same manner as skin biopsy specimens. The use of methods incorporating specific polyclonal antibodies or monoclonal antibodies allows the detection of rickettsiae in blood or other tissues. This diagnostic approach allows for confirmation of infection in patients before their seroconversion and thus permits early prescription of specific treatment. The method can also be used to diagnose rickettsial infection retrospectively in fixed tissues. This technique has been adapted to allow the immunologic detection of rickettsiae in circulating endothelial cells, which are isolated from whole blood with immunomagnetic beads coated with an endothelial cell-specific monoclonal antibody (76). A 1-ml volume of whole blood diluted 1:4 with phosphate-buffered saline is mixed with a suspension of monoclonal antibody-coated beads. Following incubation, the magnetic beads and rosetted cells are separated from other blood constituents with a magnetic particle extractor. After being washed, the rosetted cells are divided into two aliquots. One is stained with acridine orange and counted in a hemocytometer, and the other is cytocentrifuged onto a glass slide. These smears are then fixed, and bacteria are detected by immunofluorescence with polyclonal *R. conorii* antiserum. The sensitivity of this method is estimated to be 50% for acutely ill patients (118). Moreover, it has a prognostic value, because the number of circulating endothelial cells detected is directly proportional to the severity of the infection (77).

Ticks collected for attempted isolation of rickettsiae should be kept alive before being tested. If they need to be transported or kept for long periods, a humidifier box is useful. While the ticks are still alive, the hemolymph test should be performed following surface sterilization (28). In this procedure, one tick leg is broken, allowing the collection of a drop of hemolymph, which can be spread onto a slide and then subjected either to Gimenez staining (81) or to immunodetection methods. The tick should then be dissected (114, 159). Organs, including reproductive tissue, can be carefully dissected and separated for further testing. Immunological detection methods can employ polyclonal or monoclonal antibodies; the latter can be used to determine the infecting species. Immunofluorescent labels have been widely used in conjunction with these antibodies, but immunoperoxidase labels and detection systems appear to allow a better microscopic definition of cells around the detected rickettsiae (52).

PCR-Based Detection of Rickettsiae

Rickettsiae may be detected by PCR amplification from an array of samples that include blood, skin biopsy samples, and arthropod tissues. Specific sample preparation procedures must be used prior to testing samples. Blood is held at an ambient temperature until cells are sedimented and rickettsiae are sought in the leukocytic cell buffy coat. Although heparinized blood is used for cell culture, it is necessary to use blood collected in EDTA or sodium citrate for PCR amplification, because heparin inhibits PCR. The PCR amplification must be performed before the initiation of antibiotic treatment and before antibody becomes detectable. The tache noire is the most useful biopsy sample to assay although not always present. Fresh tissues are preferred for this procedure, but paraffin-embedded tissues and even slide-fixed specimens may be used (226). Tache noire samples are preferred for detecting SFG rickettsiae because more bacteria are present than in blood; several such isolates have been characterized in our laboratory by this approach (25, 178). PCR amplification of tache noire or blood samples can be very useful because infection can be detected before a cell culture is positive or seroconversion has occurred. PCR-based methods for the detection of rickettsiae are attractive as they not only circumvent the need for culture (and the biohazard risk) but also potentially offer more sensitivity and specificity. Rickettsial DNA can also be detected in ticks (72, 73), fleas, and lice by PCR-based amplification methods (99). Detection strategies based on recognition of sequences within the genes encoding the 16S rRNA gene (206, 230), a 17-kDa protein (4, 11, 12), the citrate synthase (187, 212, 263), and the outer membrane proteins rOmpA (69, 204), rOmpB (78, 207), and PS120 (215) have been developed. The complete sequence of the *R. conorii* genome has provided an important source of gene sequences for further PCR-based assays (148). Most of the PCR assays to date are not specific for individual rickettsial species, and reaction products must be further analyzed to identify the species being detected.

Recently, a PCR assay with increased sensitivity, named suicide PCR, has been developed (67a, 176, 182–184, 197). This test was mainly designed to detect DNA from blood samples as regular PCR has a poor sensitivity when applied to blood. This technique is a nested PCR using single-use primers targeting a gene never amplified previously in the laboratory. Such a procedure avoids "vertical" contamination by amplicons from previous assays. All positive PCR products are sequenced to identify the causative agent. Suicide PCR has been successful with EDTA-blood, serum, and skin and lymph node specimens. Leitner et al. have also successfully applied nested PCR to serum and tissue specimens from patients suffering from severe MSF (121).

Identification and Differentiation of Rickettsiae

Rickettsiae are poorly stained by Gram stain but retain basic fuchsin when stained by the Gimenez method (81). For many years, the differentiation of rickettsiae was based solely on immunologic methods. Initially, the toxin neutralization test was used with mice (21, 200); this was followed by complement fixation (169) and later MIF (165). The main problems with these techniques are that reference sera are needed and that each time a new isolate is tested, the test sample and all other antigens need to be screened against all antisera. Monoclonal antibodies against *R. rickettsii* (1, 3), *R. akari* (137, 267), *R. conorii* (250, 267), *R. japonica* (240), *R. massiliae* (266), *R. africae* (265, 267), *R. sibirica* (267), and *R. slovaca* (267) have been introduced. Although these are useful tools, a complete collection organized in pools is required to identify all rickettsiae. Protein analysis by SDS-PAGE has also been used to differentiate rickettsial species (158). The molecular masses of the major protein antigens, rOmpA, PS120, and rOmpB, are estimated to be 115, 120, and 155 kDa for *R. rickettsii*, respectively; although their precise masses vary among rickettsial species, these proteins determine the serospecificity in mice (15). However, since the reproducibility of SDS-PAGE is never perfect and depends on gel conditions and solubilization temperature, it is usually necessary to include all species when attempting to identify a new isolate. Furthermore, since comparison with other species or strains is needed, it is necessary to introduce all purified rickettsiae; the technique is time-consuming and laborious. Macrorestriction analysis of rickettsiae by pulsed-field gel electrophoresis is also a sensitive method for differentiating species (205). It has been a useful approach for identifying rickettsiae, but much biomass is required and it is necessary to include other rickettsiae on the gel to obtain a precise comparison of profiles. Thus, applying this approach each time a strain is isolated is almost impossible. Regnery et al. (194) described the utility of RFLP analysis of PCR-amplified fragments of the citrate synthase and rOmpA-encoding genes (204). This technique has proven to be sensitive and practical, and when it was coupled with RFLP analysis of an *ompB* gene fragment (14, 58), all Russian, European, and many Chinese isolates were identified (9, 55, 57, 270). RFLP analysis of the gene encoding a 17-kDa protein has also been used (12, 175). Species-specific RFLP profiles can be stored in a database, simplifying subsequent identifications. By sequencing the PCR amplification product, it is easy to obtain a precise identification of a new isolate. Since a databank of sequences exists, the determined sequence can be compared with those previously obtained. Sequencing part of the genes encoding the 16S rRNA, citrate synthase, 17-kDa protein, rOmpA, rOmpB, and PS120 was used to characterize rickettsia. The most useful identification of an unidentified rickettsia is based on PCR amplification followed by sequencing of fragments of the citrate synthase-encoding (*gltA*) or rOmpA-encoding (*ompA*) genes. However, the use of broad-spectrum 16S rRNA gene primers allows PCR to be used to detect rickettsiae in unexpected conditions. The 5' end of the *ompA* gene is highly variable among rickettsiae which possess this gene (i.e., most of the tick-borne rickettsiae except *R. helvetica*). Interestingly, *ompA* sequence differences have also been detected among *R. conorii* isolates which demonstrate genotypic diversity (69, 204). Differences in the *metK* gene were used to discriminate *R. montanensis* from *R. rhipicephali* in tick tissues (126, 127). In 2003, gene sequence-based criteria were proposed to facilitate the identification of new rickettsial isolates as new *Rickettsia* species or not (63a). Moreover, recently, a method based on the comparison of highly variable intergenic spacer sequences, named multispacer typing, has been developed for typing of *R. conorii* isolates (71a).

TREATMENT

Three methods have been described to test the antibiotic susceptibility of rickettsiae: (i) the inhibition of plaque-forming units, which was the first in vitro method developed (135, 185); (ii) a microplaque colorimetric assay based on the staining of intact cells with neutral red (185, 202); and (iii) a method using quantitative PCR (203). Antibiotics active against rickettsiae in vitro include tetracyclines, chloramphenicol, rifampin, fluoroquinolones, josamycin, roxithromycin, and pristinamycin (202). Newer macrolides, azithromycin, clarithromycin, and telithromycin have also demonstrated activity against these bacteria (201, 202). In contrast, beta-lactams, erythromycin, aminoglycosides, and co-trimoxazole are not active against tick-transmitted rickettsiae. Members of the *R. massiliae* group, including the pathogenic *R. aeschlimannii*, are naturally resistant to rifampin due to a mutation in the *rpoB* gene (50).

Doxycycline (200 mg per day, usually given as two divided doses) is the treatment of choice for tick-transmitted rickettsioses (100). It can be prescribed for adults and for children 8 years or older (174) but not for pregnant women or allergic patients. It is relatively contraindicated in children under 8 years. In such patients, 50 to 75 mg/kg of body weight/day of chloramphenicol or 50 mg/kg/day of josamycin may be administered. A combination of rifampin and erythromycin has also been successfully used for a pregnant woman (42). Appropriate antibiotic therapy should be prescribed early for any suspected tick-transmitted rickettsiosis.

In patients with severe forms such as malignant MSF, doxycycline should be administered intravenously and for up to 24 h after resolution of fever. The exact treatment duration is not fully determined. Usually, therapy should be continued for up to 2 or 3 days after the patient's fever has abated. However, in MSF a single dose of 200 mg of doxycycline has been shown to be sufficient. In pregnant women, josamycin has proven to be active at a dose of 3 g per day for 7 days. Fluoroquinolones and newer macrolides are as active in vitro as doxycycline but are less well proven clinically and require longer treatment (39, 202, 213). Usually, hospitalization is needed only in rare severe cases of rickettsioses, and symptomatic treatment and supportive care should be given in addition to the antibiotics. Corticosteroids have not proven useful.

CONCLUSIONS

Ten new tick-transmitted rickettsioses have been described over the last 12 years, whereas only four had been characterized prior to 1984. This dramatic increase in the number of recognized rickettsial infections has resulted from numerous circumstances. First, the role of the astute physician should be emphasized, as in the case of FISF, JSF, and Astrakhan fever. In other cases, epidemiological evidence played a major role, as for ATBF. In this case, the demonstration of the prevalence of a *Rickettsia* species in ticks led to a prospective work to detect clinical cases, and then a modification of human activities, such as tourism, amplified the importance of the disease. Finally, technological advances have allowed easier recognition of new pathogens and diagnosis of infection, as with *R. sibirica mongolotimonae*, *R. slovaca*, *R. aeschlimannii*, *R. parkeri*, and "*R. heilongjiangensis*" infections. In these cases, the identification of isolates by molecular methods or improved culture systems allowed for incrimination of a new species in human diseases.

Will there be additional tick-transmitted rickettsioses described? First, one should consider the potential candidates, which are described in the section on rickettsiae of unknown pathogenicity. It is likely that the number of rickettsiae found in ticks will increase in the coming years. If a vector is able to bite humans, rickettsiae harbored by these ticks should be considered potential pathogens, as is the case for most of the tick-transmitted rickettsiae. Second, the etiology of some human diseases whose cause is currently unknown may, in some cases, be rickettsial, such as acute cerebral vasculitis. Moreover, one may expect new diseases to be recognized in places where no spotted fevers have yet been described. It should be expected that in countries where spotted fevers are known, several may exist in the same place, making serological surveys difficult, as has occurred in southern France, Portugal, and in southern Africa. Finally, when attributing a disease to a rickettsia, the obligate intracellular nature of these bacteria sets them apart from the free-living bacteria, and thus their pathogenic role should be based only upon strong evidence.

REFERENCES

1. Anacker, R. L., R. H. List, R. E. Mann, S. F. Hayes, and L. A. Thomas. 1985. Characterization of monoclonal antibodies protecting mice against *Rickettsia rickettsii*. *J. Infect. Dis.* 151:1052–1060.

2. Anacker, R. L., R. E. Mann, and C. Gonzales. 1987. Reactivity of monoclonal antibodies to *Rickettsia rickettsii* with spotted fever and typhus group rickettsiae. *J. Clin. Microbiol.* 25:167–171.

3. Anacker, R. L., G. A. McDonald, R. H. List, and R. E. Mann. 1987. Neutralizing activity of monoclonal antibodies to heat-sensitive and heat-resistant epitopes of *Rickettsia rickettsii* surface proteins. *Infect. Immun.* 55:825–827.

4. Anderson, B. E., and T. Tzianabos. 1989. Comparative sequence analysis of a genus-common rickettsial antigen gene. *J. Bacteriol.* 171:5199–5201.

5. Anigstein, L., and D. Anigstein. 1975. A review of the evidence in retrospect for a rickettsial etiology in Bullis fever. *Tex. Rep. Biol. Med.* 33:201–211.

6. Araki, M., K. Takatsuka, J. Kawamura, and Y. Kanno. 2002. Japanese spotted fever involving the central nervous system: two case reports and a literature review. *J. Clin. Microbiol.* 40:3874–3876.

7. Babalis, T., Y. Tselentis, V. Roux, A. Psaroulaki, and D. Raoult. 1994. Isolation and identification of a rickettsial strain related to *Rickettsia massiliae* in Greek ticks. *Am. J. Trop. Med. Hyg.* 50:365–372.

8. Bacellar, F., L. Beati, A. Franca, J. Pocas, R. Regnery, and A. Filipe. 1999. Israeli spotted fever rickettsia (*Rickettsia conorii* complex) associated with human disease in Portugal. *Emerg. Infect. Dis.* 5:835–836.

9. Bacellar, F., R. L. Regnery, M. S. Nuncio, and A. R. Filipe. 1995. Genotypic evaluation of rickettsial isolates recovered from various species of ticks in Portugal. *Epidemiol. Infect.* 114:169–178.

10. Baird, R. W., M. Lloyd, J. Stenos, B. C. Ross, R. S. Stewart, and B. Dwyer. 1992. Characterization and comparison of Australian human spotted fever group rickettsiae. *J. Clin. Microbiol.* 30:2896–2902.

11. Baird, R. W., J. Stenos, R. Stewart, B. Hudson, M. Lloyd, S. Aiuto, and B. Dwyer. 1996. Genetic variation in Australian spotted fever group rickettsiae. *J. Clin. Microbiol.* 34:1526–1530.

12. Balayeva, N. M., M. E. Eremeeva, H. Tissot-Dupont, I. A. Zakharov, and D. Raoult. 1995. Genotype characterization of the bacterium expressing the male-killing trait in the ladybird beetle *Adalia bipunctata* with specific rickettsial molecular tools. *Appl. Environ. Microbiol.* 61:1341–1347.

13. Balayeva, N. M., and V. F. Ignatovich. 1991. Serological studies of patients with fever disease of unknown etiology in Astrakhan region with spotted fever group rickettsial antigens. *Zh. Microbiol. Epidemiol. Immunol.* 4:69–71.

14. Beati, L., J. P. Finidori, B. Gilot, and D. Raoult. 1992. Comparison of serologic typing, sodium dodecyl sulfate-polyacryl-amide gel electrophoresis protein analysis, and genetic restriction fragment length polymorphism analysis for identification of rickettsiae: characterization of two new rickettsial strains. *J. Clin. Microbiol.* 30:1922–1930.

15. Beati, L., P. J. Kelly, P. R. Mason, and D. Raoult. 1994. Species-specific BALB/c mouse antibodies to rickettsiae studied by Western blotting. *FEMS Microbiol. Lett.* 119:339–344.

16. Beati, L., M. Meskini, B. Thiers, and D. Raoult. 1997. *Rickettsia aeschlimannii* sp. nov., a new spotted fever group rickettsia associated with *Hyalomma marginatum* ticks. *Int. J. Syst. Bacteriol.* 47:548–554.

17. Beati, L., O. Peter, W. Burgdorfer, A. Aeschlimann, and D. Raoult. 1993. Confirmation that *Rickettsia helvetica* sp. nov. is a distinct species of the spotted fever group of rickettsiae. *Int. J. Syst. Bact.* 43:521–526.

18. Beati, L., and L. Raoult. 1993. *Rickettsia massiliae* sp. nov., a new spotted fever group rickettsia. *Int. J. Syst. Bacteriol.* 43:839–840.

19. Beati, L., V. Roux, A. Ortuno, J. Castella, F. Segura Porta, and D. Raoult. 1996. Phenotypic and genotypic characterization of spotted fever group rickettsiae isolated from catalan *Rhipicephalus sanguineus* ticks. *J. Clin. Microbiol.* 34:2688–2694.

20. Bell, E. J., G. M. Kohls, H. G. Stoenner, and D. B. Lackman. 1963. Nonpathogenic rickettsias related to the spotted fever group isolated from ticks, *Dermacentor variabilis* and *Dermacentor andersoni* from Eastern Montana. *J. Immunol.* 90:770–781.

21. Bell, E. J., and H. G. Stoenner. 1960. Immunologic relationships among the spotted fever group of rickettsias determined by toxin neutralisation tests in mice with convalescent animal serums. *J. Immunol.* 84:171–182.

22. Bitsori, M., E. Galanakis, C. E. Papadakis, and S. Sbyrakis. 2001. Facial nerve palsy associated with *Rickettsia conorii* infection. *Arch. Dis. Child.* 85:54–55.

23. Bouyer, D. H., J. Stenos, P. Crocquet-Valdes, C. Moron, P. Vsevolod, J. E. Zavala-Velasquez, L. Foil, D. Stothard, A. Azad, and D. Walker. 2001. *Rickettsia felis*: molecular characterization of a new member of the spotted fever group. *Int. J. Syst. Evol. Microbiol.* 51:339–347.

24. Bozeman, F. M., B. L. Elisberg, J. W. Humphries, K. Runcik, and D. B. Palmer, Jr. 1970. Serologic evidence of *Rickettsia canada* infection of man. *J. Infect. Dis.* 121:367–371.

25. Brouqui, P., J. R. Harle, J. Delmont, C. Frances, P. J. Weiller, and D. Raoult. 1997. African tick bite fever: an imported spotless rickettsiosis. *Arch. Intern. Med.* 157:119–124.

26. Brumpt, E. 1922. Les spirochétoses, p. 491–531. *In* H. Roger, G. W. Vidal, and P. Teissier (ed.), *Nouveau Traité de médecine*. Masson, Paris, France.

27. Brumpt, E. 1932. Longévité du virus de la fièvre boutonneuse (*Rickettsia conorii* n. sp.) chez la tique *Rhipicephalus sanguineus*. *C. R. Séances Soc. Biol. Fil.* 110:1199–1209.

28. Burgdorfer, W. 1970. Hemolymph test. A technique for detection of rickettsiae in ticks. *Am. J. Trop. Med. Hyg.* 19:1010–1014.

29. Burgdorfer, W., A. Aeschlimann, O. Peter, S. F. Hayes, and R. N. Philip. 1979. *Ixodes ricinus*: vector of a hitherto undescribed spotted fever group agent in Switzerland. *Acta Trop.* 36:357–367.

30. Burgdorfer, W., R. L. Anacker, R. G. Bird, and D. S. Bertram. 1968. Intranuclear growth of *Rickettsia rickettsii*. *J. Bacteriol.* 96:1415–1418.

31. Burgdorfer, W., and L. P. Brinton. 1975. Mechanisms of transovarial infection of spotted fever Rickettsiae in ticks. *Ann. N. Y. Acad. Sci.* 266:61–72.

32. Burgdorfer, W., L. P. Brinton, W. L. Krinsky, and R. N. Philip. 1978. *Rickettsia rhipicephali*: a new spotted fever group rickettsia from the brown dog tick *Rhipicephalus sanguineus*, p. 307–316. *In* J. Kazar, R. A. Ormsbee, and I. V.

Tarasevich (ed.), *Rickettsiae and Rickettsial Diseases*. House of the Slovak Academy of Sciences, Bratislava, Slovakia.

33. **Burgdorfer, W., R. A. Ormsbee, M. L. Schmidt, and H. Hoogstraal.** 1973. A search for the epidemic typhus agent in Ethiopian ticks. *Bull. W. H. O.* 48:563–569.

34. **Burgdorfer, W., D. J. Sexton, R. K. Gerloff, R. L. Anacker, R. N. Philip, and L. A. Thomas.** 1975. *Rhipicephalus sanguineus*: vector of a new spotted fever group rickettsia in the United States. *Infect. Immun.* 12:205–210.

35. **Burgdorfer, W., and M. G. R. Varma.** 1967. Trans-stadial and transovarial development of disease agents in arthropods. *Ann. Rev. Entomol.* 12:347–376.

36. **Burridge, M. J., L. A. Simmons, B. H. Simbi, S. M. Mahan, P. E. Fournier, and D. Raoult.** 2002. Introduction of the exotic tick *Amblyomma hebraeum* into Florida on a human host. *J. Parasitol.* 88:800–801.

37. **Burton, R.** 1992. *Bird Migration*, p. 1–160. Aurum Press Limited, London, England.

38. **Campbell, R. W., and R. Domrow.** 1974. Rickettsioses in Australia: isolation of *Rickettsia tsutsugamushi* and *R. australis* from naturally infected arthropods. *Trans. R. Soc. Trop. Med. Hyg.* 68:397–402.

39. **Cascio, A., C. Colomba, D. Di Rosa, L. Salsa, L. di Martino, and L. Titone.** 2001. Efficacy and safety of clarithromycin as treatment for Mediterranean spotted fever in children: a randomized controlled trial. *Clin. Infect. Dis.* 33:409–411.

40. **Chen, D. Q., B. C. Campbell, and A. H. Purcell.** 1996. A new rickettsia from a herbivorous insect, the pea aphid *Acyrthosiphon pisum* (Harris). *Curr. Microbiol.* 33:123–128.

41. **Chen, M., M. Y. Fan, D. Z. Bi, and J. Z. Zhang.** 1998. Sequence analysis of PCR products amplified from five strains of spotted fever group rickettsiae with Rr with Rr 190.70p and Rr 190.602n primers. *Acta Virol.* 42:91–93.

42. **Cohen, J., Y. Lasri, and Z. Landau.** 1999. Mediterranean spotted fever in pregnancy. *Scand. J. Infect. Dis.* 31:202–203.

43. **Conor, A., and A. Bruch.** 1910. Une fièvre éruptive observée en Tunisie. *Bull. Soc. Pathol. Exot. Filial.* 8:492–496.

44. **Cook, I., and R. W. Campbell.** 1965. Rickettsiosis—North Queensland tick typhus. *Rep. Queensland Inst. Med. Res.* 20:4.

45. **Cory, J., C. E. Yunker, J. A. Howarth, Y. Hokama, L. E. Hughes, L. A. Thomas, and C. M. Clifford.** 1975. Isolation of spotted fever group and *Wolbachia*-like agents from field-collected materials by means of plaque formation in mammalian and mosquito cells. *Acta Virol.* 19:443–445.

46. **de Galan, B. E., B. J. van Kasteren, A. W. van den Wall Bake, and G. Vreugdenhil.** 1999. A case of Guillain-Barré syndrome due to infection with *Rickettsia conorii*. *Eur. J. Clin. Microbiol. Infect. Dis.* 18:79–80.

47. **Drancourt, M., L. Beati, I. V. Tarasevich, and D. Raoult.** 1992. Astrakhan fever rickettsia is identical to Israeli tick typhus rickettsia, a genotype of the *Rickettsia conorii* complex. *J. Infect. Dis.* 165:1167–1168.

48. **Drancourt, M., P. Brouqui, G. Chiche, and D. Raoult.** 1992. Acute pericarditis in Mediterranean spotted fever. *Trans. R. Soc. Trop. Med. Hyg.* 85:799.

49. **Drancourt, M., P. J. Kelly, R. L. Regnery, and D. Raoult.** 1992. Identification of spotted fever group rickettsiae using polymerase chain reaction and restriction-endonuclease length polymorphism analysis. *Acta Virol.* 36:1–6.

50. **Drancourt, M., and D. Raoult.** 1999. Characterization of mutations in the *rpoB* gene in naturally rifampin-resistant *Rickettsia* species. *Antimicrob. Agents Chemother.* 43:2400–2403.

51. **Drancourt, M., D. Raoult, J. R. Harle, H. Chaudet, F. Janbon, C. Charrel, and H. Gallais.** 1990. Biological variations in 412 patients with Mediterranean spotted fever. *Ann. N. Y. Acad. Sci.* 590:39–50.

52. **Dumler, J. S., W. R. Gage, G. L. Pettis, A. F. Azad, and F. P. Kuhadja.** 1990. Rapid immunoperoxydase demonstration of *Rickettsia rickettsii* in fixed cutaneous specimens from patients with Rocky Mountain spotted fever. *Am. J. Clin. Pathol.* 93:410.

53. **Dwyer, B. W., S. R. Graves, M. I. McDonald, A. P. Yung, R. R. Doherty, and J. K. McDonald.** 1991. Spotted fever in East Gippsland, Victoria: a previously unrecognised focus of rickettsial infection. *Med. J. Aust.* 154:121–125.

54. **Eremeeva, M., N. M. Balayeva, V. Roux, V. Ignatovich, M. Kotsinjan, and D. Raoult.** 1995. Genomic and proteinic characterization of strain S, a rickettsia isolated from *Rhipicephalus sanguineus* ticks in Armenia. *J. Clin. Microbiol.* 33:2738–2744.

55. **Eremeeva, M. E., N. M. Balayeva, V. F. Ignatovich, and D. Raoult.** 1993. Proteinic and genomic identification of spotted fever group rickettsiae isolated in the former USSR. *J. Clin. Microbiol.* 31:2625–2633.

56. **Eremeeva, M. E., N. M. Balayeva, V. F. Ignatovich, and D. Raoult.** 1995. Serologic response to rickettsial antigens in patients with Astrakhan fever. *Eur. J. Epidemiol.* 11:383–387.

57. **Eremeeva, M. E., L. Beati, V. A. Makarova, N. F. Fetisova, I. V. Tarasevich, N. M. Balayeva, and D. Raoult.** 1994. Astrakhan fever rickettsiae: antigenic and genotypic of isolates obtained from human and *Rhipicephalus pumilio* ticks. *Am. J. Trop. Med. Hyg.* 51:697–706.

58. **Eremeeva, M. E., X. Yu, and D. Raoult.** 1994. Differentiation among spotted fever group rickettsiae species by analysis of restriction fragment length polymorphism of PCR-amplified DNA. *J. Clin. Microbiol.* 32:803–810.

59. **Espejo-Arenas, E., and D. Raoult.** 1989. First isolates of *Rickettsia conorii* in Spain using a centrifugation-shell vial assay. *J. Infect. Dis.* 159:1158–1159.

60. **Fan, M. Y., D. H. Walker, S. R. Yu, and Q. H. Liu.** 1987. Epidemiology and ecology of rickettsial diseases in the People's Republic of China. *Rev. Infect. Dis.* 9:823–840.

61. **Fan, M. Y., J. Z. Zhang, M. Chen, and X. J. Yu.** 1999. Spotted fever group rickettsioses in China, p. 247–257. *In* D. Raoult and P. Brouqui (ed.), *Rickettsiae and Rickettsial Diseases at the Turn of the Third Millennium*. Elsevier, Paris, France.

62. **Fenollar, F., and D. Raoult.** 1999. Diagnosis of rickettsial diseases using samples dried on blotting paper. *Clin. Diag. Lab. Immunol.* 6:483–488.

63. **Font-Creus, B., F. Bella-Cueto, E. Espejo-Arenas, R. Vidal-Sanahuja, T. Munoz-Espin, M. Nolla-Salas, A. Casagran-Borrell, J. Mercade-Cuesta, and F. Segura-Porta.** 1985. Mediterranean spotted fever: a cooperative study of 227 cases. *Rev. Infect. Dis.* 7:635–642.

63a. **Fournier, P. E., F. Gouriet, P. Brouqui, F. Lucht, and D. Raoult.** 2003. Gene sequence-based criteria for identification of new *Rickettsia* isolates and description of *Rickettsia heilongjiangensis* sp. nov. *J. Clin. Microbiol.* 41:5456–5465.

64. **Fournier, P. E., J. P. Durand, J. M. Rolain, J. L. Camicas, H. Tolou, and D. Raoult.** 2003. Detection of Astrakhan fever rickettsia from ticks in Kosovo. *Ann. N. Y. Acad. Sci.* 990:158–161.

65. **Fournier, P. E., H. Fujita, N. Takada, and D. Raoult.** 2002. Genetic identification of rickettsiae isolated from ticks in Japan. *J. Clin. Microbiol.* 40:2176–2181.

65a. **Fournier, P. E., J. S. Dumler, G. Greub, J. Zhang, Y. Wu, and D. Raoult.** Lymphangitis-associated rickettsiosis (LAR), a new rickettsiosis caused by *Rickettsia sibirica mongolotimonae*. Seven new cases and review of the literature. *Clin. Infect. Dis.*, in press.

66. **Fournier, P. E., F. Gunnenberger, B. Jaulhac, G. Gastinger, and D. Raoult.** 2000. Evidence of *Rickettsia helvetica* infec-

tion in humans, Eastern France. *Emerg. Infect. Dis.* 6:389–392.

67. Fournier, P. E., M. Jensenius, H. Laferl, S. Vene, and D. Raoult. 2002. Kinetics of antibody responses in *Rickettsia africae* and *Rickettsia conorii* infections. *Clin. Diagn. Lab. Immunol.* 9:324–328.

67a. Fournier, P. E., and D. Raoult. 2004. Suicide PCR on skin biopsy specimens for diagnosis of rickettsiosis. *J. Clin. Microbiol.* 42:3428–3434.

68. Fournier, P. E., V. Roux, E. Caumes, M. Donzel, and D. Raoult. 1998. Outbreak of *Rickettsia africae* infections in participants of an adventure race from South Africa. *Clin. Infect. Dis.* 27:316–323.

69. Fournier, P. E., V. Roux, and D. Raoult. 1998. Phylogenetic analysis of spotted fever group rickettsiae by study of the outer surface protein rOmpA. *Int. J. Syst. Bacteriol.* 48:839–849.

70. Fournier, P. E., H. Tissot-Dupont, H. Gallais, and D. Raoult. 2000. *Rickettsia mongolotimonae*: a rare pathogen in France. *Emerg. Infect. Dis.* 6:290–292.

71. Fournier, P. E., B. Xeridat, and D. Raoult. 2003. Isolation of a rickettsia from a patient in Chad which is related to Astrakhan fever rickettsia. *Ann. N. Y. Acad. Sci.* 990:152–157.

71a. Fournier, P. E., Y. Zhu, H. Ogata, and D. Raoult. 2004. Use of highly variable intergenic spacer sequences for multispacer typing of *Rickettsia conorii* strains. *J. Clin. Microbiol.* 42:5757–5766.

72. Gage, K., M. E. Schrumpf, R. H. Karstens, W. Burgdorfer, and T. G. Schwan. 1994. DNA typing of rickettsiae in naturally infected ticks using a polymerase chain reaction/restriction fragment length polymorphism system. *Am. J. Trop. Med. Hyg.* 50:247–260.

73. Gage, K. L., R. D. Gilmore, R. H. Karstens, and T. G. Schwan. 1992. Detection of *Rickettsia rickettsii* in saliva, hemolymph and triturated tissues of infected *Dermacentor andersoni* ticks by polymerase chain reaction. *Mol. Cell. Probes* 6:333–341.

74. Gear, J. H. S. 1938. South African typhus. *S. Afr. J. Med. Sci.* 3:134–160.

75. Gear, J. H. S. 1939. Complications in tick-bite fever. A survey of fifty cases. *S. Afr. Med. J.* 13:35–38.

76. George, F., C. Brisson, P. Poncelet, J. C. Laurent, O. Massot, D. Arnoux, P. Ambrosi, C. Klein-Soyer, J. P. Cazenave, and J. Sampol. 1992. Rapid isolation of human endothelial cells from whole blood using S-Endo 1 monoclonal antibody coupled to immuno-magnetic beads: demonstration of endothelial injury after angioplasty. *Thromb. Haemost.* 67:147–153.

77. George, F., P. Brouqui, M. C. Boffa, M. Mutin, M. Drancourt, C. Brisson, D. Raoult, and J. Sampol. 1993. Demonstration of *Rickettsia conorii*-induced endothelial injury in vivo by measuring circulating endothelial cells, thrombomodulin and Von Willebrand factor in patients with mediterranean spotted fever. *Blood* 82:2109–2116.

78. Gilmore, R. D., W. Cieplak, P. F. Policastro, and T. Hackstadt. 1991. The 120 kilodalton outer membrane protein (rOmpB) of *Rickettsia rickettsii* is encoded by an unusually long open reading frame. Evidence for protein processing from a large precursor. *Mol. Microbiol.* 5:2361–2370.

79. Gilot, B., M. L. Laforge, J. Pichot, and D. Raoult. 1990. Relationships between the *Rhipicephalus sanguineus* complex ecology and Mediterranean spotted fever epidemiology in France. *Eur. J. Epidemiol.* 6:357–362.

80. Gilot, B., and M. Marjolet. 1982. Contribution à l'étude du parasitisme humain par les tiques (Ixodidae et Argasidae), plus particulièrement dans le sud-est de la France. *Med. Mal. Infect.* 12:340–351.

81. Gimenez, D. F. 1964. Staining rickettsiae in yolk-sac cultures. *Stain Technol.* 39:135–140.

82. Giroud, P. 1973. Syndromes cliniques non classiques provoqués par des rickettsies et des agents proches. *Med. Mal. Infect.* 3:241–245.

83. Goldwasser, R. A., M. A. Klingberg, W. Klingberg, Y. Steiman, and T. A. Swartz. 1974. Laboratory and epidemiologic studies of rickettsial spotted fever in Israel, p. 270–275. *In Frontiers of Internal Medicine. 12th International Congress of Internal Medicine, Tel Aviv.* Karger, Basel, Switzerland.

84. Goldwasser, R. A., and C. C. Shepard. 1959. Fluorescent antibody methods in the differentiation of murine and epidemic typhus fever: specific changes resulting from previous immunization. *J. Immunol.* 82:373–380.

85. Goldwasser, R. A., Y. Steiman, W. Klingberg, T. A. Swartz, and M. A. Klingberg. 1974. The isolation of strains of rickettsiae of the spotted fever group in Israel and their differentiation from other members of the group by immunofluorescence methods. *Scand. J. Infect. Dis.* 6:53–62.

86. Gross, E. M., and P. Yagupsky. 1987. Israeli rickettsial spotted fever in children. A review of 54 cases. *Acta Trop.* 44:91–96.

87. Guardia, J., J. M. Martinez-Vazquez, A. Moragas, C. Rey, J. Vilaseca, J. Tornos, M. Beltran, and R. Bacardi. 1974. The liver in boutonneuse fever. *Gut* 15:549–551.

88. Hackstadt, T., R. Messer, W. Cieplak, and M. G. Peacock. 1992. Evidence for proteolytic cleavage of the 120-kilodalton outer membrane protein of rickettsiae: identification of an avirulent mutant deficient in processing. *Infect. Immun.* 60:159–165.

89. Halle, S., G. A. Dasch, and E. Weiss. 1977. Sensitive enzyme-linked immunosorbent assay for detection of antibodies against typhus rickettsiae, *Rickettsia prowazekii* and *Rickettsia typhi*. *J. Clin. Microbiol.* 6:101–110.

90. Hamilton, J. G. C. 1992. The role of pheromones in tick biology. *Parasitol. Today* 8:130–133.

91. Hattwick, M. A., R. J. O'Brien, and B. F. Hanson. 1976. Rocky Mountain spotted fever: epidemiology of an increasing problem. *Ann. Intern. Med.* 84:732–739.

92. Hayes, S. F., W. Burgdorfer, and A. Aeschlimann. 1980. Sexual transmission of spotted fever group rickettsiae by infected male ticks: detection of rickettsiae in immature spermatozoa of *Ixodes ricinus*. *Infect. Immun.* 27:638–642.

93. Hechemy, K. E., R. L. Anacker, N. L. Carlo, J. A. Fox, and H. A. Gaafar. 1983. Absorption of *Rickettsia rickettsii* antibodies by *Rickettsia rickettsii* antigens in four diagnostic tests. *J. Clin. Microbiol.* 17:445–449.

94. Hechemy, K. E., J. A. Fox, D. H. M. Groschel, F. G. Fayden, and R. P. Wenzel. 1991. Immunoblot studies to analyse antibody to the *Rickettsia typhi* group antigen in sera from patients with acute febrile cerebrovasculitis. *J. Clin. Microbiol.* 29:2559–2565.

95. Hechemy, K. E., D. Raoult, C. Eisemann, Y. S. Han, and J. A. Fox. 1986. Detection of antibodies to *Rickettsia conorii* with a latex agglutination test in patients with Mediterranean spotted fever. *J. Infect. Dis.* 153:132–135.

96. Hechemy, K. E., D. Raoult, J. Fox, Y. Han, L. B. Elliott, and J. Rawlings. 1989. Cross-reaction of immune sera from patients with rickettsial diseases. *J. Med. Microbiol.* 29:199–202.

97. Heinzen, R. A., S. F. Hayes, M. G. Peacock, and T. Hackstadt. 1993. Directional actin polymerization associated with spotted fever group rickettsia infection of Vero cells. *Infect. Immun.* 61:1926–1935.

98. Helmick, C. G., K. W. Bernard, and L. J. D'Angelo. 1984. Rocky mountain spotted fever: clinical, laboratory, and epidemiological features of 262 cases. *J. Infect. Dis.* 150:480–488.

99. Higgins, J. A., and A. F. Azad. 1995. Use of polymerase chain reaction to detect bacteria in arthropods: a review. *J. Med. Entomol.* 32:213–222.

100. Holman, R. C., C. D. Paddock, A. T. Curns, J. W. Krebs, J. H. McQuiston, and J. E. Childs. 2001. Analysis of risk factors for fatal rocky mountain spotted fever: evidence for superiority of tetracyclines for therapy. *J. Infect. Dis.* 184:1437–1444.

101. Hoogstraal, H. 1985. *Advances in Parasitology*, p. 135–239. Academic Press, Inc., London, England.

102. Houpikian, P., and D. Raoult. 2002. Diagnostic methods current best practices and guidelines for identification of difficult-to-culture pathogens in infective endocarditis. *Infect. Dis. Clin. North Am.* 16:377–392.

103. Huebner, R. J., W. L. Jellison, and C. Pomerantz. 1946. Rickettsialpox—a newly recognized rickettsial disease. IV. Isolation of a rickettsia apparently identical with the causative agent of rickettsialpox from *Allodermanyssus sanguineus*, a rodent mite. *Public Health Rep.* 61:1677–1682.

104. Hugues, L. E., C. M. Clifford, R. Gresbrink, L. A. Thomas, and J. E. Keirans. 1976. Isolation of a spotted fever group rickettsia from the pacific coast tick, *Ixodes pacificus*, in Oregon. *Am. J. Trop. Med. Hyg.* 25:513–516.

105. Ignatovich, V. F. 1977. Antigenic relations of *Rickettsia prowazekii* and *Rickettsia canada*, established in the study of sera of patients with Brill's disease. *J. Hyg. Epidemiol. Microbiol. Immunol.* 21:55–60.

106. Ishikura, M., H. Fujita, S. Ando, K. Matsuura, and M. Watanabe. 2002. Phylogenetic analysis of spotted fever group rickettsiae isolated from ticks in Japan. *Microbiol. Immunol.* 46:241–247.

106a. Jensenius, M., P. E. Fournier, S. Vene, T. Hoel, G. Hasle, A. Z. Henriksen, K. B. Hellum, D. Raoult, B. Myrvang, and the Norwegian African Tick Bite Fever Study Group. 2003. African tick bite fever in travelers to rural sub-Equatorial Africa. *Clin. Infect. Dis.* 36:1411–1417.

107. Jensenius, M., T. Hoel, D. Raoult, P. E. Fournier, H. Kjelshus, A. L. Bruu, and B. Myrvang. 2002. Seroepidemiology of *Rickettsia africae* infection in Norwegian travellers to rural Africa. *Scand. J. Infect. Dis.* 34:93–96.

108. Kelly, D. J., G. A. Dasch, B. L. Smoak, B. McClain, J. F. Brundage, L. Broadhurst, C. T. Chan, and R. N. Miller. 1992. Etiology of a rickettsial disease outbreak in US troops returning from deployment to Bostwana, p. 3. *In* Program and Abstracts of 10th Sequi-Annual Meeting of the American Society for Rickettsiology and Rickettsial Diseases. Rocky Mountain Laboratories, Hamilton, Mont.

109. Kelly, P. J., L. Beati, P. R. Mason, L. A. Matthewman, V. Roux, and D. Raoult. 1996. *Rickettsia africae* sp. nov., the etiological agent of African tick bite fever. *Int. J. Syst. Bacteriol.* 46:611–614.

110. Kelly, P. J., L. Beati, L. A. Matthewman, P. R. Mason, G. A. Dasch, and D. Raoult. 1994. A new pathogenic spotted fever group rickettsia from Africa. *J. Trop. Med. Hyg.* 97:129–137.

111. Kelly, P. J., and P. R. Mason. 1990. Serological typing of spotted fever group rickettsia isolates from Zimbabwe. *J. Clin. Microbiol.* 28:2302–2304.

112. Kelly, P. J., P. R. Mason, L. A. Matthewman, and D. Raoult. 1991. Seroepidemiology of spotted fever group rickettsial infections in humans in Zimbabwe. *J. Trop. Med. Hyg.* 94:304–309.

113. Kelly, P. J., L. A. Matthewman, L. Beati, D. Raoult, P. Mason, M. Dreary, and R. Makombe. 1992. African tick-bite fever: a new spotted fever group rickettsiosis under an old name. *Lancet* 340:982–983.

114. Kelly, P. J., D. Raoult, and P. R. Mason. 1991. Isolation of spotted fever group rickettsias from triturated ticks using a modification of the centrifugation-shell vial technique. *Trans. R. Soc. Trop. Med. Hyg.* 85:397–398.

115. Lackman, D. B., E. J. Bell, H. G. Stoenner, and E. G. Pickens. 1965. The Rocky mountain spotted fever group of rickettsiae. *Health Lab. Sci.* 2:135.

116. Lakos, A. 1997. Tick-borne lymphadenopathy—a new rickettsial disease? *Lancet* 350:1006.

117. Landau, Z., S. Feld, S. Kunichezly, M. Grinspan, and M. Gorbacz. 1992. Thrombosis of the mesenteric vein as a complication of mediterranean spotted fever. *Clin. Infect. Dis.* 15:1070–1071.

118. La Scola, B., and D. Raoult. 1996. Diagnosis of Mediterranean spotted fever by cultivation of *Rickettsia conorii* from blood and skin samples using the centrifugation-shell vial technique and by detection of *R. conorii* in circulating endothelial cells: a 6-year follow-up. *J. Clin. Microbiol.* 34:2722–2727.

119. La Scola, B., and D. Raoult. 1997. Laboratory diagnosis of rickettsioses: current approaches to the diagnosis of old and new rickettsial diseases. *J. Clin. Microbiol.* 35:2715–2727.

120. Le Gac, P. 1972. Multiple sclerosis and zoonoses. Importance of the role of the bovine abortion virus (pararickettsia X-14) in the etiopathogenesis of multiple sclerosis. *C. R. Acad. Sci. Paris* 275:147–148. (In French.)

121. Leitner, M., S. R. S. Yitzhaki, and A. Keysary. 2002. Polymerase chain reaction-based diagnosis of Mediterranean spotted fever in serum and tissue samples. *Am. J. Trop. Med. Hyg.* 67:166–169.

122. Li, H., and D. H. Walker. 1992. Characterization of rickettsial attachment to host cells by flow cytometry. *Infect. Immun.* 60:2030–2035.

123. Linnemann, C. C., Jr., C. I. Pretzman, and E. D. Peterson. 1989. Acute febrile cerebrovasculitis. A non-spotted fever group rickettsial disease. *Arch. Intern. Med.* 149:1682–1684.

124. Lou, D., Y. M. Wu, B. Wang, W. Wang, Z. Zhang, and X. W. Zhang. 1989. Confirmation of patients with tick-borne spotted fever caused by *Rickettsia heilongjiangi*. *Chin. J. Epidemiol.* 10:128–132.

125. Lyskovtsev, M. M. 1968. Tickborne rickettsiosis. *Misc. Publ. Entomol. Soc. Am.* 6:42–140.

126. Macaluso, K. R., D. E. Sonenshine, S. M. Ceraul, and A. F. Azad. 2001. Infection and transovarial transmission of rickettsiae in *Dermacentor variabilis* ticks acquired by artificial feeding. *Vector Borne Zoonotic Dis.* 1:45–53.

127. Macaluso, K. R., D. E. Sonenshine, S. M. Ceraul, and A. F. Azad. 2002. Rickettsial infection in *Dermacentor variabilis* (Acari: Ixodidae) inhibits transovarial transmission of a second rickettsia. *J. Med. Entomol.* 39:809–813.

128. Mahara, F. 1984. Three Weil-Felix reaction OX2 positive cases with skin eruptions and high fever. *J. Anan Med. Assoc.* 68:4–7.

129. Mahara, F. 1987. Japanese spotted fever a new disease named for spotted fever group rickettsiosis in Japan. *Annu. Rep. Ohara Hosp.* 30:83–89.

130. Mahara, F. 1997. Japanese spotted fever: report of 31 cases and review of the literature. *Emerg. Infect. Dis.* 3:105–111.

131. Mahara, F., K. Koga, S. Sawada, T. Taniguchi, F. Shigemi, T. Suto, Y. Tsuboi, A. Ooya, H. Koyama, T. Uchiyama, and T. Uchida. 1985. The first report of the rickettsial infections of spotted fever group in Japan; three clinical cases. *Kansenshogaku Zasshi* 59:1165–1172. (In Japanese.)

132. Maiden, M. C. J., J. A. Bygraves, E. Feil, G. Morelli, J. E. Russel, I. Urwin, Q. Zhang, J. Zhou, K. Zurth, D. A. Caugant, I. M. Feavers, M. Achtman, and B. G. Spratt. 1998. Multilocus sequence typing: a portable approach to the identification of clones within populations of pathogenic microorganisms. *Proc. Natl. Acad. Sci. USA* 95:3140–3145.

133. Mansueto, S., G. Tringali, and D. H. Walker. 1986. Widespread, simultaneous increase in the incidence of spotted fever group rickettsiosis. *J. Infect. Dis.* **154**:539–540.

134. Marrero, M., and D. Raoult. 1989. Centrifugation-shell vial technique for rapid detection of Mediterranean spotted fever rickettsia in blood culture. *Am. J. Trop. Med. Hyg.* **40**:197–199.

135. Maurin, M., and D. Raoult. 1997. Bacteriostatic and bactericidal activity of levofloxacin against *Rickettsia rickettsii*, *Rickettsia conorii*, "Israeli spotted fever group rickettsia" and *Coxiella burnetii*. *J. Antimicrob. Chemother.* **39**:725–730.

136. McDade, J. 1990. Evidence supporting the hypothesis that rickettsial virulence factors determine the severity of spotted fever and typhus group infections. *Ann. N. Y. Acad. Sci.* **590**:20–26.

137. McDade, J. E., C. M. Black, L. F. Roumillat, M. A. Redus, and C. L. Spruill. 1988. Addition of monoclonal antibodies specific for *Rickettsia akari* to the rickettsial diagnostic panel. *J. Clin. Microbiol.* **26**:2221–2223.

138. McKiel, Y. A., E. J. Bell, and D. B. Lackman. 1967. Rickettsia canada: a new member of the typhus group of rickettsiae isolated from Haemaphylasis leporispalustris ticks in Canada. *Can. J. Microbiol.* **13**:503–510.

138a. Mediannikov, O.Y., Y. Sidelnikov, L. Ivanov, E. Mokretsova, P. E. Fournier, I. Tarasevich, and D. Raoult. 2004. Acute tick-borne rickettsiosis caused by *Rickettsia heilongjiangensis* in Russian Far East. *Emerg. Infect. Dis.* **10**:810–817.

139. Montenegro, M. R., S. Mansueto, B. C. Hegarty, and D. H. Walker. 1983. The histology of "tâches noires" of boutonneuse fever and demonstration of *Rickettsia conorii* in them by immunofluorescence. *Virchows. Arch. A Pathol. Anat. Histopathol.* **400**:309–317.

140. Myers, W. F., and C. L. Wisseman, Jr. 1981. The taxonomic relationship of *Rickettsia canada* to the typhus and spotted fever groups of the genus *Rickettsia*, p. 313–325. *In* W. Burgdorfer and R. L. Anacker (ed.), *Rickettsiae and Rickettsial Diseases*. Academic Press, New York, N.Y.

141. Niebylski, M. L., M. E. Schrumpf, W. Burgdorfer, E. R. Fischer, K. L. Gage, and T. G. Schwan. 1997. *Rickettsia peacockii* sp. nov., a new species infecting wood ticks, *Dermacentor andersoni*, in Western Montana. *Int. J. Syst. Bacteriol.* **47**:446–452.

142. Nilsson, K., T. G. T. Jaenson, I. Uhnoo, O. Lindquist, B. Pettersson, M. Uhlen, G. Friman, and C. Pahlson. 1997. Characterization of a spotted fever group rickettsia from *Ixodes ricinus* ticks in Sweden. *J. Clin. Microbiol.* **35**:243–247.

143. Nilsson, K., O. Lindquist, and C. Pahlson. 1999. Association of *Rickettsia helvetica* with chronic perimyocarditis in sudden cardiac death. *Lancet* **354**:1169–1173.

144. Nilsson, K., C. Pahlson, A. Lukinius, L. Eriksson, L. Nilsson, and O. Lindquist. 2002. Presence of *Rickettsia helvetica* in granulomatous tissue from patients with sarcoidosis. *J. Infect. Dis.* **185**:1128–1138.

145. Obijeski, J. R., E. L. Palmer, and T. Tzianabos. 1974. Proteins of purified rickettsiae. *Microbios* **11**:61–76.

146. Ogata, H., S. Audic, C. Abergel, P. E. Fournier, and J. M. Claverie. 2002. Protein coding palindromes are a unique but recurrent feature in *Rickettsia*. *Genome Res.* **12**:808–816.

147. Ogata, H., S. Audic, V. Barbe, F. Artiguenave, P. E. Fournier, D. Raoult, and J. M. Claverie. 2000. Selfish DNA in protein-coding genes of *Rickettsia*. *Science* **290**:347–350.

148. Ogata, H., S. Audic, P. Renesto-Audiffren, P. E. Fournier, V. Barbe, D. Samson, V. Roux, P. Cossart, J. Weissenbach, J. M. Claverie, and D. Raoult. 2001. Mechanisms of evolution in *Rickettsia conorii* and R. prowazekii. *Science* **293**:2093–2098.

149. Olmer, D. 1925. Sur une infection épidémique, avec exanthème de nature indéterminée. *Mars. Méd.* **22**:1291–1293.

150. Oteo, J. A., and V. Ibarra. 2002. DEBONEL (dermacentor-borne-necrosis-erythemalymphadenopathy). A new tick-borne disease? *Enferm. Infect. Microbiol. Clin.* **20**:51–52.

150a. Paddock, C. D., J. W. Sumner, J. A. Comer, S. R. Zaki, C. S. Goldsmith, J. Goddard, S. L. F. McLellan, C. L. Tamminga, and C. A. Ohl. 2004. *Rickettsia parkeri*: a newly recognized cause of spotted fever in the United States. *Clin. Infect. Dis.* **38**:805–811.

151. Parker, R. R., G. M. Kohls, G. W. Cox, and G. E. Davis. 1939. Observations on an infectious agent from *Amblyomma maculatum*. *Public Health Rep.* **54**:1482–1484.

152. Parker, R. R., and R. R. Spencer. 1926. Rocky mountain spotted fever. A study of the relationship between the presence of rickettsia-like organisms in tick smears and the infectiveness of the same ticks. *Public Health Rep.* **41**:461–469.

153. Parola, P., L. Beati, M. Cambon, and D. Raoult. 1998. First isolation of *Rickettsia helvetica* from *Ixodes ricinus* ticks in France. *Eur. J. Clin. Microbiol. Infect. Dis.* **17**:95–100.

154. Parola, P., F. Fenollar, S. Badiaga, P. Brouqui, and D. Raoult. 2001. First documentation of *Rickettsia conorii* infection (strain Indian tick typhus) in a traveller. *Emerg. Infect. Dis.* **7**:909–910.

155. Parola, P., H. Inokuma, J. L. Camicas, P. Brouqui, and D. Raoult. 2001. Detection and identification of spotted fever group Rickettsiae and Ehrlichiae in African ticks. *Emerg. Infect. Dis.* **7**:1014–1017.

156. Parola, P., J. Jourdan, and D. Raoult. 1998. Tick-borne infection caused by *Rickettsia africae* in the West Indies. *N. Engl. J. Med.* **338**:1391.

157. Pavis, C., and N. Barré. 1993. Kinetics of male pheromone production by *Amblyomma variegatum* (Acari: Ixodidae). *J. Med. Entomol.* **30**:961–965.

158. Pedersen, C. E. Jr., and V. D. Walters. 1978. Comparative electrophoresis of spotted fever group rickettsial proteins. *Life Sci.* **22**:583–587.

159. Peter, O., D. Raoult, and B. Gilot. 1990. Isolation by a sensitive centrifugation cell culture system of 52 strains of spotted fever group rickettsiae from ticks collected in France. *J. Clin. Microbiol.* **28**:1597–1599.

160. Philip, C. B. 1950. Miscellaneous human rickettsioses, p. 781–788. *In* R. L. Pullen (ed.), *Communicable Diseases*. Lea and Febiger Co., Philadelphia, Pa.

161. Philip, C. B. 1959. Some epidemiological considerations in Rocky Mountain spotted fever. *Public Health Rep.* **74**:595–600.

162. Philip, C. B., and L. E. Hugues. 1953. Disease agents found in the rabbit tick, *Dermacentor parumapertus*, in the southwestern United States, p. 541. *In Atti del VI Congreso Internazionale di Microbiologia Roma*, Rome, Italy.

163. Philip, C. B., and R. R. Parker. 1933. Rocky mountain spotted fever. Investigation of sexual transmission in the wood tick *Dermacentor andersoni*. *Public Health Rep.* **48**:266–272.

164. Philip, R. N., E. A. Casper, R. L. Anacker, J. Cory, S. F. Hayes, W. Burgdorfer, and E. Yunker. 1983. *Rickettsia bellii* sp. nov.: a tick-borne rickettsia, widely distributed in the United States, that is distinct from the spotted fever and typhus biogroups. *Int. J. Syst. Bacteriol.* **33**:94–106.

165. Philip, R. N., E. A. Casper, W. Burgdorfer, R. K. Gerloff, L. E. Hugues, and E. J. Bell. 1978. Serologic typing of rickettsiae of the spotted fever group by microimmunofluorescence. *J. Immunol.* **121**:1961–1968.

166. Pijper, A. 1934. Tick-bite fever—a clinical lecture. *S. Afr. Med. J.* **11**:551–556.

167. Pijper, A. 1936. Etude expérimentale comparée de la fièvre boutonneuse et de la tick-bite-fever. *Arch. Inst. Pasteur Tunis* **25**:388–401.

168. Piras, M. A., G. Calia, F. Saba, C. Gakis, and G. Andreoni. 1983. Glucose-6-phosphate dehydrogenase deficiency in male patients with Mediterranean spotted fever in Sardinia. *J. Infect. Dis.* **147:**607–608.

169. Plotz, H., R. L. Reagan, and K. Wertman. 1944. Differentiation between "Fièvre boutonneuse" and Rocky Mountain spotted fever by means of complement fixation. *Proc. Soc. Exp. Biol. Med.* **55:**173–176.

170. Plotz, H., J. E. Smadel, and B. I. Bennet. 1946. North Queensland tick typhus: studies of the aetiological agent and its relation to other rickettsial diseases. *Med. J. Aust.* **2:**263–268.

171. Popivanova, N., D. Hristova, and E. Hadjipetrova. 1998. Guillain-Barré polyneuropathy associated with mediterranean spotted fever: case report. *Clin. Infect. Dis.* **27:**1549.

172. Pretorius, A. M., and R. J. Birtles. 2002. *Rickettsia aeschlimannii:* a new pathogenetic spotted fever group rickettsia, South Africa. *Emerg. Infect. Dis.* **8:**874.

172a.Pretorius, A. M., and R. J. Birtles. 2004. *Rickettsia mongolotimonae* infection in South Africa. *Emerg. Infect. Dis.* **10:**125–126

173. Pretzman, C., D. R. Stothard, D. Ralph, and A. Fuerst. 1994. A new Rickettsia isolated from the lone star tick, *Amblyomma americanum* (Ixodidae), p. 24. *In* 11th Sesqui-annual Meeting of the American Society for Rickettsiology and Rickettsial Diseases, St. Simons Island, Ga.

174. Purvis, J. J., and M. S. Edwards. 2001. Doxycycline use for rickettsial disease in pediatric patients. *Pediatr. Infect. Dis. J.* **19:**871–874.

175. Radulovic, S., J. A. Higgins, D. C. Jaworski, G. A. Dasch, and A. F. Azad. 1995. Isolation, cultivation, and partial characterization of the ELB agent associated with cat fleas. *Infect. Immun.* **63:**4826–4829.

176. Raoult, D., G. Aboudharam, E. Crubezy, G. Larrouy, B. Ludes, and M. Drancourt. 2000. Molecular identification by "suicide PCR" of *Yersinia pestis* as the agent of medieval black death. *Proc. Natl. Acad. Sci. USA* **97:**12800–12803.

177. Raoult, D., P. Berbis, V. Roux, W. B. Xu, and M. Maurin. 1997. A new tick-transmitted disease due to *Rickettsia slovaca. Lancet* **350:**112–113.

178. Raoult, D., P. Brouqui, and V. Roux. 1996. A new spotted-fever-group rickettsiosis. *Lancet* **348:**412.

179. Raoult, D., and G. A. Dasch. 1989. Line blot and western blot immunoassays for diagnosis of Mediterranean spotted fever. *J. Clin. Microbiol.* **27:**2073–2079.

180. Raoult, D., and G. A. Dasch. 1995. Immunoblot cross-reactions among *Rickettsia, Proteus* spp. and *Legionella* spp. in patients with Mediterranean spotted fever. *FEMS Immunol. Med. Microbiol.* **11:**13–18.

181. Raoult, D., P. E. Fournier, P. Abboud, and F. Caron. 2002. First documented human *Rickettsia aeschlimannii* infection. *Emerg. Infect. Dis.* **8:**748–749.

182. Raoult, D., P. E. Fournier, F. Fenollar, M. Jensenius, T. Prioe, J. J. de Pina, G. Caruso, N. Jones, H. Laferl, J. E. Rosenblatt, and T. J. Marrie. 2001. *Rickettsia africae,* a tick-borne pathogen in travelers to sub-Saharan Africa. *N. Engl. J. Med.* **344:**1504–1510.

183. Raoult, D., B. La Scola, M. Enea, P. E. Fournier, V. Roux, F. Fenollar, M. A. M. Galvao, and X. De Lamballerie. 2001. A flea-associated rickettsia pathogenic for humans. *Emerg. Infect. Dis.* **7:**73–81.

184. Raoult, D., A. Lakos, F. Fenollar, J. Beytout, P. Brouqui, and P. E. Fournier. 2002. Spotless rickettsiosis caused by *Rickettsia slovaca* and associated with *Dermacentor* ticks. *Clin. Infect. Dis.* **34:**1331–1336.

185. Raoult, D., P. Roussellier, G. Vestris, and J. Tamalet. 1987. In vitro antibiotic susceptibility of *Rickettsia rickettsii* and *Rickettsia conorii:* plaque assay and microplaque colorimetric assay. *J. Infect. Dis.* **155:**1059–1062.

186. Raoult, D., and V. Roux. 1997. Rickettsioses as paradigms of new or emerging infectious diseases. *Clin. Microbiol. Rev.* **10:**694–719.

187. Raoult, D., V. Roux, J. B. Ndihokubwaho, G. Bise, D. Baudon, G. Martet, and R. J. Birtles. 1997. Jail fever (epidemic typhus) outbreak in Burundi. *Emerg. Infect. Dis.* **3:**357–360.

188. Raoult, D., H. Tissot-Dupont, P. Caraco, P. Brouqui, M. Drancourt, and C. Charrel. 1992. Mediterranean spotted fever in Marseille: descriptive epidemiology and the influence climatic factors. *Eur. J. Epidemiol.* **8:**192–197.

189. Raoult, D., H. Tissot-Dupont, C. Chicheportiche, O. Peter, B. Gilot, and M. Drancourt. 1993. Mediterranean spotted fever in Marseille, France: correlation between prevalence of hospitalized patients, seroepidemiology, and prevalence of infected ticks in three different areas. *Am. J. Trop. Med. Hyg.* **48:**249–256.

190. Raoult, D., P. J. Weiller, A. Chagnon, H. Chaudet, H. Gallais, and P. Casanova. 1986. Mediterranean spotted fever: clinical, laboratory and epidemiological features of 199 cases. *Am. J. Trop. Med. Hyg.* **35:**845–850.

191. Raoult, D., P. J. Weiller, I. Juhan-Vague, M. Finaud, and M. Mongin. 1985. Platelet antibodies in Mediterranean tick typhus. *Trans. R. Soc. Trop. Med. Hyg.* **79:**699.

192. Raoult, D., P. Zuchelli, P. J. Weiller, C. Charrel, J. L. San Marco, H. Gallais, and P. Casanova. 1986. Incidence, clinical observations and risk factors in the severe form of Mediterranean spotted fever among patients admitted to hospital in Marseille 1983–1984. *J. Infect.* **12:**111–116.

193. Regev-Yochay, G., E. Segal, and E. Rubinstein. 2000. Glucose-6-phosphate dehydrogenase deficiency: possible determinant for a fulminant course of Israeli spotted fever. *Isr. Med. Assoc. J.* **2:**781–782.

194. Regnery, R. L., C. L. Spruill, and B. D. Plikaytis. 1991. Genotypic identification of rickettsiae and estimation of intraspecies sequence divergence for portions of two rickettsial genes. *J. Bacteriol.* **173:**1576–1589.

195. Rehacek, J. 1984. *Rickettsia slovaca,* the organism and its ecology. *Acta SC. Nat. Brno* **18:**1–50.

196. Rehacek, J., and I. V. Tarasevich. 1988. Acari-borne rickettsiae and rickettsioses in Eurasia, p. 128–145. Veda, Publishing House of the Slovak Academy of Sciences, Bratislava, Slovakia.

197. Richter, J., P. E. Fournier, J. Petridou, D. Häussinger, and D. Raoult. 2002. *Rickettsia felis* infection acquired in Europe and documented by polymerase chain reaction. *Emerg. Infect. Dis.* **8:**207–208.

198. Ricketts, H. T. 1909. Some aspects of Rocky Mountain spotted fever as shown by recent investigations. *Med. Rec.* **16:**843–855.

199. Robertson, R. G., C. L. Wiseman, Jr., and R. Traub. 1970. Tick-borne rickettsiae of the spotted fever group in west Pakistan. I. Isolation of strains from ticks in different habitats. *Am. J. Epidemiol.* **92:**382–394.

200. Robertson, R. G., and C. L. Wisseman, Jr. 1973. Tick-borne rickettsiae of the spotted fever group in west Pakistan. II. Serological classification of isolates from west Pakistan and Thailand: evidence for two new species. *Am. J. Epidemiol.* **97:**55–64.

201. Rolain, J. M., M. Maurin, A. Bryskier, and D. Raoult. 2000. In vitro activities of telithromycin (HMR 3647) against *Rickettsia rickettsii, Rickettsia conorii, Rickettsia africae, Rickettsia typhi, Rickettsia prowazekii, Coxiella burnetii, Bartonella henselae, Bartonella quintana, Bartonella bacilliformis,* and *Ehrlichia chaffeensis. Antimicrob. Agents Chemother.* **44:**1391–1393.

202. Rolain, J. M., M. Maurin, G. Vestris, and D. Raoult. 1998. In vitro susceptibilities of 27 rickettsiae to 13 antimicrobials. *Antimicrob. Agents Chemother.* **42:**1537–1541.

203. Rolain, J. M., L. Sthul, M. Maurin, and D. Raoult. 2002. Evaluation of antibiotic susceptibilities of three Rickettsial species including Rickettsia felis by a quantitative PCR DNA assay. *Antimicrob. Agents Chemother.* 46:2747–2751.

204. Roux, V., P. E. Fournier, and D. Raoult. 1996. Differentiation of spotted fever group rickettsiae by sequencing and analysis of restriction fragment length polymorphism of PCR-amplified DNA of the gene encoding the protein rOmpA. *J. Clin. Microbiol.* 34:2058–2065.

205. Roux, V., and D. Raoult. 1993. Genotypic identification and phylogenetic analysis of the spotted fever group rickettsiae by pulsed-field gel electrophoresis. *J. Bacteriol.* 175:4895–4904.

206. Roux, V., and D. Raoult. 1995. Phylogenetic analysis of the genus Rickettsia by 16S rDNA sequencing. *Res. Microbiol.* 146:385–396.

207. Roux, V., and D. Raoult. 2000. Phylogenetic analysis of members of the genus *Rickettsia* using the gene encoding the outer-membrane protein rOmpB (ompB). *Int. J. Syst. Evol. Microbiol.* 50:1449–1455.

208. Roux, V., E. Rydkina, M. Eremeeva, and D. Raoult. 1997. Citrate synthase gene comparison, a new tool for phylogenetic analysis, and its application for the rickettsiae. *Int. J. Syst. Bacteriol.* 47:252–261.

209. Ruiz, R., J. I. Herrero, A. M. Martin, F. Sanz, A. Mateos, A. Hernandez, R. Querol, and J. Portugal. 1984. Vascular permeability in boutonneuse fever. *J. Infect. Dis.* 149:1036. (Letter.)

210. Rydkina, E., V. Roux, N. Fetisova, N. Rudakov, M. Gafarova, I. Tarasevich, and D. Raoult. 1999. New *Rickettsiae* in ticks collected in territories of the former Soviet Union. *Emerg. Infect. Dis.* 5:811–814.

211. Sarov, B., A. Galil, E. Sikuler, P. Yagupsky, A. Saah, A. Gilad, L. Naggan, and I. Sarov. 1990. Prospective study on symptomatic versus asymptomatic infections and serological response to spotted fever group rickettsiae in two rural sites in the Negev (southern Israel). *Ann. N. Y. Acad. Sci.* 590:243–245.

212. Schriefer, M. E., J. B. Sacci, Jr., J. P. Taylor, J. A. Higgins, and A. F. Azad. 1994. Murine typhus: updated roles of multiple urban components and a second typhuslike rickettsia. *J. Med. Entomol.* 31:681–685.

213. Segura, F., and E. Anton. 2002. Clarithromycin for the treatment of Mediterranean spotted fever. *Clin. Infect. Dis.* 34:560.

214. Sekeyova, Z., P. E. Fournier, J. Rehacek, and D. Raoult. 2000. Characterization of a new spotted fever group Rickettsia detected in *Ixodes ricinus* (Acari: Ixodidae) collected in Slovakia. *J. Med. Entomol.* 37:707–713.

215. Sekeyova, Z., V. Roux, and D. Raoult. 2001. Phylogeny of *Rickettsia* spp. inferred by comparing sequences of 'gene D,' which encodes an intracytoplasmic protein. *Int. J. Syst. Evol. Microbiol.* 51:1353–1360.

216. Sekeyova, Z., V. Roux, W. B. Xu, J. Rehacek, and D. Raoult. 1998. *Rickettsia slovaca* sp. nov., a member of the spotted fever group rickettsiae. *Int. J. Syst. Bacteriol.* 48:1455–1462.

217. Sekeyoya, Z., E. Kovacova, P. E. Fournier, and D. Raoult. 2003. Isolation and characterization of a new rickettsia from *Ixodes ricinus* ticks collected in Slovakia. *Ann. N. Y. Acad. Sci.* 990:54–56.

218. Sexton, D. J., J. Banks, S. Graves, K. Hughes, and B. W. Dwyer. 1991. Prevalence of antibodies to spotted fever group rickettsiae in dogs from southeasthern Australia. *Am. J. Trop. Med. Hyg.* 45:243–248.

219. Sexton, D. J., B. W. Dwyer, R. Kemp, and S. Graves. 1991. Spotted fever group rickettsial infections in Australia. *Rev. Infect. Dis.* 13:876–886.

220. Sexton, D. J., G. King, and B. W. Dwyer. 1990. Fatal Queensland tick typhus. *J. Infect. Dis.* 162:779–780.

221. Shpynov, S., P. E. Fournier, N. Rudakov, and D. Raoult. 2003. "*Candidatus* Rickettsia tarasevichiae" in *Ixodes persulcatus* ticks collected in various territories of Russia. *Ann. N. Y. Acad. Sci.* 990:162–172.

222. Shpynov, S., P. Parola, N. Rudakov, I. Samoilenko, M. Tankibaev, I. Tarasevich, and D. Raoult. 2001. Detection and identification of spotted fever group rickettsiae in *Dermatocentor* ticks from Russia and central Kazakhstan. *Eur. J. Clin. Microbiol. Infect. Dis.* 20:903–905.

223. Simser, J. A., A. T. Palmer, V. Fingerle, B. Wilske, T. J. Kurtti, and U. G. Munderloh. 2002. *Rickettsia monacensis* sp. nov., a spotted fever group rickettsia, from ticks (*Ixodes ricinus*) collected in a European city park. *Appl. Environ. Microbiol.* 68:4559–4566.

224. Spencer, R. R., and R. R. Parker. 1923. Rocky mountain spotted fever: infectivity of fasting and recently fed ticks. *Public Health Rep.* 38:333–339.

225. Stackebrandt, E., W. Frederiksen, G. M. Garrity, P. A. D. Grimont, P. Kampfer, M. C. J. Maiden, X. Nesme, R. Rossello-Mora, J. Swings, H. G. Truper, L. Vauterin, A. C. Ward, and W. B. Whitman. 2002. Report of the ad hoc committee for the re-evaluation of the species definition in bacteriology. *Int. J. Syst. Evol. Microbiol.* 52:1043–1047.

226. Stein, A., and D. Raoult. 1992. A simple method for amplification of DNA from paraffin-embedded tissues. *Nucleic Acids Res.* 20:5237–5238.

227. Stenos, J., V. Roux, D. Walker, and D. Raoult. 1998. *Rickettsia honei* sp. nov., the aetiological agent of Flinders Island spotted fever in Australia. *Int. J. Syst. Bacteriol.* 48:1399–1404.

228. Stewart, R. S. 1991. Flinders Island spotted fever: a newly recognized endemic focus of tick typhus in Bass Strait. I. Clinical and epidemiological features. *Med. J. Aust.* 154:94–99.

229. Stoenner, H. G., R. Holdenreid, D. Lackman, and J. S. Orsborn, Jr. 1959. The occurrence of *Coxiella burnetii*, *Brucella* and other pathogens among fauna of the Great Lake desert in Utah. *Am. J. Trop. Med. Hyg.* 8:590.

230. Stothard, D. R., and P. A. Fuerst. 1995. Evolutionary analysis of the spotted fever and typhus groups of *Rickettsia* using 16S rRNA gene sequences. *Syst. Appl. Microbiol.* 18:52–61.

231. Takada, N., H. Fujita, Y. Yano, Y. Tsuboi, and F. Mahara. 1994. First isolation of a rickettsia closely related to Japanese spotted fever pathogen from a tick in Japan. *J. Med. Entomol.* 31:183–185.

232. Tamura, A., N. Ohashi, H. Urakami, and S. Miyamura. 1995. Classification of *Rickettsia tsutsugamushi* in a new genus, *Orientia* gen. nov, as *Orientia tsutsugamushi* comb. nov. *Int. J. Syst. Bacteriol.* 45:589–591.

233. Tarasevich, I. V., V. Makarova, N. F. Fetisova, A. Stepanov, E. Mistkarova, N. M. Balayeva, and D. Raoult. 1991. Astrakhan fever: a new spotted fever group rickettsiosis. *Lancet* 337:172–173.

234. Tarasevich, I. V., V. A. Makarova, N. F. Fetisova, A. V. Stepanov, E. D. Miskarova, and D. Raoult. 1991. Studies of a "new" rickettsiosis, "Astrakhan" spotted fever. *Eur. J. Epidemiol.* 7:294–298.

235. Tarasevich, I. V., and G. P. Somov. 1966. Comparative serological study of tick-borne typhus of northern Asia and tsutsugamushi fever. *J. Microb. Epidemiol. Immunol.* 1:83–86.

236. Teysseire, N., J. A. Boudier, and D. Raoult. 1995. *Rickettsia conorii* entry into vero cells. *Infect. Immun.* 63:366–374.

237. Teysseire, N., C. Chiche-Portiche, and D. Raoult. 1992. Intracellular movements of *Rickettsia conorii* and *R. typhi* based on actin polymerization. *Res. Microbiol.* 143:821–829.

238. Tissot-Dupont, H., P. Brouqui, B. Faugere, and D. Raoult. 1995. Prevalence of antibodies to *Coxiella burnetii*, *Rick-*

ettsia conorii, and *Rickettsia typhi* in seven African countries. *Clin. Infect. Dis.* 21:1126–1133.

239. Tissot-Dupont, H., J. P. Cornet, and D. Raoult. 1994. Identification of rickettsiae from ticks collected in the Central African Republic using the polymerase chain reaction. *Am. J. Trop. Med. Hyg.* 50:373–380.

240. Uchida, T. 1993. *Rickettsia japonica*, the etiologic agent of Oriental spotted fever. *Microbiol. Immunol.* 37:91–102.

241. Uchida, T., F. Tashiro, T. Funato, and Y. Kitamura. 1986. Immunofluorescence test with *Rickettsia montana* for serologic diagnosis of rickettsial infection of the spotted fever group in Shikoku, Japan. *Microbiol. Immunol.* 30:1061–1066.

242. Uchida, T., T. Uchiyama, K. Kumano, and D. H. Walker. 1992. *Rickettsia japonica* sp. nov., the etiological agent of spotted fever group rickettsiosis in Japan. *Int. J. Syst. Bacteriol.* 42:303–305.

243. Uchida, T., Y. Yan, and S. Kitaoka. 1995. Detection of *Rickettsia japonica* in *Haemaphysalis longicornis* ticks by restriction fragment length polymorphism of PCR product. *J. Clin. Microbiol.* 33:824–828.

244. Uchida, T., X. J. Yu, T. Uchiyama, and D. H. Walker. 1989. Identification of a unique spotted fever group rickettsia from humans in Japan. *J. Infect. Dis.* 159:1122–1126.

245. Vestris, G., J. M. Rolain, P. E. Fournier, M. L. Birg, M. Enea, J. Y. Patrice, and D. Raoult. 2003. Seven years' experience of isolation of *Rickettsia* spp. From clinical specimens using the shell vial cell culture assay. *Ann. N. Y. Acad. Sci.* 990:371–374.

246. Walker, D. H. 1989. Rocky Mountain spotted fever: a disease in need of microbiological concern. *Clin. Microbiol. Rev.* 2:227–240.

247. Walker, D. H., B. G. Cain, and P. M. Olmstead. 1978. Specific diagnosis of Rocky Mountain spotted fever by immunofluorescence demonstration of *Rickettsia rickettsii* in biopsy of skin. *Public Health Lab.* 36:96–100.

248. Walker, D. H., and D. B. Fishbein. 1991. Epidemiology of rickettsial diseases. *Eur. J. Epidemiol.* 7:237–245.

249. Walker, D. H., R. M. Gay, and M. Valdes-Dapena. 1981. The occurrence of eschars in Rocky Mountain spotted fever. *J. Am. Acad. Dermatol.* 4:571–576.

250. Walker, D. H., Q. H. Liu, X. J. Yu, H. Li, C. Taylor, and H. M. Feng. 1992. Antigenic diversity of *Rickettsia conorii*. *Am. J. Trop. Med. Hyg.* 47:78–86.

251. Wayne, L. G., D. J. Brenner, R. R. Colwell, P. A. D. Grimont, O. Kandler, M. I. Krichevsky, L. H. Moore, W. E. C. Moore, R. G. E. Murray, E. Stackebrandt, M. P. Starr, and H. G. Truper. 1987. Report of the ad hoc committee on reconciliation of approaches to bacterial systematics. *Int. J. Syst. Bacteriol.* 37:463–464.

252. Weil, E., and A. Felix. 1916. Zur Serologischen Diagnose des Fleckfiebers. *Wien. Klin. Wochenschr.* 29:33–35.

253. Weisburg, W. G., M. E. Dobson, J. E. Samuel, G. A. Dasch, L. P. Mallavia, O. Baca, L. Mandelco, J. E. Sechrest, E. Weiss, and C. R. Woese. 1989. Phylogenetic diversity of the rickettsiae. *J. Bacteriol.* 171:4202–4206.

254. Weiss, E., J. C. Coolbaugh, and J. C. Williams. 1975. Separation of viable *Rickettsia typhi* from yolk sac and L cell host components by renografin density gradient centrifugation. *Appl. Microbiol.* 30:456–463.

255. Weiss, E., and J. W. Moulder. 1984. Order I *Rickettsiales*, Gieszczkiewicz 1939, p. 687–703. *In* N. R. Krieg and J. G. Holt (ed.), *Bergey's Manual of Systematic Bacteriology*. Williams & Wilkins, Baltimore. Md.

256. Wenzel, R. P., F. G. Hayden, D. H. Groschel, R. A. Salata, W. S. Young, J. E. Greenlee, S. Newman, P. J. Miller, K. E. Hechemy, W. Burgdorfer, et al. 1986. Acute febrile cerebrovasculitis: a syndrome of unknown, perhaps rickettsial, cause. *Ann. Intern. Med.* 104:606–615.

257. Werren, J. H., G. D. Hurst, W. Zhang, J. A. J. Breeuwer, R. Stouthamer, and M. E. N. Majerus. 1994. Rickettsial relative associated with male killing in the ladybird beetle (*Adalia bipunctata*). *J. Bacteriol.* 176:388–394.

258. Williams, W. J., S. Radulovic, G. A. Dasch, J. Lindstrom, D. J. Kelly, C. N. Oster, and D. H. Walker. 1994. Identification of *Rickettsia conorii* infection by polymerase chain reaction in a soldier returning from Somalia. *Clin. Infect. Dis.* 19:93–99.

259. Winkler, H. H. 1976. Rickettsial permeability. An ADP-ATP transport system. *J. Biol. Chem.* 251:389–396.

260. Winkler, H. H., and E. T. Miller. 1982. Phospholipase A and the interaction of *Rickettsia prowazekii* and mouse fibroblasts (L-929 cells). *Infect. Immun.* 38:109–113.

261. Woese, C. R. 1987. Bacterial evolution. *Microbiol. Rev.* 51:221–271.

262. Wolbach, S. B. 1919. Studies on rocky mountain spotted fever. *J. Med. Res.* 41:1–70.

263. Wood, D. O., L. R. Williamson, H. H. Winkler, and D. C. Krause. 1987. Nucleotide sequence of the *Rickettsia prowazekii* citrate synthase gene. *J. Bacteriol.* 169:3564–3572.

264. Wu, Y. M., S. R. Yu, and D. Lou. 1994. Western-blot analysis of *Rickettsia heilongjiangi*. *J. Prev. Med. PLA* 12:28–30.

265. Xu, W. B., L. Beati, and D. Raoult. 1997. Characterization of and application of monoclonal antibodies against *Rickettsia africae*, a newly recognized species of spotted fever group rickettsia. *J. Clin. Microbiol.* 35:64–70.

266. Xu, W. B., and D. Raoult. 1997. Production of monoclonal antibodies against *Rickettsia massiliae* and their use in antigenic and epidemiological studies. *J. Clin. Microbiol.* 35:1715–1721.

267. Xu, W. B., and D. Raoult. 1998. Taxonomic relationships among spotted fever group rickettsiae as revealed by antigenic analysis with monoclonal antibodies. *J. Clin. Microbiol.* 36:887–896.

268. Yagupsky, P., and B. Wolach. 1993. Fatal Israeli spotted fever in children. *Clin. Infect. Dis.* 17:850–853.

269. Yan, Y., T. Uchiyama, and T. Uchida. 1994. Nucleotide sequence of polymerase chain reaction product amplified from *Rickettsia japonica* DNA using *Rickettsia rickettsii* 190-kilodalton surface antigen gene primers. *Microbiol. Immunol.* 38:865–869.

270. Yu, X., Y. Jin, M. Fan, G. Xu, Q. Liu, and D. Raoult. 1993. Genotypic and antigenic identification of two new strains of spotted fever group rickettsiae isolated from China. *J. Clin. Microbiol.* 31:83–88.

271. Zdrodovskii, P. F. 1949. Systematics and comparative characterization of endemic rickettsioses. *Zh. Mikrobiol. Epidemiol.* 10:19–28.

272. Zhang, J. Z., M. Y. Fan, D. Z. Bi, W. F. Cui, and Y. F. Han. 1996. Genotypic identification of three new strains of spotted fever group rickettsiae isolated in China. *Acta Virol.* 40:215–219.

273. Zhang, J. Z., M. Y. Fan, Y. M. Wu, P. E. Fournier, V. Roux, and D. Raoult. 2000. Genetic classification of "*Rickettsia heilongjiangii*" and "*Rickettsia hulinii*" two Chinese spotted fever group rickettsiae. *J. Clin. Microbiol.* 38:3498–3501

Chapter 19

Q Fever

HERBERT A. THOMPSON, DAVID T. DENNIS, AND GREGORY A. DASCH

INTRODUCTION

Q fever is a bacterial zoonosis caused by infection with *Coxiella burnetii*. Mammals, birds, and ticks are natural hosts of the agent, which they persistently shed into the environment in their secretions, wastes, and products of parturition. Humans most often become infected by inhaling contaminated aerosols, especially those associated with the birth of domesticated animals and with dried tick feces. Q fever occurs worldwide. Reliable estimates of disease incidence are unavailable owing to inadequate surveillance. Endemic infections and outbreaks occur among populations exposed to principal animal sources, especially dairy cows, sheep, and goats. Acute infections may manifest as isolated fever, pneumonia, or hepatitis or be asymptomatic. The symptomatology can be protean, and the disease is difficult to diagnose based on clinical presentation alone. Chronic disease most often occurs in immunocompromised hosts and in those with anatomical defects of heart valves or other structures of the vascular system (40). A chronic fatigue-like illness has been described, arising 1 to 10 years following initial acute Q fever infections (45). The myriad symptoms and presentations seen in human Q fever are both confusing and fascinating (8). Laboratory diagnosis usually relies on results of serologic testing.

C. burnetii has recently been reclassified into the order *Legionellales*, in the gamma subdivision of the proteobacteria. It shares significant genomic and therefore both genotypic and phenotypic characteristics with the pathogen *Legionella pneumophila*, which in natural settings is likely to be found primarily as an intracellular parasite within hydroprotozoan populations. It is not known to what extent *Coxiella* might share this ecology, but experimental studies suggest that such a parasitic association is possible (59). The microbiological and clinical similarities of *L. pneu-*

mophila and Legionnaire's disease to the *C. burnetii* organism and to acute Q fever disease led to serious consideration of Q fever in the 1976 outbreak of *Legionella* pneumonia in Philadelphia (85).

Although tick transmission of *C. burnetii* to various species of mammals is well documented, there are no confirmed occurrences of direct transmission to humans by feeding ticks. The organism is prevalent in a wide diversity of wild and domesticated animals, including sheep, goats, cattle, cats, dogs, and birds, and in the ticks that parasitize them (137, 142). Several researchers have proposed that the continued maintenance of infections in domestic animals might depend upon introductions by tick species that act as bridging vectors from wild animal cycles (70).

Much of the data on the occurrence of *C. burnetii* in ticks and vertebrate hosts, and on transmission between them, dates to descriptions of the ecology of Q fever published in the mid-20th century. One purpose of this review is to refocus on these observations. More detailed discussions of common transmission routes for *Coxiella*, pathogenesis and clinical descriptions of Q fever, and general microbiology of the organism have been presented recently in other reviews (79, 81, 88, 104).

HISTORY OF DISCOVERY

The disease was recognized first in Australia by Derrick (28), who in 1935 and 1936 investigated outbreaks of "abattoir fever" among employees at the Cannon Hill meat packing plant in Brisbane, Australia. Derrick described the disease characteristics and likely transmission and made the index isolate by passage of human blood in guinea pigs. But for some time the nature of the etiologic agent remained undefined, and hence the name "Query" or Q fever. Burnet and Freeman employed guinea pig spleens received

Herbert A. Thompson and Gregory A. Dasch • Viral and Rickettsial Zoonoses Branch, Division of Viral and Rickettsial Diseases, National Center for Infectious Diseases, Centers for Disease Control and Prevention, Atlanta, GA 30333. **David T. Dennis** • Division of Vector-Borne Infectious Diseases, National Center for Infectious Diseases, Centers for Disease Control and Prevention, Fort Collins, CO 80522.

from Derrick; after passage of these tissues through mice, they were able to visualize the agent, to study its infectivity and immunity characteristics in the laboratory, and to suggest its rickettsial rather than viral nature (14). The organism was named *Rickettsia burnetii*.

In the United States, tick studies of spotted fever at the Rocky Mountain Laboratory, National Institutes of Health (NIH), conducted by R. R. Parker and G. E. Davis and others revealed that a pool of *Dermacentor andersoni* ticks collected on Nine Mile Creek in Montana contained a filter-passing agent that, unlike the agent of spotted fever, did not cause scrotal swelling and necrosis when inoculated into guinea pigs (26, 97). The agent and the disease observed in guinea pigs remained an exotic curiosity until a human laboratory infection occurred (34). Dyer, an NIH scientist from Washington, D.C., visited the Hamilton, Montana, laboratory to investigate the recent claim by H. Cox that he could culture rickettsiae in chicken embryos. While there, Dyer was exposed to the Nine Mile agent in the laboratory and fell ill with fever after returning to the eastern United States. Dyer was aware of the Australian discovery of Q fever by Burnet and Freeman (14) and had secured the organism and guinea pig antiserum from Burnet. Given the rickettsial nature of the Nine Mile fever organism and similarities in the features of the two human diseases, Dyer followed his suspicions and used Burnet's reagents to prove that the agent of Australian Q fever was the same as that causing Nine Mile fever (34). In 1948, the organism was renamed *Coxiella burnetii* (100, 101) to recognize contributions of both scientists in the discovery of the agent.

Although the discoveries by both Australian and NIH researchers are well recognized, some give Hideo Noguchi credit for the first published description of *C. burnetii*. His description of what is believed to have been *C. burnetii*, a filter-passing "virus" isolated from *D. andersoni* from Sawtooth Canyon, Montana, was published in 1926 (94).

Allied forces experienced Q fever outbreaks in Italy and other Mediterranean countries during the close of hostilities in World War II, and the similarity of these outbreaks to the features of "Balkan grippe" was appreciated by J. E. Smadel and others (106, 107). Q fever was, however, considered an unlikely cause of disease in North America. This view persisted until the explosive outbreaks of Q fever in abattoirs in Texas, Chicago, and elsewhere in the late 1940s (134). Soon thereafter, the disease was described in Great Britain (72) and in several other countries (summarized by Babudieri) (5), and it was recognized as an occupational hazard in the southern California dairy (52) and northern California sheep (60) industries.

The Prototype Strain: Isolation and Early Transmission Studies

The first isolate was obtained by Davis and Cox in Hamilton, Mont., in 1937 (26), from a pool of 200 *D. andersoni* ticks. The tick pool was divided into four groups of 50 ticks each, and each group was placed in feeding capsules and attached to the bellies of guinea pigs. One of the pigs became febrile and eventually died. Blood from this pig was passaged subsequently into two other guinea pigs, both of which succumbed to the infection. The infection was maintained in guinea pigs by intraperitoneal injection of blood or spleen tissue. Further tick transmission studies of this infection were immediately carried out by Parker and Davis (97). In these studies, *D. andersoni* larvae were fed on infected guinea pigs and recovered. A single surviving nymph that molted from these larvae was placed on a second guinea pig. This host became febrile on the 12th day after infestation. Spleen and blood from this infection were further passaged to demonstrate the infectivity and to fulfill Koch's postulates. In another set of experiments, transovarial passage in *D. andersoni* was demonstrated. The agent was initially named *Rickettsia diaporica* because of its ability to pass through bacteria-blocking filters, and the disease it caused was called Nine Mile fever (26). Almost certainly, the ability of infectivity to pass through filters was due to the small size of the "dust-like" particles observed by Kordova and Rosenberg (56, 108) and confirmed years later as the sporelike forms of the organism (82). The sporelike forms accumulate at the end of a growth cycle (19a).

Studies of Australian Strains

After his initial clinical and laboratory descriptions, Derrick worked with D. W. J. Smith in solving the epidemiology of Q fever. This led to the discovery of the organism in Australian ticks (30, 119), especially in *Haemaphysalis humerosa*, which was known as a common ectoparasite of the bandicoot, an insectivorous marsupial. This tick was found on many of the mammals of the eastern and northern seaboards of Australia. Although the sources of known human outbreaks were clearly domestic animals, the Australian group soon began looking for wild animal reservoirs and in 1939 published on the infection of bandicoots and the high seroprevalence in this species (29). Soon to follow were several other tick experiments, including one in which *H. humerosa*, not known to naturally feed on humans, was induced to feed on a human subject in the Australian laboratory. Further work by Smith (115) showed that larval, nymphal, and adult stages of the tick *H. humerosa* could be infected while feeding on febrile guinea pigs. He further showed that the feces of the ticks were infectious by applying feces to abraded or unabraded guinea pig skin (115). Subsequent studies led to the famous finding of a high infection rate of bandicoots on Moreton Island off the coast of Australia (29, 30). Six isolates of *Coxiella* were obtained from *H. humerosa* ticks that had been removed from bandicoots captured on Moreton Island. These ticks were allowed to feed on guinea pigs and thereby transmitted the disease. Isolates were also made directly from bandicoot blood. It was concluded that the bandicoot-tick cycle was important for natural conservation of the disease and might be a source of infection to cattle. Tick transmission to cattle was supported by the observation that cattle ticks could become infected by feeding on an infected calf (31, 32). Although *H. humerosa* ticks were induced to feed on humans in the laboratory, they were never implicated as natural vectors of infection to humans.

MICROBIOLOGY

C. burnetii is a small, pleomorphic organism, measuring 0.2 to 0.3 μm wide by 0.6 to 1.0 μm long. It is an obligate parasite in eukaryotic hosts. It stains gram variable but possesses a cell wall and envelope structure resembling those of gram-negative bacteria (83). The organism undergoes a life cycle that includes DNA-containing endospore-like structures and cells which differ remarkably in ultrastructure, size, and density (82, 83, 84, 139). These stages differ sharply in protein composition and therefore in gene regulatory pattern (47, 112). It is presently accepted that the smaller dense cells with spore-like attributes explain the environmental stability and high (and unusual) spectra of chemical resistance (111). The organism possesses lipopolysaccharides (LPSs) (109), which are believed to be associated with its outer membrane (15). Wild-type LPS appears to have the classical gram-negative structure comprising a lipid A, a heptose-rich inner core, other core sugars primarily composed of mannose and mannose derivatives, and an outer O-antigen repeat structure. The arrangement and stereochemistry of the latter component are not completely established but do consist of mannose, hexose amino sugars, and the branched sugars virenose and dihydrohydroxy-streptose (3, 109, 133). These sugars are rare in nature but appear to be key immunogenic determinants (53, 109, 132, 133).

Some strains or isolates appear to be prone to antigenic variation associated with repeated passages in nonimmune laboratory hosts. The best-understood example occurs in the Nine Mile strain, which reverts to antigenic phase II after dozens of sequential passages in embryonated eggs. These initial observations on phase variation were made by Stoker and Fiset (124), who noted that sera obtained early after infection of guinea pigs were reactive with organisms passaged several times in eggs but not with organisms found in spleens of guinea pigs or in early egg passage. Late convalescent-phase serum from the animals, however, reacted well with animal-passaged strains, the so-called phase I stage. We now know that this antigenic transition is explained by changes in LPS structure concomitant with passage. Phase I organisms possess a full LPS, whereas phase II organisms possess a much simpler structure, comprising lipid A and core sugars (3, 132) and lacking both virenose and streptose sugars. This change is analogous to the smooth-to-rough transition seen in gram-negative enteric bacteria. In the transition studied in the Nine Mile strains, a chromosomal rearrangement (136) explained by a large chromosomal deletion occurs (50). The deleted DNA primarily contains genes homologous to LPS biosynthesis and O-antigen assembly and secretion. Plasmids are present in both phase I and phase II organisms; plasmid types ranging in length from 36 to 56 kb have been described (81, 121).

However, this large chromosomal deletion does not accompany all phase II or phase II-like strains. Notably, the M-44 Grita strain, which has a truncated LPS very similar to Nine Mile phase II and lacks the signature O-antigen sugars (3), does not have a DNA deletion in the LPS region (128). The Nine Mile RSA 514 strain, which was obtained from a guinea pig placenta more than 300 days after infection, also has deleted DNA in a region which overlaps that of Nine Mile phase II. This interesting isolate (called the Crazy strain) possesses an LPS which is intermediate in size between wild-type phase I and phase II, is intermediate in animal virulence (92), and lacks virenose but not dihydrohydroxystreptose (3). However, the Australian QD strain, which has a long egg passage history and an LPS with characteristics similar to that of RSA 514, does not have a comparable DNA deletion (128). Thus the explanation for antigenic phase transition and changes in animal virulence seems to correlate with LPS changes, including truncation and a loss of smoothness, but the genetic explanation for these changes in LPS structure is not consistent.

C. burnetii was shown by Hackstadt and Williams to be an acidophilic bacterium (43). The organism has a glucose- or hexose-based metabolism (43), possesses many Embden-Meyerhof-Parnas pathway enzymes for glucose metabolism (20, 96, 113), and depends primarily on proton-driven transport of nutrients for metabolic activity, which can be measured in axenic media at lower pHs of 4 to 5 (44). During long-term in vitro incubations at pH 4.5 in the presence of all 20 naturally occurring amino acids including glutamate, nucleosides, and glucose, the organisms can be induced to increase protein biomass by over 50% and to replicate DNA (18). But this host cell-free environment is incomplete, and biomass increases fall short of a single cell division cycle (18, 146). The acidophilic biochemistry of the organism (43) matches its environment in phagocytes and fibroblasts, where the organism is known to reside in acidified vacuoles, probably in some stage of phagolysosomes (2, 15, 80).

Complete sequencing of the Nine Mile phase I strain genome revealed both surprises and confirmations (113). Several repeat sequences resembling eukaryotic ankyrin genes and a complete set of type IV secretion apparatus genes quite like those of *Legionella* were among the most notable findings. An overly large contingent of genes purportedly functioning as transporters, permeases, and toxin pumps was another. The organism lacks enzymes for the biosynthesis of nearly half the required amino acids and thus must transport these from host pools. As is seen in many acidophiles, over 40% of *Coxiella*'s proteins possess an isoelectric point (pI) between pH 8 and pH 10 (113). It is speculated that those proteins can help control the intracellular pH by titrating excessive protons which would leak from the acidic environment. Finally, the organism possesses many remnant and existing enzymes for the synthesis of macrolide-like antibiotics (113). These observations suggest that *Coxiella*'s ancestors resided within acidic soils or water and developed compounds to counter competing microbes.

Studies to locate origins of chromosome replication (125) led to the discovery of an autonomous replication sequence that was useful in development of shuttle plasmids that could be used to genetically transform *C. burnetii* via electroporation methods (126). However, the method has been applied only once to introduce green fluorescent protein into the organism (64). Several plasmids observed in various strains may be associated with as-yet-undefined virulence factors (81).

NATURAL HISTORY AND ECOLOGY

The finding of the Nine Mile fever agent in *D. andersoni* ticks in Montana was the first in a series of tick infection discoveries. Davis (23) made similar isolations in 1939 from *D. andersoni* ticks captured in southeastern Wyoming and concluded that these isolates were essentially identical to the Montana Nine Mile isolate. Parker and Kohls (98) isolated a filter-passing agent from *Amblyomma americanum* ticks collected in eastern Texas; by repeated guinea pig passages, they determined that this tick isolate was also similar to the Nine Mile strain. Davis (25) used the

Wyoming strain he isolated in 1939 to infect guinea pigs, upon which he fed the argasid ticks *Ornithodoros moubata* and *Ornithodoros hermsi*. The former is an African species, whereas the latter is common in western and northwestern states. Transmission from the infected animals to adult ticks occurred, and transovarial transmission to progeny ticks was observed in each of the ticks. Similarly, transmission of the Q fever agent to or by a number of Australian ticks was proven. Smith (116, 117) proved transmission by *Rhipicephalus sanguineus* and by the paralysis tick, *Ixodes holocyclus*. He also showed that *Haemaphysalis bispinosa* and *Ornithodoros* species could be experimentally infected and that the former could transmit infection while feeding on guinea pigs (118). De Rodaniche (27) did similar guinea pig experiments to show transmission by *Amblyomma cajennense*. As early as 1949, at least six species of ticks from the United States, Australia, and Algeria had been found to be naturally infected: *D. andersoni*, *A. americanum*, *Dermacentor occidentalis*, *H. humerosa*, *Hyalomma savignyi*, and *Ornithodoros turicata* (24, 52).

Bandicoot-Tick Cycle

The bandicoot is a nocturnal marsupial that feeds on grubs and insects on and in the forest floor. It roots and digs for its food. The pouch is inverted (opens to the rear) to prevent filling up with dirt and debris during rooting and burrowing. Within a few years of the discovery of Q fever in Australia, a significant amount of evidence was obtained to support an animal-tick cycle of *Coxiella* involving the bandicoot and the slender-bodied tick *H. humerosa* (1, 29, 30, 119). It was soon determined that bandicoots, especially the ones located on Moreton Island, Australia, were hosts for *H. humerosa* ticks infected with *Coxiella* (30). The bandicoots, sometimes as many as 20% of them, were also infected, although apparently without ill effects. Experimental infections of captured bandicoots were carried out with some Australian *C. burnetii* strains isolated from the abattoir outbreaks, also resulting in nonapparent carrier states. In autopsied bandicoots, the only obvious pathology was enlargement of the triangular spleen (29). Because *H. humerosa* ticks could also be found in significant numbers on cattle, it was suggested that the bandicoot-tick cycle could help maintain Q fever infection in cattle herds, but this has not been proven (33, 115).

Kangaroo-Tick Cycle

More recently, *Amblyomma triguttatum*, the ornate kangaroo tick, was reported to harbor *C. burnetii*

(86, 102). *A. triguttatum* is extremely common in western Australia, and *C. burnetii* was readily isolated from kangaroos infested with this tick, as well as from the ticks themselves (102). Human cases of Q fever are prevalent in regions of western Australia (68). Because this tick species also infests sheep, goats, and wallabies, a cycle between natural and domestic hosts has been considered. However, studies have failed to show transstadial or transovarial maintenance of *C. burnetii* in *A. triguttatum*, and this tick's role in maintaining infection in animal populations is unlikely.

Kangaroo Rat–Deer Mice–Tick Cycles

Shortly after World War II, the U.S. Department of the Army funded several studies to determine the ecology and parasitism of animals living in and around the Dugway chemical testing grounds west of Salt Lake City, Utah. The first of these studies was carried out by Stoenner and colleagues in 1959 (123) from the NIH. Later, scientists from the University of Utah (135) took over these studies and turned up a surprising list of wild mammal species infected with *C. burnetii*. The organism was isolated from over a dozen different rodent species, coyotes, foxes, raccoons, and deer. Because isolates of the organism were readily made from kangaroo rats and deer mice, as well as from the *Dermacentor parumapertus* ticks which infest these rodents, a rodent-tick cycle was suggested. Again, however, there are no data supporting transstadial or transovarial transmission of the organism within ticks.

The Dugway strains of *C. burnetii* have low pathogenicity for guinea pigs and cannot be recovered by sequential spleen passage. These are the only known natural isolates that possess this avirulence characteristic. The prototypic Dugway strain (sometimes called the rodent strain) of *C. burnetii* derives from one of these isolates. It is believed to be nonpathogenic for humans and possesses an unusual plasmid type (69).

Deer Mice- and/or Brush Mice-Tick Cycles

A serostudy made in Mendocino County, northern California, confirmed the widespread distribution of the Q fever organism among wild rodents, deer, grey foxes, coyotes, and raccoons (37). Isolates of *C. burnetii* were made from locally collected *D. occidentalis* by injecting tick extracts into guinea pigs and mice. The organism was also obtained from several of the mammalian species trapped in this study. Because of a seasonal correlation of appearance of antibodies within captured rodents and tick feeding, the existence of a small animal-tick cycle was suggested. A total of 3,035 ectoparasites obtained from wild animals in an area shared with livestock herds were investigated. Ticks were pooled according to species, extracted, and inoculated into laboratory animals (mice, hamsters, and guinea pigs). Although seven species of ticks were studied, *C. burnetii* was isolated from only two species, *D. occidentalis* and the soft tick *Ornithodoros coriaceus*. The former were picked from deer, grey foxes, and raccoons. In this same area, deer (*Odocoileus hemionus columbianus*) and grey foxes had high seroprevalence rates (22 and 55%, respectively) and a high rate of successful isolation (9 and 10%, respectively). Thus, a correlation between wildlife infection and the occurrence of *Coxiella* within their tick ectoparasites was established (37). However, since only one pool from each kind of tick yielded isolates and since the antibody prevalence in the animals did not increase during the tick season, the authors concluded that ticks could not be a major factor in transmission and maintenance of Q fever in these populations. An exception to this observation was that seropositive results were obtained from various rodents (wood rats, kangaroo rats, and grey squirrels) collected during the first part of the year (January to June), the season of high tick activity in Mendocino County and the season during which the ticks found harboring the agent were also collected. Thus, it was speculated that the rodents and their ticks could represent a tick-wildlife cycle separate from that of domestic animals (37). Evidence for transmission from local ticks to humans was not found.

European Sheep- and/or Wildlife-Tick Cycles

In Europe, it was proposed that the original endemic zones for Q fever were defined by a region comprising the Mediterranean countries, the Balkans, and much of the southern European parts of the former Soviet Union. This region was rather precisely defined on its northern boundary by the annual 10°C isotherm. Because this margin corresponded closely to the northern end of the range for the tick *Dermacentor marginatus*, it was proposed that this tick was important for the maintenance of *C. burnetii* throughout central Europe (62). The possible role of this tick in the cycle of the Q fever agent has been particularly well studied in Germany in both the south and central portions, because Q fever disease is well recognized there, especially in areas of concentrated sheep husbandry. Very high parasitism of sheep by this tick, up to 200 ticks per animal, is common. Since the *Coxiella* organisms are found in both the tick and sheep, it is considered likely that a sheep-tick cycle is responsible for maintaining the agent at a high rate of prevalence. Outbreaks of Q fever in persons associated with sheep shearing have been reported (48, 62). *D. marginatus* prefers to locate and feed on the back of the head and neck of sheep, and the feces of large numbers of ticks blackens the wool in these places, making infestations easy to spot. *C. burnetii* within the tick feces is aerosolized during the agitation of shearing. Researchers in Germany and border countries have implicated several other tick species as potential vectors. These are *Haemaphysalis punctata, Ixodes ricinus, R. sanguineus, Rhipicephalus bursa, Hyalomma marginatum,* and *Hyalomma anatolicum* (62). Active control of Q fever in sheep is practiced in Germany by animal immunization, washes with microbial disinfectants, acaricides, and culling of infected animals.

Despite a lack of evidence for any substantial role of direct tick transmission of *C. burnetii* to humans, some countries emphasize the importance of tick-domestic animal or tick-wild animal cycles in the epidemiology of the disease. Recently published recommendations for control of human Q fever in Germany aim at preventing human contact with potentially infectious dust in animal fur and products of conception; in areas where *D. marginatus* infection is endemic, acaricides are recommended to control the transmission of infection from ticks to animals (48).

Other Animal-Tick Cycles

Places where other natural tick-borne cycles have been suspected include Nova Scotia in Canada, involving cats and rodents; Japan, where isolates have been made from ticks captured in dairy pastures; Russia; and France. In Nova Scotia, infected rodents include the meadow vole (*Microtus pennsylvanicus*), the red-backed vole (*Clethrionomys gapperi*), and the meadow jumping mouse (*Zapus hudsonius*), all of which are hosts of the dog tick *Dermacentor variabilis*. Since cats but not dogs were found to be seropositive, it was suggested that ticks other than *D. variabilis* may be serving as vectors (78).

In Japan, 12 isolates of *C. burnetii* were made from raw milk, aborted bovine fetuses, bovine mammary gland samples, and ticks from two separate dairy pastures. Four out of 15 ticks yielded two isolates (pooled ticks). The protein profiles of these isolates resembled the prototypical Nine Mile strain (49).

In Russia and some Eastern European countries, ticks have been considered to be important in the ecology of the Q fever agent (90, 143), especially various ixodid ticks. Evidence has been gathered to suggest that ticks there are both reservoirs and vectors for *C. burnetii*. The findings through 1988 have been summarized by Rehacek and Tarasevich (105) and implicate several tick species, including *D. marginatus, Hyalomma plumbeum, R. bursa, Ornithodoros lahorensis, Dermacentor nuttalli,* and *Argas persicus*. In addition to ecological studies, the biology of infection of ticks has been described. The course of infection in ticks has been traced, originating in the intestinum. Most of the replication occurs in midgut epithelial cells. Organisms then penetrate the gut wall from which the organisms spread to all organs, including salivary glands, with spread occurring via invaded hemocytes (105). During periods of multiplication, ticks are said to be capable of transmission by feeding. Up to 10^{11} organisms were found in salivary glands from a single *Hyalomma asiaticum* tick, and it was determined that up to 10^9 organisms could be secreted in saliva from experimentally infected *Hyalomma dromedarii* ticks. Considerable quantities are shed in feces as well, and the stability of Q fever organisms in tick feces is high. Dry, powdered feces can be transmitted by wind. During a Q fever outbreak in Hamburg, *O. moubata* ticks were used to aid in isolations of *C. burnetii* from humans. Similar studies were conducted in Switzerland, with similar results (105). Transfer of organisms from larvae to nymphs and from nymphs to adults was found to be common (105), and transovarial transmission was observed. *H. asiaticum* and *Rhipicephalus turanicus* were able to transmit infection on to progeny; *Dermacentor reticulatus* and *Ixodes persulcatus* were not.

In Cyprus, the presence of *C. burnetii* in *R. sanguineus* and *Hyalomma* spp. has been shown by PCR techniques (120) and by the shell vial technique of isolation.

EPIDEMIOLOGY

Sources of Infection

Q fever is a zoonosis in which humans are incidental hosts. The reservoir of *C. burnetii* is extensive, including many wild and domestic animals and ticks (5). Domesticated livestock, especially cattle, sheep, and goats, are considered the most frequent source of infection to humans. Pregnancy stimulates the growth of organisms in reproductive and mammary gland tissues of many mammalian species (5, 127, 140, 141). Extensive shedding of organisms in fluids and tissues occurs during birthing, and large numbers of organisms are found as well in urine, feces, and milk of affected animals. Infected cows have been shown to shed the organism in milk for up to 32 months, and sheep pass the organism in feces for 11 to 18 days postpartum. As noted in a review by Marrie, placental tissues of infected sheep can contain 10^9 organisms per g (77). Domestic pets, especially cats and dogs, can also become infected and disperse large numbers of organisms during the birthing process (13, 58). *C. burnetii* has been isolated from chickens, pigeons, ducks, geese, and turkeys (6), and infective organisms from birds can be dispersed in contaminated fomites (5). *C. burnetii* has also been isolated from more than 40 species of ticks; tick saliva, body fluids, and feces may be sources of infection (6). Exposures to domestic animals and their products, wastes, and secretions (including hides, products of parturition, animal bedding material such as straw and hay, and dust in buildings and shelters that previously housed animals) have been described as important risk factors for infection in humans (5). Dairy cows are more important sources of infection than beef cattle, which are rarely infected; *C. burnetii* introduced into a dairy herd spreads rapidly, so that 80% of cows are infected within a few months of its appearance (65, 66).

Routes of Transmission to Humans

C. burnetii is readily dispersed into the air in resistant and highly infectious spore forms, and the principal mode of transmission of infection to humans is inhalation of airborne organisms from fresh or desiccated livestock tissues, fluids, and wastes, especially those associated with the birthing process and its products (38, 74, 77, 78, 79, 81). Infection by inhalation of organisms from other mammals, birds, and tick feces may also occur but is less common. Zdrodovskii and Golinevich considered ticks to be major reservoirs of *C. burnetii* and the bite wounds of infected ticks to be portals of entry (143), even though epidemiological evidence for this is lacking. Infection by ingesting raw milk and milk products has been suggested, but this mode has not been borne out by experimental studies with humans (79).

Major Epidemiologic Features as Determined by Outbreak Investigations

An understanding of the epidemiology of Q fever has greatly broadened since the early descriptions by Derrick of the disease as an exotic disease risk to abattoir workers in eastern Australia (33). Q fever was recognized as a serious occurrence among Allied forces in Italy during the Second World War, where outbreaks involving approximately 1,000 cases were identified. In one outbreak, large numbers of troops came down with the disease following exposures to dust in a barn converted into a makeshift theater; laboratory personnel processing specimens from this outbreak were also affected (106). It was concluded that inhalation of contaminated dust was the likely infective exposure and that arthropod transmission was not a factor. It was further noted that although the attack rate was high (greater than 30%) and morbidity was consider-

able, the disease was not fatal. The disease was not recognized in the local population, even though surveys showed a high seroprevalence of *C. burnetii* antibodies (38).

An outbreak of fever was described among U.S. military troops at Camp Bullis, Tex., in 1943 (57). The Bullis fever episode featured many cases among troops who where heavily infested, some with over 100 ticks each, with *A. americanum*. *A. americanum* ticks collected as part of the investigation were found to be infected with a rickettsial organism, called the Bullis fever agent (4, 7). This agent was subsequently determined to be *C. burnetii* by scientists at the Rocky Mountain Laboratory (57, 122).

Following these military experiences, several outbreaks were identified and described in civilian populations in the United States. In 1946, aerosol-generated outbreaks were described among workers at meat-packing plants in Amarillo, Tex., and Chicago, Ill. (38, 134). Next, the disease was reported among dairy workers in both northern and southern California, extensive investigations of which provided a much expanded understanding of the epidemiology and ecology of the disease. Q fever was recognized to be endemic in California. In northern California, sheep and goats were described as the main sources of infection. Importantly, it was shown that recrudescence of infection in animals occurred during periods of gestation, leading to extraordinary contamination of the environment with *C. burnetii* during birthing. Although most sheep shed organisms only after their first lambing, about a third shed organisms twice, and a few shed during three successive birthings (10, 52, 60). It was further demonstrated that the organisms could be isolated from the air of contaminated premises. In southern California, dairy herds were identified as major sources of infection of humans. Among dairy herds studied, the seroprevalence was about 10%, and infection did not appear to have an observable pathogenic effect on the animals. The seroprevalence among the general population of Los Angeles was found to be about 1.4%. In groups of human subjects selected for exposure to livestock, the rate was positively associated with closeness of the contact: the seroprevalence of workers in packing plants where few or no dairy cows were slaughtered was about 4% versus a rate of 11% where dairy cattle were routinely slaughtered. Among dairy workers it was 23%. Among raw-milk drinkers, seroprevalence was 12% versus 1.2% in non-raw-milk drinkers (38, 51). Most infections in humans were found to be mild or asymptomatic.

An outbreak among workers at a wool- and hair-processing plant was attributed to airborne exposure (114). Several outbreaks associated with sheep used in perinatal research were described in the United States and Canada; in these outbreaks, cases occurred not only in persons with direct exposure to infected animals but also in persons working in buildings through which infected animals had been transported (38).

Transmission of infection to humans by inhalation of contaminated dusts and aerosols can occur over considerable distances (46). In Australia, where the vaccination of at-risk personnel is a common practice, it is noted that small outbreaks of Q fever often occur among unvaccinated individuals who have no known direct contact with contaminated animals (19). Investigations of a recent large outbreak of Q fever in a rural community in Germany identified exposure to airborne fomites from sheep flocks at the time of lambing as the most likely source of infection, with highest seroprevalence among persons with activities taking them closest to where the herds were pastured (67). Community outbreaks have been described in Britain among persons exposed to contaminated straw, manure, or dust disseminated by farm vehicles moving along country roads; elsewhere in Europe, outbreaks occur in populations exposed to sheep herds being driven through small villages (38, 79). Distant and delayed exposures can be explained by the extreme stability of the organism in the environment, survival for indefinite lengths of time in soils and on fomites, and the ability of the fomites to be dispersed by wind (46, 131). C. burnetii forms life cycle stages, including a small-cell variant and a spore-like particle (47), which probably explains the organism's high resistance to osmotic stress and to physical and chemical agents (82, 83, 111). This is an unusual, perhaps unique, trait for a gram-negative organism. The stability enables airborne transmission during dry periods, sometimes over miles from a source, coinciding with an increased disease incidence above background levels (46, 131).

C. burnetii is highly infectious, with an infective dose in humans of less than 10 organisms (129, 130). The ability of infective Q fever particles to be dispersed over wide areas and their high infectiousness have been considered in designating C. burnetii as a category B select agent of concern as a potential weapon of terrorism (16).

Although airborne spread from parturient animals and products accounts for most transmission of Q fever to humans, dispersal of dried tick feces has also been considered potentially important as a source of infection in some settings and is cited as an occupational hazard of sheep shearers (48, 62). C. burnetii can be concentrated in extremely high numbers in tick feces, and infection of humans by inhalation or cutaneous inoculation of dried material is possible (101, 105).

Ingestion of unpasteurized (or improperly pasteurized) milk or milk products is considered another possible source of infection (39, 71, 73). As noted above, infected California dairy herds were identified as important sources of Q fever in humans in the 1950s and 1960s (10, 52). How much disease in humans occurred due to ingestion of contaminated unpasteurized products is unknown, but a causal association was suggested (71, 73). The standards for pasteurization of milk in the United States and elsewhere are set according to the times and temperatures required to kill C. burnetii, rather than mycobacterial or other milk-borne bacterial species (36, 55).

Person-to-person transmission of Q fever is extremely rare, even though respiratory infection is a common form of disease. Maurin and Raoult (81) described a case of Q fever pneumonia in an obstetrician who performed an abortion on an infected mother. Recrudescence of infection during pregnancy has been recognized in several women who had Q fever illness 2 to 3 years previously (127), and it is surprising that transmission to obstetrical staff is not more common. There are two reports of infection in persons attending autopsies and mentions of accidental infections arising from needle stick and from transfusions (81). Sexual transmission has also been described in humans, but it is thought to be rare (91).

Direct transmission to humans by infective tick bite or by inoculation of tick feces through the bite wound is also considered to be rare. Anecdotal cases have, however, been described. Beaman and Hung (9) reported on a western Australian well digger who had five kangaroo ticks (A. triguttatum) removed from his iliac crest region and who developed acute Q fever with pericarditis within 14 days. His phase II antibody titer rose from 1:10 at hospital admission to 1:640 8 days later. However, no isolates were made from the recovered ticks. Eklund, Parker, and Lackman (35) reported a patient from Montana who encountered a large number of ticks while hiking a canyon, which he crushed with his fingers. Within 13 days, he had onset of an illness with retroorbital headache, sweating, chills, and weight loss. The patient developed a complement-fixing antibody titer of 512 within 4 weeks of onset. C. burnetii was isolated by guinea pig passage. Janbon et al. (54) reported two patients who were each simultaneously infected with Mediterranean spotted fever (Rickettsia conorii) and Q fever. Both had maculopapular eruptions on day six of the disease, pneumonia, and high fever. One of them had an eschar. Serology performed by indirect immunofluorescence assay (IFA) showed elevated titers for both spotted fever and Q fever, with titers for the latter reaching 1:800 in one case and 1:1,600 in the other. Since Mediterranean spotted fever is spread by ticks, these authors concluded that both organisms were likely transmitted simultaneously by tick bite to these patients, who reported illness simultaneously in time and place (54). A more recent report likewise describes concomitant infections (107a). Dyer (34) reported on a laboratory-acquired infection in which the mode of transmission was thought to be the handling of ticks in the laboratory. *R. diaporica (C. burnetii)* was isolated by guinea pig passage of the patient's blood.

Descriptive Epidemiology of Q Fever in the United States

Q fever is considered enzootic among livestock throughout the United States, and human infections have been reported from almost every state (89). Seroprevalence studies have shown an average antibody prevalence to *C. burnetii* of 7.8% among traditionally high-risk groups and an average antibody prevalence of 0.8% among the general population (89).

Between 1948 and 1977, 1,168 cases of Q fever in humans were reported by 26 state health departments (mean, 58.4 cases/year) (22). Between 1978 and 1999, a total of 430 cases of Q fever in humans were identified by state health departments (mean, 35.8 cases/year) (17). Q fever was made nationally notifiable in 1999 (21); however, reporting requirements vary by state. In 2001, only 38 states considered Q fever in humans a reportable disease (17). In 2000 and 2001, 48 cases of Q fever in humans were reported to the Centers for Disease Control and Prevention (17).

Calculated average annual incidence of Q fever in humans for the period 1978 to 2001 varied by state. The highest annual incidence was reported from the upper-Midwest states of North Dakota (1.3 persons per million), Wyoming (0.89), Colorado (0.88), and Nebraska (0.68) (17). Far-Western states typically reported more moderate ranges of incidence (0.11 to 0.50 cases per million population), while Eastern states reported lower rates. When considering calculated average annual incidence, it is important to bear in mind that reporting periods varied by state and that some states provided less than 2 years of accumulated data. In addition, data such as these largely rely on passive surveillance mechanisms. The protean clinical signs associated with acute Q fever and generally self-limiting nature of infection often interfere with an appropriate diagnosis. Physicians must request appropriate diagnostic tests and report positive findings to a state health department for cases to be confirmed. Thus, the number of reported cases likely greatly underestimates the true Q fever disease burden in the United States.

CLINICAL FINDINGS

The incubation period for the onset of acute disease is variable and may be dependent upon the infect-

ing dose and the health status of the patient. Most often, it is about 20 days (range, 14 to 39 days) (77, 129, 130). Q fever cases present in a number of ways. Atypical pneumonia, hepatitis, and neurological manifestations are the more common clinical presentations. In a review of over 1,300 cases in Europe, 77% of cases studied were classified as acute, and presentation frequencies were as follows: acute hepatitis, 40%; pneumonia, 17%; both hepatitis and pneumonia, 20%; isolated fever without apparent organ involvement, 14% (104). Age may be a factor, with adults more likely to develop pneumonia and children more typically presenting with a nonspecific febrile illness with myalgia, anorexia, and headache. Patients often complain of night sweats, recurrent or intermittent fevers with sweating, intense frontal or retroorbital headache, photophobia, myalgia, arthralgia, and mild coryza. In protracted untreated cases, weight loss is common, along with moderate to severe fatigue. In pneumonic cases, chest radiographs may show rounded pulmonary infiltrates of various sizes and multiple opacities. Auscultation may be clear, even when opacities are present, but inspiratory rales or crackles are often present. Occasionally, the patient will have a more serious picture, showing large pleural effusions. Pleuritic chest pain may be present, especially in older patients (77). Histologic examination of the lung tissue of patients with pneumonia may reveal inflammatory exudates consisting of lymphocytes and macrophages filling the alveoli, with hyperplasia of alveolar lining cells (Color Plate 16A) (77, 138). Patients with liver involvement may present either with manifestations similar to granulocytic hepatitis or with only mild abnormalities in liver function tests. Biopsies of patients with granulocytic hepatitis reveal doughnut-shaped granulomas consisting of a fibroid ring around a central space (138), and noncaseating granulomas are commonly seen in bone marrow biopsies (Color Plate 16B). Guinea pigs with experimental infections show a marked deposition of fats in the liver (11, 95), and a milder form of fatty infiltration has been observed in humans, along with Kupffer cell hyperplasia (138). Neurologic manifestations include severe headache, encephalitis, and aseptic meningitis. *C. burnetii* has been isolated from the cerebrospinal fluid of patients with these symptoms, including those with headache only, thereby suggesting that such cases represent actual infection of the central nervous system. Various degrees of dementia, vision impairment, and psychosis may also be found. Although less common, acute disease may also present as osteomyelitis, pericarditis, or myocarditis.

Chronic Q fever is defined as disease occurring 6 months or more after the onset of acute Q fever. The most common form is endocarditis, which most often occurs in persons with some valvulopathy which predisposes towards hemodynamic disturbances, fibrin deposits, and eventual infection and immunopathology (Color Plate 16C). Q fever endocarditis patients, as with those having endocarditis from more common etiologies such as *Streptococcus* or *Klebsiella* infections, may show finger clubbing, purpuric rash, fever, splenomegaly, hepatomegaly, cardiac murmur, congestive heart disease, or cardiac failure. Unlike classic culturable endocarditis, Q fever endocarditis will usually lack large vegetations detectable by ultrasonography (81). To the experienced pathologist, the resected valves will also differ histologically from those seen in other (bacterial) endocarditis cases, in that they will appear smooth, more typical of inflammatory or degenerative valve disease typified by immunopathological rather than infective causes (61). Q fever accounts for a large portion of prosthetic valve endocarditis. Other forms of chronic Q fever are vascular disease with infection (40), osteoarticular infections, pulmonary infections, hepatitis, and postinfection fatigue syndrome (45). Identification of *C. burnetii* DNA within bone marrow is commonly found in the fatigue syndrome (45).

Q fever must be distinguished from other atypical pneumonias caused by chlamydias, *Legionella* species, and mycoplasmas; from other febrile diseases such as viral hepatitis, brucellosis, relapsing fevers, and tularemia; and from causes of infective cardiovascular disease of a chronic nature.

LABORATORY DIAGNOSIS OF Q FEVER

The organism is an obligate parasite of host cells, where it resides and multiplies within acidic phagosomes. It is therefore necessary to culture the organism on tissue cultures, where it grows slowly and generally without cytopathic effects. Culture is not a useful method upon which to base a diagnosis, because primary isolates may take weeks to grow. Furthermore, blood specimens from humans should be taken within 2 to 3 days of the onset of symptoms and prior to antibiotic therapy (81, 129). Assay for organisms by the shell vial technique is one method commonly used for culture of blood and tissue extracts (93). It is possible to detect *Coxiella* in the patient's blood by PCR techniques. Usually the buffy coat (leukocyte) layer obtained from gradient centrifugation is extracted for DNA. Primers directed at the *C. burnetii* superoxide dismutase (121), the surface protein Com1 (144, 145), and the multiple-copy IS1111 insertion sequences (63) have been employed, among others (41).

Serology is generally the most useful and predictable method of confirming infection. Complement fixation tests employing a whole-cell phase II antigen are still used, but enzyme-linked immunosorbent assay and IFA methods are more common. When paired serum samples are available, a fourfold increase in either phase I or phase II antibody levels in the convalescent sample is considered indicative of recent infection. Usually the early immunoglobulin M (IgM) and IgG responses, which become detectable between 10 and 14 days after clinical onset, are reactive with phase II (surface protein) antigen, whereas in later infection and in chronic disease such as endocarditis antibodies are reactive primarily to the phase I (LPS) antigen (99). Elevated liver enzymes are also common, such as alkaline phosphatase and glutamine transferase (77). Other indicators include thrombocytopenia and (in the case of endocarditis) indicators of inflammatory disease such as elevated C-reactive protein and rheumatoid factor levels.

Culture-negative endocarditis may on occasion be caused by *C. burnetii*. These infections are hard to detect and are generally characterized by valvulopathy that features a smooth or lumpy valve surface devoid of vegetative lesions; histochemical examinations reveal granulomas containing foamy monocytic cells in which organisms may be visualized with immunohistochemistry (Color Plate 16C). The patient may or may not appear critically ill and may even be afebrile. Anemia, hematuria, increased erythrocyte sedimentation rate, thrombocytopenia, and elevated rheumatoid factor and C-reactive protein levels are common findings in Q fever endocarditis (77, 81). Chronic Q fever patients will have elevated liver transaminase and elevated alkaline phosphatase levels. Most endocarditis patients form very high IgG and IgA titers to phase I antibody. In most situations, chronic Q fever disease is characterized by a high titer of IgG and IgA antibody to phase I antigen and a lower titer to phase II antigen. Often, the antiphase I IgG titer will be >100,000 (61, 99).

TREATMENT, PROPHYLAXIS, PREVENTION, AND DECONTAMINATION

Acute Q fever is usually treated successfully with tetracyclines, preferably doxycycline. Standard doses of doxycycline for adults are 100 to 200 mg twice daily for 10 to 14 days (81, 87); alternative treatment includes a quinolone or rifamycin. Cotrimoxazole is an alternative to tetracyclines in the treatment of pregnant women and young children. Chronic disease, in particular Q fever endocarditis, is difficult to treat and requires long regimens of combination therapy. The most promising combination employs doxycycline (100 mg twice daily) and hydroxychloroquine (200 mg three times daily) for 18 months or more (81, 103). Hydroxychloroquine is believed to alkalinize the vacuoles in which the acidophilic organism metabolizes and multiplies, thereby inhibiting growth. Combinations of doxycycline and a quinolone for 18 months have also been effective against endocarditis (103), but development of antibiotic resistance to quinolones remains a possibility (92a).

An efficacious vaccine, QVax, prepared by CSL in Australia, is composed of formalin-killed Henzerling phase I cells and is given to those in Australia at occupational risk; it is not licensed for use in other countries (42, 75, 76). Because individuals who have preexposure to this antigen(s) may suffer extreme local reactions to this vaccine, a skin test and antibody assay are used to screen individuals (75). The U.S. Army has a very similar Henzerling strain phase I formalin-killed cellular vaccine classed as Investigational New Drug 610 by the U.S. Food and Drug Administration. It may be available on special request through the Department of Defense's Special Immunizations Program. Vaccination of animals is sometimes done in Europe, especially in Germany (12), but is rarely done in the United States (65).

Surface decontamination with *C. burnetii* is effectively carried out by a 5% solution (vol:vol in water) of Microchem Plus for a period of 30 min. Microchem Plus is a formulation of two quaternary ammonium compounds produced by National Chemical Laboratories, Philadelphia, Pa., and is essentially the same product as Envirochem, which was found efficacious by Scott and Williams (111). Also effective in some applications is 70% ethanol. Chlorine bleach diluted 1:10 with water is less effective. Formalin solutions may also be less than 100% effective. Formaldehyde vapors properly mixed with water vapor are used for space decontamination (111). Routine inactivation of the organism in the laboratory can be accomplished by incubating small (1-cc) volumes of dilute suspensions of the organism at 80°C for 1 hour. Most cellular reagent antigens are inactivated by cobalt source (gamma) irradiation employing 2×10^6 rads (110).

REFERENCES

1. **Abinanti, F. R.** 1959. The varied epidemiology of Q fever infections, p. 9–14. *In* J. Smadel (ed.), *Symposium on Q Fever*. Medical science publication no. 6. Walter Reed Army Institute of Research, Government Printing Office, Washington, D.C.
2. **Akporiaye, E. T., J. D. Rowatt, A. A. Aragon, and O. G. Baca.** 1983. Lysosomal response of a murine macrophage-like cell line persistently infected with *Coxiella burnetii. Infect. Immun.* **40:**1155–1162.
3. **Amano, K.-I, J. C. Williams, S. R. Missler, and V. N. Reinhold.** 1987. Structure and biological relationships of *Coxiella burnetii* lipopolysaccharides. *J. Biol. Chem.* **262:**4740–4747.
4. **Anigstein, L., and M. N. Bader.** 1943. Investigation on rickettsial diseases in Texas. 4. Experimental study of Bullis fever. *Tex. Rep. Biol. Med.* **1:**389–409.
5. **Babudieri, B.** 1959. Q fever: a zoonosis. *Adv. Vet. Sci.* **5:**81–182.
6. **Baca, O. G., and D. Paretsky.** 1983. Q fever and *Coxiella burnetii*: a model for host-parasite interactions. *Microbiol. Rev.* **47:**127–149.
7. **Bader, M. N., and L. Anigstein.** 1944. Specificity of Bullis fever rickettsia. *Tex. Rep. Biol. Med.* **2:**405–412.
8. **Bartlett, J. G.** 2000. Commentary. Questions about Q fever. *Medicine* **79:**124–125.
9. **Beaman, M., and J. Hung.** 1989. Pericarditis associated with tick-borne Q fever. *Aust. N. Z. J. Med.* **19:**254–256.
10. **Bell, J. A., M. D. Beck, and R. J. Huebner.** 1950. Epidemiologic studies of Q fever in Southern California. *JAMA* **142:**868–872.
11. **Bernier, R. D., T. Haney, and D. Paretsky.** 1974. Changes of lipid in liver and plasma during Q fever. *Acta Virol.* **18:**75–80.
12. **Bryne, W. R.** 1997. Q fever. p. 523–537. *In* F. R. Sidell, E. T. Takafuji, and D. R. Franz (ed.), *Textbook of Military Medicine: Medical Aspects of Chemical and Biological Warfare*. Borden Institute, Walter Reed Army Medical Center, Washington D.C. www.vnh.org/MedAspChemBioWar.
13. **Buhariwalla, F., B. Cann, and T. J. Marrie.** 1996. Dog-related outbreak of Q fever. *Clin. Infect. Dis.* **23:**753–755.
14. **Burnet, F. M., and M. Freeman.** 1937. Experimental studies of the virus of "Q" fever. *Med. J. Aust.* **2:**299–305.
15. **Burton, P. R., N. Kordova, and D. Paretsky.** 1971. Electron microscopic studies of the rickettsia *Coxiella burnetii*: entry, lysosomal response and fate of rickettsial DNA in L cells. *Can. J. Microbiol.* **17:**143–150.
16. **Centers for Disease Control and Prevention.** 2000. Biological and chemical terrorism: strategic plan for preparedness and response. Recommendations of the CDC Strategic Planning Workgroup. *Morb. Mortal. Wkly. Rep.* **49**(RR-4):1–14.
17. **Centers for Disease Control and Prevention.** Unpublished data.
18. **Chen, S.-Y., M. H. Vodkin, H. A. Thompson, and J. C. Williams.** 1990. Isolated *Coxiella burnetii* synthesizes DNA during acid activation in the absence of host cells. *J. Gen. Microbiol.* **136:**89–96.
19. **Chong, A. K. H., J. La Brooy, R. Norton, and J. Masson.** 2003. Q fever: a recent 'outbreak' in Townsville. *Int. Med. J.* **33:**208–210.
19a. **Coleman, S. A., E. R. Fischer, D. Howe, D. J. Mead, and R. A. Heinzen.** 2004. Temporal analysis of *Coxiella burnetii* morphological differentiation. *J. Bacteriol.* **186:**7344–7352.
20. **Consigli, R. A., and D. Paretsky.** 1962. Oxidation of glucose-6-phosphate and isocitrate by *Coxiella burnetii. J. Bacteriol.* **83:**206–207.
21. **Council of State and Territorial Epidemiologists.** 1999. Placing Q fever (*Coxiella burnetii*) under national surveillance in the United States under the National Public Health Surveillance System (NPHSS). CSTE position statement 1999-ID1. http://www.cste.org/ps/1999/1999-id-01.htm.
22. **D'Angelo, L. J., E. F. Baker, and W. Schlosser.** 1979. Q fever in the United States, 1948–1977. *J. Infect. Dis.* **139:**613–615.
23. **Davis, G. E.** 1939. *Rickettsia diaporica*: recovery of three strains from *Dermacentor andersoni* collected in southeastern Wyoming. I. Their identity with Montana strain. *Public Health Rep.* **54:**2219–2227.
24. **Davis, G. E.** 1940. *Rickettsia diaporica*: its persistence in the tissues of *Ornithodoros turicata*. *Public Health Rep.* **55:**1862.
25. **Davis, G. E.** 1943. American Q fever: experimental transmission by the argasid ticks *Ornithodoros moubata* and *Ornithodoros hermsi*. *Public Health Rep.* **58:**984–987.

26. Davis, G. E., and H. Cox. 1938. A filter-passing infectious agent isolated from ticks. I. Isolation from *Dermacentor andersoni*, reaction in animals, and filtration experiments. *Public Health Rep.* **53**:2259–2267.

27. De Rodaniche, E. C. 1949. Experimental transmission of Q fever by *Amblyomma cajennense*. *Am. J. Trop. Med.* **29**:711–714.

28. Derrick, E. H. 1937. "Q" fever, a new fever entity: clinical features, diagnosis, and laboratory investigation. *Med. J. Aust.* **2**:281–299.

29. Derrick, E. H., D. J. W. Smith, H. E. Brown, and M. Freeman. 1939. The role of the bandicoot in the epidemiology of "Q" fever: a preliminary study. *Med. J. Aust.* **1**:150–155.

30. Derrick, E. H., and D. J. W. Smith. 1940. Studies in the epidemiology of Q fever. 2. The isolation of three strains of *Rickettsia burnetii* from the bandicoot, *Isodon torosus*. *Aust. J. Exp. Biol. Med. Sci.* **18**:99–102.

31. Derrick, E. H., D. J. W. Smith, and H. E. Brown. 1940. Studies in the epidemiology of Q fever. VI. The susceptibility of various animals. *Aust. J. Exp. Biol. Med. Sci.* **18**:409–413.

32. Derrick, E. H., D. J. W. Smith, and H. E. Brown. 1942. Studies in the epidemiology of Q fever. IX. The role of the cow in the transmission of human infection. *Aust. J. Exp. Biol. Med. Sci.* **20**:105–110.

33. Derrick, E. H. 1944. The epidemiology of Q fever. *J. Hyg.* **43**:357–361.

34. Dyer, R. E. 1938. A filter-passing agent isolated from ticks. IV. Human infection. *Public Health Rep.* **53**:2277–2282.

35. Ecklund, C. M., R. R. Parker, and D. B. Lackman. 1947. A case of Q fever probably contracted by exposure to ticks in nature. *Public Health Rep.* **62**:1413–1416.

36. Enright, J. B., W. W. Sadler, and R. C. Thomas. 1957. Thermal inactivation of *Coxiella burnetii* and its relation to the pasteurization of milk. Public Health monograph No. 47, Public Health Service Publication No. 517. U.S. Government Printing Office, Washington, D.C.

37. Enright, J. B., C. E. Franti, D. E. Behymer, W. M. Longhurst, V. J. Dutson, and M. E. Wright. 1971. *Coxiella burnetii* in a wildlife-livestock environment. Distribution of Q fever in wild animals. *Am. J. Epidemiol.* **94**:79–90.

38. Fiset, P., and T. E. Woodward. 1998. Q fever, p. 583–593. *In* A. S. Evans and P. S. Brachman (ed.), *Bacterial Infections of Humans: Epidemiology and Control*, 3rd ed. Plenum Medical Book Co., New York, N.Y.

39. Fishbein, D. B., and D. Raoult. 1992. A cluster of *Coxiella burnetii* infections associated with exposure to vaccinated goats and their unpasteurized dairy products. *Am. J. Trop. Med. Hyg.* **47**:35–40.

40. Fournier, P. E., J. P. Casalta, P. Piquet, P. Tournigand, A. Branchereau, and D. Raoult. 1998. *Coxiella burnetii* infection of aneurysms or vascular grafts: report of seven cases and review. *Clin. Infect. Dis.* **26**:116–121.

41. Fraser, M. E., L. P. Mallavia, J. E. Samuel, and O. G. Baca. 1990. DNA probes for the identification of *Coxiella burnetii* strains. *Ann. N. Y. Acad. Sci.* **590**:445–448.

42. Gilroy, N., N. Formica, M. Beers A. Egan, S. Conaty, and B. P. Marmion. 2001. Abattoir-associated Q fever: a Q fever outbreak during a Q fever vaccination program. *Aust. N. Z. J. Public Health* **25**:362–367.

43. Hackstadt, T., and J. C. Williams. 1981. Biochemical stratagem for obligate parasitism of eukaryotic cells by *Coxiella burnetii*. *Proc. Natl. Acad. Sci. USA* **78**:3240–3244.

44. Hackstadt, T. 1983. Estimation of the cytoplasmic pH of *Coxiella burnetii* and effect of substrate oxidation on proton motive force. *J. Bacteriol.* **154**:591–597.

45. Harris, R. J., P. A. Storm, A. Lloyd, M. Arens, and B. P. Marmion. 2000. Long-term persistence of *Coxiella burnetii* in the host after primary Q fever. *Epidemiol. Infect.* **124**:543–549.

46. Hawker, J. I., J. G. Ayers, I. Blair, M. R. Evans, D. L. Smith, E. G. Smith, P. S. Burge, M. J. Carpenter, E. O. Caul, B. Coupland, U. Desselberger, I. D. Farrell, P. J. Saunders, and W. J. Wood. 1998. A large outbreak of Q fever in the West Midlands: windborne spread into a metropolitan area? *Commun. Dis. Public Health* **1**:180–187.

47. Heinzen, R. A., T. Hackstadt, and J. E. Samuel. 1999. Developmental biology of *Coxiella burnetii*. *Trends Microbiol.* **7**:149–154.

48. Hellenbrand, W., T. Breuer, and L. Petersen. 2001. Changing epidemiology of Q fever in Germany, 1947–1999. *Emerg. Infect. Dis.* **7**:789–796.

49. Ho, T., K. K. Htwe, N. Yamasaki, G. Q. Zhang, M. Ogawa, T. Yamaguchi, H. Fukushi, and K. Hirai. 1995. Isolation of *Coxiella burnetii* from dairy cattle and ticks, and some characteristics of the isolates in Japan. *Microbiol. Immunol.* **39**:663–671.

50. Hoover, T. A., D. W. Culp, M. H. Vodkin, J. C. Williams, and H. A. Thompson. 2002. Chromosomal DNA deletions explain phenotypic characteristics of two antigenic variants, phase II and RSA 514 (Crazy), of the *Coxiella burnetii* Nine Mile strain. *Infect. Immun.* **70**:6726–6733.

51. Huebner, R. J., and J. A. Bell. 1951. Q fever studies in southern California: summary of current results and discussion of possible control measures. *JAMA* **145**:301–305.

52. Huebner, R. J., W. J. Jellison, and D. M. Beck. 1949. Q fever—a review of current knowledge. *Ann. Intern. Med.* **30**:495–509.

53. Hussein, A., E. Kovacova, and R. Toman. 2001. Isolation and evaluation of *Coxiella burnetii* O-polysaccharide antigen as an immunodiagnostic reagent. *Acta Virol.* **45**:173–180.

54. Janbon, F., D. Raoult, J. Reynes, and A. Bertrand. 1989. Concomitant human infection due to *Rickettsia conorii* and *Coxiella burnetii*. *J. Infect. Dis.* **160**:354–355.

55. Kazar, J., and R. Brezina. 1991. Control of rickettsial diseases. *Eur. J. Epidemiol.* **7**:282–286.

56. Kordova, N. 1959. Filterable particles of *Coxiella burnetii*. *Acta Virol.* **3**:25–36.

57. Lackman, D. B., R. N. Philip, E. A. Casper, J. F. Bell, J. B. Enright, and E. G. Pickens. 1967. Q fever immunity in man. *Health Lab. Sci.* **4**:236–244.

58. Langley, J. M., T. J. Marrie, A. Covert, D. M. Waag, and J. C. Williams. 1988. Poker player's pneumonia; an urban outbreak of Q fever following exposure to a parturient cat. *New Engl. J. Med.* **319**:354–356.

59. LaScola, B., and D. Raoult. 2001. Survival of *Coxiella burnetii* within the free-living amoeba *Acanthamoeba castellanii*. *Clin. Microbiol. Infect.* **7**:75–79.

60. Lennette, E. H., and W. H. Clark. 1951. Observations of the epidemiology of Q fever in Northern California. *JAMA* **145**:306–309.

61. Lepidi, H., P. Houpikian, Z. Liang, and D. Raoult. 2003. Cardiac valves in patients with Q fever endocarditis: microbiological, molecular, and histologic studies. *J. Infect. Dis.* **187**:1097–1106.

62. Liebisch, A. 1979. Ecology and distribution of Q-fever rickettsiae in Europe with special reference to Germany, p. 225–231. *Recent Advances in Acarology*, vol. 2. Academic Press, New York, N.Y.

63. Lorenz, H., C. Jager, H. Willems, and G. Baljer. 1998. PCR detection of *Coxiella burnetii* from different clinical specimens, especially bovine milk, on the basis of DNA preparation with a silica matrix. *Appl. Environ. Microbiol.* **64**:4234–4237.

64. Lukacova, M., D. Valkova, M. Q. Diaz, D. Perecko, and I. Barak. 1999. Green fluorescent protein as a detection marker for *Coxiella burnetii* transformation. *FEMS Microbiol. Lett.* **175**:255–260.

65. Luoto, L., J. F. Winn, and R. J. Huebner. 1952. Q fever studies in southern California. XIII: Vaccination of dairy cattle against Q fever. *Am. J. Hyg.* **55**:190–202.

66. Luoto, L., and E. G. Pickens. 1961. A resume of recent research seeking to define the Q fever problem. *Am. J. Hyg.* **74**:43–49.

67. Lyytikainen, O., T. Ziese, B. Schwartlander, P. Matzdorff, C. Kuhnen, C. Jager, and L. Petersen. 1998. An outbreak of sheep-associated Q fever in a rural community in Germany. *Eur. J. Epidemiol.* **14**:193–199.

68. Mak, D. B., D. E. Fry, and M. K. Bulsara. 2003. Prevalence of the Q fever exposure in the Kimberley, Western Australia. *Commun. Dis. Intell.* **27**:267–271.

69. Mallavia, L. P. 1991. Genetics of rickettsiae. *Eur. J. Epidemiol.* **7**:213–221.

70. Marchette, N. J. 1982. *Coxiella burnetii*: its origin and distribution. p. 65–95. *In* N. Marchette and D. Stiller (ed.), *Ecological Relationships and Evolution of the Rickettsiae*, vol. 2. CRC Press, Boca Raton, Fla.

71. Marmion, B. P., and M. S. Harvey. 1956. The varying epidemiology of Q fever in the south-east area of Great Britain. I. In an urban area. *J. Hyg. (Cambridge)* **54**:533–546.

72. Marmion, B. P., and M. G. P. Stoker. 1950. Q fever in Great Britain. Epidemiology of an outbreak. *Lancet* **2**:611–616.

73. Marmion, B. P., and M. G. P. Stoker. 1958. The epidemiology of Q fever in Great Britain. *Br. Med. J.* **5100**:809–816.

74. Marmion, B. P., M. G. P. Stoker, C. B. V. Walker, and R. G. Carpenter. 1956. Q fever in Great Britain-epidemiological information from a serological survey of healthy adults in Kent and East Anglia. *J. Hyg.* **54**:118–140.

75. Marmion, B. P., R. A. Ormsbee, M. Krykou, J. Wright, D. A. Worsick, S. Cameron, A. Esterman, and B. Feery. 1984. Vaccine prophylaxis of abattoir associated Q fever. *Lancet* **8417**:1411–1414.

76. Marmion, B. P., R. A. Ormsbee, M. Krykou, J. Wright, D. A. Worsick, A. A. Izzo, A. Esterman, B. Feery, and R. A. Shapiro. 1990. Vaccine prophylaxis of abattoir-associated Q fever: eight years experience in South Australian abattoirs. *Epidemiol. Infect.* **104**:275–287.

77. Marrie, T. J., and D. Raoult. 2005. *Coxiella burnetii* (Q fever), p. 2296–2301. *In* G. Mandell, J. Z. Bennett, and R. Dolin (ed.) *Principles of Infectious Diseases*. Elsevier Churchill Livingstone, Philadelphia, Pa.

78. Marrie, T. J., J. Van Buren, J. Fraser, E. V. Haldane, R. S. Faulkner, J. C. Williams, and R. T. Kwan. 1985. Seroepidemiology of Q fever among domestic animals in Nova Scotia. *Am. J. Public Health* **75**:763–766.

79. Marrie, T. J., and D. Raoult. 1997. Q fever—a review and issues for the next century. *Int. J. Antimicrob. Agents* **8**:145–161.

80. Maurin, M., P. Benoliel, P. Bongrand, and D. Raoult. 1992. Phagolysosomes of *Coxiella burnetii*-infected cell lines maintain an acidic pH during persistent infection. *Infect. Immun.* **60**:5013–5016.

81. Maurin, M., and D. Raoult. 1999. Q fever. *Clin. Microbiol. Rev.* **12**:518–553.

82. McCaul, T. F., and J. C. Williams. 1981. Developmental cycle of *Coxiella burnetii*: structure and morphogenesis of vegetative and sporogenic differentiations. *J. Bacteriol.* **147**: 1063–1076.

83. McCaul, T. F. 1991. Developmental cycle of *Coxiella burnetii*, p. 223–258. *In* J. C. Williams and H. A. Thompson (ed.), *Q Fever: The Biology of Coxiella burnetii*. CRC Press, Boca Raton, Fla.

84. McCaul, T. F., J. C. Williams, and H. A. Thompson. 1991. Electron microscopy of *Coxiella burnetii* in tissue culture. Induction of cell types as products of developmental cycle. *Acta Virol.* **35**:545–556.

85. McDade, J. E., C. C. Shephard, D. W. Fraser, T. R. Tsai, M. A. Redus, and W. R. Dowdle. 1977. Legionnaire's disease: isolation of a bacterium and demonstration of its role in other respiratory disease. *New Engl. J. Med.* **297**:1197–1203.

86. McDiarmid, L., T. Petney, B. Dixon, and R. Andrews. 2000. Range expansion of the tick *Amblyomma triguttatum triguttatum*, an Australian vector for Q fever. *Int. J. Parasitol.* **30**:791–793.

87. McQuiston, J. H., and H. A. Thompson. 2003. *Coxiella burnetii* (Q fever), p. 911–913. *In* S. S. Long, L. K. Pickering, and C. G. Prober (ed.), *Principles and Practice of Pediatric Infectious Diseases*, 2nd ed. Churchill Livingstone, New York, N.Y.

88. McQuiston, J. H., J. E. Childs, and H. A. Thompson. 2002. Zoonoses update: Q fever. *J. Am. Vet. Assoc.* **221**:796–799.

89. McQuiston, J., and J. E. Childs. 2002. Q fever in humans and animals in the United States. *Vector Borne Zoonotic Dis.* **2**:179–191.

90. Mediannikov, O., L. Ivanov, M. Nishikawa, R. Saito, Y. N. Sidelnidov, N. I. Zdanovskaya, I. V. Tarasevich, and H. Suzuki. 2003. Molecular evidence of a *Coxiella*-like microorganism harbored by *Haemaphysalis concinnae* ticks in the Russian Far East. *Ann. N. Y. Acad. Sci.* **990**:226–228.

91. Milazzo, A., R. Hall, P. A. Storm, R. J. Harris, W. Winslow, and B. P. Marmion. 2001. Sexually transmitted Q fever. *Clin. Infect. Dis.* **33**:399–402.

92. Moos, A., and T. Hackstadt. 1987. Comparative virulence of intra- and interstrain lipopolysaccharide variants of *Coxiella burnetii* in the guinea pig model. *Infect. Immun.* **55**: 1144–1150.

92a. Musso, D., M. Drancourt, S. Osscini, and D. Raoult. 1996. Sequence of quinolone resistance-determining region of the *gyrA* gene for clinical isolates and for an in vitro-selected quinolone-resistant strain of *Coxiella burnetii*. *Antimicrob. Agents Chemother.* **40**:870–873.

93. Musso, D., and D. Raoult. 1995. *Coxiella burnetii* blood cultures from acute and chronic Q-fever patients. *J. Clin. Microbiol.* **33**:3129–3132.

94. Noguchi, H. 1926. A filter-passing virus obtained from *Dermacentor andersoni*. *J. Exp. Med.* **44**:1–10.

95. Paretsky, D. 1990. The biology of *Coxiella burnetii* and the pathobiochemistry of Q fever and endotoxicosis. *Ann. N. Y. Acad. Sci.* **590**:416–421.

96. Paretsky, D., R. A. Consigli, and C. M. Downs. 1962. Studies on the physiology of rickettsiae. III. Glucose phosphorylation and and hexokinase activity in *Coxiella burnetii*. *J. Bacteriol.* **83**:538–543.

97. Parker, R. R., and G. E. Davis. 1938. A filter-passing infectious agent isolated from ticks. II. Transmission by *Dermacentor andersoni*. *Public Health Rep.* **53**:2267–2270.

98. Parker, R. R., and G. M. Kohls. 1943. American Q fever: the occurrence of *Rickettsia diaporica* in *Amblyomma americanum* in Eastern Texas. *Public Health Rep.* **58**:1510–1511.

99. Peacock, M. G., R. N. Philip, J. C. Williams, and R. S. Faulkner. 1983. Serological evaluation of Q fever in humans: enhanced phase I titers of immunoglobulins G and A are diagnostic for Q fever endocarditis. *Infect. Immun.* **41**:1089–1098.

100. Philip, C. B. 1943. Nomenclature of the pathogenic rickettsiae. *Am. J. Hyg.* **37**:301–309.

101. Philip, C. B. 1948. Comments on the name of the Q fever organism. *Public Health Rep.* **63**:58.

102. Pope, J. H., W. Scott, and R. Dwyer. 1960. *Coxiella burnetii* in kangaroos and kangaroo ticks in Western Queensland. *Aust. J. Exp. Biol.* **38**:17–28.

103. Raoult, D., P. Houpikian, H. Tissot Dupont, J. M. Riss, J. Arditi-Djiane, and P. Brouqui. 1999. Treatment of Q fever endocarditis. Comparison of 2 regimens containing doxycycline and ofloxacin or hydroxychloroquine. *Arch. Intern. Med.* **159**:167–173.

104. Raoult, D., H. Tissot-Dupont, C. Foucalt, J. Gouvernet, P. E. Fournier, E. Bernit, A. Stein, M. Nesri, J. R. Harle, and P. J. Weiller. 2000. Q fever 1985–1998. Clinical and epidemiological features of 1,383 infections. *Medicine* **79**:109–123.

105. Rehacek, J., and I. V. Tarasevich. 1988. *Coxiella burnetii*, p. 204–343. *In Acari-Borne Rickettsiae and Rickettsioses in Eurasia.* Veda Publishing House, Slovak Academy of Sciences, Bratislava, Slovakia.

106. Robbins, F. C., R. L. Gauld, and F. B. Warner. 1946. Q fever in the Mediterranean area: report of its occurrence in allied troops. II. Epidemiology. *Am. J. Hyg.* **44**:23–50.

107. Robbins, F. C., R. Rustigian, M. J. Snyder, and J. E. Smadel. 1946. Q fever in the Mediterranean area: report of its occurrence in Allied troops. III. The etiological agent. *Am. J. Hyg.* **44**:51–63.

107a. Rolain, J. M., F. Gourier, P. Brouqui, D. Larrey, F. Jaubon, S. Vene, V. Jernestr, and D. Raoult. 2005. Concomitant or consecutive infection with *Coxiella burnetii and* tickborne diseases. *Clin. Infect. Dis.* **40**:82–88.

108. Rosenberg, M., and N. Kordova. 1960. Study of intracellular forms of *Coxiella burnetii* in the electron microscope. *Acta Virol.* **4**:52–55.

109. Schramek, S., J. Radziejewska-Lebrecht, and H. Mayer. 1985. 3-C-Branched aldoses in lipopolysaccharide of phase I *Coxiella burnetii* and their role as immunodominant factors. *Eur. J. Biochem.* **148**:455–461.

110. Scott, G. H., T. F. McCaul, and J. C. Williams. 1989. Inactivation of *Coxiella burnetii* by gamma irradiation. *J. Gen. Microbiol.* **135**:3263–3270.

111. Scott, G. H., and J. C. Williams. 1990. Susceptibility of *Coxiella burnetii* to chemical disinfectants. *Ann. N. Y. Acad. Sci.* **590**:291–296.

112. Seshadri, R., L. R. Hendrix, and J. E. Samuel. 1999. Differential expression of translational elements by life cycle variants of *Coxiella burnetii*. *Infect. Immun.* **67**:6026–6033.

113. Seshadri, R., I. T. Paulsen, J. A. Eisen, T. D. Read, K. E. Nelson, W. C. Nelson, N. L. Ward, H. Tettelin, T. M. Davidsen, M. J. Beanan, R. T. Deboy, S. C. Daugherty, L. M. Brinkac, R. Madupu, R. J. Dodson, H. M. Khouri, K. H. Lee, H. A. Carty, D. Scanlan, R. A. Heinzen, H. A. Thompson, J. E. Samuel, C. M. Fraser, and J. F. Heidelberg. 2003. Complete genome sequence of *Coxiella burnetii*. *Proc. Natl. Acad. Sci. USA* **100**:5455–5460.

114. Sigel, M. M., T. F. M. Scott, and W. Henle. 1950. Q fever in a wool and hair processing plant. *Am. J. Public Health* **40**:424–532.

115. Smith, D. J. W. 1940. Studies in epidemiology of Q fever. III. The transmission of Q fever by the tick *Haemaphysalis humerosa*. *Aust. J. Exp. Biol. Med. Sci.* **18**:103–118.

116. Smith, D. J. W. 1941. Studies in the epidemiology of Q fever. VIII. The transmission of Q fever by the tick, *Rhipicephalus sanguineus*. *Aust. J. Exp. Biol. Med. Sci.* **19**:133–136.

117. Smith, D. J. W. 1942. Studies in the epidemiology of Q fever. X. The transmission of Q fever by the tick *Ixodes holocyclus* (with notes on the paralysis in bandicoots). *Aust. J. Exp. Biol. Med. Sci.* **20**:213–217.

118. Smith, D. J. W. 1942. Studies in the epidemiology of Q fever. XI. Experimental infection of the ticks, *Haemaphysalis bispinosa* and *Ornithodoros* sp., with *Rickettsia burnetii*. *Aust. J. Exp. Biol. Med. Sci.* **20**:295–296.

119. Smith, D. J. W., and E. H. Derrick. 1940. Studies in the epidemiology of Q fever. 1. The isolation of six strains of *Rickettsia burnetii* from the tick *Haemaphysalis humerosa*. *Aust. J. Exp. Biol. Med. Sci.* **18**:1–8.

120. Spyridaki, I., A. Psaroulaki, F. Loukaides, M. Antoniou, C. Hadjichristodolou, and Y. Tselentis. 2002. Isolation of *Coxiella burnetii* by a centrifugation shell-vial assay from ticks collected in Cyprus: detection by nested PCR and by PCR-restriction fragment length polymorphism analyses. *Am. J. Trop. Med. Hyg.* **66**:86–90.

121. Stein, A., and D. Raoult. 1992. Detection of *Coxiella burnetii* by DNA amplification using the polymerase chain reaction. *J. Clin. Microbiol.* **30**:2462–2466.

122. Steinhaus, E. A., and R. R. Parker. Unpublished observations, 1943–1944. Unpublished data.

123. Stoenner, H. G., R. Holdenreid, D. Lackman, J. S. Orsborn, Jr. 1959. The occurrence of *Coxiella burnetii*, *Brucella*, and other pathogens among fauna of the Great Salt Lake Desert in Utah. *Am. J. Trop. Med. Hyg.* **8**:590–596.

124. Stoker, M. G. P., and P. Fiset. 1956. Phase variation in the Nine Mile and other strains of *Rickettsia burnetii*. *Can. J. Microbiol.* **2**:310–321.

125. Suhan, M., S.-Y. Chen, H. A. Thompson, T. A. Hoover, A. Hill, and J. C. Williams. 1994. Cloning and characterization of an autonomous replication sequence from *Coxiella burnetii*. *J. Bacteriol.* **176**:5233–5243.

126. Suhan, M., S.-Y. Chen, and H. A. Thompson. 1996. Transformation of *Coxiella burnetii* to ampicillin resistance. *J. Bacteriol.* **178**:2701–2708.

127. Syrucek, L., O. Sobeslavsky, and I. Gutvirth. 1958. Isolation of *Coxiella burnetii* from human placentas. *J. Hyg. Epidemiol.* **2**:29–35.

128. Thompson, H. A., T. A. Hoover, M. H. Vodkin, and E. I. Shaw. 2003. Do chromosomal deletions in the lipopolysaccharide biosynthetic regions explain all cases of phase variation in *Coxiella burnetii* strains? *Ann. N. Y. Acad. Sci.* **990**:664–670.

129. Tigertt, W. D. 1959. Studies on Q fever in man, p. 39–46. *In* J. Smadel (ed.), *Symposium on Q fever*. Medical science publication no. 6. Commission on Rickettsial Diseases, Walter Reed Army Institute of Research, Washington, D.C.

130. Tigertt, W. D., A. S. Benenson, and W. S. Gochenour. 1961. Airborne Q fever. *Bacteriol. Rev.* **25**:285–293.

131. Tissot-Dupont, H., S. Torres, M. Nezri, and D. Raoult. 1999. Hyperendemic focus of Q fever related to sheep and wind. *Am. J. Epidemiol.* **150**:67–74.

132. Toman, R. 1999. Lipopolysaccharides from virulent and low-virulent phases of *Coxiella burnetii*, p. 84–91. *In* D. Raoult and P. Brouqui (ed.), *Rickettsiae and Rickettsial Diseases at the Turn of the Third Millennium*. Elsevier Press, Amsterdam, The Netherlands.

133. Toman, R., L. Skultety, P. Ftacek, and M. Hricovini. 1998. NMR study of virenose and dihydrohydroxystreptose isolated from *Coxiella burnetii* phase I lipopolysaccharide. *Carbohydr. Res.* **306**:291–296.

134. Topping, N. H., C. C. Shepard, and J. V. Irons. 1947. Q fever in the United States. I. Epidemiologic studies of an outbreak among stock handlers and slaughterhouse workers. *JAMA* **133**:813–815.

135. Vest, E. D., D. L. Lundgren, D. D. Parker, D. E. Johnson, E. L. Morse, J. B. Bushman, R. W. Sidwell, and B. D. Thorpe.

1965. Results of a five-year survey for certain enzootic diseases in the fauna of western Utah. *Am. J. Trop. Med. Hyg.* **14:**124–135.

136. **Vodkin, M. H., and J. C. Williams.** 1986. Overlapping deletion in two spontaneous phase variants of *Coxiella burnetii. J. Gen. Microbiol.* **132:**2587–2594.

137. **Waag, D. M., J. C. Williams, M. G. Peacock, and D. Raoult.** 1991. Methods of isolation, amplification, and purification of *Coxiella burnetii,* p. 84–91. *In* J. C. Williams and H. A. Thompson, (ed.), *Q Fever: The Biology of Coxiella burnetii.* CDC Press, Boca Raton, Fla.

138. **Walker, D. H.** 1988. Pathology of Q fever, p. 17–27. *In* David Walker (ed.), *Biology of Rickettsial Diseases,* vol. 2. CRC Press, Boca Raton, Fla.

139. **Weibe, M., P. R. Burton, and D. M. Shankel.** 1972. Isolation and characterization of two cell types of *Coxiella burnetii* phase I. *J. Bacteriol.* **110:**368–377.

140. **Welsh, H. H., E. H. Lennette, F. R. Abinanti, and J. F. Winn.** 1951. Q fever in California. IV. Occurrence of *Coxiella burnetii* in the placenta of naturally infected sheep. *Public Health Rep.* **66:**1473–1477.

141. **Welsh, H. H., E. H. Lennette, and F. R. Abinanti.** 1958. Airborne transmission of Q fever: the role of parturition in the generation of infective aerosols. *Ann. N. Y. Acad. Sci.* **70:**528–540.

142. **Williams, J. C.** 1991. Infectivity, virulence, and pathogenicity of *Coxiella burnetii* for various hosts, p. 21–71. *In* J. C. Williams and H. A. Thompson (ed.), *Q Fever: The Biology of Coxiella burnetii.* CDC Press, Boca Raton, Fla.

143. **Zdrodovskii, P. F., and H. M. Golinevich.** 1960. Q fever, p. 372–423. *In The Rickettsial Diseases,* Pergamon Press, New York, N.Y.

144. **Zhang, G. Q., S. V. Nguyen, H. To, M. Ogawa, A. Hotta, T. Yamaguchi, H. J. Kim, H. Fukushi, and K. Hirai.** 1998. Clinical evaluation of a new PCR assay for detection of *Coxiella burnetii* in human serum samples. *J. Clin. Microbiol.* **36:**77–80.

145. **Zhang, G. Q., H. To, T. Yamaguchi, H. Fukushi, and K. Hirai.** 1997. Differentiation of *Coxiella burnetii* by sequence analysis of the gene (*com1*) encoding a 27-kDa outer membrane protein. *Microbiol. Immunol.* **41:**871–877.

146. **Zuerner, R. L., and H. A. Thompson.** 1983. Protein synthesis by intact *Coxiella burnetii* cells. *J. Bacteriol.* **156:**186–191.

Tick-Borne Diseases of Humans
Edited by Jesse L. Goodman et al.
© 2005 ASM Press, Washington, D.C.

Chapter 20

Human Babesiosis

MARY J. HOMER AND DAVID H. PERSING

Babesial organisms are tick-transmitted intra-erythrocytic parasites that are collectively called piroplasms, because they form pear-shaped figures within infected red blood cells. The piroplasms are almost universally transmitted by ixodid ticks and are capable of infecting a wide variety of vertebrate hosts that serve as reservoirs within the transmission cycle. To date, there are several species of *Babesia* that can infect humans, *Babesia microti* being the most prevalent and best studied. Infection with *Babesia* species generally follows regional distributions; cases in the United States are caused primarily by *B. microti*, whereas cases in Europe are usually caused by *Babesia divergens* or a recently described *Babesia odocoilei*-like parasite. The spectrum of human babesiosis, like that for other tick-borne diseases, is broad and ranges from a clinically silent infection, evidenced only by seroconversion, to fulminant hemolytic anemia that may be fatal. Severe, treatment-refractory infections occur in the very elderly and in patients who are immunocompromised. Because *B. microti* and perhaps other species may be present in the blood without symptoms, the disease can be transmitted by blood transfusion and represents an emerging threat to blood safety. Recent advances in the development of diagnostic tests and in approaches to treatment have resulted in earlier recognition and more effective management of the disease.

INTRODUCTION

Babesiosis is caused by infection with intraerythrocytic parasites of the genus *Babesia*. It is one of the most common infections of free-living animals worldwide and is gaining increasing interest as an emerging zoonosis of humans. All babesial parasites described to date are transmitted from ixodid ticks to vertebrate hosts. The parasites replicate in the host red blood cells and are called piroplasms, due to their pear-shaped

appearance within infected cells (67, 142). Most of what is known about the natural history of babesial infections comes from observations of vertebrate hosts other than humans, although the advent of new diagnostic tools has resulted in recent recognition of human babesiosis as an important tick-borne zoonosis.

Phylogenetic Classification

Human babesiosis may be caused by several species that have distinct geographic distributions based on the presence of competent hosts. In North America, babesiosis is caused predominantly by *B. microti* (105, 137), a rodent-borne piroplasm, and occasionally by a newly recognized species, the so-called WA1 piroplasm and its relatives (109, 119, 147). In Europe, where clinically evident babesiosis is considerably rarer but apparently more lethal, most cases have been attributed to *B. divergens* (15, 40, 44, 57), although the discovery of a *B. odocoilei*-like agent in recent European cases calls into question the cause of some of the earlier cases that had been assumed to be due to *B. divergens* (86). However, the geographic separation of cases might not be as strict as previously thought, given that *B. divergens*-like pathogens have now been recognized in cases in the United States (9, 51, 52), and seroreactivity to *B. microti* and WA1 has been demonstrated in patients in Europe (39, 62, 70).

The taxonomic classification of *Babesia* species places them in the phylum *Apicomplexa* (also *Sporozoa*), class *Aconoidasida* (*Piroplasmea*), and the order *Piroplasmida* (83, 84, 94). Piroplasms are characterized by intraerythrocytic forms which can be pear shaped (83). They have apical complex organelles (including rhoptries and micronemes), a merogonic stage within the vertebrate host erythrocytes, and sexual development and sporozoite formation within the invertebrate host (which in the case of *Babesia* has only been described in ticks) (67, 142). Two of the families within

Mary J. Homer • Infectious Disease Research Institute, Seattle Life Sciences Center, 1124 Columbia St., Seattle, WA 98104. **David H. Persing** • Corixa Corporation, 1900 9th Ave., Seattle, WA 98101, and Infectious Disease Research Institute, Seattle Life Sciences Center, 1124 Columbia St., Seattle, WA 98104.

the order *Piroplasmorida* are *Babesia* and *Theileria*; the primary distinction is usually defined as the absence of a preerythrocytic cycle in *Babesia* and the absence of transovarial transmission in *Theileria* (67, 121, 145).

Over 100 known species of *Babesia* have been identified to date (83, 145). Babesial organisms infect many mammalian and several avian species (67, 83, 145), and reservoir specificity has, in the past, been used in their classification. Additionally, *Babesia* species have been grouped informally by size: the small *Babesia* species (trophozoites of 1.0 to 2.5 μm; species include *Babesia gibsoni*, *B. microti*, and *Babesia rodhaini*) and large *Babesia* species (2.5 to 5.0 μm; species include *Babesia bovis*, *Babesia caballi*, and *Babesia canis*). However, reservoir specificity has proven to be an unreliable means of classification, and morphological characteristics can vary with the status of the host, so recent phylogenetic analysis based on genetic distance has led to some surprising insights (57, 69, 108, 130, 152). In general, however, it can be said that morphological classifications are concordant with phylogenetic characterization, based on nuclear small subunit rRNA genes (nss-rRNA) and heat shock protein gene sequences which show that the large and small *Babesia* species generally fall into distinct clusters (Fig. 1).

VECTORS AND HOSTS

Members of the genus *Babesia* are among the most ubiquitous blood parasites in the world, based on numbers and distribution of species in animals, second only to the trypanosomes (84, 145). They generally

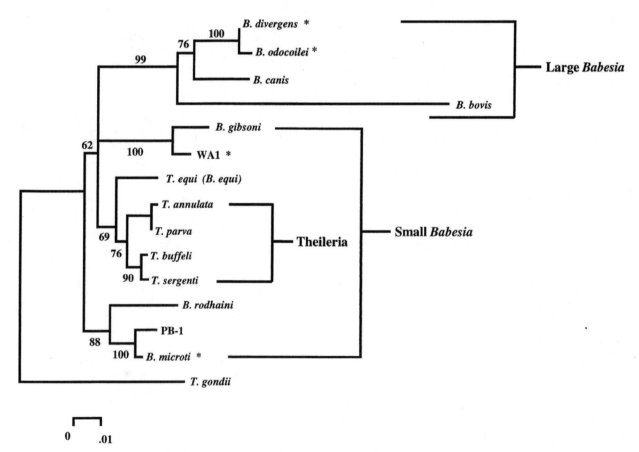

Figure 1. Phylogenetic tree representation of a neighbor-joining analysis of several species of piroplasms. Five hundred nucleotides of the nss-rRNA were aligned using the Pileup program (Genetics Computer Group, University of Wisconsin). Phylogenetic analysis of the alignment was performed as described previously (101) using the Molecular Evolutionary Genetics Analysis (MEGA) computer program, version 1.01 (108), to make a Jukes-Cantor distance measurement and perform a neighbor-joining analysis with 500 bootstrap replicates. The Phylogenetic Analysis Using Parsimony (PAUP) computer program, version 3.1.1, was used to confirm the order observed by the neighbor-joining analysis (using a branch-and-bound algorithm with 100 bootstrap replicates). The percentage of neighbor-joining bootstrap replications (>50%) is shown above each node. This tree is consistent with previously published analyses. Species known to infect humans are marked with asterisks. The groups of large and small *Babesia* species are bracketed and labeled.

have both an invertebrate and a vertebrate host. The maintenance of *Babesia* is dependent on both hosts; a specific tick vector (invertebrate host) must feed on a vertebrate reservoir that is competent in maintaining the organisms in an infectious state. Therefore, *B. microti* presents itself as an emerging infection of humans only in areas where there is both a competent tick vector and a primary competent vertebrate reservoir.

Almost any mammal that serves as a host for a *Babesia*-infected tick is a potential reservoir (145). The host ranges of *B. microti* and *B. divergens* vary from small terrestrial mammals (14, 33, 137), to nonhuman primates (98, 129), to humans (for *B. microti*). Cattle, various rodent species, and humans are all competent to host *B. divergens* or its relatives (27, 89, 102).

To date, only ixodid ticks have been identified as vectors for *Babesia*, except for one report that identified *Ornithodoros erraticus* as a reservoir for *Babesia meri* (47). The ecology and life cycle of *B. microti* and its interaction with *Ixodes scapularis*, (138) is the best understood among *Babesia* species (145) (Fig. 2). It is believed that the tick responsible for transmission of *B. divergens* to humans is *Ixodes ricinus* (42, 142). The tick vectors for the more recently discovered species WA1 (119), CA1-4 (109), and MO1 (51) are currently unknown.

Life Cycle

Apicomplexans and/or sporozoans (including *Babesia* and its close relative *Theileria*) generally go through at least three stages of reproduction (Fig. 2) (67): (i) gamogony, or formation and fusion of gametes inside the tick gut; (ii) sporogony, or asexual reproduction in salivary glands; and (iii) merogony, or asexual reproduction in the vertebrate host (reviewed in more detail in references 57 and 67). Much of what has been learned about the life cycle of *Babesia* in the tick has been from studies of *B. microti* (145).

Similar to the situation for Lyme disease, the length of time that the tick is attached to the vertebrate host directly affects the efficacy of sporozoite transmission to hamsters and white-footed mice (113) (i.e., the longer the tick is attached, the more likely it is that transmission of the sporozoites will occur). If the tick is allowed to feed to repletion, infection rates approach 100% (113). Once in the vertebrate, the transmitted sporozoites seem to infect erythrocytes directly, except in the case of *Theileria* and some *Babesia* species, where invasion of lymphocytes occurs first. Within the host erythrocytes, most merozoites become trophozoites and divide by binary fission (Fig. 2); this asexual reproduction produces more merozoites which lyse the cell (or are released during splenic destruction) and then go on to infect additional erythro-

cytes. Four parasites may form at the same time, giving rise to a Maltese cross form (Fig. 2). Rapid reproduction destroys the host cell and leads to hemolytic anemia with hemoglobinuria, classical clinical hallmarks of acute babesiosis.

Clinical and Historical Considerations

In general, the clinical spectrum of babesiosis is broad, ranging from silent infection to a fulminant, malaria-like disease resulting, in some cases, in death. Various host-specific determinants influence the severity of disease manifestation, including advanced age, immunodeficiency, splenic function, and coinfection with other pathogenic agents. Babesial infections have probably influenced the lives of humans since antiquity, primarily through the infections of domestic livestock (108, 135). Only recently in the latter half of this century have these infections become a documented threat to human health, earning the legitimate title of an emerging zoonosis.

The genus was not formally recognized until the work of Victor Babes (8), who studied the cause of febrile hemoglobinuria in cattle in the late 1800s. Shortly thereafter, it was discovered that ticks provided the mode of transmission of *Babesia bigemina*, the cause of Texas cattle fever (135). The first documented case of human babesiosis was in 1957 when a splenectomized farmer in Yugoslavia was diagnosed as having a *B. bovis* infection (133). Given the subsequent observation that most cases in Europe are due to *B. divergens*- or *B. odocoilei*-like organisms and the difficulty of discriminating among babesial species on blood smears, it is difficult to be certain as to the species causing this first case. Subsequently, there have been several cases of human babesiosis in Europe, most in splenectomized individuals and often resulting in fatality (42). Most cases have been attributed to *B. divergens*, but more recent and nonlethal cases have been attributed to a *B. odocoilei*-like agent.

Human babesiosis in the United States is most often caused by *B. microti* (145), but other distinct piroplasms are emerging as causative agents (108). *B. microti* was described in the white-footed mouse, *Peromyscus leucopus*, in the 1930s, but the latter was not identified as the primary reservoir until 1976 (50). Babesiosis was one of the first zoonoses in the United States to be identified definitively as a tick-transmitted disease. It was considered a common infection in many animals but not a threat to human health until the 1960s, when a series of *B. microti* infections (termed Nantucket fever) were identified in residents of Nantucket Island (50, 114, 126, 128, 137). Indeed, *B. microti* was an early candidate under consideration as the causative agent of Lyme disease after its initial

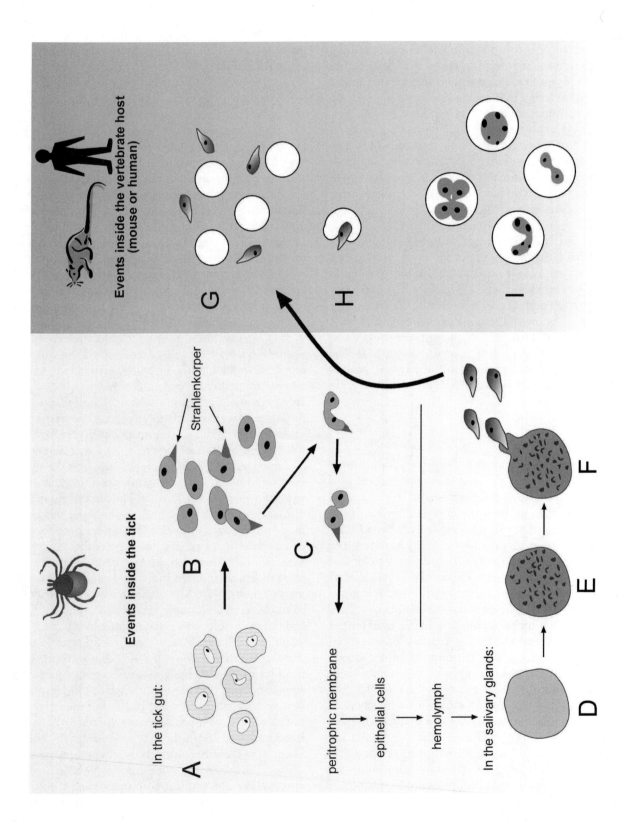

description in the 1970s, and some Lyme disease patients were found to be seroreactive to *B. microti*, thus only complicating the matter (A. Spielman, personal communication). Since then, babesiosis has been recognized as a relatively common cause of acute febrile illness following tick bite in regions of the coastal northeast and upper midwestern United States where the disease is endemic.

In eastern North America, *B. microti* is transmitted by *I. scapularis*, the same tick that transmits both Lyme disease and human granulocytic ehrlichiosis (92, 107, 137). A novel *Bartonella* species cosegregates with *B. microti* in *P. leucopus*, but its zoonotic potential is not known at present (56). *P. leucopus* is a vertebrate reservoir for at least three of the known pathogens (50, 56, 82, 144) and is itself commonly coinfected (6, 7, 56, 144). A field study of *P. leucopus* populations in areas of Lyme disease endemicity found that *Borrelia burgdorferi*-infected mice often had coinfections of *B. microti*, *Bartonella* spp., or both but that mice were not usually infected with *B. microti* or *Bartonella* in the absence of *B. burgdorferi* (7, 56). Humans are apparently susceptible to infection with a combination of these agents, which may influence both the clinical course and the choice of therapies, especially in the acute setting (see below).

CLINICAL PRESENTATION

Epidemiological Considerations

Epidemiological information should weigh heavily in considering the diagnostic possibility of babesiosis. Most cases in normosplenic, immunocompetent persons are acquired in areas of Lyme disease endemicity in the northeastern and upper-midwestern United States and are due to *B. microti*. The actual frequency of *B. microti* or WA1 infection in the United States is probably much higher than the number of reported cases (136 cases in New York between 1970 and 1991 and 160 cases in Nantucket between 1969 and 1998), because babesiosis is self-limiting and mild in most persons. Serosurveys have been the primary technique to ascertain the prevalence of babesial infection. Most

surveys have been performed in areas where clinically apparent cases have occurred. Surveys of blood donors in areas of endemicity have shown from 3 to 8% seroprevalence of *B. microti*, but the lack of standardized test methods makes the interpretation of these data difficult. One survey in California showed as much as a 16% prevalence of antibodies against WA1-like organisms (109), but high seroprevalence rates in blood donors from areas where the disease is apparently nonendemic suggest that the WA1 serologic test lacks specificity.

Babesiosis appears to be relatively rare in Europe, with only 29 reported cases. However, when diagnosed it is very serious, as a 42% case fatality rate has been described in the cases reported (42). Most European cases have been reported from France and the British Isles, but this may represent heightened medical and scientific awareness and interest in those areas rather than the actual distribution of infection (42). A few cases have been described in other parts of the world, including China (42), Taiwan (131), Egypt (96), South Africa (18), and Mexico (42). Recently, *B. microti* or a related organism has been reported in areas of Lyme disease endemicity in Europe, and serosurveys have shown higher-than-expected seroprevalence rates (39, 44, 62, 70). As mentioned above, *B. odocoilei*, a pathogen usually found in white-tailed deer, has been implicated in recent human cases of sublethal infection (86).

Over 40 cases of transfusion-acquired babesiosis have been reported in the United States and 1 has been reported in Japan (54). Most of these cases have involved the transmission of *B. microti* from an asymptomatic donor (35, 43, 91, 97, 115, 134); the implicated blood units had been stored from 5 to 35 days and include one case of transmission by frozen deglycerolized blood (32, 43, 115). The incubation period for appearance of the infection after transfusion varied from 17 days to 8 weeks (97, 134). There has also been one case of transfusion-acquired WA1 infection (53) and one recent case of transfusion-acquired neonatal infection due to a related parasite from a donor presumably infected in California (68). The not-infrequent transmission of *B. microti* by blood transfusions from asymptomatic donors has raised the possibility of screening blood donors for clinically inapparent

---

Figure 2. Life cycle of *Babesia* spp. in the tick and vertebrate hosts. Events in the tick begin with the parasites still visible in consumed erythrocytes. (A) Some are beginning to develop Strahlenkörper forms. (B) The released gametes begin to fuse (note that only one of the proposed mechanisms is pictured; one gamete has a Strahlenkörper form whereas the other does not). (C) The zygote then goes on to infect other tissues within the tick and migrates to the salivary glands. (D) Once a parasite has infected the salivary acini, a multinucleate but undifferentiated sporoblast is formed. (E) After the tick begins to feed, the specialized organelles of the future sporozoites form. (F) Finally, mature sporozoites bud off from the sporoblast. (G) As the tick feeds on a vertebrate host, these sporozoites are inoculated into the host. (H) Sporozoites (or merozoites) contact a host erythrocyte and begin the process of infection by invagination. (I) The parasites become trophozoites and can divide by binary fission within the host erythrocyte, creating the various ring forms and crosses seen on stained blood smears.

B. microti infection, especially when blood products are earmarked for immunocompromised or elderly recipients (60, 81).

Symptoms of Human Babesiosis

The clinical manifestations of human babesiosis are caused primarily by the presence of the asexual reproductive stage in host erythrocytes and their subsequent lysis. Consequently, there is a wide spectrum of disease severity that is probably directly related to the level of parasitemia. The incubation period from the time of tick transmission to the appearance of symptoms typically varies from 1 to 6 weeks but may be as long as months to years (10). In one well-documented case of *B. microti* infection, asymptomatic seroconversion was followed by persistent parasitemia (as evidenced by PCR positivity) for over 2 years before the disease became clinically apparent (74). Thus, nearly all naturally infected individuals are antibody positive for immunoglobulin G (IgG) and/or IgM at the time of presentation.

At the extreme end of the disease spectrum is a fulminant, often fatal, infection; symptoms may include malaise, chills, myalgia, anemia, fatigue, and fever as high as 40°C. Some patients also may develop nausea, emesis, night sweats, weight loss, and hematuria, which are believed to be associated with a higher level of parasitic burden (10, 108). Hepatomegaly and splenomegaly may also be present. Hemolytic anemia that lasts for several days to a few months can occur in clinically severe cases, most commonly in asplenic, severely immunocompromised, or elderly hosts. Complications of babesiosis are more likely in immunocompromised patients and may include severe hemolysis requiring exchange transfusion and respiratory distress syndrome requiring respiratory support. Patients older than 70 years of age generally present with a much greater severity of infection than younger patients. In the United States, the mortality rate for clinically apparent infections of *B. microti* is about 5% (95). However, this is almost certainly an overestimate, since most infections are asymptomatic, and clinically apparent cases almost certainly comprise an overrepresentation of individuals predisposed to poor outcomes by factors such as age and immunodeficiency.

The initial symptoms of both babesiosis and Lyme disease often overlap. In the absence of the characteristic rash (erythema migrans), Lyme disease, like babesiosis, may present only with nonspecific symptoms including fever and fatigue (79). It is important to note that the antibiotic therapy typically used for the treatment of Lyme disease is ineffective against *B. microti*. A coinfected patient treated only for Lyme disease could, therefore, still harbor a persistent babesial infection after therapy. Management of patients with persistent symptoms, fever in particular, after appropriate therapy for Lyme disease should therefore include an evaluation of other tick-transmitted agents.

Babesiosis cases attributed to *B. divergens* reported in Europe are usually more severe than those caused by *B. microti*. The onset of symptoms usually occurs within 1 to 3 weeks of the implicated tick bite (42). In contrast to cases reported in the United States, almost all reported cases in Europe have had a history of prior splenectomy which probably increases the likelihood of disease expression and subsequent recognition. In these cases, the disease generally appears suddenly, with hemoglobinuria due to severe hemolysis as the presenting symptom, followed by jaundice. In the most severe cases, patients develop a shock-like picture with renal failure and pulmonary edema (42). Little information is available regarding the possibility of subclinical infection among nonsplenectomized, immunocompetent persons exposed to *B. divergens*.

The magnitude of most laboratory abnormalities generally depends on the level of parasitemia (116). Clinically apparent cases may develop high levels of serum transaminase, alkaline phophatase, unconjugated bilirubin, and lactic dehydrogenase. Normochromic normocytic anemia, reticulocytosis, thrombocytopenia, and occasionally leukopenia may also be present. Some laboratory manifestations, such as abnormal hepatic function and depressed platelets or leukocytes, may be due to tumor necrosis factor (TNF)-mediated inflammation, as occurs in severe malarial infections. However, in light of the recent recognition of coinfection in humans with multiple tick-transmitted agents, it is also possible that some of the more variable manifestations of the disease may, in some patients, also be associated with coinfection with these other pathogens (see below).

Susceptibility Factors

There are probably many host characteristics that affect the severity of babesiosis. As mentioned, the most severe infections occur predominantly in the elderly and in splenectomized or immunocompromised hosts (10, 127). Patients reported to have been infected with *B. microti* have ranged in age from 3 weeks to 86 years, with the majority of clinically apparent cases occuring in 50- to 60-year-olds (79). This finding was most striking in a recent study of the persistence of parasitemia after acute babesiosis; the mean age of patients with mild or asymptomatic infection was approximately 30 years less than those seen with severe cases (74). Similarly, resistance to *B. divergens* is seen in young cattle (16). Some evidence also exists in animal models of immunosenescence relative to babesial infection. It has been observed that adult *P. leucopus* mice are more often persistently parasitemic than juveniles (139). Another study showed that older laboratory mice (BALB/c) had reduced and delayed peak parasitemias compared to juvenile mice but that the older mice could not clear the parasites and experienced episodic parasitemia until their death (49). Recent studies by Vannier et al. (148) showed that in DBA/2 mice, early and persistent parasitemias increased with age at infection. Unlike immunocompetent mice, SCID mice developed high, persistent levels of parasitemia that were reduced by transfer of naive BALB/c or DBA/2 splenocytes. BALB/c cells reduced the persistent parasitemia to a greater extent than did age-matched DBA/2 cells. As predicted by the experiments with DBA/2 mice, there was an age-associated loss of protection by cells of both strains (148).

Additional factors affecting the severity of babesiosis are asplenia and coinfection with other infectious agents (36, 106, 134, 142, 146). Almost all the cases of *B. divergens* infection in Europe (~83%) were severe and almost always involved patients who had been splenectomized prior to infection (42). In contrast, most of the cases in North America caused by *B. microti* were less severe and occurred in normosplenic patients. The exceptions are cases in the western United States, which are generally caused by piroplasms other than *B. microti*, notably the WA1 parasite and its relatives (119, 147), CA1 (66, 108), and MO1 (51). As expected, human immunodeficiency virus (HIV) infection may also exacerbate the severity of babesial infection, and several relatively treatment-resistant cases have been described (12, 36, 106). Coinfection with other tick-transmitted infectious agents can also result in more severe manifestations (79) (see below). For instance, patients with coinfection of *B. burgdorferi* and *B. microti* appear to experience increased disease severity (79).

Host Immunity to Babesial Infection

Most of what is known about immunity to babesiosis comes from animal models; a schematic of the course of infection and host immune responses is shown in Fig. 3. All mammalian hosts examined to date develop immunity to *Babesia* species either after infection and recovery or after prophylactic immunization. However, the efficacy of the immune response varies widely. In the initial dissemination phase after the tick bite, sporozoites are free in the plasma for a brief period; at this stage, preexisting IgG antibodies in immune individuals can prevent infection by binding and neutralizing sporozoites before they succeed in invading target erythrocytes. The second, more-refractory, and yet-critical stage begins when babesial

organisms establish intraerythrocytic infection. The elimination of infected erythrocytes is mediated by a number of factors including splenic destruction of deformed erythrocytes and cellular immune responses largely mediated by nitric oxide (NO). At this stage, the cycle of splenic or peripheral erythrocyte destruction, sporozoite release, and reinfection of red blood cells is responsible for the maintenance of parasitemia. In animal models, unrestrained levels of parasitemia during this initial expansion phase often precede a poor clinical outcome.

Cells of the innate immune system are largely responsible for controlling the initial hematogenous spread and expansion of the parasite population. In the absence of macrophages and natural killer (NK) cells, a high degree of parasitemia develops within a short time period; the control parasitemia is most likely accomplished by the production of soluble factors such as nitric oxide and reactive oxygen species (ROS) by macrophages. An important role for NK cells was first proposed after observation of NK cell activity and resistance to *B. microti* in inbred strains of mice (34). NK cells might mediate protection in the early stages of infection (136). Other studies have found high levels of NK cell activity during peak parasitemia and the recovery phase (65). Evidence of NK activity has also been observed in acute human babesiosis (11). Macrophages are also important in the innate response; depleting them with silica suppresses protection against *B. microti* (5, 104). A defining characteristic of macrophages and NK cells is their ability to produce soluble effector molecules in response to a variety of microbial stimuli, presumably via activation of toll-like receptors. This could be of primary importance in babesiosis, since activation of innate immune responses via unrelated stimuli can confer resistance to infection (23, 25, 26, 31, 80, 153), and a nonspecific soluble mediator is thought to be responsible for the protection. These data have been largely supported by recent studies (5), in which mice genetically deficient in gamma interferon (IFN-γ)-mediated responses (IFNGR2KO mice) and interleukin-12 (IL-12)-mediated responses (Stat4KO mice) were infected with *Babesia* WA1 and observations were made on the course of infection and cytokine responses. The increased susceptibility observed in both IFNGR2KO and Stat-4KO mice suggested that the early IL-12- and IFN-γ-mediated responses are involved in protection against acute infection and that resistance appears to correlate with an increase in nitric oxide (NO) production. Mice genetically deficient in B lymphocytes or CD4$^+$ T lymphocytes were able to mount protective responses comparable to those of immunosufficient mice. In contrast, depletion of macrophages or NK cells in vivo resulted in elevated susceptibility to infection.

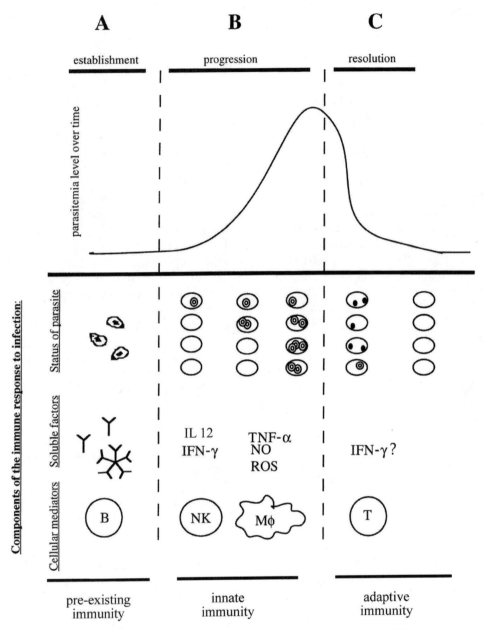

Figure 3. Model of the cells and effector molecules involved in immunity to *Babesia* species. Different immune mechanisms contribute to resistance during each stage of the babesial infection. (A) During the establishment stage antibodies (IgG) play a role in preventing erythrocyte infection by binding the free sporozoites. (B) During the progression stage the *Babesia* organisms succeed in invading the erythrocyte, and the resulting merozoites proliferate and lyse the infected cell. After lysis has occurred, parasites reach the bloodstream again to initiate a new round of invasion. Several rounds of this cycle cause parasitemia levels to increase. Cells of the innate immune system, especially NK cells and macrophages, have been implicated in antibabesial activity and are thought to control the growth rate of the merozoites. The inhibition seems to rely on the production of soluble factors: IFN-γ by NK cells, and TNF-α, nitric oxide (NO), and ROS by macrophages. (C) In the resolution stage parasitemia reaches a maximum and then declines. The decrease in parasites seems to be due at least in part to intracellular degeneration inside the erythrocyte, as evidenced by the appearance of "crisis forms." T lymphocytes seem to be the cells responsible for parasite clearance, specifically the subpopulation of CD4+ IFN-γ producers, although the specific role of IFN-γ is uncertain.

The humoral component of the immune system is currently considered of limited importance, except perhaps during the initial dissemination of infection. It has been demonstrated that antibodies in the serum neutralize extracellular babesial sporozoites or mero-zoites (1, 55, 120, 149). Passive transfer of immune serum to immunodeficient mice infected with *B. microti* does not confer the ability to resolve infection (93). However, some degree of immunity to *B. microti* can be transferred to cattle and mice with serum containing anti-babesial antibodies (90), and immune serum delays the onset of *B. rodhaini* parasitemia. Yet neither prevents the development of infection nor protects infected mice from death (1). Overall, the protective effect of antibody seems restricted to a brief period of exposure of sporozoite or merozoite to the bloodstream, while in transit to a new target cell.

In contrast to humoral adaptive responses, cell-mediated adaptive responses are critical in the resolution of infection. In most murine models, parasitemia achieves a plateau and then begins to decline approximately 10 days after infection. The decrease in parasitemia is due to *Babesia* degeneration inside the erythrocyte and clearance by the hyperactive spleen; the infection resolves, and the disease subsides. The contribution of T cells has been examined with thymus-deficient animals. Infecting congenic athymic mice (24, 125) with *B. microti* results in both increased and persistent parasitemia, in contrast to the transient parasitemia observed in normal mice. Further, the transfer of purified T lymphocytes from immune animals is sufficient to confer immunity to *B. microti* naïve mice (125), and the transfer of immune thymocytes to immunodeficient mice confers the ability to resolve *B. microti* infection (93). Mice depleted of $CD4^+$ T helper cells are more susceptible to *B. microti* infection than normal mice (63, 132), while susceptibility to infection is unaffected (63, 132) or even decreased (132) in mice depleted of CD8 cytotoxic T cells. Collectively, these data indicate that the $CD4^+$ T cells are critical in resistance to babesiosis and that specific cell-mediated immunity plays a major role in the resolution of infection (124). Intraerythrocytic killing during this resolution stage requires T lymphocytes, specifically a TH1 $CD4^+$ effector population. It has been proposed that IFN-γ is directly responsible for intraerythrocytic parasite degradation, but such direct involvement has not been proven. More recent studies suggest that loss of IFN-γ function affects initial susceptibility, rather than disease resolution (28).

Potential Immunological Effects of Coinfection with Other Pathogens

Multiple simultaneous infections with distinct pathogens in the same host may affect each other through alterations in host immune responses. The role of helper T cells and their differentiation into Th1, Th2, and regulatory T-cell subsets has been the focus of recent studies attempting to elucidate the mechanisms involved in the apparently synergistic inflammatory effects observed during coinfection. Similar to the immunologic effects seen during infection with unrelated pathogens in the experiments conducted by Clark et al. in the 1970s, it is possible that immuno-

logic interactions occur within the Lyme disease transmission cycle involving combinations of agents within the mouse reservoir; currently, the list includes *Ehrlichia*, *Babesia*, *Borrelia*, and *Bartonella*. It is reasonable to hypothesize that an immune response to one organism may have adjuvant effects related to the infectious processes due to coinfecting agents, and that these effects could be either synergistic or antagonistic. Immune suppression is a documented characteristic of some parasitic infections (46, 103, 140). There are several lines of evidence that demonstrate the immunosuppressive effects of *B. microti* infections relative to coinfection; *B. microti* infections in mice can impair the ability of the host to reject *Trichuris muris* (nematode) infections (111), prolong and enhance *Trypanosoma musculi* infections (103), result in decreased *Trypanosoma*-specific antibody production (103), and decrease the murine immune response to sheep red blood cells (2, 118).

One potential effect of *B. microti* infection could be to skew T-cell differentiation towards a Th1 response, thereby enhancing inflammatory responses to *B. burgdorferi*. This finding has been validated experimentally in mouse models, in which coinfection of BALB/c mice with *B. microti* and *B. burgdorferi* resulted in significant increases in arthritis severity, despite the fact that there were no apparent differences in spirochetal burden compared to mice infected with *B. burgdorferi* alone (101). Coinfected mice had reduced levels of the anti-inflammatory cytokine IL-10, which correlated with increased arthritis severity. An alternative scenario is also possible, in which *B. burgdorferi* or *Bartonella* could enhance babesial infection; this could be consistent with recent field survey results in which *B. microti* was found primarily in mice that were also infected with *B. burgdorferi* and a novel *Bartonella* species (7, 56).

Genetic Susceptibility and Gender Dimorphism

A study examining the susceptibility of various mouse strains to *B. microti* found profound differences in peak parasitemia levels between strains, with the C3H and A strains highly susceptible and C57BL/6 most resistant (123). The data also suggested that resistance was a dominant trait and not due to a specific major histocompatibility complex (MHC) haplotype (34). A more recent study examined WA1 infection of several inbred and congenic strains encompassing five different haplotypes. Differences within each haplotype were observed, demonstrating that the susceptible phenotype was independent of the MHC haplotype and attributable instead to the genetic background (100). An interesting characteristic of the WA1 model is that differences in susceptibility are manifested not only in differing parasitemia levels but also in dramatically polarized outcomes of infection: full recovery or death. Resistance is conferred in part by a small number of autosomal dominant genes (99). The *scid* mutation showed little effect in genetically susceptible C3H mice and did not decrease the inherent resistance of C57BL/6 mice, suggesting that innate immunity plays a central role in determining the course of infection in these strains (4). In contrast, the *scid* mutation dramatically impaired resistance in moderately susceptible BALB/c mice, suggesting that T cells play an important role in resolving infection when the initial innate response is suboptimal. An interesting gender dimorphism was also noted: in comparison to their female counterparts, male mice of several genetic backgrounds manifested increased resistance to the infection, indicating that the gender of the host may influence protection against babesiosis (4). To date, however, there is no indication of such gender dimorphism in humans, although large-scale population-based information is not available.

Diagnosis of Babesiosis

The diagnosis of babesiosis should begin with a patient's history, which should include appropriate clinical manifestations, history of travel to an area where babesiosis is endemic, tick bite or potential exposure to ticks, recent blood transfusion, or splenectomy. A subsequent analysis should include examination of stained blood smears (described below), as well as serologic evaluation with indirect fluorescent antibody tests (IFAT) (21), recombinant immunoassays, and possibly PCR (73, 75, 110). In severe cases, morphological changes in the spleen (hypertrophy, sometimes with necrotic foci) may be identified by magnetic resonance imaging (MRI) or computerized tomography (CT) scan. Other laboratory abnormalities (liver enzyme elevation and evidence of hemolysis) described below usually depend directly on the level of parasitemia in the patient and are likely to be within normal ranges for clinically mild or silent cases. In most instances, an accurate patient history, clinical presentation, and observation of characteristic organisms on blood smear evaluation are sufficient to establish a diagnosis. However, a large number of cases have been described that are negative by smear but positive by PCR; these cases generally would have been missed with an exclusive reliance on blood smears.

Before the development of a PCR-based assay for *B. microti*, inoculation of hamsters with patient blood was the most sensitive method of detecting *B. microti* (108). The organisms require several weeks or longer to establish a detectable infection, and the results may be unreliable due to factors such as host adaptation,

isolate variation, and dose of inoculum (14, 33). There have also been cases of infection with novel *Babesia* species (119) that could not be isolated via hamster inoculation and were eventually identified via broad-range PCR (108, 109). Hamster inoculation has been very useful for detecting and monitoring persistent infection (for up to 7 months) in asplenic hosts, but improved sensitivity is a necessity for detection of the very low levels of parasitemia characteristic of normosplenic persons (74). Thus, PCR is rapidly becoming the test of choice for confirmation of ongoing infection in antibody-reactive persons and/or for monitoring therapeutic responses (see below). However, great care must be taken to avoid contamination by PCR methods, which can lead to false-positive results (110). Thus, PCR data should be corroborated by immunologic testing whenever possible. Because of the long latency period of *B. microti* infections, nearly all persons who are PCR positive will also be antibody positive at the time of clinical presentation (74). The exception may be HIV-positive subjects who present with persistent fevers (12).

Hematologic Evaluation

The technique most frequently used to diagnose human babesiosis is manual microscopic examination of thin blood smears to demonstrate the presence of parasites within erythrocytes (17, 33, 42, 127). Automated blood analyzers cannot detect babesial organisms in blood. Peripheral blood smears are typically stained with Wright's or Giemsa stain; acridine orange can also be used. The organisms are apparent within red blood cells as darkly staining ring forms with light blue cytoplasm or as brightly staining fluorescent inclusions with acridine orange (Color Plate 17). *B. microti* merozoites are approximately 1.5 to 2 μm in size (67); *B. divergens* merozoites are variable in size (1 to 3 μm), depending on which host they have infected (42). Morphologically, there is great variation in the forms seen (Color Plate 17A to C): simple rings (annular), paired or single pear-shaped trophozoites (pyriform), or the rarely seen but often-described Maltese cross. *B. microti* infection can cause levels of parasitemia that vary from undetectable on microscopy to levels as high as 85% on peripheral blood smears. The duration of detectable parasitemia on blood smears varies from 3 to 12 weeks (127), with the longest reported duration of smear positivity of 7 months in samples from a splenectomized patient (141). In general, the analysis of blood smears is a subjective process, the accuracy of which depends on the intensity of parasitemia, the experience of the observer, and the time spent examining the smear. The necessity of discriminating the subtleties of babesial morphology coupled with often low levels of parasitemia may result in inaccurate diagnoses. In studies of well-defined cases of nonspecific febrile illness after tick bite, we recently found that of 29 acute babesiosis patients defined by PCR positivity, 25 patients had positive smears as evaluated by an experienced technologist who spent more than 5 min evaluating slides based on a high index of suspicion (83% sensitivity). Acridine orange staining and fluorescent microscopy may assist in detection of low levels of parasitemia (Color Plate 17D).

There are some points of caution with respect to blood smear analyses. The ring forms visible within erythrocytes can vary greatly and may be confused with those of *Plasmodium falciparum*; however, the absence of the pigment hemozoin should help diagnose babesiosis (116), although early stages of *P. falciparum* may also lack pigment (142). There have been several cases in which patients with babesiosis have initially been misdiagnosed as having malaria, resulting in potentially life-threatening delays of appropriate treatment. The parasitology testing program of the College of American Pathologists offers a proficiency panel that occasionally includes a babesia sample. After initial misidentification of the organism as *Plasmodium* spp., participants become facile with identification of *B. microti* and its discrimination from malaria.

Serology and Immunology

Serological testing with IFAT is both specific and sensitive and is the currently recommended serologic method (21) for diagnosing *B. microti* infections, particularly chronic infections (142). This test uses hamster-derived *B. microti* antigen. The cutoff titer for a positive result varies from laboratory to laboratory; some laboratories report that titers above 1:64 are diagnostic (77). In general, higher cutoff titers (1:128 to 1:256) are associated with greater specificity. In our experience, titers of 1:128 to 1:256 are rarely associated with false positivity, but screening of blood donor populations at a 1:64 titer may result in occasional false-positive results. In the acute phase of infection, antibody titers often rise 10- to 20-fold above the cutoff, with a steady decline afterwards over weeks to months (116). Antibody is usually detectable when patients present clinically with *B. microti* infection (142). In smear-negative or smear-inconclusive cases, the IFAT is still sensitive and specific (14).

Antibody titers can remain elevated for several years after infection (108). Although persistence of antibody does not necessarily indicate persistent infection (74, 128), levels of IgG antibody decline less rapidly in persistently infected patients (as measured by levels of *B. microti* DNA detectable in blood) than in those patients whose parasitemia resolves in <3 months (74).

Persistence of infection correlates with persistently elevated antibody levels in *B. gibsoni* infections in dogs (30). One theoretical drawback to serologic testing is that other protozoal parasites could elicit cross-reactivity, generating false-positive results by *B. microti* or WA1 IFAT procedures, especially when IgM is the antibody class being detected. Patients with connective tissue disorders such as systemic lupus erythematosus or rheumatoid arthritis (109) may also have false-positive results by other mechanisms. Conversely, samples from immunosuppressed patients or patients from whom samples are collected early in the course of the infection may generate false negatives (12, 106). HIV-infected and splenectomized patients generally have very low titers (143); if the disease is suspected in such patients, repeated examination of blood smears and PCR testing may be appropriate even in antibody-negative individuals.

B. divergens infections are usually too acute and severe to allow time for serological diagnosis, as *B. divergens* antibodies do not become detectable in sera until 7 to 10 days after the onset of hemoglobinuria (42). IFAT can be used, however, to distinguish among infections due to different *Babesia* species, since *B. microti*, WA1, and *B. divergens* have almost no serologic cross-reactivity.

By using recombinant serologic expression cloning, a set of diagnostically useful antigens was identified that may lead to the development of a more standardized diagnostic test (58, 60, 85). Recently, a recombinant immunoassay has been developed that demonstrates good sensitivity and specificity (60). A combination of two complementary immunodominant peptides detected 98 of 107 IgG blot-positive sera taken after documented infection. Reactives included all 12 samples that were PCR positive at the time of collection and 6 sera from smear-negative patients that were confirmed positive by PCR, immunoblotting, or IFAT. Of the IgG blot-positive specimens that were equivocal (four specimens) or nonreactive (nine specimens) by enzyme immunoassay (EIA), most had low IFAT titers consistent with exposure in the remote past. Of 38 IFAT-positive blood donor samples, 35 were positive by peptide EIA. The three EIA-negative sera were also Western blot negative. Therefore, *B. microti*-specific peptide EIA shows a high correlation with IFAT, PCR, and *B. microti* immunoblotting results in confirmed cases and may be a suitable test for blood donor screening if testing for *B. microti* is recommended in the future (54, 81, 86).

Homer et al. identified seven families of antigens by using a technique tailored specifically to detect *B. microti* antigens that are secreted or shed into the cytoplasm of red blood cells and then released into the serum after red blood cell lysis. Initial serological data obtained with recombinant proteins and a patient serum panel demonstrated that several of the proteins may be useful in developing diagnostic tests for detection of *B. microti* antibodies and antigens in serum (59).

Molecular Diagnostic Approaches

Although clinically apparent cases are usually diagnosed by blood smears and/or serology, patients with milder infections often remain undiagnosed and, therefore, untreated. Detection of these mild cases of babesiosis requires more sensitive techniques than the ones described thus far. With the evolution of more sensitive PCR-based techniques, the molecular diagnosis and monitoring of even mild cases of babesiosis have become possible.

Development of PCR-based assays for both *B. microti* (3, 45, 54, 58, 71, 73, 110) and *B. divergens* (105) has been previously described. Studies have shown these assays to be more sensitive and equally specific for the detection of acute cases when compared to blood smear evaluation and hamster inoculation (109, 110, 147). These assays typically rely on the amplification of highly conserved sequences (with species-informative regions within the conserved sequence) such as nss-rRNA or multicopy targets (58, 74, 79, 110). Broad-range PCR can be used for detection of a wide range of babesial species, as previously described (51, 109), and subsequent sequence analysis of the amplified fragments and comparison to a database of known sequences allow for definitive identification of the infecting agent. However, the sensitivity of the broad-range approach as a front-line diagnostic procedure is unproven at present and is more likely to encounter problems of specificity than methods based on unique sequences. As mentioned, patients with detectable babesial DNA in their blood are likely to be parasitemic, since loss of reactivity over time is correlated with antibabesial therapy, clinical response, and lack of transmissibility of parasites by blood transfusion (74). PCR is fast becoming the test of choice for confirmation of serologic testing and monitoring the course of infection during and after therapy.

Novel multicopy targets have recently been identified which may provide certain sensitivity advantages. Homer et al. performed immunoscreening of an expression library of genomic DNA from a human isolate of *B. microti* (strain MN1). Among 17 unique immunoreactive clones, 9 were identified from a related family of genes, with little sequence homology to other known sequences but with an architecture resembling that of several surface proteins of *Plasmodium*. Within this family, one member (BMN1-6) comprising a tandem array of degenerate six-amino-acid repeats was found in various lengths between relatively well-conserved segments at the N and C termini. To examine within-clone variation, a PCR protocol was developed allowing for direct recovery of specific BMN1-6 homologues directly from 30 human blood isolates, 4 corresponding hamster isolates, and 5 geographically corresponding *P. leucopus* (white-footed mouse) isolates. Isolates from the hamsters had the same sequences as those found in the corresponding human blood, suggesting that genetic variation of BMN1-6 does not occur during passage. Moreover, it was found that strains that were closely related geographically were also closely related at the sequence level; nine patients, all from Nantucket Island, Mass., harbored clones that were indistinguishable from each other but distinct from those found in other northeastern or upper-midwestern strains. However, clones from different patients were often substantially different from each other with regard to the number and location of the degenerate repeats within the BMN1-6 homologue. It was concluded from this study that considerable genetic and antigenic diversity exists among isolates of *B. microti* from the United States and that distinct sequence variants map to different United States locations (58).

TREATMENT

Most cases of *B. microti* infection are mild and usually resolve without treatment. Standard therapy with a combination of clindamycin and quinine has been administered in more severe cases. This therapeutic regimen was discovered by Wittner et al. during the management of a case of presumed transfusion-acquired malarial infection (151). Initially, chloroquine was used but proved to be unsuccessful. The patient was then treated with quinine and clindamycin, which successfully eradicated the organisms. Subsequent studies with animals supported the usefulness of this combination of agents (122). The duration of *B. microti* DNA detection in patients treated with quinine and clindamycin is shorter than in untreated patients (74).

The potential toxicities of clindamycin and quinine are significant (29) and include hearing loss, tinnitus, syncope, hypotension, gastrointestinal discomfort, diarrhea, and antibiotic-associated colitis. This limits the use of this regimen to serious cases, even if patients are proven to be persistently parasitemic. More recent studies have pointed to a potentially more effective and less toxic regimen combining atovaquone and azithromycin (71, 72). This regimen merits further investigation, as it may widen the scope of patients who could be considered for therapy, since for mild cases, treatment with the standard regimen of quinine and clindamycin may be worse than the disease itself. Several studies have shown the activity of atovaquone in treating *B. microti* infections (48, 61, 150); and atovaquone may be more effective than imidocarb in treating *B. divergens* infections (117). Even though they are apparently less toxic, broad use of atovaquone and azithromycin should generally be limited to patients with a confirmed diagnosis of active infection with *B. microti*. Another interesting recent development has been the recognized activity of certain antifungals in the treatment of babesial infection in animal models; ketoconazole was found to be especially effective (13). If proven effective in humans, available treatment options may be expanded further.

As in malarial infection, in very serious cases, particularly when very high levels of parasitemia and acute hemolysis are present, anti-infective therapy may not be sufficient; procedures such as erythrocyte exchange transfusion can be beneficial or even lifesaving (20, 35, 41, 64). In addition, patients who are immunosuppressed (19), are HIV infected (88), or merely have a severe babesial infection sometimes do not respond to standard antimicrobial therapy and require additional or more prolonged treatment courses. Patients with *B. divergens* infections are treated as medical emergencies and often require prompt treatment that may include erythrocyte exchange transfusion along with intravenous clindamycin and oral quinine to arrest hemolysis and prevent renal failure (42, 142).

Consideration of Coinfection

Therapeutic consideration must be given to the possibility of coinfection of *B. microti* and other tick-borne pathogens, particularly *B. burgdorferi*, the causative agent of Lyme disease (see Chapter 11), and *Anaplasma phagocytophila*, the causative agent of human granulocytic anaplasmosis-ehrlichiosis (see Chapter 13). It is estimated from serosurveys that as many as 13% of Lyme disease patients in areas where babesiosis is endemic are coinfected with *B. microti* (10, 76, 79). Furthermore, it has been suggested that the increase in *B. microti* seropositivity seen during the past 30 years is consistent with the increase in incidence of Lyme disease (79). Since the clinical features of early Lyme disease, *A. phagocytophila* infection, and babesiosis may overlap and because the treatment of babesiosis is generally ineffective for Lyme disease or anaplasmosis, definitive diagnostic information is extremely useful in areas where these infections can occur simultaneously. Recently, a combination of three tests (PCR for *A. phagocytophila* and *B. microti* and IgM capture EIA for *B. burgdorferi*) has been offered to physicians in the Cape Cod area for the diagnosis of acute febrile illnesses in the spring, summer, or fall.

Approximately 20 to 30% of such cases are infected with at least one of the three agents; in the 2003 transmission season, nearly one-third of the acute Lyme disease patients were found to be coinfected with *B. microti* (Victor Berardi, personal communication). Thus, the availability of accurate diagnostic information in a timely manner relative to treatment decisions may be critical to the successful treatment of coinfected patients.

Persistent Infection—Implications for Blood Safety

The potential of *B. microti* and other *Babesia* species to cause chronic asymptomatic parasitemia is of potential importance to blood safety. The existence of such chronic asymptomatic carrier states in babesial infections of domestic and wild animals has been recognized for many years (30, 37, 87, 128, 145); consequently, most information about the chronic carrier state is derived from animal models. Dogs infected with *B. gibsoni*, for instance, can remain chronic carriers after clinical symptoms have resolved (30). Chronically infected animals maintain elevated antibody titers, and some develop signs of chronic infection such as pathologic evidence of liver disease, chronic membranoproliferative glomerulonephritis, or both (30). Hamsters display an initial parasitemia that evolves to a carrier state in which the parasites can only infrequently be detected. The carrier state can last 2 or more years, but in the last month of life, the animals show signs of relapse, characterized by a rise in parasitemia, ascites, anorexia, and lethargy (87). There have also been studies that have demonstrated chronic infection in primates (129). The widely infected *B. microti* reservoir host, *P. leucopus*, seems to maintain a chronic carrier state, generally harboring low-level parasitemia (33, 56, 112, 139). Indeed, the chronic asymptomatic carrier state is probably an essential component of the *B. microti* transmission cycle that contributes significantly to the overall prevalence of infections. The ubiquity of infection of free-living creatures, coupled with the frequent observation of chronic infection, has even led to the suggestion that there could be some immunologic or other benefit conferred on the host (57), such as protection against infection by more pathogenic *Plasmodium* spp. (22).

Less is known about the chronic carrier state in humans. Until recently, the actual duration of infection with *Babesia* and *Babesia*-like organisms in humans has been difficult to determine because the tests lacked sensitivity. With the advent of PCR, however, serial studies of patient blood have shown that a chronic carrier state can occur and last for months to years (54, 74). The best evidence that an asymptomatic carrier state exists is provided by the over 40 cases of transfusion-transmitted babesiosis (35, 43, 91, 97, 115, 134). Several serosurveys have suggested that exposure to *B. microti* (38, 78, 126) and perhaps other species (68, 109) occurs in much greater numbers than the reported number of clinically apparent cases. However, these intriguing findings await confirmation of babesial infection by subinoculation of animals or PCR, and much work must be done to better define the specificity of the methods used to detect babesial antibody in humans and to correlate antibody levels with the persistence of infection. Nonetheless, the surprising prevalence of chronic infections may become an increasing concern for blood safety in areas where babesiosis is endemic. Unfortunately, behavioral screening (such as inquiries about history of tick bites and travel to areas of endemicity) may not be sensitive or specific enough to eliminate true carriers from becoming blood donors (81). Serologic or PCR-based screening tests may eventually become important for blood donor screening in areas of high endemicity (60).

CONCLUSIONS

Human babesiosis was first described only in 1957 but is now known to have a worldwide distribution. The increase in reported cases is likely due to both increases in actual incidence and increased awareness of the disease. Despite improved understanding of the disease, babesiosis continues to have significant medical impact. It can also be a confounding variable in the diagnosis and treatment of Lyme disease and as a potential threat to the blood supply, especially in the United States. Diagnostic advances, including the development of PCR assays, have resulted in increased sensitivity of detection as well as the discovery and characterization of new babesial species. Further studies using the molecular tools available and those under development will lead to a better understanding of the natural history of this disease and its pathogenesis in humans.

REFERENCES

1. Abdalla, H. S., H. S. Hussein, and J. P. Kreier. 1978. Babesia rodhaini: passive protection of mice with immune serum. *Tropenmed. Parasitol.* 29:295–306.
2. Adachi, K., H. Kawano, and S. Makimura. 1993. Suppressed antibody response to sheep erythrocytes in experimentally Babesia rodhaini-infected mice. *J. Vet. Med. Sci.* 55:189–190.
3. Aguero-Rosenfeld, M. E. 2003. Laboratory aspects of tick-borne diseases: Lyme, human granulocytic ehrlichiosis and babesiosis. *Mt. Sinai J. Med.* 70:197–206.
4. Aguilar-Delfin, I., M. J. Homer, P. J. Wettstein, and D. H. Persing. 2001. Innate resistance to *Babesia* infection is influenced by genetic background and gender. *Infect. Immun.* 69:7955–7958.
5. Aguilar-Delfin, I., P. J. Wettstein, and D. H. Persing. 2003. Resistance to acute babesiosis is associated with interleukin-12- and gamma interferon-mediated responses and requires macrophages and natural killer cells. *Infect. Immun.* 71:2002–2008.
6. Anderson, J. F., R. C. Johnson, L. A. Magnarelli, F. W. Hyde, and J. E. Myers. 1986. *Peromyscus leucopus* and *Microtus pennsylvanicus* simultaneously infected with *Borrelia burgdorferi* and *Babesia microti*. *J. Clin. Microbiol.* 23:135–137.
7. Anderson, J. F., E. D. Mintz, J. J. Gadbaw, and L. A. Magnarelli. 1991. *Babesia microti*, human babesiosis, and *Borrelia burgdorferi* in Connecticut. *J. Clin. Microbiol.* 29:2779–2783.
8. Babes, V. 1888. Sur l'hemoglobinurie bacterienne du boeuf. *C. R. Acad. Sci.* 107:692–694.
9. Beattie, J. F., M. L. Michelson, and P. J. Holman. 2002. Acute babesiosis caused by Babesia divergens in a resident of Kentucky. *N. Engl. J. Med.* 347:697–698.
10. Benach, J. L., and G. S. Habicht. 1981. Clinical characteristics of human babesiosis. *J. Infect. Dis.* 144:481.
11. Benach, J. L., G. S. Habicht, and M. I. Hamburger. 1982. Immunoresponsiveness in acute babesiosis in humans. *J. Infect. Dis.* 146:369–380.
12. Benezra, D., A. E. Brown, B. Polsky, J. W. Gold, and D. Armstrong. 1987. Babesiosis and infection with human immunodeficiency virus (HIV). *Ann. Intern. Med.* 107:944. (Letter.)
13. Bork, S., N. Yokoyama, T. Matsuo, F. G. Claveria, K. Fujisaki, and I. Igarashi. 2003. Clotrimazole, ketoconazole, and clodinafop-propargyl as potent growth inhibitors of equine Babesia parasites during in vitro culture. *J. Parasitol.* 89:604–606.
14. Brandt, F., G. R. Healy, and M. Welch. 1977. Human babesiosis: the isolation of *Babesia microti* in golden hamsters. *J. Parasitol.* 63:934–937.
15. Brasseur, P., and A. Gorenflot. 1992. Human babesiosis in Europe. *Mem. Inst. Oswaldo Cruz* 87(Suppl. 3):131–132.
16. Brocklesby, D. W., E. Harness, and S. A. Sellwood. 1971. The effect of age on the natural immunity of cattle to Babesia divergens. *Res. Vet. Sci.* 12:15–17.
17. Bruce-Chwatt, L. J. 1985. *Essential Malariology.* John Wiley & Sons, Inc., New York, N.Y.
18. Bush, J. B., M. Isaacson, A. S. Mohamed, F. T. Potgeiter, and D. T. de Waal. 1990. Human babesiosis—a preliminary report of 2 suspected cases in South Africa. *S. Afr. Med. J.* 78:699.
19. Cahill, K. M., J. L. Benach, L. M. Reich, E. Bilmes, J. H. Zins, F. P. Siegel, and S. Hochweis. 1981. Red cell exchange: treatment of babesiosis in a splenectomized patient. *Transfusion* 21:193–198.
20. Callow, L. L. 1976. Tick-borne livestock diseases and their vectors. III. The Australian methods of vaccination against anaplasmosis and babesiosis. *World Anim. Rev.* 18:9–15.
21. Chisholm, E. S., T. K. Ruebush, A. J. Sulzer, and G. R. Healy. 1978. Babesia microti infection in man: evaluation of an indirect immunofluorescent antibody test. *Am. J. Trop. Med. Hyg.* 27:14–19.
22. Clark, I. A. 2001. Heterologous immunity revisited. *Parasitology* 122(Suppl.):S51–S59.
23. Clark, I. A. 1979. Resistance to *Babesia* spp. and *Plasmodium* sp. in mice pretreated with an extract of *Coxiella burnetii*. *Infect. Immun.* 24:319–325.
24. Clark, I. A., and A. C. Allison. 1974. Babesia microti and Plasmodium berghei yoelii infections in nude mice. *Nature* 252:328–329.

25. Clark, I. A., A. C. Allison, and F. E. Cox. 1976. Protection of mice against Babesia and Plasmodium with BCG. *Nature* **259:**309–311.

26. Clark, I. A., F. E. Cox, and A. C. Allison. 1977. Protection of mice against Babesia spp. and Plasmodium spp. with killed Corynebacterium parvum. *Parasitology* **74:**9–18.

27. Clarke, C. S., E. T. Rogers, and E. L. Egan. 1989. Babesiosis: under-reporting or case-clustering? *Postgrad. Med. J.* **65:**591–593.

28. Clawson, M. L., N. Paciorkowski, T. V. Rajan, C. La Vake, C. Pope, M. La Vake, S. K. Wikel, P. J. Krause, and J. D. Radolf. 2002. Cellular immunity, but not gamma interferon, is essential for resolution of *Babesia microti* infection in BALB/c mice. *Infect. Immun.* **70:**5304–5306.

29. Clyde, D. F., R. H. Gilman, and V. C. McCarthy. 1975. Antimalarial effects of clindamycin in man. *Am. J. Trop. Med. Hyg.* **24:**369–370.

30. Conrad, P., J. Thomford, I. Yamane, J. Whiting, L. Bosma, T. Uno, H. J. Holshuh, and S. Shelly. 1991. Hemolytic anemia caused by Babesia gibsoni infection in dogs. *J. Am. Vet. Med. Assoc.* **199:**601–605.

31. Cox, F. E. 1978. Heterologous immunity between piroplasms and malaria parasites: the simultaneous elimination of Plasmodium vinckei and Babesia microti from the blood of doubly infected mice. *Parasitology* **76:**55–60.

32. Eberhard, M. L., E. M. Walker, and F. J. Steurer. 1995. Survival and infectivity of Babesia in blood maintained at 25 C and 2–4 C. *J. Parasitol.* **81:**790–792.

33. Etkind, P., J. Piesman, T. K. Ruebush, A. Spielman, and D. D. Juranek. 1980. Methods for detecting Babesia microti infection in wild rodents. *J. Parasitol.* **66:**107–110.

34. Eugui, E. M., and A. C. Allison. 1980. Differences in susceptibility of various mouse strains to haemoprotozoan infections: possible correlation with natural killer activity. *Parasitol. Immunol.* **2:**277–292.

35. Evenson, D. A., E. Perry, B. Kloster, R. Hurley, and D. F. Stroncek. 1998. Therapeutic apheresis for babesiosis. *J. Clin. Apheresis* **13:**32–36.

36. Falagas, M. E., and M. S. Klempner. 1996. Babesiosis in patients with AIDS: a chronic infection presenting as fever of unknown origin. *Clin. Infect. Dis.* **22:**809–812.

37. Figueroa, J. V., L. P. Chieves, G. S. Johnson, and G. M. Buening. 1992. Detection of Babesia bigemina-infected carriers by polymerase chain reaction amplification. *J. Clin. Microbiol.* **30:**2576–2582.

38. Filstein, M. R., J. L. Benach, D. J. White, B. A. Brody, W. D. Goldman, C. W. Bakal, and R. S. Schwartz. 1980. Serosurvey for human babesiosis in New York. *J. Infect. Dis.* **141:**518–521.

39. Foppa, I. M., P. J. Krause, A. Spielman, H. Goethert, L. Gern, B. Brand, and S. R. Telford III. 2002. Entomologic and serologic evidence of zoonotic transmission of Babesia microti, eastern Switzerland. *Emerg. Infect. Dis.* **8:**722–726.

40. Gelfand, J. A., and M. V. Callahan. 2003. Babesiosis: an update on epidemiology and treatment. *Curr. Infect. Dis. Rep.* **5:**53–58.

41. Gorenflot, A., P. Brasseur, G. Bonmarchand, D. Laneele, and D. Simonin. 1990. 2 Cases of severe human babesiosis treated successfully. *Presse Med.* **19:**335. (Letter.) (In French.)

42. Gorenflot, A., K. Moubri, E. Precigout, B. Carcy, and T. P. Schetters. 1998. Human babesiosis. *Ann. Trop. Med. Parasitol.* **92:**489–501.

43. Grabowski, E. F., P. J. Giardina, D. Goldberg, H. Masur, S. E. Read, R. L. Hirsch, and J. L. Benach. 1982. Babesiosis transmitted by a transfusion of frozen-thawed blood. *Ann. Intern. Med.* **96:**466–467.

44. Gray, J., L. V. von Stedingk, and M. Granstrom. 2002. Zoonotic babesiosis. *Int. J. Med. Microbiol.* **291:**108–111.

45. Gray, J., L. V. von Stedingk, M. Gurtelschmid, and M. Granstrom. 2002. Transmission studies of *Babesia microti* in *Ixodes ricinus* ticks and gerbils. *J. Clin. Microbiol.* **40:**1259–1263.

46. Greenwood, B. M., J. H. L. Playfair, and G. Torrigiani. 1971. Immunosuppression of murine malaria. I. General characteristics. *Clin. Exp. Immunol.* **8:**467–478.

47. Gunders, A. E. 1977. Piroplasmal sporozoites in the argasid Ornithodoros eraticus (Lucas). *Experientia* **33:**892–893.

48. Gupta, P., R. W. Hurley, P. H. Helseth, J. L. Goodman, and D. E. Hammerschmidt. 1995. Pancytopenia due to hemophagocytic syndrome as the presenting manifestation of babesiosis. *Am. J. Hematol.* **50:**60–62.

49. Habicht, G. S., J. L. Benach, K. D. Leichtling, B. L. Gocinski, and J. L. Coleman. 1983. The effect of age on the infection and immunoresponsiveness of mice to Babesia microti. *Mech. Ageing Dev.* **23:**357–369.

50. Healy, G. R., A. Speilman, and N. Gleason. 1976. Human babesiosis: reservoir in infection on Nantucket Island. *Science* **192:**479–480.

51. Herwaldt, B., D. H. Persing, E. A. Precigout, W. L. Goff, D. A. Mathiesen, P. W. Taylor, M. L. Eberhard, and A. F. Gorenflot. 1996. A fatal case of babesiosis in Missouri: identification of another piroplasm that infects humans. *Ann. Intern. Med.* **124:**643–650.

52. Herwaldt, B. L., G. de Bruyn, N. J. Pieniazek, M. Homer, K. H. Lofy, S. B. Slemenda, T. R. Fritsche, D. H. Persing, and A. P. Limaye. 2004. Babesia divergens-like infection, Washington State. *Emerg. Infect. Dis.* **10:**622–629.

53. Herwaldt, B. L., A. M. Kjemtrup, P. A. Conrad, R. C. Barnes, M. Wilson, M. G. McCarthy, M. H. Sayers, and M. L. Eberhard. 1997. Transfusion-transmitted babesiosis in Washington State: first reported case caused by a WA1-type parasite. *J. Infect. Dis.* **175:**1259–1262.

54. Herwaldt, B. L., D. F. Neitzel, J. B. Gorlin, K. A. Jensen, E. H. Perry, W. R. Peglow, S. B. Slemenda, K. Y. Won, E. K. Nace, N. J. Pieniazek, and M. Wilson. 2002. Transmission of Babesia microti in Minnesota through four blood donations from the same donor over a 6-month period. *Transfusion* **42:**1154–1158.

55. Hines, S. A., T. F. McElwain, G. M. Buening, and G. H. Palmer. 1989. Molecular characterization of Babesia bovis merozoite surface proteins bearing epitopes immunodominant in protected cattle. *Mol. Biochem. Parasitol.* **37:**1–9.

56. Hofmeister, E. K., C. P. Kolbert, A. S. Abdulkarim, J. M. Magera, M. K. Hopkins, J. R. Uhl, A. Ambyaye, S. R. Telford III, F. R. Cockerill III, and D. H. Persing. 1998. Cosegregation of a novel Bartonella species with Borrelia burgdorferi and Babesia microti in Peromyscus leucopus. *J. Infect. Dis.* **177:**409–416.

57. Homer, M. J., I. Aguilar-Delfin, S. R. Telford III, P. J. Krause, and D. H. Persing. 2000. Babesiosis. *Clin. Microbiol. Rev.* **13:**451–469.

58. Homer, M. J., E. S. Bruinsma, M. J. Lodes, M. H. Moro, S. Telford III, P. J. Krause, L. D. Reynolds, R. Mohamath, D. R. Benson, R. L. Houghton, S. G. Reed, and D. H. Persing. 2000. A polymorphic multigene family encoding an immunodominant protein from *Babesia microti*. *J. Clin. Microbiol.* **38:**362–368.

59. Homer, M. J., M. J. Lodes, L. D. Reynolds, Y. Zhang, J. F. Douglass, P. D. McNeill, R. L. Houghton, and D. H. Persing. 2003. Identification and characterization of putative secreted antigens from *Babesia microti*. *J. Clin. Microbiol.* **41:**723–729.

60. Houghton, R. L., M. J. Homer, L. D. Reynolds, P. R. Sleath, M. J. Lodes, V. Berardi, D. A. Leiby, and D. H. Persing. 2002. Identification of Babesia microti-specific immunodominant epitopes and development of a peptide EIA for detection of antibodies in serum. *Transfusion* **42:**1488–1496.

61. Hughes, W. T., and H. S. Oz. 1995. Successful prevention and treatment of babesiosis with atovaquone. *J. Infect. Dis.* **172:**1042–1046.

62. Hunfeld, K. P., R. Allwinn, S. Peters, P. Kraiczy, and V. Brade. 1998. Serologic evidence for tick-borne pathogens other than Borrelia burgdorferi (TOBB) in Lyme borreliosis patients from midwestern Germany. *Wien. Klin. Wochenschr.* **110:**901–908.

63. Igarashi, I., S. Waki, M. Ito, Y. Omata, A. Saito, and N. Suzuki. 1994. Role of CD4$^+$ T cells in the control of primary infection with Babesia microti in mice. *J. Protozool. Res.* **4:**164–171.

64. Jacoby, G. A., J. V. Hunt, K. S. Kosinski, Z. N. Demirjian, C. Huggins, P. Etkind, L. C. Marcus, and A. Spielman. 1980. Treatment of transfusion-transmitted babesiosis by exchange transfusion. *N. Engl. J. Med.* **303:**1098–1100.

65. James, M. A. 1988. Immunology of babesiosis, p. 119–130. *In* M. Ristic (ed.), *Babesiosis of Domestic Animals and Man.* CRC Press, Boca Raton, Fla.

66. Jerant, A. F., and A. D. Arline. 1993. Babesiosis in California. *West J. Med.* **158:**622–625.

67. Kakoma, I., and •••. 1994. Babesia of domestic animals, p. 141–216. *In* J. P. Kreier (ed.), *Parasitic Protozoa*, 2nd ed., vol. 7. Academic Press, San Diego, Calif.

68. Kjemtrup, A. M., B. Lee, C. L. Fritz, C. Evans, M. Chervenak, and P. A. Conrad. 2002. Investigation of transfusion transmission of a WA1-type babesial parasite to a premature infant in California. *Transfusion* **42:**1482–1487.

69. Kjemtrup, A. M., J. Thomford, T. Robinson, and P. A. Conrad. 2000. Phylogenetic relationships of human and wildlife piroplasm isolates in the western United States inferred from the 18S nuclear small subunit RNA gene. *Parasitology* **120:**487–493.

70. Krampitz, H. E. 1979. Babesia microti: morphology, distribution and host relationship in Germany. *Zentralbl. Bakteriol. Orig. A* **244:**411–415.

71. Krause, P. J. 2003. Babesiosis diagnosis and treatment. *Vector Borne Zoonotic Dis.* **3:**45–51.

72. Krause, P. J., T. Lepore, V. K. Sikand, J. Gadbaw, Jr., G. Burke, S. R. Telford III, P. Brassard, D. Pearl, J. Azlanzadeh, D. Christianson, D. McGrath, and A. Spielman. 2000. Atovaquone and azithromycin for the treatment of babesiosis. *N. Engl. J. Med.* **343:**1454–1458.

73. Krause, P. J., K. McKay, C. A. Thompson, V. K. Sikand, R. Lentz, T. Lepore, L. Closter, D. Christianson, S. R. Telford, D. Persing, J. D. Radolf, and A. Spielman. 2002. Disease-specific diagnosis of coinfecting tickborne zoonoses: babesiosis, human granulocytic ehrlichiosis, and Lyme disease. *Clin. Infect. Dis.* **34:**1184–1191.

74. Krause, P. J., A. Spielman, S. R. Telford III, V. K. Sikand, K. McKay, D. Christianson, R. J. Pollack, P. Brassard, J. Magera, R. Ryan, and D. H. Persing. 1998. Persistent parasitemia after acute babesiosis. *N. Engl. J. Med.* **339:**160–165.

75. Krause, P. J., S. Telford III, A. Spielman, R. Ryan, J. Magera, T. V. Rajan, D. Christianson, T. V. Alberghini, L. Bow, and D. Persing. 1996. Comparison of PCR with blood smear and inoculation of small animals for diagnosis of Babesia microti parasitemia. *J. Clin. Microbiol.* **34:**2791–2794.

76. Krause, P. J., S. R. Telford III, R. J. Pollack, R. Ryan, P. Brassard, L. Zemel, and A. Spielman. 1992. Babesiosis: an underdiagnosed disease of children. *Pediatrics* **89:**1045–1048.

77. Krause, P. J., S. R. Telford III, R. Ryan, P. A. Conrad, M. Wilson, J. W. Thomford, and A. Spielman. 1994. Diagnosis of babesiosis: evaluation of a serologic test for the detection of Babesia microti antibody. *J. Infect. Dis.* **169:**923–926.

78. Krause, P. J., S. R. Telford III, R. Ryan, A. B. Hurta, I. Kwasnik, S. Luger, J. Niederman, M. Gerber, and A. Spielman. 1991. Geographical and temporal distribution of babesial infection in Connecticut. *J. Clin. Microbiol.* **29:**1–4.

79. Krause, P. J., S. R. Telford III, A. Spielman, V. Sikand, R. Ryan, D. Christianson, G. Burke, P. Brassard, R. Pollack, J. Peck, and D. H. Persing. 1996. Concurrent Lyme disease and babesiosis. Evidence for increased severity and duration of illness. *JAMA* **275:**1657–1660.

80. Kurtzhals, J., B. J. Andersen, and N. O. Christensen. 1988. Effects on in vitro growth of Babesia microti by cells and serum from B. microti and Schistosoma mansoni infected mice. *Acta Vet. Scand.* **29:**357–362.

81. Leiby, D. A., A. P. Chung, R. G. Cable, J. Trouern-Trend, J. McCullough, M. J. Homer, L. D. Reynolds, R. L. Houghton, M. J. Lodes, and D. H. Persing. 2002. Relationship between tick bites and the seroprevalence of Babesia microti and Anaplasma phagocytophila (previously Ehrlichia sp.) in blood donors. *Transfusion* **42:**1585–1591.

82. Levine, J. F., M. L. Wilson, and A. Spielman. 1985. Mice as reservoirs of the Lyme disease spirochete. *Am. J. Trop Med. Hyg.* **34:**355–360.

83. Levine, N. D. 1971. Taxonomy of the piroplasms. *Trans. Am. Microsc. Soc.* **90:**2–33.

84. Levine, N. D., J. O. Corliss, F. E. Cox, G. Deroux, J. Grain, B. M. Honigberg, G. F. Leedale, A. R. Loeblich III, J. Lom, D. Lynn, E. G. Merinfeld, F. C. Page, G. Poljansky, V. Sprague, J. Vavra, and F. G. Wallace. 1980. A newly revised classification of the protozoa. *J. Protozool.* **27:**37–58.

85. Lodes, M. J., R. L. Houghton, E. S. Bruinsma, R. Mohamath, L. D. Reynolds, D. R. Benson, P. J. Krause, S. G. Reed, and D. H. Persing. 2000. Serological expression cloning of novel immunoreactive antigens of *Babesia microti. Infect. Immun.* **68:**2783–2790.

86. Lux, J. Z., D. Weiss, J. V. Linden, D. Kessler, B. L. Herwaldt, S. J. Wong, J. Keithly, P. Della-Latta, and B. E. Scully. 2003. Transfusion-associated babesiosis after heart transplant. *Emerg. Infect. Dis.* **9:**116–119.

87. Lykins, J. D., M. Ristic, and R. M. Weisiger. 1975. Babesia microti: pathogenesis of parasite of human origin in the hamster. *Exp. Parasitol.* **37:**388–397.

88. Machtinger, L., S. R. Telford III, C. Inducil, E. Klapper, S. Pepkowitz, and D. Goldfinger. 1993. Treatment of babesiosis by red blood cell exchange in an HIV-positive, splenectomized patient. *J. Clin. Apheresis* **8:**78–81.

89. Mahoney, D. F. 1977. Babesia of domestic animals, p. 1–52. *In* J. P. Krier (ed.), *Parasitic Protozoa*, vol. 5. Academic Press, San Francisco, Calif.

90. Mahoney, D. F. 1967. Bovine babesiosis: the passive immunization of calves against Babesia argentina with special reference to the role of complement fixing antibodies. *Exp. Parasitol.* **20:**119–124.

91. Marcus, L. C., J. M. Valigorsky, W. L. Fanning, T. Joseph, and B. Glick. 1982. A case report of transfusion-induced babesiosis. *JAMA* **248:**465–467.

92. Mather, T. N., and M. E. Mather. 1990. Intrinsic competence of three ixodid ticks (Acari) as vectors of the Lyme disease spirochete. *J. Med. Entomol.* **27:**646–650.

93. Matsubara, J., M. Koura, and T. Kamiyama. 1993. Infection of immunodeficient mice with a mouse-adapted substrain of the gray strain of Babesia microti. *J. Parasitol.* **79:**783–786.

94. Mehlhorn, H., W. Peters, and A. Haberkorn. 1980. The formation of kinetes and oocysts in Plasmodium gallinaceum and considerations on phylogenetic relationships between Haemosporidia, Piroplasmida, and other Coccidia. *Protistologica* 16:135–154.

95. Meldrum, S. C., G. S. Birkhead, D. J. White, J. L. Benach, and D. L. Morse. 1992. Human babesiosis n New York State: an epidemiological description of 136 cases. *Clin. Infect. Dis.* 15:1019–1023.

96. Michael, S. A., T. A. Morsy, and M. F. Montasser. 1987. A case of human babesiosis (preliminary case report in Egypt). *J. Egypt. Soc. Parasitol.* 17:409–410. (Letter.)

97. Mintz, E. D., J. F. Anderson, R. G. Cable, and J. L. Hadler. 1991. Transfusion-transmitted babesiosis: a case report from a new endemic area. *Transfusion* 31:365–368.

98. Moore, J. A., and R. E. Kuntz. 1981. Babesia microti infections in nonhuman primates. *J. Parasitol.* 67:454–456.

99. Moro, M., and I. Aguilar-Delfin. 1999. Unpublished results.

100. Moro, M. H., C. S. David, J. M. Magera, P. J. Wettstein, S. W. Barthold, and D. H. Persing. 1998. Differential effects of infection with a *Babesia*-like piroplasm, WA1, in inbred mice. *Infect. Immun.* 66:492–498.

101. Moro, M. H., O. L. Zegarra-Moro, J. Bjornsson, E. K. Hofmeister, E. Bruinsma, J. J. Germer, and D. H. Persing. 2002. Increased arthritis severity in mice coinfected with Borrelia burgdorferi and Babesia microti. *J. Infect. Dis.* 186:428–431.

102. Murphy, T. M., J. S. Gray, and R. J. Langley. 1986. Effects of rapid passage in the gerbil (Meriones unguiculatus) on the course of infection of the bovine piroplasm Babesia divergens in splenectomised calves. *Res. Vet. Sci.* 40:285–287.

103. Murray, P. K., F. W. Jennings, M. Murray, and G. M. Urquhart. 1974. The nature of immunosuppression in Trypanosome brucei infections in mice. 2. The role of the T and B lymphocytes. *Immunology* 27:825–840.

104. Mzembe, S. A., S. Lloyd, and E. J. Soulsby. 1984. Macrophage mediated resistance to Babesia microti in Nematospiroides dubius-infected mice. *Z. Parasitenkd.* 70:753–761.

105. Olmeda, A. S., P. M. Armstrong, B. M. Rosenthal, B. Valladares, A. del Castillo, F. de Armas, M. Miguelez, A. Gonzalez, J. A. Rodriguez Rodriguez, A. Spielman, and S. R. Telford III. 1997. A subtropical case of human babesiosis. *Acta Trop.* 67:229–234.

106. Ong, K. R., C. Stravropoulos, and R. Inada. 1990. Babesiosis, asplenia, and AIDS. *Lancet* 336:112. (Letter.)

107. Pancholi, P., C. P. Kolbert, P. D. Mitchell, K. D. Reed, Jr., J. S. Dumler, J. S. Bakken, S. R. Telford III, and D. H. Persing. 1995. Ixodes dammini as a potential vector of human granulocytic ehrlichiosis. *J. Infect. Dis.* 172:1007–1012.

108. Persing, D. H., and P. A. Conrad. 1995. Babesiosis: New insights from phylogenetic analysis. *Infect. Agents Dis.* 4:182–195.

109. Persing, D. H., B. L. Herwaldt, C. Glaser, R. S. Lane, J. W. Thomford, D. Mathiesen, P. J. Krause, D. F. Phillip, and P. A. Conrad. 1995. Infection with a babesia-like organism in northern California. *N. Engl. J. Med.* 332:298–303.

110. Persing, D. H., D. Mathiesen, W. F. Marshall, S. R. Telford, A. Spielman, J. W. Thomford, and P. A. Conrad. 1992. Detection of Babesia microti by polymerase chain reaction. *J. Clin. Microbiol.* 30:2097–2103.

111. Phillips, R. S., and D. Wakelin. 1976. Trichuris muris: effect of concurrent infections with rodent piroplasms on immune expulsion from mice. *Exp. Parasitol.* 39:95–100.

112. Piesman, J., T. N. Mather, G. J. Dammin, S. R. Telford III, C. C. Lastavica, and A. Spielman. 1987. Seasonal variation

113. Piesman, J., T. N. Mather, R. J. Sinsky, and A. Spielman. 1987. Duration of tick attachment and *Borrelia burgdorferi* transmission. *J. Clin. Microbiol.* 25:557–558.

114. Piesman, J., and A. Spielman. 1980. Human babesiosis on Nantucket Island: prevalence of *Babesia microti* in ticks. *Am. J. Trop.Med. Hyg.* 29:742–746.

115. Popovsky, M. A. 1991. Transfusion-transmitted babesiosis. Transfusion 31:296–298. (Editorial.)

116. Pruthi, R. K., W. F. Marshall, J. C. Wiltsie, and D. H. Persing. 1995. Human babesiosis. *Mayo Clin. Proc.* 70:853–862.

117. Pudney, M., and J. S. Gray. 1997. Therapeutic efficacy of atovaquone against the bovine intraerythrocytic parasite, Babesia divergens. *J. Parasitol.* 83:307–310.

118. Purvis, A. C. 1977. Immunodepression in Babesia microti infections. *Parasitology* 75:197–205.

119. Quick, R. E., B. L. Herwaldt, J. W. Thomford, M. E. Garnett, M. L. Eberhard, M. Wilson, D. H. Spach, J. W. Dickerson, S. R. Telford III, and K. R. Steingart. 1993. Babesiosis in Washington State: a new species of babesia? *Ann. Intern. Med.* 119:284–290.

120. Reduker, D. W., D. P. Jasmer, W. L. Goff, L. E. Perryman, W. C. Davis, and T. C. McGuire. 1989. A recombinant surface protein of Babesia bovis elicits bovine antibodies that react with live merozoites. *Mol. Biochem. Parasitol.* 35:239–247.

121. Riek, R. F. 1968. Babesiosis. *In* D. Weinman and M. Ristic (ed.), *Infectious Blood Diseases of Man and Animals*, vol. 2. Academic Press, New York, N.Y.

122. Rowin, K. S., H. B. Tanowitz, and M. Wittner. 1982. Therapy of experimental babesiosis. *Ann. Intern. Med.* 97:556–558.

123. Ruebush, M. J., and W. L. Hanson. 1979. Susceptibility of five strains of mice to Babesia microti of human origin. *J. Parasitol.* 65:430–433.

124. Ruebush, M. J., and W. L. Hanson. 1980. Thymus dependence of resistance to infection with Babesia microti of human origin in mice. *Am. J. Trop. Med. Hyg.* 29:507–515.

125. Ruebush, M. J., and W. L. Hanson. 1980. Transfer of immunity to Babesia microti of human origin using T lymphocytes in mice. *Cell. Immunol.* 52:255–265.

126. Ruebush, T. D., D. D. Juranek, E. S. Chisholm, P. C. Snow, G. R. Healy, and A. J. Sulzer. 1977. Human babesiosis on Nantucket Island. Evidence for self-limited and subclinical infections. *N. Engl. J. Med.* 297:825–827.

127. Ruebush, T. K., P. B. Cassaday, H. J. Marsh, S. A. Lisker, D. B. Voorhees, E. B. Mahoney, and G. R. Healy. 1977. Human babesiosis on Nantucket Island. Clinical features. *Ann. Intern. Med.* 86:6–9.

128. Ruebush, T. K., D. D. Juranek, A. Spielman, J. Piesman, and G. R. Healy. 1981. Epidemiology of human babesiosis on Nantucket Island. *Am. J. Trop. Med. Hyg.* 30:937–941.

129. Ruebush, T. K., J. Piesman, W. E. Collins, A. Spielman, and M. Warren. 1981. Tick transmission of Babesia microti to rhesus monkeys (Macaca mulatta). *Am. J. Trop. Med. Hyg.* 30:555–559.

130. Ruef, B. J., T. J. Ward, C. R. Oxner, P. G. Conley, W. C. Brown, and A. C. Rice-Ficht. 2000. Phylogenetic analysis with newly characterized Babesia bovis hsp70 and hsp90 provides strong support for paraphyly within the piroplasms. *Mol. Biochem. Parasitol.* 109:67–72.

131. Shih, C. M., L. P. Liu, W. C. Chung, S. J. Ong, and C. C. Wang. 1997. Human babesiosis in Taiwan: asymptomatic infection with a *Babesia microti*-like organism in a Taiwanese woman. *J. Clin. Microbiol.* 35:450–454.

132. Shimada, T., S. Shikano, R. Hashiguchi, N. Matsuki, and K. Ono. 1996. Effects of depletion of T cell subpopulations

on the course of infection and anti-parasite delayed type hypersensitivity response in mice infected with Babesia microti and Babesia rodhaini. *J. Vet. Med. Sci.* **58:**343–347.

133. Skrabalo, Z., and Z. Deanovic. 1957. Piroplasmosis in man. Report of a case. *Doc. Med. Geogr. Trop.* **9:**11–16.

134. Smith, R. P., A. T. Evans, M. Popowsky, L. Mills, and A. Spielman. 1986. Transfusion-acquired babesiosis and failure of antibiotic treatment. *JAMA* **256:**2726–2727.

135. Smith, T. 1893. Investigations into the nature, causation, and prevention of Texas or Southern cattle tick fever. *USDA Bull. Anim. Ind.* **1:**177–304.

136. Solomon, J. B., M. G. Forbes, and G. R. Solomon. 1985. A possible role for natural killer cells in providing protection against Plasmodium berghei in early stages of infection. *Immunol. Lett.* **9:**349–352.

137. Spielman, A. 1976. Human babesiosis on Nantucket Island: transmission by nymphal Ixodes ticks. *Am. J. Trop. Med. Hyg.* **25:**784–787.

138. Spielman, A., C. M. Clifford, J. Piesman, and M. D. Corwin. 1979. Human babesiosis on Nantucket Island, USA: description of the vector, Ixodes dammini. *J. Med. Entomol.* **15:**218–234.

139. Spielman, A., P. Etkind, J. Piesman, T. K. Ruebush, D. D. Juranek, and M. S. Jacobs. 1981. Reservoir hosts of human babesiosis on Nantucket Island. *Am. J. Trop. Med. Hyg.* **30:**560–565.

140. Strickland, G. T., R. A. Voller, L. E. Pettit, and D. G. Fleck. 1972. Immunodepression associated with concomitant Toxoplasma and malarial infections in mice. *J. Infect. Dis.* **126:**54–60.

141. Sun, T., M. J. Tenenbaum, J. Greenspan, S. Teichberg, R. T. Wang, T. Degnan, and M. H. Kaplan. 1983. Morphologic and clinical observations in human infection with Babesia microti. *J. Infect. Dis.* **148:**239–248.

142. Telford, S., III, and A. Speilman. 1998. Babesiosis of humans, p. 349–359. *In* L. Collier, A. Balows, and M. Sussman (ed.), *Topley and Wilson's Microbiology and Microbial Infections*, 9th ed. Arnold, London, England.

143. Telford, S. R. 1999. Unpublished observations.

144. Telford, S. R., J. E. Dawson, P. Katavolos, C. K. Warner, C. P. Kolbert, and D. H. Persing. 1996. Perpetuation of the agent of human granulocytic ehrlichiosis in a deer tick-rodent cycle. *Proc. Natl. Acad. Sci. USA* **93:**6209–6214.

145. Telford, S. R., A. Gorenflot, P. Brasseur, and A. Spielman. 1993. Babesial infections in humans and wildlife, p. 1–47. *In* J. P. Krier (ed.), *Parasitic Protozoa*, 2nd ed., vol. 5, Academic Press, San Diego, Calif.

146. Teutsch, S. M., P. Etkind, E. L. Burwell, K. Sato, M. M. Dana, P. R. Fleishman, and D. D. Juranek. 1980. Babesiosis in post-splenectomy hosts. *Am. J. Trop. Med. Hyg.* **29:**738–741.

147. Thomford, J. W., P. A. Conrad, S. R. Telford III, D. Mathiesen, B. H. Bowman, A. Spielman, M. L. Eberhard, B. L. Herwaldt, R. E. Quick, and D. H. Persing. 1994. Cultivation and phylogenetic characterization of a newly recognized human pathogenic protozoan. *J. Infect. Dis.* **169:**1050–1056.

148. Vannier, E., I. Borggraefe, S. R. Telford III, S. Menon, T. Brauns, A. Spielman, J. A. Gelfand, and H. H. Wortis. 2004. Age-associated decline in resistance to Babesia microti is genetically determined. *J. Infect. Dis.* **189:**1721–1728.

149. Winger, C. M., E. U. Canning, and J. D. Culverhouse. 1989. A monoclonal antibody-derived antigen of Babesia divergens: characterization and investigation of its ability to protect gerbils against virulent homologous challenge. *Parasitology* **3:**341–348.

150. Wittner, M., J. Lederman, H. B. Tanowitz, G. S. Rosenbaum, and L. M. Weiss. 1996. Atovaquone in the treatment of Babesia microti infections in hamsters. *Am. J. Trop. Med. Hyg.* **55:**219–222.

151. Wittner, M., K. S. Rowin, H. B. Tanowitz, J. F. Hobbs, S. Saltzman, B. Wenz, R. Hirsch, E. Chisholm, and G. R. Healy. 1982. Successful chemotherapy of transfusion babesiosis. *Ann. Intern. Med.* **96:**601–604.

152. Yamasaki, M., M. Tajima, K. W. Lee, J. R. Jeong, O. Yamato, and Y. Maede. 2002. Molecular cloning and phylogenetic analysis of Babesia gibsoni heat shock protein 70. *Vet. Parasitol.* **110:**123–129.

153. Zivkovic, D., J. E. Speksnijder, H. Kuil, and W. Seinen. 1984. Immunity to Babesia in mice. II. Cross protection between various Babesia and Plasmodium species and its relevance to the nature of Babesia immunity. *Vet. Immunol. Immunopathol.* **5:**359–368.

III. Color Atlases

Color Maps

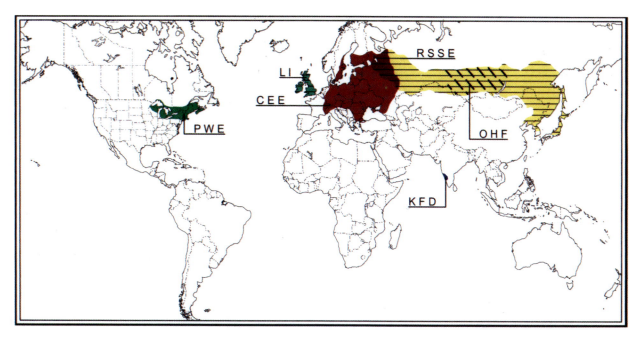

Color Map 1. Approximate geographic distributions of tick-borne encephalitides caused by Central European encephalitis virus (CEE) (red), Kyasanur Forest disease virus (KFD) (blue), louping ill virus (LI) (green with horizontal lines), Omsk hemorrhagic fever virus (OHF) (back slashes), Powassan encephalitis virus (PWE) (green), and Russian spring-summer encephalitis virus (RSSE) (yellow with horizontal lines).

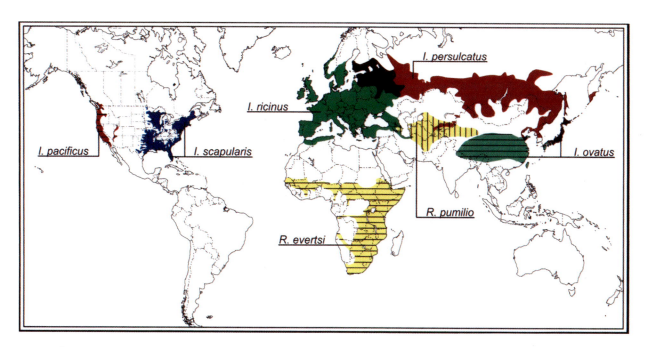

Color Map 2. Approximate geographic distributions of *I. ovatus* (green with horizontal lines). *I. pacificus* (red with horizontal lines), *I. persulcatus* (red), *I. ricinus* (green), *I. scapularis* (blue), *R. evertsi* (yellow with horizontal lines), and *R. pumilio* (yellow with vertical lines).

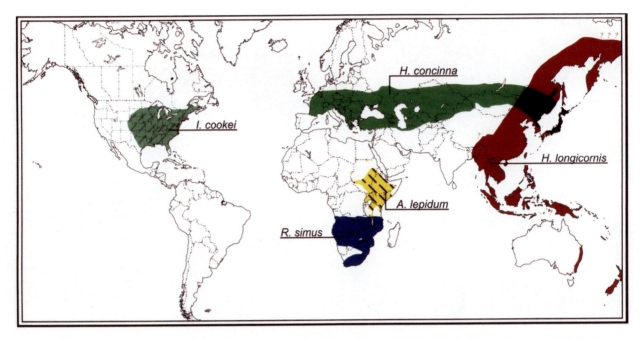

Color Map 3. Approximate geographic distributions of *A. lepidum* (yellow with black slashes), *H. concinna* (green), *H. longicornis* (red), *I. cookei* (green with forward slashes), and *R. simus* (blue).

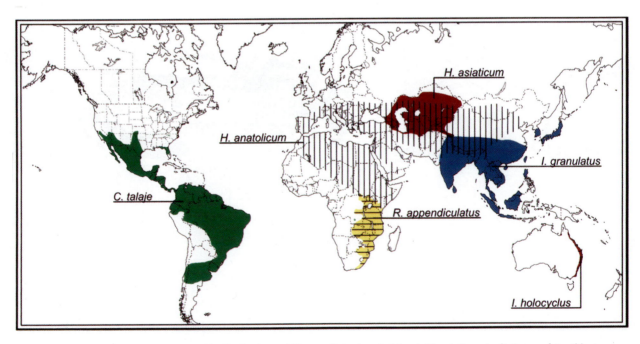

Color Map 4. Approximate geographic distributions of *H. anatolicum* (vertical lines), *H. asiaticum* (red). *I. granulatus* (blue), *I. holocyclus* (red with horizontal lines), *R. appendiculatus* (yellow with horizontal lines), and *C. talaje* (green).

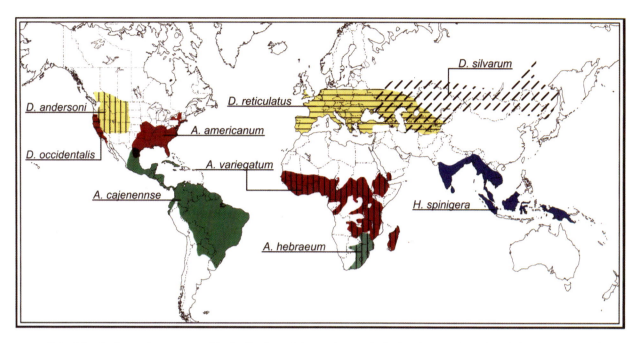

Color Map 5. Approximate geographic distributions of *A. americanum* (red), *A. cajenennse* (green), *A. hebraeum* (green with vertical lines), *A. variegatum* (red with vertical lines), *D. andersoni* (yellow with vertical lines), *D. occidentalis* (red with horizontal lines), *D. reticulatus* (yellow with horizontal lines), *D. silvarum* (forward slash), and *H. spinigera* (blue).

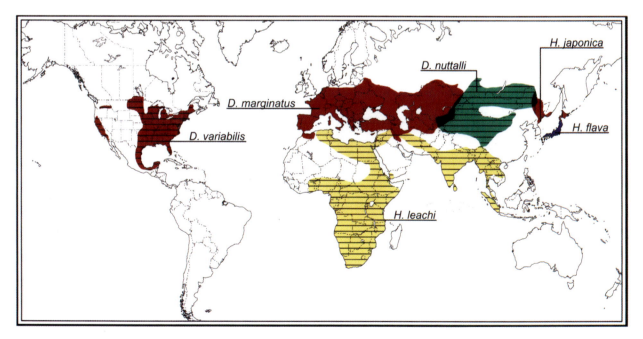

Color Map 6. Approximate geographic distributions of *D. marginatus* (red), *D. nuttalli* (green with horizontal lines), *D. variabilis* (red with horizontal lines), *H. flava* (blue), *H. japonica* (red with vertical lines), and *H. leachi* (yellow with horizontal lines).

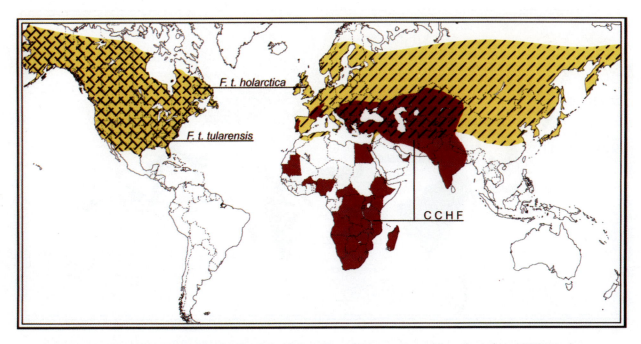

Color Map 7. Approximate geographic distributions of human cases of Crimean-Congo hemorrhagic fever (CCHF) (red), type A tularemia caused by *F. tularensis tularensis* (back-slashed lines), and type B tularemia caused by *F. tularensis holarctica* (yellow with forward-slashed lines).

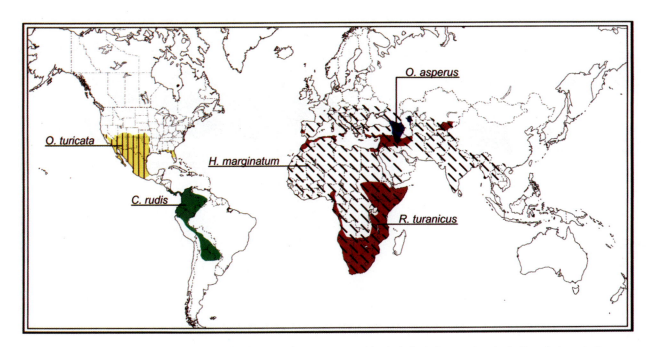

Color Map 8. Approximate geographic distributions of *H. marginatum* (back slashes), *R. turanicus* (red), *C. rudis* (green), *O. asperus* (blue), and *O. turicata* (yellow with vertical lines).

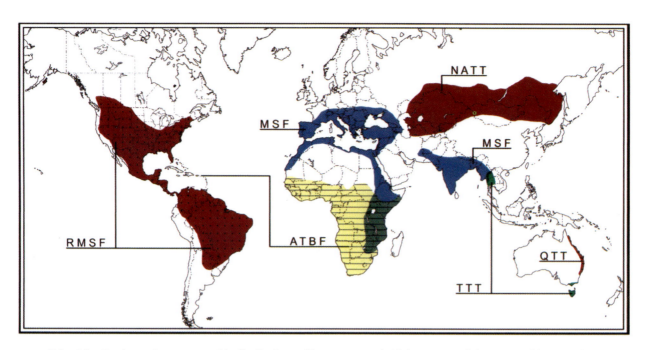

Color Map 9. Approximate geographic distributions of human cases of tick-borne spotted fevers caused by *R. rickettsii* (Rocky Mountain spotted fever [RMSF]) (red with spots), *R. conorii* (Mediterranean spotted fever [MSF]) (blue), *R. sibirica* (North Asian tick typhus [NATT]) (red), *R. africae* (African tick bite fever [ATBF]) (yellow with horizontal lines), *R. honei* (Flinder's Island-Thailand tick typhus [TTT] (green), and *R. australis* (Queensland tick typhus [QTT]) (red with horizontal lines).

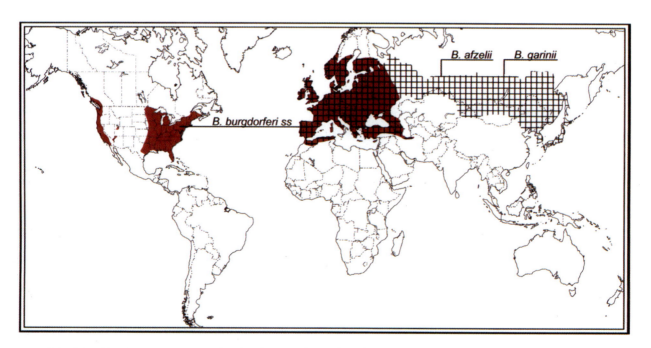

Color Map 10. Approximate geographic distributions of Lyme borreliosis caused by *B. burgdorferi* sensu stricto (ss) (red), *B. afzelii* (horizontal lines), and *B. garinii* (vertical lines) (*B. garinii* overlaps *B. afzelii*).

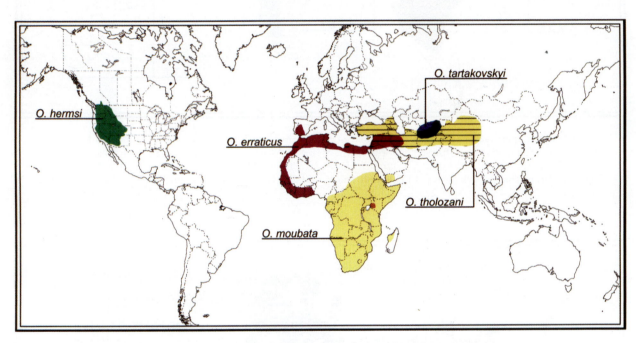

Color Map 11. Approximate geographic distributions of *O. erraticus* (red), *O. hermsi* (green), *O. moubata* (yellow), *O. tartakovskyi* (blue), and *O. tholozani* (yellow with horizontal lines).

Color Plates

Clinical and Pathologic Atlas of Tick-Borne Diseases

J. STEPHEN DUMLER AND CHRISTOPHER D. PADDOCK

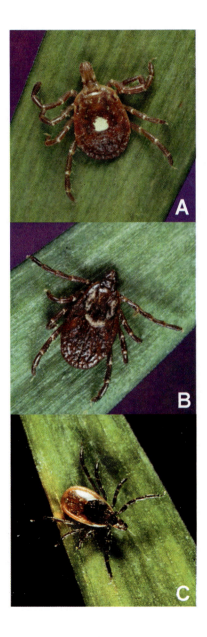

Color Plate 1. (A) Adult female lone star tick (*A. americanum*). The lone star tick is broadly distributed throughout the southeastern quadrant of the United States, with range extensions into New England and midwestern states. All three stages bite humans. *A. americanum* is a recognized vector of several pathogens that cause diseases in humans, including ehrlichioses caused by *E. chaffeensis* and *E. ewingii*, and has been implicated as a vector of southern tick-associated rash illness believed to be caused by "*B. lonestari.*" Other pathogens or potential pathogens have been detected in this tick, including various spotted fever group rickettsiae, *F. tularensis*, and *C. burnetii*, although the role of *A. americanum* in the transmission of these agents to humans is not well characterized. (B) Adult female American dog tick (*D. variabilis*). This tick is abundant in the southeastern United States and coastal New England, with limited distribution in several midwestern states, southern Canada, and western coastal regions. The tick is best known as the primary vector of Rocky Mountain spotted fever in the eastern United States. (C) Adult female blacklegged or deer tick (*I. scapularis*). As a member of the greater *I. persulcatus* group that also includes *I. pacificus*, *I. ricinus*, and *I. persulcatus*, this tick is an important vector of several infectious agents that cause disease in humans, including Lyme borreliosis, (granulocytic) anaplasmosis, and babesiosis. *I. persulcatus* ticks elsewhere in the world may also transmit tick-borne flaviviruses capable of causing encephalitis, encephalomyelitis, and even hemorrhagic fevers (including tick-borne encephalitis virus, louping ill virus, Russian spring-summer encephalitis virus, Powassan virus, Kyasanur Forest disease virus, and Langat virus). Images courtesy of G. Maupin.

J. Stephen Dumler • Division of Medical Microbiology, Department of Pathology, The Johns Hopkins University, Baltimore, MD 21205. Christopher D. Paddock • Infectious Disease Pathology Activity, Centers for Disease Control and Prevention, Atlanta, GA 30333.

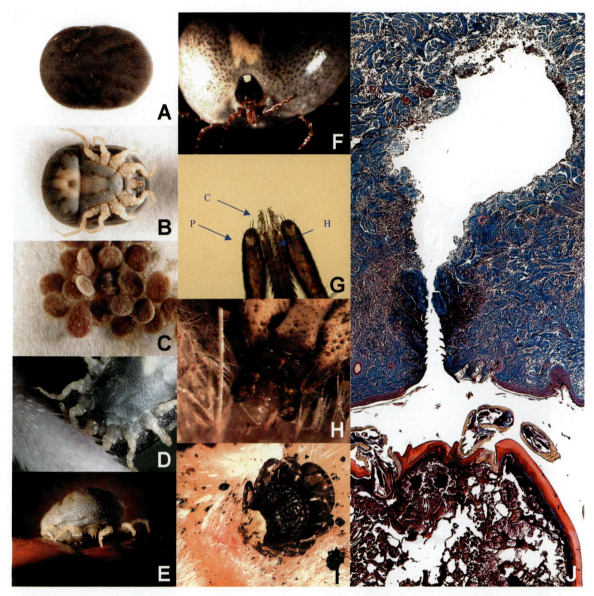

Color Plate 2. (A to E) **Soft tick morphology.** (A) The soft tick *O. moubata* is long lived and feeds repeatedly on humans and other mammals. (A and E) Dorsal aspect of an engorged female: the cuticle has a leather-like texture, lending to the name "Lederzecke" (leather tick), the German vernacular for argasid ticks. (B, C, and D) The capitulum is located in a subterminal, ventral position. The unfed argasid ticks are flat and highly mobile. When inactive, they hide in cracks and crevices. Each blood meal takes minutes to a few hours. In contrast, adult ixodid females feed for several days. (F to I) **Hard tick morphology.** (F) Engorged female *A. americanum* tick. (G) Closeup of mouthparts *I. scapularis* nymph. C, chelicerae; P, palps; H, hypostome. The mobile distal cheliceral teeth reach beyond the hypostome. (H) During feeding, the palps are splayed laterally (female *D. andersoni* tick). (I) A feeding *D. andersoni* couple; the female tick is in front. (J) **Tick feeding lesion.** Adult *I. scapularis* female (below) feeding on a sensitized rabbit (above). Predominantly mixed inflammatory infiltrate cells line the feeding cavity. Discrete dermal swelling and dilated venules are found in the proximity. The mouthparts are anchored deep into the dermis, just reaching the cavity from which the tick feeds as indicated by the imprint of the hypostome contours (trichrome stain). Photographs courtesy of S. Archibald and E. Denison.

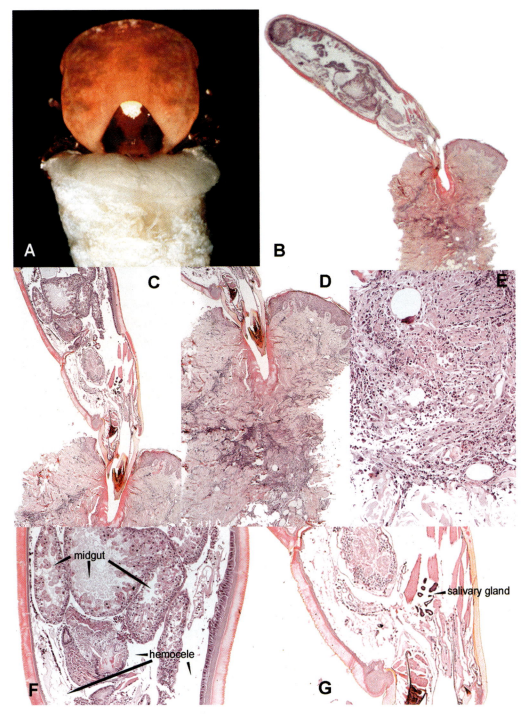

Color Plate 3. Anatomy of a tick bite. This series of images was obtained from a single feeding adult female *A. americanum* tick removed by biopsy from a patient in Maryland. The images show the partially engorged tick embedded in the skin (A) and the tick and skin sectioned en block (B) (hematoxylin and eosin [H&E] stain; original magnification, ×8). (C to E) Positioning of the tick capitulum and hypostome with relation to the epidermis (H&E stain; original magnification ×16) (C and D), the positioning of the hypostome into the dermis with the inflammatory vascular pool at its distal end (H&E stain; original magnification, ×16) (E), and the inflammation and edema present in the dermal blood pool upon which the tick feeds (H&E stain; original magnification, ×40). (F) Anatomical structures of importance in acquisition and transmission of pathogens by ticks with subsequent molts include the midgut into which pathogens pass with the blood meal and the hemocele into which pathogens pass after penetration of the midgut epithelium (H&E stain; original magnification, ×40). (G) Pathogens that are transmitted by tick bite gain access to the tick salivary gland before passing into the dermal vascular pool in tick saliva (H&E stain; original magnification, ×40). Not shown is the tick ovary, into which some pathogens may invade to allow transovarian transmission.

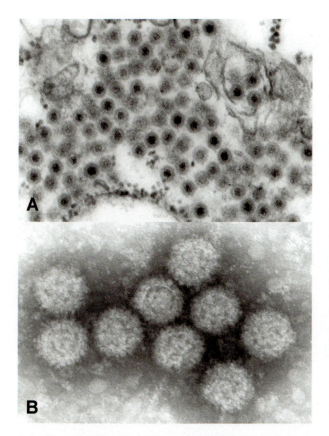

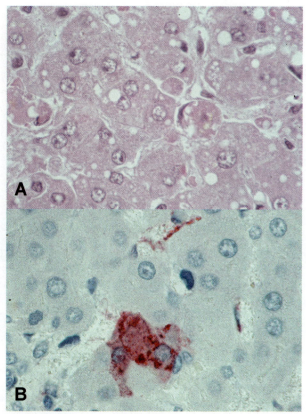

Color Plate 4. Colorado tick fever virus (family *Reoviridae*) (see Chapter 8) propagated in BHK-21 cells produces viral particles approximately 80 nm in diameter with a 50-nm core. (A) Thin-section electron microscopy; original magnification, ×30,500; (B) negative stain electron microscopy, original magnification, ×118,800. Images courtesy of F. A. Murphy.

Color Plate 5. (A) Crimean-Congo hemorrhagic fever virus (family *Bunyaviridae*) (CCHF) (see Chapter 10) causes liver injury characterized by diffuse microvesicular steatosis and hepatocyte necrosis (H&E stain; original magnification, ×133). (B) Immuno-histochemistry for CCHF virus demonstrates localization of viral antigens to the cytoplasm of swollen, degenerating hepatocytes and to endothelial cells lining hepatic sinusoids (original magnification, ×133). Images courtesy of S. R. Zaki.

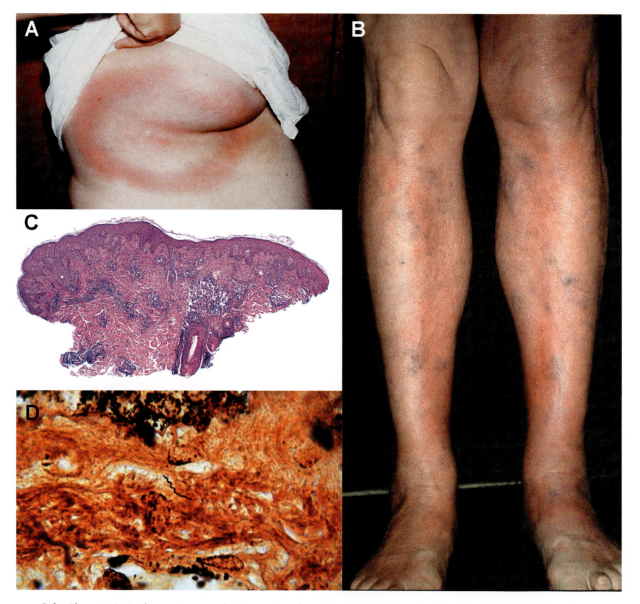

Color Plate 6. (A) Erythema migrans rash in Lyme borreliosis (Chapter 11). Note the distinctive and well-defined erythematous border of this large lesion. Also, note the relative central clearing and central punctate ("bull's eye") lesion at the site of tick attachment. Image courtesy of P. G. Auwaerter. (B) Acrodermatitis chronica atrophicans, a late skin manifestation of *B. afzelii* infection, shown affecting the legs of an elderly woman where the skin has become thinned and atrophic. Image courtesy of R. Muellegger. (C) Photomicrograph of skin biopsy of erythema migrans lesion (as seen in panel A) from a patient with early-stage Lyme disease (H&E stain), showing perivascular lymphocytic and plasma cell inflammatory infiltrates. (D) Modified Dieterle silver stain of *B. burgdorferi* spirochete in perivascular area of an erythema migrans lesion. Images in panels C and D courtesy of B. Berger.

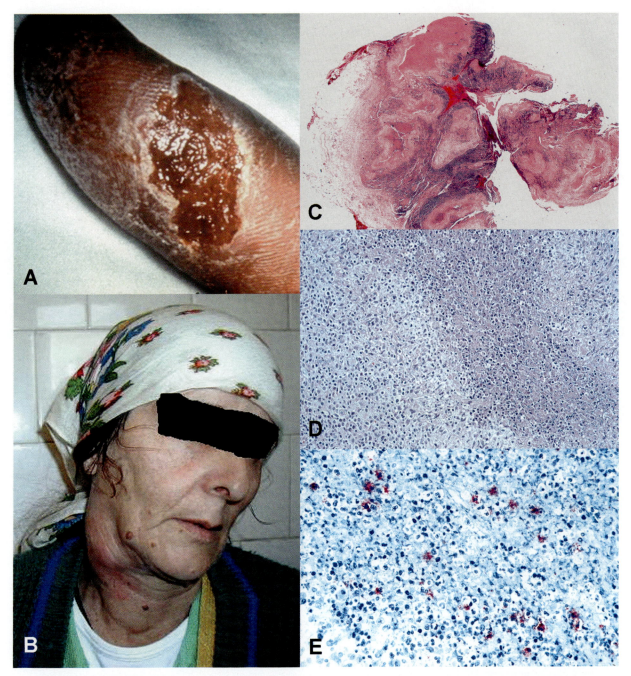

Color Plate 7. The ulceroglandular form of tularemia (see Chapter 12) may present with a striking ulcer, such as that seen here on a finger (A) or with lymphadenitis, which may also occur independently without evidence of an ulcer (so-called glandular tularemia) or in oropharyngeal tularemia (B). (C) Affected lymph glands are characterized by multiple granulomas and geographic necrotizing inflammation (H&E stain; original magnification, ×12.5). (D) The lymph node shows granulomas and granulomatous inflammation with palisaded histiocytes surrounding an extensive central region of suppurative and necrotizing inflammation (H&E stain; original magnification, ×100). (E) *F. tularensis* can be demonstrated by immunohistochemistry within histiocytes in the necrotic tissue (original magnification, ×100). Images in panels D and E courtesy of S. R. Zaki.

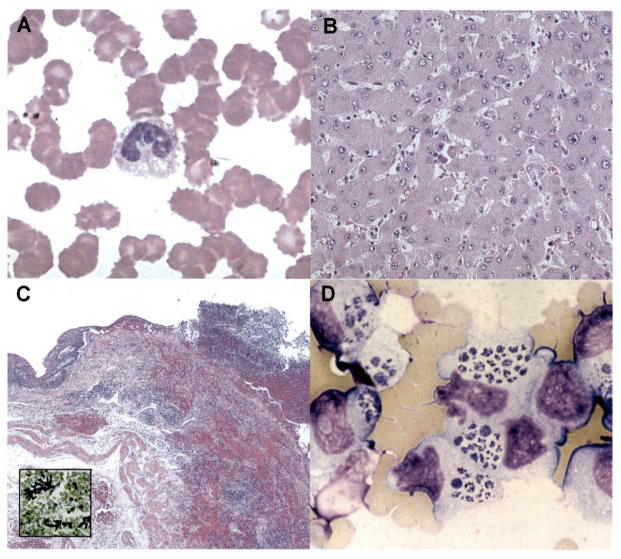

Color Plate 8. Human granulocytic anaplasmosis (HGA, formerly known as human granulocytic ehrlichiosis or HGE) (see Chapter 13) caused by *A. phagocytophilum*. (A) A cluster of bacteria, called a morula, is visible in the cytoplasm of a peripheral blood neutrophil (Wright stain; original magnification, ×400). The morula is differentiated from other leukocyte inclusions by the presence of dark blue to violaceous punctate staining, confined to one or few vacuoles. (B) Mild to moderate liver injury is frequent, and the underlying histopathology illustrates the frequent presence of mild lobular hepatitis with focal inflammatory lesions, apoptotic hepatocytes, and Kupffer cell hyperplasia (H&E stain; original magnification, ×40). (C) Opportunistic infections may occur as severe complications of HGA (H&E stain; original magnification, ×8); in this case, a gastroesophageal ulcer caused by *Candida albicans* infection occurred, resulting in fatal gastrointestinal bleeding (panel C inset, Gomori methenamine silver stain; original magnification, ×160). (D) Photomicrograph of Giemsa-stained HL-60 cells infected in vitro with *A. phagocytophilum* isolated directly from the blood of a patient with HGA. Note multiple colonies of organisms in the cytoplasm of infected cells. Image courtesy of J. L. Goodman.

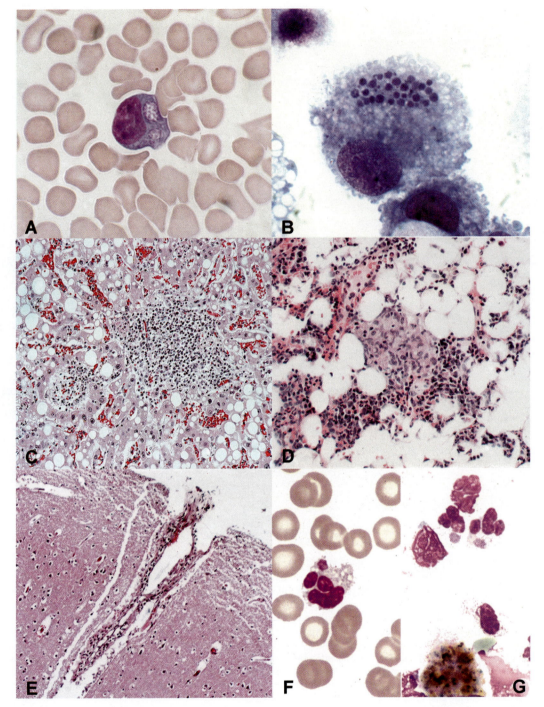

Color Plate 9. *Ehrlichia* spp. infections include human monocytic ehrlichiosis (HME) (*E. chaffeensis*) (see Chapter 14) and infection by *E. ewingii* (see Chapter 15). (A) Typical *E. chaffeensis* morula with pale blue violaceous bacteria in a circulating blood monocyte (Wright stain; original magnification, ×400). Image courtesy of Aileen Marty. (B) Morulae of *E. chaffeensis* isolated from the blood of a patient with HME growing in the DH82 canine macrophage cell line. (C) As with human granulocytic anaplasmosis (HGA), HME frequently involves the liver and may be severe. The image shows necrosis and moderate lobular hepatitis (H&E; original magnification, ×16). (D) Small noncaseating granulomas typical of those frequently seen in tissues of patients with HME, including the bone marrow (H&E stain; original magnification, ×16). (E) Meningitis and meningoencephalitis occur in approximately 20% of patients with HME but are rare in HGA. Shown is a mild infiltration of the meninges by lymphocytes and histiocytes in a patient who died after contracting HME (H&E; original magnification, ×16). (F) As with *A. phagocytophilum*, *E. ewingii* propagates in neutrophils in peripheral blood (modified Wright's stain; original magnification, ×400); (G) it may also occasionally be identified in inflammatory infiltrates in various organs, as in this bronchoalveolar lavage specimen of a patient with pulmonary manifestations associated with *E. ewingii* infection (modified Wright's stain, original magnification, ×400).

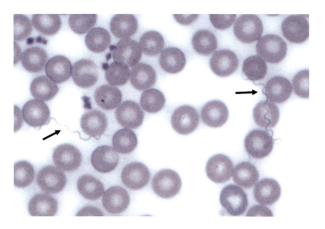

Color Plate 10. Relapsing fever borreliae (*B. hermsii*) (see Chapter 16) in peripheral blood can accumulate to quantities as high as 10^7 to 10^8/ml, sufficient for easy identification on Romanovsky-stained films (Wright-Giemsa stain; original magnification, ×336). Note the long (15 to 30 μm) and narrow (0.2 to 0.5 μm) spiral shape (arrows), typical of *Borrelia* and other spirochetes. Blood smear courtesy of T. G. Schwan.

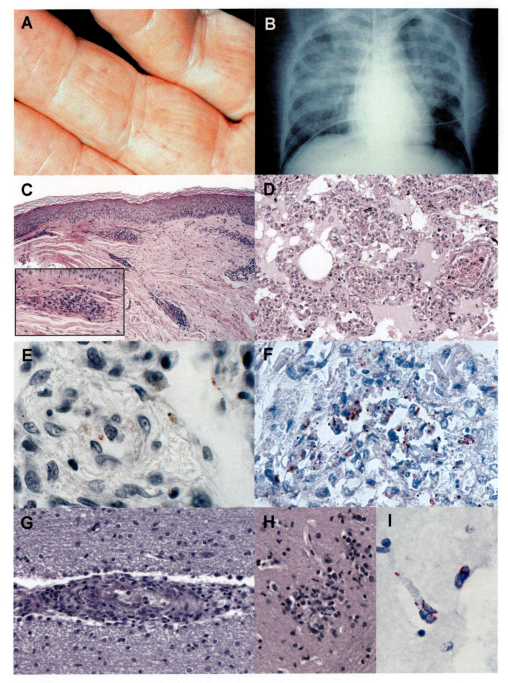

Color Plate 11. Rocky Mountain spotted fever (RMSF). *R. rickettsii* infects and damages endothelial cells and may cause profound vascular leakage. A macular or maculopapular rash that blanches with pressure is typically detected in the first several days of illness. (A) Petechiae frequently develop as the rash evolves, as a result of extravasation of erythrocytes into the dermis where vasculitis (C) may also be observed (H&E stain; original magnification, ×8). (C, inset) The rickettsiae alone are sufficient to cause vascular leakage, but their presence also elicits lymphohistiocytic and leukocytoclastic vasculitis, occasionally associated with fibrin deposition or non-occlusive thrombus formation (H&E stain; original magnification, ×16). (E) Vasculitis may involve all organs, and the most significant complications include pulmonary and central nervous system involvement (*R. rickettsii* immunohistochemistry; original magnification, ×260). (B) Pulmonary involvement may lead to bilateral interstitial infiltrates seen on chest radiographs. (D) Markedly increased microvascular permeability in the lung, believed to be due to rickettsia-mediated endothelial cell damage (H&E stain; original magnification, ×16) may lead to noncardiogenic pulmonary edema (*R. rickettsii* immunohistochemistry in skin; original magnification, ×260) (F). Meningoencephalitis and rickettsia-induced endothelial cell damage and inflammation can lead to cerebral edema and herniation. (G to I) Meningeal vasculitis (H&E stain; original magnification, ×100) (G) and one of many scattered mononuclear inflammatory cell infiltrates in the brain called microglial or typhus nodules (H&E stain; original magnification, ×100) (H). Immunohistochemical staining for *R. rickettsii* shows widespread rickettsial infection of cerebral microvascular endothelial cells (original magnification, ×160) (I).

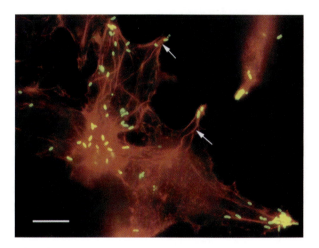

Color Plate 12. Double-stained (F-actin and spotted fever group rickettsiae) immunofluorescence photomicrograph of *Rickettsia monacensis* utilizing actin tail formation for mobility in and cell-to-cell spread between mouse (L-929) host cells. Image created by dual excitation of appropriate wavelengths for Texas red phalloidin and fluorescein isothiocyanate-conjugated antibodies to *R. monacensis*. Bar, 10 μm. Image courtesy of J. A. Simser and T. J. Kurtti.

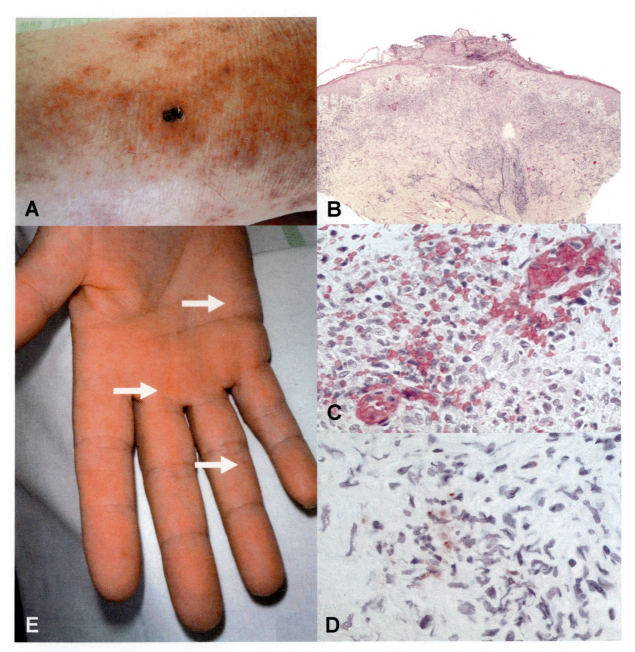

Color Plate 13. Mediterranean spotted fever (MSF) (boutonneuse fever) caused by *R. conorii* (see Chapter 18). (A) The hall-mark lesion of MSF is an eschar (tache noir) at the site of tick attachment. Image provided courtesy of P. E. Fournier and D. Raoult. (B and C) The tache noir is characterized by epidermal and dermal necrosis with extensive mixed inflammation, dominated by lymphocytes and histiocytes, with admixed endothelial cell injury, vasculitis, edema, and fibrin deposition or thrombosis. H&E stain; original magnification, ×8 (B) and ×100 (C). (D) Immunohistochemical staining for *R. conorii* shows the scattered presence of organisms in cells in areas of necrosis and inflammation (original magnification, ×160). (E) In disseminated MSF, vasculitis and maculopapular skin lesions similar to those seen in Rocky Mountain spotted fever can be observed. Image courtesy of P. E. Fournier and D. Raoult.

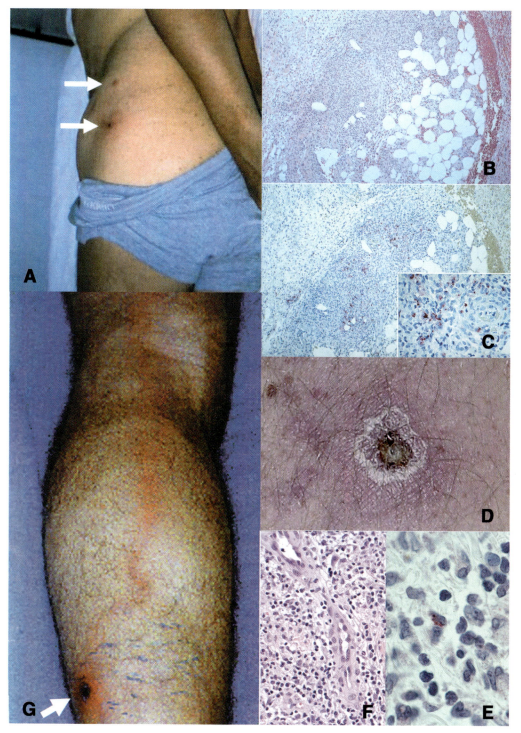

Color Plate 14. Other spotted fever group rickettsiae frequently elicit eschars at the site of tick bites. (A) African tick-bite fever caused by *R. africae* (see Chapter 18) is associated with one or more eschars, but the disease is often milder than Mediterranean spotted fever (MSF) and may include vesicular skin lesions. Image courtesy of P. E. Fournier and D. Raoult. (B) Similar to the histopathologic changes in MSF, *R. africae* eschars demonstrate an intense lymphohistiocytic infiltrate in the deep dermis extending into the panniculus (H&E stain; original magnification, ×25). (C) Immunohistochemical staining identifies intact rickettsiae and rickettsial antigens (red) in the infiltrate, distributed predominantly in perivascular locations (original magnification, ×25; inset original magnification, ×158). Panels B and C courtesy of R. Zaki. (D) Although rarely recognized, *R. parkeri*, a close relative of *R. africae*, is a proven cause of eschars in the Americas (see Chapter 17). Image courtesy of C. A. Ohl. (E) In this case, immunohistochemical staining (original magnification, ×250) demonstrates *R. parkeri* in the cytoplasm of a mononuclear cell. (F) This infected cell was identified subjacent to the eschar in the intense perivascular lymphohistiocytic infiltrate surrounding a dermal vessel with swollen endothelial cells (H&E stain; original magnification. ×158). Images in panels E and F courtesy S. R. Zaki. (G) Eschar and lymphangitis observed in a febrile patient in Marseille, France, possibly due to *R. sibirica* (*R. mongolotimonae*) (see Chapter 18).

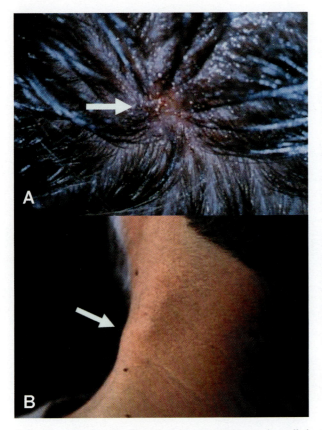

Color Plate 15. Tick-borne lymphadenitis (TIBOLA) (also called wood scar or *Dermacentor*-borne necrosis-erythema lymphadenopathy [DEBONEL]), likely due to *R. slovaka* (see Chapter 18). Inoculation eschar to the scalp (arrow) (A) and resultant enlarged cervical lymph nodes (B, arrow) in a patient with TIBOLA (see Chapter 18).

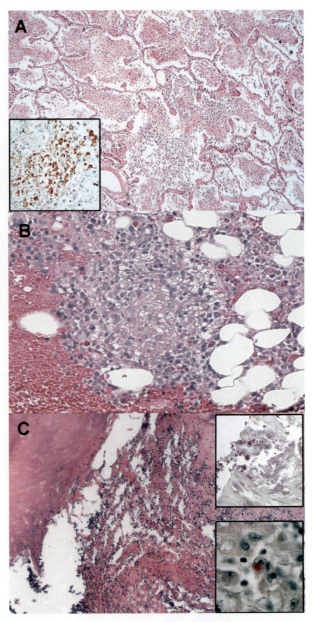

Color Plate 16. *C. burnetii* causes both acute and chronic Q (query) fever (see Chapter 19). While typically transmitted via the respiratory route, it is rarely transmitted to humans by ticks. Acute manifestations range from moderate to severe pneumonia with airspace involvement and mild interstitial pneumonitis (A) (H&E stain; original magnification, ×16). (Inset) *C. burnetii* replicates to enormous levels in infected macrophages that often are localized within alveolar spaces (*C. burnetii* immunohistochemistry; original magnification, ×100). (B) Acute *C. burnetii* infection can result in dissemination and formation of noncaseating granulomas in many organs, including the liver and bone marrow (H&E stain; original magnification, ×40). Chronic Q fever, usually manifested as endocarditis (C) or infection of vascular prostheses, does not typically cause an immune response that results in granulomas. Q fever endocarditis progresses slowly resulting in cardiac valves dominated by lymphohistiocytic inflammation with necrosis and fibrin deposition (H&E stain; original magnification, ×16). (Insets) *C. burnetii* can be visualized within macrophages of the inflammatory infiltrate of the damaged valve (*C. burnetii* immunohistochemistry; original magnification, ×16 and ×100).

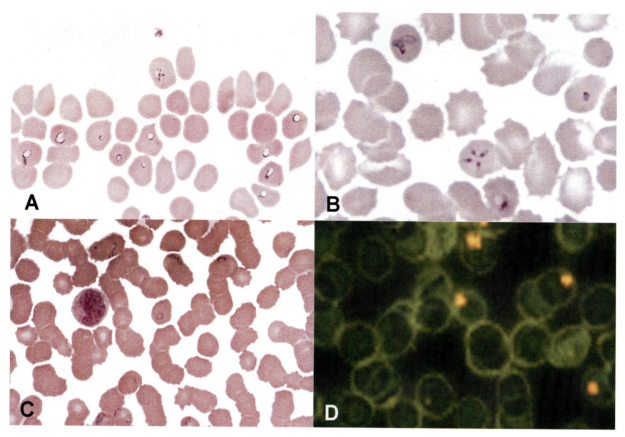

Color Plate 17. Human babesiosis (see Chapter 20) can be caused by several different protozoan species in the genus *Babesia*. In North America, most cases of human babesiosis are caused by *B. microti*. (A) *B. microti* forms pleomorphic and amoeboid intraerythrocytic rings that can be difficult to differentiate from other babesial species and from *Plasmodium* spp. (Wright stain, original magnification, ×160). (B) Rare examples of infection by *B. gibsoni*-like piroplasms called WA-1 (Wright stain; original magnification, ×160) have been documented in the Pacific northwest and in California. Image courtesy of D. H. Persing. (C) *B. divergens*-like piroplasms are found in Europe and have also been observed in an infected person in Missouri in the south-central United States (Wright stain; original magnification, ×160). Image courtesy of E. Masters. When present, a helpful finding differentiating *Babesia* spp. from *Plasmodium* spp. is the presence of tetrads of merozoites, termed Maltese crosses (B). (D) *B. microti* in a peripheral blood smear from an infected patient detected by acridine orange staining and fluorescent microscopy. Image courtesy of D. H. Persing.

Chapter 21

Geographic Distributions of Tick-Borne Diseases and Their Vectors

Richard N. Brown, Robert S. Lane, and David T. Dennis

INTRODUCTION

This chapter reviews information on the geographic distributions of tick-borne diseases and their primary tick vectors. In the first section, "Tick-Borne Diseases," we address tick-borne encephalitis (TBE); Crimean-Congo hemorrhagic fever (CCHF); Colorado tick fever (CTF); tularemia; the tick-borne rickettsioses, including the rickettsial spotted fevers, tick typhuses, and Q fever; human granulocytic anaplasmosis (HGA) (previously called human granulocytic ehrlichiosis), human monocytotropic ehrlichiosis (HME), and ehrlichiosis caused by *Ehrlichia ewingii*; the tick-borne borrelioses, including Lyme borreliosis (LB) and tick-borne relapsing fever (TBRF); and babesiosis. Causative agents are identified, and principal ecological and epidemiological determinants of the diseases are outlined, providing information on vectors and vertebrate hosts, as well as features of the diseases useful in understanding exposures and spread and in framing case definitions. Modes of transmission other than tick bite are noted. In the following section, "Primary Vectors of Tick-Borne Diseases," brief descriptions are given of primary tick vectors and their distributions. We specifically address 35 ixodid species and 10 argasid species of the 867 recognized species of ticks that commonly bite people.

Maps are provided (Color Map section preceding this chapter) showing distributions of major disease groupings and primary tick vectors. Although correlations between the two are high, inconsistencies may result when there is diversionary feeding of primary vectors on incompetent vertebrate hosts, when competent vertebrate reservoirs are absent in an area, when modes of transmission other than tick bite are dominant, or when there is poor detection and reporting of human cases.

Risk of transmission to humans in foci of tick-borne diseases is determined by such factors as the density of competent vectors and reservoir hosts, infection thresholds of the pathogens, and the behaviors of humans that place them at risk of bites by infective ticks. At a local scale, the force of transmission is influenced by biotic factors (e.g., habitat characteristics, including changes in landscape and land use) and abiotic factors (e.g., climate and soil characteristics) that affect population and community dynamics of vectors and hosts. Expanding distributions may result from introduction of vectors or pathogens by movements of wildlife (including migrating birds), people, pets, and livestock.

The accuracy of our maps reflects the information available, determined in part by such variables as the public health and economic importance of the diseases, the time elapsed since emergence or recognition, and the region and country from which the disease is reported. Our literature search has been biased towards publications and reports written in English. We have not attempted to comprehensively examine primary data on either the diseases or tick species, and the maps presented are meant to be only close approximations of actual distributions. More detailed information may be available in individual disease chapters in this book and in other review publications on this subject (130, 141). Readers are encouraged to seek primary data sources and to contact public health authorities regarding up-to-date information on the local prevalence of vectors and the occurrence of the diseases they transmit within their jurisdictions.

TICK-BORNE DISEASES

TBE

Agents and distribution of human cases of TBE

TBE is caused by a complex of related flaviviruses associated with regionally defined diseases known

Richard N. Brown • Department of Wildlife, Humboldt State University, Arcata, CA 95521-8222. **Robert S. Lane** • Department of Environmental Science, Policy, and Management, Division of Insect Biology, University of California, Berkeley, CA 94720. **David T. Dennis** • Division of Vector-Borne Infectious Diseases, National Center for Infectious Diseases, Centers for Disease Control and Prevention, P.O. Box 2087, Fort Collins, CO 80522.

as Central European tick-borne encephalitis (CEE), Russian spring-summer encephalitis (RSSE), louping ill (LI), Negishi viral encephalitis (NEG), Powassan encephalitis (PWE), Kyasanur Forest disease (KFD), Omsk hemorrhagic fever (OHF), Alkhurma disease (ALK), and Langat encephalitis.

TBE is endemic throughout much of Europe, the Middle East, and Asia, and rare cases occur in North America (Color Map 1). CEE occurs in Europe, western Russia, and the Balkan states. RSSE occurs from the Ural Mountains of northeastern Europe through northern Asia to Japan. Rare cases of PWE occur sporadically in the northeastern United States and adjacent Canada, and cases have been reported recently from Russia. More localized TBEs include LI in the United Kingdom and Norway (the agent also has been identified in sheep in Spain, Turkey, and Bulgaria) (34); NEG, which is closely related to the LI virus, in Japan; OHF throughout the forest-steppe zones of western Siberia (34); KFD in southwestern India (34); ALK, for which the causative virus is most closely related to KFD virus, from Saudi Arabia; and Langat encephalitis from Southeast Asia.

Vectors of TBE

The primary vectors of the viruses causing CEE and RSSE include *Ixodes ricinus* (Color Map 2) in western and central Europe and *Ixodes persulcatus* (Color Map 2) in northern Asia, as well as *Haemaphysalis* spp. (Color Map 3) in the Khabarovsk region near the Sea of Japan (98). Other species that maintain enzootic transmission or amplify infection beyond enzootic cycles include *Ixodes arboricola*, *Ixodes hexagonus*, and *Ixodes trianguliceps* (49, 126). *Ixodes ovatus* (Color Map 2) was implicated recently as a vector of infection to humans in Japan (134). *I. ricinus* is the vector of LI in the United Kingdom, and *I. persulcatus* is the vector of NEG in Japan, but the mechanisms limiting LI virus endemicity to the United Kingdom and NEG virus to Japan remain unexplained. Moreover, *I. ricinus* occurs in the United Kingdom without transmitting CEE virus. Langat encephalitis appears to be transmitted by *Ixodes granulatus* (Color Map 4). The PWE virus has been isolated from a variety of tick species including *Ixodes scapularis* (Color Map 2), *Ixodes cookei* (Color Map 3), and *Ixodes marxi* in the northeastern United States, *Dermacentor andersoni* (Color Map 5) and *Ixodes spinipalpis* in the western United States; and *I. persulcatus*, *Dermacentor silvarum* (Color Map 5), and *Haemaphysalis neumanni* in Russia. *I. spinipalpis* and *I. marxi* may be important to the enzootic maintenance of PWE virus, but neither tick commonly bites people. OHF virus is transmitted by *Dermacentor reticulatus* (Color Map 5)

in the northern forest-steppe region of the Omsk district of western Siberia. Another Central Asian species, *Ixodes apronophorus*, is considered important in the enzootic maintenance of OHF virus among voles in the grassy marshes of the western Siberian lowlands (34) but does not feed on people. Additionally, *I. persulcatus* and *Dermacentor marginatus* (Color Map 6) appear to be important vectors in the southern forest steppe of western Siberia (48, 72, 98). KFD virus has been isolated from a variety of tick species, but most human infections appear to be transmitted by *Haemaphysalis spinigera* (Color Map 5) and *Haemaphysalis turturis* (98, 130).

Epidemiology, ecology, and alternate routes of transmission of TBE

Several thousand cases of TBE are reported annually in Europe and Russia. Areas with the highest incidence of CEE are found in Germany, Poland, the Czech Republic, Slovakia, some Baltic states, and western and far-eastern Russia (112). Cases in Austria, where incidence is generally high, have fallen dramatically over the past 20 years, due to government promotion of vaccination of persons who consider themselves to be at risk. CEE is generally manifest as a mild meningoencephalitis; severe motor dysfunction and permanent disability occur only rarely, and the case fatality ratio is less than 2%. RSSE is generally a more severe disease than CEE. In the form found in far-eastern Russia, severe meningoencephalitis and residual damage are much more frequent and the case fatality rate is 20 to 30% (128).

Small mammals (hedgehogs and rodents) serve as reservoirs of most TBE viruses. Reservoirs of CEE and RSSE are diverse and their roles are complex, but European hedgehogs (*Erinaceus europaeus*), field mice (*Apodemus* spp.), and voles (*Clethrionomys* spp.) appear to be important hosts throughout Europe and Asia. Prevalence of TBE virus in tick populations is aggregated, rather than consistently homogeneous across the range of the primary vectors, creating local foci of elevated risk (98). Nuttall and Labuda (98) suggest that microfoci develop due to the clumped distribution of questing larval ticks, enhanced transmission among cofeeding ticks, and drop-off of large numbers of fed females in animal bedding areas. However, this does not explain the clumped distribution of TBE cases across the landscape. Randolph and collaborators (113, 114) have attributed recent changes in the incidence of cases of CEE in Latvia, Lithuania, Poland, Belarus, Estonia, Germany, the Czech Republic, Slovakia, Russia, Switzerland, Sweden, Finland, Slovenia, and Croatia, along with the first cases in Norway, to climate-based changes. Changes in local weather patterns associated with global warming alter the seasonal overlap of larval and nymphal *I. ricinus*, affecting the amplification of infections through the tick populations and altering the associated risk of transmission to people. The role of birds in the maintenance of TBE foci has yet to be resolved (98). Species of ticks other than those mentioned above and other bloodsucking arthropods may be involved with occasional transmission of these viruses. Turrel and Durden (137) recently transmitted Langat virus to *Ornithodoros sonrai* as an illustration of this point.

LI virus causes disease in domestic sheep, red grouse (*Lagopus lagopus*), and occasionally in people in northern England, Scotland, Wales, and Ireland. Although it has been associated with willow grouse and ptarmigan, sheep appear to be the reservoir of this virus (47, 112). LI virus or closely related viruses have been associated with disease in sheep in Norway, Spain, Greece, Bulgaria, and Turkey, as well as the United Kingdom (47).

PWE virus is a rare cause of encephalitis in forested areas of northeastern North America that occurs mostly in spring and summer months. The disease has a high case fatality rate of approximately 50%. It is maintained enzootically in three regionally distinct cycles (34). These include a cycle in the northeastern United States and southeastern Canada among tree squirrels (*Tamiasciurus hudsonicus* and *Sciurus carolinensis*) and *I. marxi,* a parallel cycle in the northeastern United States among woodchucks (*Marmota monax*) and *I. cookei,* and a cycle in the northwestern United States among rodents and rabbits maintained by *I. spinipalpis* and *D. andersoni.* Since neither *I. spinipalpis* nor *I. marxi* commonly feeds on people, North American PWE occurs mostly within the range of the human-biting *I. cookei* and potentially within the range of *D. andersoni.* Although PWE virus has been isolated from *I. persulcatus, D. silvarum* (Color Map 5), and *H. neumanni* in Russia, the distribution and ecological maintenance of this virus within the ranges of these vectors have yet to be thoroughly described.

KFD occurs in a limited focus in forested areas of southwestern India, with the number of cases reported annually ranging from 50 to more than 1,000. KFD causes gastrointestinal hemorrhage as well as encephalitis and has a case fatality rate of 3 to 10%. The disease occurs with greatest frequency in the dry season of February through June, and adults are more often affected than children, reflecting exposures during harvesting of forest products (82). KFD affects monkeys (including the black-faced langur *Presbytis entellus* and the bonnet macaque *Macaca radiata,* hence the local name of monkey fever) and humans. Putative reservoirs include shrews (*Suncus murinus*), forest rats

(*Rattus rattus*), and Indian crested porcupines (*Hystrix indica*), but the virus has been isolated from a fairly large number of vertebrates including bats and birds (98). Secondary vectors may also play important roles in both maintenance and occasional transmission of KFD virus; as an example, an infected soft tick (*Ornithodoros tholozani*) accidentally transmitted the virus to a human (98). Some have suggested that disturbance of native forest habitat related to wood collection and eventual local deforestation have led to greater numbers of the primary vectors as well as greater exposure of people to tick bites (98, 130). The ixodids responsible for most of the transmission of tick-borne human diseases are generalists that thrive in disturbed habitats.

OHF is restricted to the mixed forest-steppe region of western Siberia. The disease resembles KFD, with an incubation period of 3 to 7 days followed by fever in two distinct waves. During the first febrile period of 5 to 12 days there may be signs of bronchopneumonia and gastrointestinal hemorrhage, while mild encephalitic signs appear during a second period of 2 to 7 days of fever. The case fatality rate is less than 5% (82). Water voles (*Microtus gregalis* and *Arvicola* spp.) are considered important reservoirs of OHF. Water vole populations are prone to wide fluctuations in density. When vole numbers are high, tick populations also expand and the prevalence of OHF virus in the tick population is strongly correlated with tick densities. Muskrats (*Ondatra zibethicus*) serve as amplifying hosts and are quite susceptible to OHF, and epizootics of high mortality in muskrats are common. Muskrats are not native to Asia but were first introduced to western Siberia around 1930 to support a growing fur trade. The annual number of human cases, sometimes exceeding 100 cases, was greatest when muskrat trapping was most intense in the middle part of the 20th century. The number of cases has since dropped dramatically, probably due to the decreasing importance of trapping of these rodents. Most human cases of OHF occur during autumn and winter among hunters and trappers who handle muskrats and their tissues (98, 130).

Although principally tick borne, the various TBE viruses may be transmitted by diverse routes, including handling of infectious materials, ingestion of contam-inated milk and milk products, or bites by arthropods other than ticks. The viruses causing CEE, RSSE, and LI have been contracted by humans from ingestion of nonpasteurized milk products; KFD virus has been transmitted experimentally via milk to monkeys; and PWE virus has been demonstrated in milk from experimentally infected goats. Hawks have become infected with TBE virus after feeding on infected small mammals, and OHF virus has been isolated from the urine and feces of infected muskrats, prompting some to suggest a water-borne route of transmission, most likely during peak periods of epizootics (98). The PWE virus has been isolated from mosquitoes. Like OHF, ALK has been contracted by butchers exposed to carcasses of infected animals (sheep in the case of ALK virus and primarily muskrats in the case of OHF); the likelihood of a tick vector of ALK virus is speculated because of its close relationship to other TBE-associated viruses. All tick species that commonly feed on both sheep and people in Saudi Arabia should be considered potential ALK vectors until the ecological maintenance of ALK is understood. It is also possible that ALK virus could be transmitted to humans in sheep milk and its products.

Crimean-Congo Hemorrhagic Fever

Agents and distribution of human cases of CCHF

CCHF is caused by a virus in the genus *Nairovirus* (family *Bunyaviridae*), has the largest geographic distribution of any of the tick-borne viral diseases (Color Map 7), and is known in Portugal, France, Greece, Yugoslavia, Hungary, Bulgaria, Moldovia, Russia, Turkey, Armenia, Azerbaijan, Iran, Turkmenistan, Kazakhstan, Uzbekistan, Tadzhikistan, Afganistan, Pakistan, Iraq, India, China, United Arab Emirates, Kuwait, Egypt, and Mauritania and sub-Saharan Africa (85, 130).

Vectors of CCHF

The CCHF virus is exceptional in the large number of tick species from which it has been isolated, including seven genera of ixodids and two species of argasids (*Argas lahorensis* and *Argas persicus*) (85); Sonenshine (130) noted 25 species of competent vectors. However, the distribution of human disease correlates well with that of its main vector, *Hyalomma marginatum* (Color Map 8). *I. ricinus*, *D. marginatus*, and several species of *Rhipicephalus* that potentially serve as important secondary vectors (85).

Epidemiology, ecology, and alternate routes of transmission of CCHF

CCHF is one of the most virulent hemorrhagic fevers. Following an incubation period of 2 to 9 days, there is sudden onset of fever and nonspecific symptoms, followed in 3 to 7 days by gastrointestinal and other hemorrhages, often with severe blood loss. The blood and secretions of these patients are highly infectious, and transmission to caregivers by direct exposure of mucous membranes or skin breaks to blood or saliva of a viremic host is a serious problem. Human cases also spread as a result of inhalation of aerosols containing virus (85). Case fatality rates range from 15 to 25%. Patients may experience neurological problems during acute illness, and occasionally patients experience peripheral neuritis, emotional disturbances, or both for months or even years after the acute illness (82).

Ticks are considered the principal reservoir of the virus in nature. However, since transovarial transmission of the virus in primary vectors occurs only in a small proportion of infected ticks, ticks are thought to be unable to perpetuate infection without amplification by feeding on viremic hosts. Lagomorphs (rabbits and hares) and hedgehogs are important sources of virus and serve as important hosts for vectors in most areas. In addition, increases in the local abundance of hares can result in explosive increases in tick populations, accompanied by an increased risk of disease transmission to humans. Large mammals may be important in maintaining cycles of infection in areas where their densities are high, such as eastern and southern Africa, and livestock that feed large numbers of *H. marginatum* in enzootic areas amplify the risk to people (85, 130). Most rodents appear to be incompetent hosts for CCHF virus and mostly play an inconsequential role in maintaining the virus in nature. The multimammate mouse (*Mastomys natalensis*) is an exception, having been shown to serve as a reservoir in Senegal (130). Immature *H. marginatum* ticks feed on birds as well as mammals, and birds may play an important role in the dissemination of infected ticks. The role of birds as potential reservoirs of infection remains unclear; with the exception of ostriches that can circulate virus for several days, avian viremias are transient. Nonviremic transmission between cofeeding ticks on birds has been demonstrated (see Chapter 10). Onsets of human cases correlate with activity patterns of adult *H. marginatum*; peak activity occurs during April to October in Europe and during January and February in South Africa (85, 130).

The distribution of human cases correlates with suitability of the environment for *H. marginatum*. Thus, CCHF is typically associated with xeric habitats, savannas, tropical grasslands, semideserts, dry forest-steppe regions, and lowland foothill environments with long dry seasons and mild winters (85, 130). Exceptions to this include foci in the deciduous forests of Moldavia and on Madagascar. In Moldavia, *H. marginatum* is uncommon, possibly related to cattle ranching practices, and human infections are transmitted by *I. ricinus* and *D. marginatus*. On the island of Madagascar, CCHF virus has been isolated from *Boophilus microplus*, a non-human-biting, one-host tick (85).

Colorado Tick Fever

Agents and distribution of human cases of CTF

CTF is caused by a coltivirus in the family *Reoviridae*. In North America, CTF virus (CTFV) has been isolated from ticks and rodents at elevations above 1,200 m in Rocky Mountain regions of the United States and Canada and from coastal foothills in California (75), but most human cases have been reported from Colorado (9, 69, 132). A related virus causes Eyach fever in northern Europe, including France, Germany, and Czechoslovakia (69).

Vectors of CTF

The Rocky Mountain wood tick, *D. andersoni* (Color Map 5), is the principal vector maintaining CTFV in the enzootic cycle and the primary vector to humans in the western United States and southwestern Canada. However, the virus also has been isolated from *Dermacentor albipictus*, *Dermacentor occidentalis* (Color Map 5), *Dermacentor parumapertus*, *Haemaphysalis leporispalustris*, *Ixodes sculptus*, *I. spinipalpis*, and *Ornithodoros lagophilus* (132). Of these potential secondary vectors, only *D. occidentalis*, the Pacific Coast tick, commonly bites people, and there have been only a few cases of CTF from the range of *D. occidentalis* (36, 75). The other species noted may be important as enzootic maintenance vectors or in amplifying transmission during local epizootics. Eyach fever virus has been isolated from *I. ricinus* and *Ixodes ventalloi* in France and Germany (132), but little has been reported concerning the ecological maintenance of the virus or the relative competence of these two vectors.

Epidemiology, ecology, and alternate routes of transmission of CTF

CTF is not nationally notifiable in the United States, and not all states where CTF is endemic require reporting. Recently, fewer than 75 cases have been reported annually, although the true incidence is likely much higher. Infections are typically acquired during recreational and occupational activities in natural settings that place humans at risk of bites by *D. andersoni*, such as hiking, camping, foresting, and maintaining trails and communication lines (9). Young adult males appear most likely to be diagnosed with CTF; cases involving males outrank females by 2:1 (69) to 25:1 (132). Infections occur from early spring to October but are highest during May and June, the peak feeding period for adult *D. andersoni* ticks. Following an incubation period of 3 to 6 days, there is an abrupt onset of a biphasic illness characterized by fever and chills, headache, prostration, gastrointestinal com-plaints, leukopenia, and thrombocytopenia. Rash occurs in 5 to 10% of cases and may lead to confusion of the illness with Rocky Mountain spotted fever (RMSF). Rare complications include meningitis, encephalitis, carditis, and orchitis (69, 128).

In a hyperendemic focus in Rocky Mountain National Park, Colorado, *D. andersoni* is most abundant on rocky south-facing slopes at elevations ranging from 1,200 to 3,000 m. Important hosts of CTFV vary somewhat within the range of *D. andersoni*. Regionally important hosts include least chipmunks (*Tamias minimus*), golden-mantled ground squirrels (*Spermophilus lateralis*), porcupines (*Erethizon dorsatum*), bushy-tailed woodrats (*Neotoma cinerea*), and deer mice (*Peromyscus maniculatus*) (9). Sonenshine et al. (132) noted that rabbits (e.g., *Sylvilagus nuttalli*) are apparently incompetent hosts of CTFV. This is unexplained in light of the fact that four of the seven listed potential secondary vectors (*D. parumapertus*, *H. leporispalustris*, *I. spinipalpis*, and *O. lagophilus*) feed heavily on rabbits and hares, suggesting that further evaluation of other species of lagomorphs as hosts for CTFV is warranted. Moreover, Lane et al. (75) isolated a CTF-like virus from the black-tailed jackrabbit, *Lepus californicus*, from California.

Rare case reports suggest that CTV may be acquired by direct contact exposure to fluids of crushed infected ticks, and at least one case of transfusion-associated illness has been reported (9).

Tularemia

Agents and distribution of human cases of tularemia

Tularemia is caused by infection with *Francisella tularensis*, of which several subspecies cause human illness. The agent is a pleomorphic, non-spore-forming, aerobic, gram-negative bacillus that is a facultative intracellular organism. *F. tularensis* is capable of invading most tissues in its vertebrate hosts as well as in its tick vectors (130). Tularemia is widely distributed in the Northern Hemisphere, from the Arctic to subtropical regions, including North America, Europe, Scandinavia, Russia, Tunisia, Turkey, Israel, Iran, China, and Japan (1). Pathogenic *Francisella tularensis* subsp. *tularensis* (type A) strains have been described only from North America (Color Map 7); they are generally more virulent than *Francisella tularensis* subsp. *holarctica* (type B) strains, which are found throughout the Holarctic region (Color Map 7).

Vectors of tularemia

Tularemia is transmitted by ticks and biting flies, including tabanids and mosquitoes. Many species of ticks are competent biological vectors, and ticks are a significant interepizootic reservoir (1). *F. tularensis* is vertically transmitted from one stage of tick to another, but transovarial transmission is infrequent and unimportant in its maintenance. The rabbit tick, *H. leporispalustris*, is an important enzootic vector throughout the Holarctic, and tick transmission to people is typically associated with bridging vectors, including *Dermacentor variabilis* (Color Map 6), *D. andersoni*, *D. occidentalis*, and *Amblyomma americanum* (Color Map 5) in North America and *I. apronophorus* and *D. reticulatus* in Europe and Asia (60, 131). Mechanical transmission of *F. tularensis* by deer flies (*Chrysops* spp.) and horse flies (*Tabanus* spp.) is important in some arid areas of the western United States, and mechanical transmission by mosquitoes is important in Scandinavia and the Baltic region. In sub-Arctic and Arctic regions beyond the northern distributions of human-biting ticks, transmission depends on either water-borne or mosquito-borne sources (2, 129). Because tularemia is so widely distributed and because there are so many potential routes of transmission, we have not attempted to review the distributions of the vectors in relation to the distribution of human cases.

Epidemiology, ecology, and alternate routes of transmission of tularemia

F. tularensis is one of the most infectious bacterial disease agents, requiring exposure to less than 10 organisms of type A to regularly cause disease in humans (28). Although highly infectious, the agent is not known to be transmitted from person to person. The typical incubation period for tularemia is 3 to 5 days (range, 1 to 14 days), followed by an acute febrile viral-like illness that may take several forms depending on the route of infection. Although *F. tularensis* subsp. *tularensis* is considered more virulent than *F. tularensis* subsp. *holarctica*, both cause a similar spectrum of illness (59). The most common clinical forms are ulceroglandular and glandular tularemia, characterized by fever and regional lymphadenitis, with or without an ulcerative lesion at the site of cutaneous inoculation. More severe forms include blood-borne systemic illness (typhoidal form), pleuropneumonia, and meningitis. Case fatality rates are generally less than 2%, but untreated severe forms may have fatality rates of 30% or more.

The number of cases that occur worldwide is unknown. In the United States, the number of reported cases has fallen over the past 60 years from >1,000 to <200 per year (18, 25). Incidence is highest in the southcentral and western regions, but notable small aerosol-borne outbreaks have occurred repeatedly on small islands off the coast of Massachusetts (39, 59).

Outbreaks associated with inhalation and other environmental exposures have occurred in Scandinavia and elsewhere in Europe that have numbered in the hundreds, and even thousands, of cases (58).

Reservoir hosts include principally rodents (*Microtus* spp., *Arvicola* spp., *Apodemus* spp., *O. zibethica*, and *Castor* spp.) and lagomorphs (*Sylvilagus* and *Lepus* spp.), but a large number of vertebrates and arthropods (>100 species each) have been found naturally infected (1, 130). Transmission between animals occurs through contaminated environmental sources and arthropod bites and by predation and cannibalism.

In addition to infective tick bite exposures, people become infected from direct contact with infectious tissues of rodents, rabbits, or hares and less frequently by the bites of bloodsucking flies (including mosquitoes, black flies, horse flies, and deer flies) (1, 130). Cases also occur after ingesting contaminated water or foodstuffs or inhaling infectious aerosols, sometimes resulting in large common-source outbreaks (25, 35). In the United States, cases most frequently resulted in the past from direct contact with infectious carcasses during hunting, trapping, and skinning rabbits, squirrels, beavers, or muskrats. However, contact transmission has markedly diminished as fewer people hunt and trap these animals, and the relative importance of tick transmission has increased. A seasonally biphasic incidence of disease onset occurs in the United States, associated with arthropod bites in the spring and summer and the handling of trapped and hunted animals in the late fall and winter. Cases in Europe occur most commonly in the summer months, related to contamination of the environment by rodents and hares and by mosquito or tick bites. *F. tularensis* is a hazard to laboratory workers because it is easily aerosolized, is highly infectious, and causes severe disease, a combination of traits that also makes it an important potential biological weapon (28).

Spotted Fever Group Rickettsioses

The recognized tick-borne rickettsial agents causing illness in humans are included in Table 1. Readers are advised that there is a rapidly growing list of rickettsial species associated with human-biting ticks that either are nonpathogenic or have yet to be associated with human disease.

Agents and distribution of human cases of the spotted fever group rickettsiae

Tick-borne disease agents of the genus *Rickettsia* occur worldwide. The principal members of the spotted fever group of rickettsial pathogens include *Rick-*

Table 1. Tick-borne rickettsial species associated with human disease

Human disease (agent)	Primary vector(s)	Geographical region
RMSF (*R. rickettsii*)	*D. variabilis, D. andersoni, R. sanguineus, A. cajennense*	Western Hemisphere
MSF, Mediterranean tick typhus, boutonneuse fever, Kenyan tick typhus, Indian tick typhus, Astrakhan fever, tick bite fever, Israeli tick typhus (*R. conorii* complex)	*R. sanguineus, D. marginatus, D. reticulatus, I. hexagonus, I. ricinus, R. pumilio, R. turanicus, A. variegatum, A. hebraeum, H. leachi, H. marginatum, R. appendiculatus*	Southern Europe, Mediterranean and sub-Saharan Africa, Middle East, Asia
North Asian tick typhus, Siberian tick typhus (*R. sibirica*)	*D. nuttalli, D. marginatus, D. silvarum, D. reticulatus, D. pictus, H. asiaticum, H. concinna, H. japonica, H. punctata*	Widespread through central Russia, Siberia, China, Mongolia, Japan, Central Asian republics, Czech Republic, Lithuania, Pakistan, and Afghanistan
JSF, Oriental spotted fever (*R. japonica*)	*H. longicornis, H. flava, D. taiwanensis, I. ovatus*	Japan and Korea
Czechoslovakian tick typhus (*R. slovaca*)	*D. marginatus*	Southern, central, and eastern Europe
ATBF, South African tick typhus (*R. africae*)	*A. hebraeum, A. variegatum, A. lepidum*	Southern Africa, Mali, Niger, Sudan, Central African Republic, Kenya, Guadeloupe, and French West Indies
QTT (*R. australis*)	*I. holocyclus*	Coastal eastern Queensland, Australia
TTT (*R. honei*)	*I. granulatus, I. cornuatus, A. hydrosauri, A. cajennense(?)*	Flinders Island, Tasmania, and eastern Victoria, Australia, and Thailand
Mongolian tick typhus (*R. mongolotimonae*)	*H. asiaticum*	Inner Mongolia, southern France, Niger
"Unnamed" tick typhus (*R. helvetica*)	*I. ricinus*	France, Switzerland, Japan, possibly Thailand
"Unnamed" tick typhus (*R. aeschlimannii*)	*H. marginatum*	Morocco, Zimbabwe, Niger, Mali, and Okinawa
"Unnamed" tick typhus (*R. massiliae*)	*R. turanicus*	Portugal, France, Greece, Central African Republic, and Okinawa
HGA (*A. phagocytophilum*)	*I. ricinus, I. scapularis, I. pacificus*	Europe, eastern and far-western United States
HME (*E. chaffeensis*)		Eastern seaboard and upper midwestern United States
Ehrlichiosis (*E. ewingii*)		Southern and eastern United States
Q fever (*C. burnetti*)	Fomites of infectious dusts and aerosols from infected sheep, goats, and cattle; isolated from many species of ticks; found in tick feces	Worldwide with the exception of New Zealand and Antarctica

ettsia rickettsii (the cause of RMSF), *Rickettsia conorii*-complex (the cause of Mediterranean spotted fever [MSF] and related infections), *Rickettsia sibirica* (the cause of North Asian tick typhus [NATT]), and *Rickettsia australis* (the cause of Queensland tick typhus

[QTT]). Fevers caused by *R. rickettsii* are limited to the Western Hemisphere from Canada to Argentina, with most cases recorded in the United States. MSFs occur throughout the Mediterranean and Black Sea regions, the Middle East, much of Africa and the Indian subcontinent. NATT occurs in Siberia, Central Asia, China, Mongolia, and Pakistan. QTT occurs only along the eastern coast of Australia (Color Map 9).

Vectors and enzootic maintenance of RMSF

R. rickettsii occurs from southern Canada through much of the United States, Mexico, Central America, Colombia, Brazil, and Argentina (Color Map 9) (130). Reservoirs of *R. rickettsii* include various rodents, rabbits, and hares; enzootic cycles are maintained by ticks that feed heavily on these hosts, including the rabbit tick, *H. leporispalustris* (45). Humans are infected by bridging vectors that feed on small mammals as well as people. The American dog tick, *D. variabilis*, is the most important vector of *R. rickettsii* in its eastern and southern range, but it has not been confirmed as a vector in the far-western United States. The Rocky Mountain wood tick, *D. andersoni*, transmits RMSF throughout the Rocky Mountain regions of Canada and the United States, the mountains of the Great Basin region, and in northeastern California (130). *D. variabilis* (Color Map 6) and *D. andersoni* (Color Map 5) both appear to be important as enzootic vectors as well as the principal vectors to people. The Pacific Coast tick, *D. occidentalis* (Color Map 5), also appears to be a potential vector of RMSF in California (75, 108), but cases throughout most of its distribution are rare. The brown dog tick, *Rhipicephalus sanguineus*, is known to be a vector of RMSF in Mexico, but it has not been associated with cases elsewhere. The cayenne tick, *Amblyomma cajennense* (Color Map 5), ranges from the southern United States through Argentina, and it has been associated with cases in humans in both Central America and South America; *R. rickettsii* DNA was recently amplified from *Amblyomma cooperi* removed from a capybara in Brazil (24). Although RMSF is well known in Central and South America, studies proving vector competence of *A. cajennense* or *A. cooperi* have not been reported. Early studies implicated *A. americanum* as a potential vector of RMSF in the southern United States, but follow-up studies have failed to substantiate this (20, 130). A recent finding that *R. rickettsii* causes mortality in infected *D. andersoni* (95) indicates a mechanism that might limit prevalence in vectors. However, *R. rickettsii* has been maintained in laboratory colonies of *D. andersoni* and *D. variabilis* simply through transovarial and transstadial transmission, demonstrating that the vector-killing potential of *R. rickettsii* may depend on specific combinations of rickettsial strains and tick populations.

Although RMSF is known only from the Americas, *R. rickettsii* DNA was amplified recently from *Haemaphylis longicornis* (Color Map 3) in Korea (139).

Epidemiology, ecology, and alternate routes of transmission of RMSF

In North America, most cases arise in the southern Atlantic southwest-central states, in a much smaller incidence in the Rocky Mountain and far-western regions of both the United States and Canada, and in Mexico. Typically, 500 or so cases of RMSF have been reported annually in the United States, although long-term trends over the past 40 years have shown sustained periods of higher or lower levels (30). The incidence of infection peaks during late spring and summer. Persons most at risk are those exposed occupationally or recreationally to habitats infested by the vectors *D. variabilis* and *D. andersoni*.

Illness usually begins abruptly 2 to 12 days after tick exposure. Untreated, a high, persistent fever of 2 to 3 weeks' duration, severe headache, myalgias, and a characteristic maculopapular rash are typical; nausea and vomiting, abdominal pain, and conjunctivitis frequently occur. The rash usually does not appear before the third day of illness. It starts on the ankles and wrists, rapidly spreads to the rest of the body, and may become petechial or ecchymotic in character. Complications of the systemic inflammatory response syndrome and death may intervene if appropriate antibiotic treatment is not begun in a timely fashion. Untreated, the fatality ratio is about 20%; overall, the fatality ratio is about 5% in the United States. In addition to tick bite, transmission can occur from accidental inoculation of fluids of crushed ticks through breaks in the skin or mucous membranes.

Vectors and enzootic maintenance of MSF group rickettsiae

The *R. conorii* complex (*R. conorii* sensu lato) includes related rickettsiae causing classical MSF, Kenyan tick typhus, Indian tick typhus, Israeli tick typhus, Astrakhan fever, and African tick-bite fever (ATBF). Human cases occur throughout southern Europe, Russia, the Middle East, South Asia (including India and along the Thailand-Myanmar border), the Mediterranean, and sub-Saharan Africa (Color Map 9). In most areas, *R. sanguineus* has been identified as the primary vector (42, 111, 130, 140), but several species have been implicated as regionally important. These include *D. marginatus*, *D. reticulatus*, *H. marginatum*, *I. hexagonus*, *I. ricinus*, and *Rhipicephalus turanicus* (Color Map 8) in Europe (5, 130); *Haemaphysalis leachi* (Color Map 6) in India (130); *Rhipicephalus pumilio* (Color Map 2) in the Astrakhan region of Russia (37); and *Rhipicephalus appendiculatus* (Color Map 4), *Rhipicephalus evertsi* (Color Map 2), *Amblyomma hebraeum* (Color Map 5), *Amblyomma variegatum* (Color Map 5), and

H. leachi in Africa (31, 98, 130, 147). In addition, serologic data from patients suggest the occurrence of *R. conorii* infections in South America (29).

Natural cycles of *R. conorii* involve a variety of small mammals that are fed upon by immature stages of the various vectors. Immature brown dog ticks feed opportunistically on rodents, hedgehogs, lagomorphs, and other small mammals. Adults feed on a variety of wild carnivores, ungulates (including livestock), dogs, and people. Dogs are important hosts in MSF cycles for several reasons: unlike with RMSF, dogs are competent reservoir hosts, they move infective vectors from sylvatic habitats into yards and homes, and they provide blood meals for large numbers of the primary vector in kennels, barns, homes, and other areas generally frequented by people and dogs (130).

Epidemiology, ecology, and alternative routes of transmission of MSF group rickettsiae

Human infections with *R. conorii* and closely related organisms occur throughout southern Europe, Russia, the Middle East, South Asia (including India and along the Thailand-Myanmar border), the Mediterranean, and sub-Saharan Africa (Color Map 9). In the Middle East, incidence is highest adjacent to the Mediterranean, Black, and Caspian Seas. The disease has been spreading northward in Europe, possibly because of transport of the brown dog tick by pet dogs. The incidence of MSFs is unknown. Serological studies indicate that most cases in areas of endemicity are probably mild, self-limited, and unrecognized, although a severe, sometimes fatal, form has been described (117). In Africa, risk of exposure to vector ticks is greatest in the bush, and MSF is increasingly recognized as a cause of fever in travelers returning from safari; *R. conorii* is the most common rickettsial infection in southern Africa. In temperate areas, the disease occurs most commonly in the summer months.

The incubation period of MSF is usually 5 to 7 days. The illness is characterized by sudden onset of fever (>39°C), headache, myalgia, and arthralgia. A primary lesion (tache noir) commonly occurs at the site of the infective tick bite and is often present at the onset of fever. It is characterized by an ulcer, 2 to 5 mm in diameter, with a black scab and erythematous halo. A generalized maculopapular skin rash that appears on the fourth or fifth day of fever and often involves the palms and soles gives the illness its common name in the Mediterranean region, boutonneuse fever. Without treatment, the illness may persist for a few days to as long as 2 weeks. A small proportion of patients may experience a malignant form accompanied by a petechial rash and neurological, cardiac, or renal complications (117).

Vectors and enzootic maintenance of NATT

R. sibirica naturally infects a variety of ticks (19, 86), including tick species in the genera *Dermacentor*, *Haemaphysalis*, and *Hyalomma* (Table 1). Sonenshine (130) listed the four most common vectors as *Dermacentor nuttalli* (Color Map 6) (122), *D. marginatus*, *D. silvarum*, and *D. reticulatus*. As with other members of the spotted fever disease group, ticks serve as reservoirs as well as vectors. Rodents (*Apodemus* spp., *Clethrionomys* spp., *Rattus* spp., and *O. zibethica*), hedgehogs, and other small mammals commonly fed upon by these tick species serve both as vehicles of transmission between ticks and as reservoir hosts. Primary vectors of NATT are associated with agricultural areas, and people engaged in farming appear to be at greatest risk of infective bites (130).

Vectors and enzootic maintenance of Japanese (or Oriental) spotted fever (JSF)

Rickettsia japonica causes spotted fever in Japan and Korea (83, 88, 125). Several putative vectors have been identified, including *H. longicornis* in both countries (83, 139) and *Haemaphysalis flava* (Color Map 6) (43, 61, 65), *I. ovatus* (65), and *Dermacentor taiwanensis* (43, 61) in Japan. Small mammals likely supplement the tick reservoir in both countries, but the details of enzootic maintenance have not been elucidated.

Vectors and enzootic maintenance of Czechoslovakian tick typhus

Rickettsia slovaca is known from Portugal, Spain, France, Germany, Switzerland, Austria, Hungary, Slovakia, Bulgaria, and Armenia. In these areas, *D. marginatus* is most commonly associated with the agent and the disease (4–7, 119, 123).

Vectors and enzootic maintenance of ATBF

Rickettsia africae is widespread throughout sub-Saharan Africa and has been introduced in Guadeloupe in the West Indies. *A. hebraeum* and *A. variegatum* have been implicated as primary vectors in West (101), Central (101), and East (31, 87) Africa; and in southern Africa and on Guadeloupe (66, 104), respectively (Color Map 5). Small mammals that are commonly fed upon by immature ticks are thought to be the most important mammalian hosts, but adults of both species feed on wild carnivores, ungulates, and many other mid- and large-sized mammals, including livestock, dogs, and people. *A. variegatum* is an introduced exotic species on Guadeloupe, where 27% of ticks were recently found infected with *R. africae* (104). This illustrates the potential for globalization of rickettsial organisms with accidental introductions of ticks or infected reservoir hosts.

Vectors and enzootic maintenance of QTT

R. australis occurs along the eastern coast of Australia. *Ixodes holocyclus* (Color Map 4) is the primary vector to humans, but other species of ticks may contribute to the overall reservoir. The habitat supporting *I. holocyclus* correlates well with the zones of risk for transmission to humans; specifically, tall grasslands adjacent to or interspersed with rain forest (130). Antibodies to *R. australis* have been detected in bandicoots and other rodents trapped in northeastern Queensland.

Vectors and enzootic maintenance of Thai or Flinder's Island tick typhus (TTT)

Rickettsia honei occurs in Thailand and in Gippsland, Victoria, and Flinder's Island, Tasmania, in southeastern Australia (51, 52, 121). In Thailand, *R. honei* was first identified in a pool of larval *Ixodes* spp. and *Rhipicephalus* spp. and recently in *I. granulatus* removed from a black rat (*Rattus rattus*) (51, 71). In Australia, *Ixodes cornuatus* removed from both people and dogs were found to be infected, and serologic assays indicated that bush rats (*Rattus fuscipes*) had been exposed. A reptile-feeding tick, *Aponomma hydrosauri*, collected from blue-tongue lizards (*Tiliqua nigrolutea*), tiger snakes (*Notechis ater humphreysi*), and copperhead snakes (*Austrelaps superbus*) was demonstrated by PCR to be infected (51). Although many species of ticks are hosts to rickettsiae, this appears to be the first rickettsial pathogen of humans that was shown to be maintained in reptiles and their ticks. This pathogen has also recently been identified in *A. cajennense* removed from cattle in the state of Texas (51).

Vectors associated with Mongolian tick typhus

Rickettsia mongolotimonae has been identified recently as a cause of tick typhus in France (44), and infected *Hyalomma asiaticum* (Color Map 4) and *Hyalomma truncatum* have been found infected in Mongolia and Niger, respectively (101). Thus, although only newly recognized as a human pathogen, this agent spans a large area covering three continents. Little else about its ecological maintenance is known (103).

Vectors associated with *Rickettsia* spp. causing "unnamed" tick typhus

At least three additional rickettsial organisms have been clearly associated with human diseases. These are *R. helvetica*, *R. aeschlimannii*, and *R. massiliae*. Enzootic cycles for each of these agents remain relatively unstudied. *R. helvetica* probably occurs widely, including throughout southern Europe, having been recognized as causing disease or recovered from ticks in France (44, 102), Italy (124), Switzerland (116, 119), Japan (61, 124), and along the Thailand-Myanmar border (103). *R. helvetica* has been recovered from *I. ricinus* in Europe (124), and *I. ovatus*, *I. persulcatus*, and *Ixodes monospinosus* in Japan (124).

R. aeschlimannii has been associated with human cases of tick typhus in South Africa (110, 115). Ticks from which *R. aeschlimannii* DNA has been amplified include *A. variegatum* from Mali, Niger, and Burundi (101); *Amblyomma lepidum* (Color Map 3) from the Sudan; and six species from Spain (40). Within a large number of Spanish ticks sampled, *H. marginatum* was the species most commonly infected (5.9%) while <2% of the other five species (*I. ricinus*, *Haemaphysalis punctata*, *Rhipicephalus bursa*, *R. sanguineus*, and *R. turanicus*) were infected (40). These findings indicate that *R. aeschlimanni* is widespread at least in Spain and several regions of Africa.

R. massiliae is another widespread pathogen of which little is known. A recent serosurvey of suspected MSF patients from Europe revealed high titers to *R. massiliae*, but the agent has not been isolated, nor has its DNA been PCR amplified, from human patients. *R. massiliae* has been identified in *Rhipicephalus muhsamae* from Mali (101), otherwise-unidentified "ticks" from the Central African Republic (31), *R. turanicus* and *R. sanguineus* from Portugal (5), and *R. sanguineus* from Spain (16), Greece (3, 111), and Russia (122).

HGA and Ehrlichiosis

Agents and distribution of HGA and ehrlichioses

The agents of HGA, ehrlichiosis caused by *E. ewingii*, and HME are small, obligate, intracellular, gram-negative bacteria that grow in cytoplasmic vacuoles in characteristic clusters called morulae. These morulae are aggregates of two bacterial forms, larger reticulate forms and smaller forms with condensed central masses. *Anaplasma phagocytophilum* is the causative agent of HGA and is distinguished by 16S RNA and other gene sequence differences from *Ehrlichia chaffeensis* (the agent causing HME) and *E. ewingii*. These diseases are reported mostly from the United States and Europe but likely are distributed throughout the Holarctic region. In the United States, HME occurs mostly in the south-central, southeastern, and mid-Atlantic regions, while HGA is most frequent in the northeastern and upper north-central regions, with clusters in coastal New England and adjacent areas of Minnesota and Wisconsin. A few hundred cases each of HME and HGA are reported annually in the United States, but the diseases are considerably underreported. Although relatively few cases of HGA have been described from Pacific coastal states, surveys suggest that exposures in wildlife, horses, and dogs are relatively common in coastal and foothill habitats of California (41).

Vectors and enzootic maintenance of HGA

The primary vectors of *A. phagocytophilum* are ticks of the *I. ricinus* complex (Color Map 2). In the northeastern and upper-midwestern United States, *I. scapularis* serves as the enzootic maintenance vector in cycles involving the white-footed mouse (*Peromyscus leucopus*), raccoons (*Procyon lotor*), and eastern gray squirrels (*S. carolonensis*), and it is also the primary vector to people (84, 92, 142, 143). In the western United States, *Ixodes pacificus* (Color Map 2) serves as the primary vector to people, and enzootic maintenance cycles likely involve both *I. pacificus* and *I. spinipalpis* among reservoir hosts, including woodrats (*Neotoma* spp.) and possibly other rodents (73). In Europe, *I. ricinus* has been implicated as the primary vector to people, and enzootic maintenance vectors among various small mammal reservoirs (*Clethrionomys glareolus*, *Apodemus* spp., and *Sorex araneus*) include *I. ricinus* and *I. trianguliceps* (8, 10). *A. phagocytophilum* DNA has been amplified from *I. persulcatus* in both northeastern China and Korea (15, 67) and from *H. longicornis* in Korea (67), suggesting that this agent is more widespread in northern and central Asia than currently documented.

Vectors and enzootic maintenance of HME

E. chaffeensis is transmitted by the lone star tick, *A. americanum*. In the United States, DNA associated with *E. chaffeensis* has been found in ticks from 15 states along the eastern seaboard and from the midwestern region (21). The agent has been most often associated with the white-tailed deer (*Odocoileus virginianus*), dogs, people, and lone star ticks. Since immature *A. americanum* feed heavily on birds as well as mammals, birds may facilitate translocation of the agent.

DNA sequences similar to those of *E. chaffeensis* have been amplified from *I. persulcatus* in Russia (118) and Korea (67); from *I. ovatus*, *Amblyomma testudinarium*, and *Haemaphysalis yeni* in southern China (14, 146); from *I. ovatus* in Japan (127); and from *Haemaphysalis hystricis* in Vietnam (100). Although such findings do not prove the existence of stable enzootic cycles, they should alert medical workers to the potential for cases beyond the range of *A. americanum*.

Vectors and enzootic maintenance of ehrlichiosis caused by *E. ewingii*

E. ewingii is transmitted primarily by lone star ticks in the southern and eastern regions of the United States (21), but natural infections in *R. sanguineus* and *D. variabilis* have been documented. Like *E. chaffeensis*, this organism infects white-tailed deer, dogs, and people. Although additional species may eventually be found to be important hosts of the agent, white-tailed deer appear to be the most likely reservoir because they are infected commonly and serve as hosts for large numbers of *A. americanum* ticks (148). Birds may facilitate spread of the agent as described for *E. chaffeensis* (21).

Epidemiology and alternate routes of transmission of HGA, HME, and ehrlichiosis caused by *E. ewingii*

In the United States, *A. phagocytophilum* shares similar reservoir hosts and vectors with the agents of LB and human babesiosis. Not surprisingly, coinfections of humans by these pathogens sometimes occur, and the emergence of each of these diseases is driven by the increasing density and expanding range of *I. scapularis*. HME also is emerging in the United States, and this emergence is correlated with the distribution and increasing density of the lone star tick, *A. americanum*, in the southcentral, southeastern, and mid-Atlantic regions. The incubation period is usually 7 to 21 days, followed by an acute onset of fever, headache, myalgia, and anorexia. Nausea and vomiting are common. Thrombocytopenia and mild disturbances of liver function are typical. A macular rash is more often seen with HME and ehrlichiosis caused by *E. ewingii* than with HGA. When it does occur, the rash can lead to confusion with RMSF. About a third of patients require hospitalization the mortality rate is about 2%. Most cases have onsets in the late spring and summer months when vector tick bites are most frequent, although cases of HME also occur commonly in the fall.

Q Fever

Agent and distribution of human cases of Q fever

Q fever results from infection with *Coxiella burnetii*, a small, spore-forming, gram-negative bacterium that exists in two antigenic forms, phase I and phase II. The phase I form is highly infectious and exists in humans and other animals; phase II is avirulent. Q fever is widespread on every inhabited continent, and its distribution is closely correlated with populations of its principal reservoir hosts, including goats, sheep, bovines, and other ungulates (20, 21); an exception is that it appears to be absent from New Zealand (56). *C. burnetii* causes persistent infections and may be shed in feces, urine, oral-nasal discharges, blood, milk, placental tissues, and aborted fetuses of its hosts. The spore form is highly resistant to harsh environments. It can remain viable for long periods as spore forms in desiccated tissues and fluids, and in contaminated dusts (56, 130).

Vectors and enzootic maintenance of Q Fever

Many species of ticks, both argasids and ixodids, have been incriminated as vectors of *C. burnetii* in its wild animal cycles, but such involvement is secondary to respiratory and direct contact exposures (130). Tick-borne maintenance of *C. burnetii* in herds of livestock has been proposed but remains unproven. The control of vector ticks on wildlife and livestock may, however, reduce the force of transmission in animal cycles and thus reduce the risk of human exposures to infection, even though ticks rarely if ever transmit infection to humans. Geographic distributions are not considered further herein because the disease is found on every inhabited continent, aggregated by locations where herding of livestock and dairy farming are most common. Moreover, because tick-borne transmission is secondary to other modes of spread, the large number of tick species found infected provides little useful information on the relative risk of transmission.

Epidemiology and alternate routes of transmission of Q fever

Most transmission of *C. burnetii* to humans is thought to occur from exposure to airborne infectious aerosols and dusts related to birthing of lambs and other livestock, sheep shearing, manure processing, and dry summer winds that carry spores beyond ranch lands (56, 130). A low infective dose of *C. burnetii* and the long survivability in the environment of spores facilitate airborne transmission. Spores can remain viable in aerosols for up to 2 weeks and in soil for months.

Tick-Borne Borrelioses

LB

Agents and distribution of human cases of LB. LB is caused by a group of related spirochetes known collectively as *Borrelia burgdorferi* sensu lato. This group includes at least 11 genospecies, and more are likely to be identified. Genospecies associated clearly with human disease include *B. burgdorferi* sensu stricto, *Borrelia afzelii*, and *Borrelia garinii* (Color Map 10). *B. burgdorferi* sensu stricto ranges through-out large areas of the United States, focal areas of temperate Canada, and most of Europe, while *B. afzelii* and *B. garinii* occur throughout most of Europe and temperate Asia (Color Map 10). *Borrelia bissettii* occurs in North America and Europe, but pathogenicity to humans remains equivocal. Several other borreliae, including *Borrelia valaisiana*, *B. tanukii*, *B. turdi*, *B. andersonii*, and several genospecies that have yet to be named are transmitted by ixodid ticks, but infection of humans has yet to be demonstrated.

In the United States, cases of human LB occur mostly in the northeastern and upper-midwestern regions and at a lower incidence in the Pacific coastal areas of California and Oregon. Small numbers of cases occur in Canada, mostly in the southern parts of Ontario and British Columbia. In Eurasia, cases occur mostly in western and central Europe. Relatively small numbers of cases occur in southern Europe, far-eastern Russia, some central Asian states, northeastern China, Korea, and Japan. No cases have been confirmed by the isolation of spirochetes in Africa, Central or South America, the Caribbean, or any areas of the Southern Hemisphere.

Vectors of LB. Most cases of human borreliosis are acquired from the bites of four related *I. ricinus* complex species (*I. ricinus* in Europe, *I. persulcatus* in eastern Europe and Asia, *I. scapularis* in eastern North America, and *I. pacificus* in western North America) (Color Map 2). The Holarctic distribution of cases of LB closely matches the distribution of these four species. An important exception occurs in the southern United States, where *I. scapularis* is widely distributed but where lizards apparently serve as important zooprophylactic (diversionary) hosts, resulting in a relatively low risk of infection to humans. Enzootic maintenance cycles may be complicated by the occurrence in an area of multiple genospecies of borreliae, involvement of more than one vector species, and many potential species of vertebrate hosts.

Epidemiology, ecology, and alternate routes of transmission of LB. LB may be present as early localized, early, or late disseminated stages of disease. The characteristic marker of early infection is erythema migrans, a distinctive large red expanding annular cutaneous lesion. This first appears 3 to 30 days after an infective tick bite at the site of inoculation. Blood-borne dissemination may result in invasion of various target tissues, usually manifested within a few weeks of exposure as multiple erythema migrans rashes, meningitis, cranial or peripheral neuritis, or carditis. Arthritis of large, weight-bearing joints is common in untreated cases and usually makes its first appearance 3 or more months after exposure. Although many cases go undetected or unreported, tens of thousands of cases of LB are recorded annually in the United States and in Europe, making it the most frequently reported vector-borne disease in temperate regions of the Northern Hemisphere. In the United States, where LB reporting has been mandatory and standardized since 1991, there is a clear trend of increasing numbers of cases and continuous geographic expansion of enzootic infection and human disease (17, 27, 109).

LB is a disease of place, determined by the distribution of its vectors and by competent reservoir hosts, which are mostly small rodents and birds. Humans are infected primarily by the nymphal stage of feeding *Ixodes* spp., which mostly feed during late spring and early summer months; the Asian vector, *I. persulcatus*, appears to be an exception because most transmission appears to result from the bites of adult female ticks. In the eastern United States, persons are at most risk during periresidential activities in suburban or rural neighborhoods where mixed forest habitats support large numbers of deer and rodent reservoirs (27, 48, 53, 109). Recreational or occupational activities in parks and other natural areas can also pose a risk. In California, the state with the most cases in the western United States, exposures to nymphal ticks are most likely to occur in woodlands where ample leaf litter provides a favorable moist habitat for vectors (22, 135). In all areas except eastern Russia, onsets of early stage illness correlate with the greatest periods of feeding of nymphal ticks. In the United States, age groups at highest risk are children less than 15 years old and adults aged 35 years or older because of their outdoor activity patterns (27, 53). Modes of transmission of LB other than tick bites, such as transfusion, sexual or transplacental transmission, or through breast milk, have not been proven. If transmission by these modes does occur, it must be so rare as to be epidemiologically inconsequential.

Most *I. ricinus* complex ticks, including the four primary vectors of LB, are nonnidicolous species whose larvae and nymphs feed on a variety of small mammals, birds, and reptiles and whose adults feed on medium-sized or large mammals (33). Transovarial transmission (through female tissues to her eggs and subsequent larvae) rarely occurs, and is unimportant in the epidemiology and ecology of maintenance. Habitats in which people are most commonly infected vary between regions, but all species thrive in disturbed mixed forests (second-growth forest with saplings, brush, adequate leaf litter, and sunlight), mixed grasslands, mixed woodlands, fields allowed to revert naturally, and ecotones between grasslands and brush zones. Seasonality of peak periods of activity of different stages

is important to the maintenance of *B. burgdorferi. I. scapularis* and *I. persulcatus* nymphs tend to feed prior to the peak in larval feeding on reservoir hosts. Such reversed phenology amplifies prevalence in vector populations because naïve larvae become infected when feeding on hosts recently infected by feeding nymphs (33, 72, 109, 133). Larval *I. pacificus* and *I. ricinus* ticks tend to feed prior to nymphal activity, so prevalence is not amplified in this manner.

Several species may serve as secondary vectors, and possibly as minor primary vectors, including *I. hexagonus, I. trianguliceps, Ixodes uriae, I. ovatus, Ixodes columnae, I. granulatus, Ixodes nipponensis, Ixodes tanuki, Ixodes turdus, Ixodes minor, Ixodes muris, I. spinipalpis, Ixodes dentatus, Ixodes angustus,* and *Ixodes jellisoni* (33). The importance of these vectors varies considerably, depending on their proclivity to feed on people and competent reservoir hosts, local vector densities, and the strains of borreliae being transmitted. Ecological cycles maintaining these borreliae in nature may be quite complex. In the northeastern United States, where enzootic maintenance appears to be the most simple, cycles involving *B. burgdorferi* sensu stricto transmitted by *I. scapularis* among white-footed mice (*P. leucopus*) and eastern chipmunks (*Tamias striatus*) are complicated by parallel cycles involving *I. dentatus*, varying habitat-related host and vector community dynamics, and trends in host population densities that influence transmission risks. The late-20th-century white-tailed deer expansion (with contemporary overabundance) appears to be the principal driving force in the emergence of LB in the eastern United States, since, as primary maintenance hosts, their presence determines the distribution and densities of *I. scapularis* populations (109). *Peromyscus* spp. reservoir populations experience considerable year-to-year variation in abundance associated, in part, with changes in availability of their major food sources of acorns and gypsy moths (62, 64).

In the far-western United States, cycles are complicated by multiple species of coexisting borreliae (*B. burgdorferi* sensu stricto, *B. bissettii*, and several unnamed strains of unknown pathogenicity to people) that are transmitted by at least four species of vectors (*I. pacificus, I. spinipalpis, I. angustus,* and *I. jellisoni*) through a combined reservoir that involves dusky-footed woodrats (*Neotoma fuscipes*) and other small mammals (11, 12, 77, 78, 80, 106, 107). Another complexity of transmission cycles in this region is presented by locally abundant lizards (including *Sceloporus occidentalis* and *Elgaria multicarinata*) that have borrelicidal factors in their blood (74, 81). Since large numbers of immature *I. pacificus* feed on these hosts and because spirochetes in infected ticks that feed on lizards are killed, lizards serve a zooprophylactic role;

prevalence of borreliae is thought to be lower in quest-ing populations of *I. pacificus* nymphs and adults due to immature ticks feeding on lizards (81, 109). The role of lizards in influencing transmission risks cor-relates well with the general pattern of prevalence of borreliae in North American tick populations; pre-valence is relatively high in the northeastern United States, where lizards are absent or rare, and relatively low in the southeastern and far-western United States, where lizards are relatively common (109). Bites by *A. americanum* in the southern and southeastern coastal United States have been associated with a self-limited rash illness similar to erythema migrans, called southern tick-associated rash illness (STARI). Persons with STARI do not react serologically to major anti-gens specific to *B. burgdorferi*. An uncultivable borre-lial spirochete, provisionally named *Borrelia lonestari* and phylogenetically related to *Borrelia miyamotoi* and *Borrelia theileri*, has been identified in *A. ameri-canum* by PCR amplification of borrelial DNA, but it has yet to be shown to be a cause of STARI (27, 109).

Cycles in Europe are still more complicated by additional species of human pathogenic borreliae (most importantly *B. afzelii* and *B. garinii*) as well as cycles involving secondary vectors (*I. hexagonus, I. uriae,* and *I. trianguliceps*). Cycles in Asia include a larger list of potential borrelial pathogens (including *B. burg-dorferi* sensu stricto, *B. afzelii, B. garinii, Borrelia japonica, Borrelia lusitaniae, B. tanukii, B. turdi,* and *B. valaisiana*) and a large number of potential sec-ondary vectors (including *I. columnae, I. granulatus, I. nipponensis, I. ovatus, I. tanuki,* and *I. turdus*) (72, 93). Lastly, the ranges of *I. persulcatus* and *I. ricinus* overlap broadly through eastern Europe and western Russia (33, 48, 72). Although the existence of parallel cycles in these two primary Eurasian systems appears not to increase the prevalence in vectors above those noted from areas beyond the zone of sympatry, addi-tional complexity of risk factors must develop with the overlap of these two competent vectors. Several authors have discussed the potential role of birds as borrelial reservoirs or transport hosts (48, 72, 93, 109), and *B. garinii* is associated with avian reservoirs in Eurasia. However, even when birds are not compe-tent reservoir hosts, their roles as transport hosts for ticks infected with *B. burgdorferi* sensu lato may be important to the geographic movements of these agents.

TBRF

Agents and distribution of human cases of TBRF.
TBRFs are caused by a large number of closely related species of borrelial spirochetes. These spirochetes are distinguished by the ability to change their outer sur-face antigenic character in their human hosts, thereby allowing immunological escape and relapsing waves of spirochetemia and fever alternating with asympto-matic periods when the suppressed agent is unde-tectable in the blood. The species of TBRF borreliae historically have been named for the principal argasid tick vectors responsible for maintaining enzootic in-fections and for transmitting infection to humans (Table 2). Little is known about many of these borre-liae, and the importance of some of them as a cause of human disease has yet to be established. TBRF is widely distributed throughout the world; although re-liable statistics are unavailable, most cases are thought to occur in rural areas of Africa, the Middle East, and central Asia. One of the most important TBRF agents in Africa, *Borrelia duttonii*, has no known enzootic vertebrate reservoir. The agents causing TBRF in hu-mans in the United States are *Borrelia hermsii, Borre-lia turicatae,* and (reported once) *Borrelia parkeri* (32). In the United States, TBRF is endemic only in the western region, with most cases occurring in forested mountainous areas of the Rocky Mountains, Cas-cades, and Sierra Nevada Range (usually at eleva-tions above 1,500 m), where *B. hermsii* is the princi-pal cause of TBRF. Sporadic small clusters of cases of TBRF caused by *B. turicatae* have been reported from Texas, Oklahoma, and Kansas, especially in persons exposed to rodent-infested limestone caves. The en-zootic *B. parkeri* distribution overlaps that of *B. hermsii*, but it occurs at lower elevations.

Vectors of TBRF.
The TBRF borreliae are trans-mitted by soft ticks (family Argasidae) of the genera *Ornithodoros* and *Carios* (Color Maps 8 and 11). In contrast to ixodids, argasids molt through multiple nymphal stages, feed multiple times as adults, oviposit multiple clutches of eggs, feed rapidly (often requiring 30 min or less for a complete blood meal), and survive several years of starvation if necessary. Most relapsing fever spirochetes demonstrate consid-erable specificity for their vectors (13, 132), so foci of transmission risk tend to be ecologically restricted.

Although they may be opportunistic feeders, many argasids are habitat specialists found most commonly near the nests, tree cavities, burrows, bird roosts, and rest sites of their main hosts. Ticks that transmit re-lapsing fever spirochetes typically show rodent host specificity, and, with the exception of *B. duttonii*, these rodents serve as the reservoirs of relapsing fever borreliae. Because most of these vectors live in the burrows or nests of their typical hosts, enzootic foci tend to be ecologically restricted to those specific hosts and habitat associations, and most human cases occur as sporadic events related to individuals or

Table 2. Agents, vectors, and regional distributions of tick-borne borrelioses

Human disease and *Borrelia* species	Primary vector(s)	Geographical region
LB		
B. burgdorferi sensu lato	*I. ricinus* complex	Holarctic
B. burgdorferi sensu stricto	*I. ricinus, I. scapularis, I. pacificus*	North America and Europe
B. afzelii	*I. ricinus, I. persulcatus*	Eurasia
B. garinii	*I. ricinus, I. persulcatus*	Eurasia
TBRF		
B. caucasica	**O. asperus**	Former Soviet Union, Iraq, Armenia, Azerbaijan, Georgia, Caucasia
B. crocidurae, B. dipodilli, B. merionesi, B. microti	**O. erraticus** sensu lato (including *O. erraticus* sensu stricto, *O. alactagalis, O. graingeri, O. sonrai*)	**North African coast from Morocco to Egypt; probably much of rural West Africa, including Senegal, Kenya; Greece; Cyprus; Turkey; Armenia; Azerbaijan; Turkmenistan; Iran**
B. duttonii	*O. moubata*	Central, eastern, and southern Africa
B. hermsii	*O. hermsi*	Western North America
B. hispanica	**O. erraticus** sensu lato (including *O. macrocanus*)	**Portugal, Spain, Greece, Cyprus, and North African coast**
B. latyschewii	*O. tartakovskyi*	Central Asian republics and Iran
B. persica	*O. tholozani*	Former Soviet Union, Middle East, northeast Africa, and India
B. mazzottii	*C. talaje*	Southern United States, Mexico, Central America, South America
B. turicatae	*O. turicata*	Western United States and Mexico
B. venezuelensi	*C. rudis*	Central and South America to northern Peru, Bolivia, western Brazil
STARI		
B. lonestari	*A. americanum*	Mid-Atlantic and southern United States

small groups of people who expose themselves to the vectors. *Ornithodoros parkeri* (Color Map 11) has been recovered most often from the burrows of ground squirrels and other rodents and is a relative specialist, feeding only opportunistically on non-burrow-dwelling hosts and only rarely on people. In contrast, *Ornithodoros hermsi* (Color Map 11), which occurs at higher elevations, feeds more broadly, including on ground squirrels (*Spermophilus* spp.), deer mice (*P. maniculatus*), and chipmunks (*Tamias* spp.) (46). *O. hermsi* occupies a wider habitat, having been recovered from tree cavities, downed woody debris, and rodent-inhabited cabins, as well as from rodent burrows. Another possible exception may be *Borrelia coriaceae*, which appears to be maintained in cycles involving *Ornithodoros coriaceus* and Columbian black-tailed deer in California (79).

O. tholozani (Color Map 11), an important vector of TBRF in the Middle East, is a fairly indiscriminate feeder. It is commonly associated with caves and rock outcrops, as well as houses and barns, where it feeds opportunistically on livestock and people as well as on its normal rodent hosts.

As noted earlier, *B. duttonii*, which is transmitted by *Ornithodoros moubata* (Color Map 11) in equatorial Africa, is an exception to the other TBRF spirochetes in that it has no known rodent or other animal

reservoir. The tick vector normally inhabits cracks in the floors, walls, and roofs of mud and thatch houses.

Borreliae are able to penetrate many tissues in their tick vectors, including salivary glands and coxal glands of some species. As ticks feed, they concentrate blood in their gut and excrete excess fluids through their coxal glands; coxal fluid excretion is most pronounced in large-bodied, adult argasids that feed to full repletion in as little as 30 min. Coxal fluids may contain spirochetes, and infections may result via excreted borreliae at the site of the tick bite; this appears to be an important route of transmission from *O. moubata* sensu stricto to people.

Readers are advised that the taxonomy of the family Argasidae was revised recently (70) and that some historic associations of borreliae with the genus *Ornithodoros* are now associated with the genus *Carios*; e.g., the designations of *Carios rudis* (Color Map 8) and *Carios talaje* (Color Map 4) have replaced *Ornithodoros rudis* and *Ornithodoros talaje*, respectively.

Epidemiology, ecology, and alternate routes of transmission of TBRF. Following a typical incubation period of about 7 days (range, 2 to 18 days), patients with TBRF experience a sudden onset of acute, severe illness with symptoms of high fever, headache, shaking chills and sweats, myalgias, and arthralgias, rapidly leading to prostration (26). It is characterized by relapsing periods of fever and spirochetemia (mean duration, 5 days) interspersed with remissions lasting days or weeks. It can be complicated by bleeding, especially epistaxis and sometimes petechiation, gastrointestinal bleeding, meningitis, cranial nerve palsies, and Jarisch-Herxheimer reactions precipitated by rapid spirochete clearance. In sub-Saharan Africa, TBRF is an important fetal-threatening complication of pregnancy (63), and the overall case-fatality rate for TBRF in Africa may be as high as 5%. In the United States, fatalities from TBRF are rare (32).

In contrast to epidemic louse-borne relapsing fever, TBRF is an endemic, mostly sporadic infection of humans. Because many tick vectors inhabit human dwellings, cases often occur in familial clusters. Outbreaks can occasionally occur when many persons share infested dwellings, such as guest houses or groups of cabins (105). The number of cases occurring worldwide is unknown, but many thousands of cases of relapsing fever caused by B. duttonii probably occur each year.

The relapsing fever borreliae are not known to be transmitted directly from person to person, except by transplacental passage, infective blood exposure of infants during parturition, and the rare infective exposure of health workers to contaminated blood. Transmission by blood transfusion is possible but has not been documented.

In the United States, 30 to 50 cases of TBRF are reported annually, almost entirely due to B. hermsii infection, and most humans are exposed when they stay in rustic, rodent-infested cabins in forested mountainous areas in far-western states (32). Risk to humans is increased when the rodents that normally inhabit these structures are killed by rodenticides or experience natural die-offs and their ticks seek alternate human hosts. Control can be achieved by removing rodent nests, applying acaricides, and rodent-proofing dwellings (105).

Babesiosis

Agents and distribution of human cases of babesiosis

Babesiosis is caused by infection with several species of intraerythrocytic sporozoan parasites of the genus Babesia. Immunocompromised persons, especially splenectomized individuals, are at greatest risk of acquiring the disease. Babesia bovis and Babesia divergens are parasites of cattle that have caused rare cases of human babesiosis in Europe. More recently, Babesia microti, a parasite of small rodents in the United States, has been found to be an important emerging in-

fection of persons living in areas endemic for I. scapularis, especially coastal New England, New York, and the north-central states of Wisconsin and Minnesota (50, 68). A few cases of babesiosis have been reported also from Washington State and California. The parasites involved in these western cases (identified by case numbers WA1, WA2, CA1, etc.) are only distantly related to B. microti.

Vectors and enzootic maintenance of babesiosis

B. divergens in central Europe is transmitted by I. ricinus (50, 68). Cases have also been reported from Mexico, the Canary Islands, Egypt, South Africa, Mozambique, China, and Taiwan (50, 68). In these areas, enzootic maintenance and primary vectors are unknown. I. scapularis is the only identified vector of B. microti to humans. Although B. microti occurs in Europe, where it is transmitted enzootically by I. trianguliceps, I. trianguliceps does not commonly feed on people, and no human cases of this parasite have been reported from Europe. The vectors of Babesia in the western United States are not known. Although enzootic maintenance also remains unexplained, parasites isolated from natural infections of mule deer, Odocoileus hemionus, and bighorn sheep, Ovis canadensis, were genetically quite similar to those from human cases in California (68).

Epidemiology, ecology, and alternate routes of transmission of babesiosis

Illness caused by infection with B. microti ranges from a mild, self-limiting, viral-like febrile illness to a severe and sometimes fatal hemolytic anemia, depending mostly on the immune status of the host. In the United States, several hundred cases of babesiosis caused by B. microti have been reported over the relatively short period since its recognition in the 1980s. There has been an emerging trend of increasing numbers of reported cases and slow geographic expansion in the New England coastal focus into New York and New Jersey (57). The ecology of B. microti in the northeastern United States is similar to that of B. burgdorferi and A. phagocytophilum, with which it shares its reservoir rodent hosts and tick vectors. However, the emergence of babesiosis has been much slower and less intense than that of Lyme borreliosis; cases mostly occur on islands off the coast of Connecticut, Rhode Island, and Massachusetts. Because babesia parasites are intraerythrocytic and cause chronic and sometimes mild or subclinical infection, it is not surprising that transmission of infection through transfusion of blood products is an important problem in babesiosis-endemic areas (91).

PRIMARY VECTORS OF TICK-BORNE DISEASES

Primary vectors are those species most responsible for transmitting the tick-borne agents to people. In some cases, tick-borne pathogens are vector specialists (such as some of the TBRF spirochetes); in these cases, the enzootic maintenance vector also serves as the primary vector to humans. However, there are some species of ticks that transmit pathogens between animals but that do not feed on people, occur in populations of low density relative to the primary vectors, or have a restricted host or geographic range. These species are considered secondary vectors. In some cases, however, the maintenance of the agent in natural foci may depend on secondary vectors, and the role of the primary vector may be mainly that of bridging natural cycles to humans. As examples, competent secondary vectors of *B. burgdorferi* sensu lato include *I. angustus* (a rodent parasite in northeastern Asia and cool regions of North America), *I. muris* (which feeds mainly on rodents in the northeastern and midwestern United States), *I. minor* (a rodent parasite distributed from the southeastern United States through Central America and into South America), *I. jellisoni* (a specialist parasite of heteromyid rodents, including *Dipodomys californicus*, in the coastal mountains of California), *I. hexagonus* (a vector of *B. burgdorferi* sensu stricto and encephalitis viruses in Europe and northern Africa), and *I. spinipalpis* (a vector of Powassan encephalitis virus, *A. phagocytophilum*, *B. burgdorferi* sensu stricto, and *B. bissettii* in the western United States) (33). In Colorado, *I. spinipalpis* maintains enzootic cycles of *B. bissettii* involving the Mexican woodrat (*Neotoma mexicana*), but this spirochete has not been established as a human pathogen; due to the absence of *I. ricinus* complex ticks in this region, there is little risk of human exposure (90). The potential of several other *I. ricinus* complex ticks as secondary vectors of *B. burgdorferi* sensu lato, including *I. trianguliceps* in Europe and Asia and *I. granulatus*, *I. nipponensis*, and *I. ovatus* in the Far East, is still under investigation. The ecological roles of secondary vectors may be important in maintaining infection in nature, but because they do not pose a direct threat to humans they are not considered further in this chapter.

Ixodidae

Most species of ixodids are three-host ticks; larvae and nymphs drop off of their hosts after feeding and then find another host for subsequent blood meals. *R. evertsi* and some populations of *H. marginatum* are two-host ticks; larvae do not drop off of their host after feeding but instead molt on the host and feed again on the same host as nymphs. Such life history characteristics have obvious impacts on the potential of a vector to transmit agents among different hosts.

Amblyomma americanum

A. americanum (the lone star tick) is a vector of *E. chaffeensis*, *E. ewingii*, *C. burnetti*, and *F. tularensis*. It has been discussed as a potential vector of *R. rickettsii* (21) and found to be infected with *B. lonestari*. This species is distributed from Iowa eastward throughout the southeastern United States, along the Atlantic seaboard north to Maine and southward into northeastern Mexico (Color Map 5). It is associated generally with woodlands throughout its range and is most commonly found in disturbed hardwood forests with young trees and dense brush. *A. americanum* is a non-nidicolous, three-host species that feeds on a wide variety of hosts. Immature stages feed widely on birds and mammals of all sizes, and adults feed on medium-sized and large mammals (including carnivores, livestock, deer, and humans), but they are especially dependent upon white-tailed deer (94). Seasonality varies with latitude, but nymphal and adult lone star ticks feed most actively during spring, and larvae are most active during early to midsummer.

Amblyomma cajennense

A. cajennense (the cayenne tick) is a vector of the agent causing RMSF. The species ranges from southern Texas, through Mexico and Central America (including Cuba and Jamaica) and throughout South America to southern Brazil and northern Argentina (Color Map 5). This species is found most commonly in dry tropical habitats and lower elevations of subtropical highlands; it is especially associated with hilly agricultural areas frequented by livestock and people. *A. cajennense* is a non-nidicolous, three-host species that feeds on a wide variety of hosts; although adults are most commonly found on livestock, all stages feed aggressively on people. Cayenne ticks are encountered throughout the year but may be relatively less active during midwinter in the extreme northern and southern regions of their distribution, and they are most commonly encountered during the dry season in relatively wet tropical regions (38, 49, 55).

Amblyomma hebraeum

A. hebraeum (the bont tick) is a vector of the agents causing MSF and ATBF. This species occurs widely in southern Africa from central Zimbabwe, western Botswana, southern Mozambique, and much of northern, eastern, and southern South Africa; there are also sporadic reports from Zambia (Color Map 5). Like the tropical bont tick (*A. variegatum*), *A. hebraeum* feeds on a variety of mammals; adults feed heavily on large ungulates, including livestock, and all stages will bite people. At its northern distribution in Zambia, this species occurs sporadically in areas that receive 60 to 130 cm of rain annually; however, Tandon suggested that the species has not yet established stable populations in that country (136). The bont tick lacks obvious seasonality; all stages may be active throughout the year (96).

Amblyomma lepidum

A. lepidum is a vector of the agent causing MSF in East Africa. The distribution includes eastern Sudan (with isolated populations in the north and patchily through the south of that country), Ethiopia, southern Somalia, Kenya, Uganda, and northern and central Tanzania (Color Map 3). This three-host tick thrives under arid and semiarid conditions of 22 to 80 cm of precipitation per year, but it also occurs in areas of Uganda where annual precipitation exceeds 130 cm of rain annually. Although typically found at elevations of less than 1,500 m, it has been recorded from elevations ranging from sea level to 2,500 m in xeric habitats, including woodlands, acacia scrublands, and mixed scrub grasslands (89, 144). Cattle and wild ungulates are the typical hosts of all stages, but immature ticks are found on small mammals, and adults occasionally feed on carnivores. This is a hardy species with broad tolerance limits, and the factors limiting its geographic distribution are not understood (97). These ticks feed on cattle throughout the year (89).

Amblyomma variegatum

A. variegatum (the tropical bont tick) transmits the agents causing CCHF, MSF, and, putatively, ATBF. This species occurs in Yemen, West and East Africa south of the Sahel (excepting the Central Democratic Republic of Congo and all but the northwestern tip of Somalia), and extends southward into northern Botswana, the Caprivi Strip of Namibia, northern Zimbabwe, Mozambique, and the island of Madagascar. Lastly, this species has been introduced to the islands of Guadeloupe, Martinique, Marie-Galante, and Antigua in the Caribbean (Color Map 5) (98, 130). It is replaced by the bont tick, *A. hebraeum*, a closely related species, along the southern border of its distribution (96). *A. variegatum* is a three-host tick that feeds on a large variety of small and large mammals, birds, and lizards as immature ticks. Adults feed heavily on cattle, as well as on wild ungulates and occasionally humans. In Kenya, the majority of ticks are

collected from moist forests, scrublands, and mixed scrub grasslands that typically receive greater than 18 cm of rain annually and in Uganda from areas receiving 65 to 190 cm of rain annually (89, 144). Tolerance to xeric environments is apparently greater than that of the bont tick (138), but less than that of *A. lepidum*. This species lacks obvious seasonality; all stages may be active throughout the year.

Dermacentor andersoni

D. andersoni (the Rocky Mountain wood tick) is a vector of the agents of CTF, RMSF, Powassan encephalitis, and tularemia, and it is an important cause of paralysis in livestock, wildlife, and humans. The distribution of this species includes southern regions of British Columbia, Alberta, and Saskatchewan; the western Great Plains of the United States; and across the Rocky Mountain and Great Basin regions to the Modoc Plateau and the east slope of the Sierra Nevada Range in California (Color Map 5) (46, 49, 54). It is encountered in a variety of wooded and brushy habitats in the Rocky Mountains with elevations above 1,000 m to over 3,000 m. This non-nidicolous, three-host tick feeds on small mammals, including ground squirrels, chipmunks, woodrats, and mice in its immature stages; adult ticks feed on medium-sized to large mammals, including carnivores, deer, livestock, and people. This general pattern of immature stages feeding on small mammals and adults feeding on medium to large mammals is repeated throughout the genus *Dermacentor*. Adults are active during spring and early summer, and larvae are active somewhat later during midsummer.

Dermacentor marginatus

D. marginatus (the ornate sheep tick) is a vector of the agents causing CEE, OHF, MSF, Czechoslovakian tick typhus (*R. slovaca*), NATT, Q fever, and tularemia. This species occurs throughout Europe from the Iberian Peninsula, central France, Germany, and Poland and eastward to Iran and central Russia (Color Map 6) in habitats as varied as lowland forest, semidesert regions, scrub steppe, alpine steppe, and grasslands. Immature stages feed on various small mammals, and occasionally on birds, and adults feed on medium to large mammals, including dogs, sheep, and people. Larvae typically feed in early summer, nymphs feed during mid- to late summer, and adults are active during autumn and early spring (49).

Dermacentor nuttalli

D. nuttalli is a vector of the agents causing NATT and tularemia in Asia (Color Map 6). This species occurs throughout Siberia and south through central Asia, northern Mongolia, and China. Immature *D. nuttalli* feed on small mammals such as mice, rats, hamsters, marmots, rabbits, cats, and dogs during summer, and adults feed on large mammals including dogs, livestock, and humans during spring. It is a common species of grasslands and steppe regions and thrives in pastures and other agricultural areas; it is reportedly uncommon in dense forests and woodlands (49).

Dermacentor occidentalis

D. occidentalis (the Pacific Coast tick) is a potential vector of the agents causing CTF and RMSF. This species occurs in a variety of wooded and brushy habitats from northern Baja California in Mexico and north through most of California and western Oregon in the United States (Color Map 5). Immature stages feed most heavily on small and medium-sized mammals (including rabbits, rodents, and small carnivores), and adults feed on medium-sized to large mammals (including deer, carnivores, livestock, and people). All stages are most active during spring and summer (46).

Dermacentor reticulatus

D. reticulatus (the ornate cow tick) is a vector of the agents causing OHF, MSF, NATT, and Q fever. The distribution includes Wales and southwest England, central Europe through Russia, and the northern forest-steppe region of the Omsk district of western Siberia (Color Map 5). Adults feed on large mammals, including people, during spring and autumn. Unlike many other *Dermacentor* species that feed on a variety of small mammals, immature *D. reticulatus* ticks in Europe feed predominately on water voles, other rodents, and occasionally birds.

Dermacentor silvarum

D. silvarum is a vector of the agents causing NATT and the recently identified "*Rickettsia heilongjiangii*." This species occurs from eastern Europe and eastward through the steppes of central Asia, Mongolia, and northern China to Japan (Color Map 5). Hosts of immature ticks include a variety of small mammals, and adults feed on medium-sized to large mammals, including humans. All stages of *D. silvarum* feed during the summer months. Like the Rocky Mountain wood tick in the Western Hemisphere, this species is associated with disturbed forests with shrubs and young second-growth trees, including areas of taiga forest cleared for cultivation.

Dermacentor variabilis

D. variabilis (the American dog tick) is a vector of the agents causing RMSF, HME, and tularemia, and it causes tick paralysis in dogs and people. This tick occurs throughout the southeastern United States east of central Texas and the Mississippi River basin, with an important northward extension along the Atlantic seaboard to Nova Scotia (Color Map 6) (130). Disjunct populations occur also in the midwestern states, parts of southern Canada as far west as Saskatchewan, and south through central Mexico to the Yucatan Peninsula, as well in California and Oregon (49, 130). These ticks thrive in disturbed (second-growth) forests, along roads, in brushy areas around homes, and along the edges of fields and forests. The American dog tick is a non-nidicolous, three-host tick that feeds in its immature stages on a variety of small mammals including deer mice, rice rats, voles, chipmunks, and tree squirrels and on medium and large mammals as adults. It is an aggressive human-biter and is most active during the late spring and summer months (49, 130).

Haemaphysalis concinna

H. concinna (the relict tick) is a vector of the agents causing RSSE, NATT, and tularemia. The distribution includes much of Europe eastward through Asia to China, Japan, and Vietnam (Color Map 3). Habitat associations include hardwood, taiga, and mixed forests; tussock swamps; and birch-aspen groves. Yamaguti et al. (149) reported that optimal conditions occur in the oak forests and mountain valleys where vegetation keeps humidity high. All stages are active from spring to autumn, with peak activity occurring in June and July. Larvae and nymphs feed on small mammals, birds, and reptiles; adults feed on large mammals, including deer and livestock; and all stages reportedly bite humans (49).

Haemaphysalis flava

H. flava is a vector of the agents causing JSF and tularemia. The distribution includes most of Japan and the southern tip of South Korea (Color Map 6). Immature stages feed on small to large mammals and birds and are found on hares during all seasons. Adult ticks feed most commonly on dogs and hares during autumn, winter, and spring but are absent in summer (149).

Haemaphysalis japonica

H. japonica is a vector of the agent causing NATT. The distribution includes the Hokkaido, Aomori, and Nagano prefectures of Japan; North and South Korea; Siberia; and northern China (Color Map 6). Habitats include foothills and valleys with thick grass and shrubs. The ticks are rare on more exposed slopes. Immature stages feed on small and medium mammals and birds during summer. Adults feed on various mammals, including hedgehogs, deer, dogs, and people, with peak activity in June and July (149).

Haemaphysalis leachi

H. leachi (the yellow dog tick) is a vector of *R. conorii*, the agent causing MSF. This species occurs throughout much of sub-Saharan Africa, with collections also from Libya, Algeria, Sudan, Egypt, and India (Color Map 6). Larvae and nymphs feed on rodents including reservoirs of *R. conorii*, and adults feed most commonly on dogs, civets, jackals, and large felids. All stages of this species are active from spring through autumn (49, 130). *H. leachi* occurs from sea level to elevations of over 2,500 m in all life zones receiving 65 to over 200 cm of rain annually (89). These ticks may survive in considerably drier regions by benefiting from the higher humidity of commonly used animal bedding areas (138).

Haemaphysalis longicornis

H. longicornis is a vector of the agents causing JSF and Q fever. The distribution includes Australia, New Zealand, New Caledonia, Fiji, Tonga, the Friendly Islands, Efate Island, New Hebrides, Japan, South Korea, North Korea, northern China (near Beijing), and Siberia (Color Map 3) (120, 149). It parasitizes birds and mammals such as cattle, deer, marsupials, rodents, hares, and people. Parthenogenetic populations occur on the northern islands of Japan. Oki Island apparently has both sexual and parthenogenetic populations, and females from sexually reproducing laboratory colonies will readily convert to parthenogenesis when deprived of males (149).

Haemaphysalis spinigera

H. spinigera is a vector of the virus causing KFD. The species is distributed throughout central and southern India and Sri Lanka; east through South Asia, Malaysia, and Indonesia; and east as far as Papua New Guinea (Color Map 5). This species is common in the dense forests of the Karnataka state in southwestern India. Larvae feed on small mammals and birds during October and November. Nymphs and adults feed on larger mammals, including cattle, monkeys, and people, during November to June, and July and August, respectively. It appears to flourish in disturbed areas of the forest; as disturbance increases, tick populations continue to expand, facilitating transmission of the virus to susceptible monkeys and people (49, 132).

Hyalomma anatolicum

H. anatolicum (the small Anatolian hyalomma) is a vector of the virus causing CCHF. The species ranges from the United Kingdom, east through southern Russia and the western border of China, northwestern India, and the Middle East; and through North Africa, Sudan, Somalia, and Kenya (Color Map 4). All stages are most active during summer months. This tick has adapted well to arid environments where it overwinters by aestivating in cracks in floors and walls of wooden structures and in rodent burrows.

Hyalomma asiaticum

H. asiaticum (the asiatic hyalomma) is a vector of the agent causing NATT and of *R. mongolotimonae*. The distribution covers arid steppes and semideserts of central Asia, including southern Russia, Kazakhstan, Uzbekistan, Turkmenistan, western China, Mongolia, Pakistan, Afganistan, Iran, and Iraq (Color Map 4). Immature ticks feed on small and medium-sized mammals and adults feed on large mammals such as camels, cattle, sheep, and goats and on people; all stages are active during spring and summer. In southern Russia, enzootic foci of NATT occur in the southern steppes and arid foothills where jirds (*Meriones* sp.) occur along overgrown, dry irrigation canals (49, 132).

Hyalomma marginatum

H. marginatum is the primary vector of the virus causing CCHF and transmits *R. aeschlimanni* and the agents causing OHF, MSF, and tularemia. This species is widespread throughout southern Europe, Africa, the Middle East, India, and Southeast Asia; its northern border includes northern Europe, where immature stages have been found on migratory birds, but adults have not been established, southern Russia, and southern China (Color Map 8). Immature ticks feed opportunistically on available mammals, but most feed on small mammals and birds. Adults feed on larger mammals, and all stages are aggressive human biters. Different populations have life cycles utilizing either two or three hosts. Like the other species of *Hyalomma* mentioned, this species is adapted to arid environments of steppe regions, dry woodlands, semideserts, and grasslands where precipitation varies from 15 to >100 cm annually (89, 144). These ticks are most active during summer and inactive during winter (49, 132).

Ixodes cookei

I. cookei is a vector of the virus causing PWE. This North American species is distributed throughout southeastern Canada and the United States east of the Rocky Mountains (Color Map 3). *I. cookei* feeds on a variety of wild mammals, including woodchucks (*M. monax*), skunks (*Mephitis* spp.), and foxes (*Vulpes vulpes*), as well as livestock and people. Woodchucks appear to be an important reservoir of PWE in the northeastern United States and southern Canada, and most cases of PWE in North America are within the range of *I. cookei* (34).

Ixodes granulatus

I. granulatus is a vector of the agents causing Langat, MSF, TTT, and *Rickettsia thailandi*. It occurs in Japan from central Honshu southward to Okinawa, South Korea, Thailand, Luzon Island in the Philippines, Malaysia, and India (Color Map 4). Although this species primarily feeds on rodents, adult ticks have been removed from a bird and a human (149).

Ixodes holocyclus

I. holocyclus (the Australian paralysis tick) is the vector of *R. australis*, the agent causing QTT, as well as a primary cause of tick paralysis. This species is distributed along the eastern coastline of Australia where it occurs in heavily vegetated rain forests (Color Map 4). It feeds on a wide variety of mammals and birds including livestock, dogs, and people, but bandicoots (*Perameles nasuta* and *Isoodon* spp.), various possums (*Trichosurus* spp.), rats (*Rattus* spp.), and rabbits (*Oryctolagus cuniculus*) are important wild hosts (120). *I. holocyclus* is active throughout the year, but peak larval activity occurs during summer and autumn, nymphs are most common during winter and early spring, and adults are most numerous during spring (October and November).

Ixodes ovatus

I. ovatus is a vector of the agents causing RSSE, JSF, tularemia, and (putatively) LB. This species is found in the Russian Far East (2), China, the northern islands of Japan, Nepal, Sikkim, and Burma (Color Map 2) (149). Immature forms of this species feed on wild rodents, and adults feed most commonly on hares and large mammals, including livestock and people.

Ixodes pacificus

I. pacificus (the western black-legged tick) is a vector of the agents causing LB, HGA, and babesiosis. This species is distributed throughout the Pacific Coast region of the United States from southern British Columbia through coastal southern California and into the mountains of northern Baja California, Mexico,

as well as in isolated populations in Arizona, Utah, and Nevada (Color Map 2). Western black-legged ticks thrive in revegetated, disturbed forest and chaparral habitats with adequate humidity and appear to be widely distributed across habitat types of the Far West; *I. pacificus* is limited by mountains and arid lands to the east of its range. Seasonality varies with latitude and habitat, but adults are active generally from the autumn until spring, larvae are active in spring and early summer, and nymphs are most active during mid- to late spring (99). This is a non-nidicolous, three-host species whose immature forms feed on a variety of mammals (mostly small mammals), birds, and lizards, and whose adults feed commonly on medium and large mammals including Columbian black-tailed deer, carnivores, and people. As with *I. ricinus* and *I. scapularis*, *I. pacificus* nymphs appear to be the most significant vectors of agents causing human diseases (22, 76).

Ixodes persulcatus

I. persulcatus (the taiga tick) is a vector of the agents that cause PWE, OHF, RSSE, HGA, LB, and tularemia. The taiga tick is distributed widely over the southern forests of Russia (Color Map 2). The distribution (Color Map 2) extends from Estonia and Latvia, through most of southern Russia to the tip of the Kamchatka Peninsula, far-eastern Kazakhstan, the forests of the Tien Shan of Kyrgyzstan and northwestern China, northern Mongolia, Inner Mongolia, Manchuria, North Korea, and northern Japan (72, 149). The taiga tick is a non-nidicolous, three-host tick that feeds heavily on small vertebrates (rodents, rabbits, hares, and birds) in larval and nymphal stages and on a variety of medium and large mammals as adults. Seasonality varies between regions, but immature ticks are generally active during late spring and early summer. Importantly, like *I. scapularis* in North America, nymphs tend to feed earlier in the year than larvae, intensifying enzootic transmission which ultimately increases human risk (33). In contrast to *I. pacificus*, *I. scapularis* and *I. ricinus* (for which nymphs are the most important primary vectors of *B. burgdorferi* sensu lato and probably other zoonotic agents), adult female *I. persulcatus* appears to present the greatest risk for people. Adult ticks may be active throughout the year in some regions but tend to be encountered most commonly during spring and autumn.

Ixodes ricinus

I. ricinus (the castor bean or common sheep tick) is a vector of the agents causing CEE, LI, Eyach fever, HGA, LB, babesiosis, tularemia, Q fever, and *R. helvetica*. The sheep tick (Color Map 2) occurs from

Iceland throughout southern Scandinavia and all of Europe east to the Ural Mountains of Russia, along the Mediterranean region of North Africa, Turkey, Cyprus, Georgia, Armenia, and northern Iran (48, 72). Its typical habitat includes deciduous, mixed, and coniferous forests; heathlands; moorlands; and tall grasslands that support the humid microclimates necessary for high densities of *I. ricinus*. Immature ticks feed on mammals (such as rabbits, rodents, and hedgehogs), birds, and reptiles, and most adults feed on medium and large mammals. Seasonality varies between regions, but bimodal peaks of activity in spring and autumn are reported for all stages; larger numbers of adults are active in spring and more larvae are active during autumn (48). Importantly, in most situations, nymphal activity does not precede larval activity, and enzootic transmission is not intensified by this mechanism, as are some agents maintained by *I. persulcatus* and *I. scapularis* (33).

Ixodes scapularis

I. scapularis (the black-legged or deer tick [includes *Ixodes dammini*]) is a vector of the agents causing PWE, HGA, LB, babesiosis, and tularemia. This species occurs in North America from southeastern Canada along the Atlantic coast and as far west as Saskatchewan, through the eastern half of the United States to eastern Texas and Florida (Color Map 2). The species is something of a habitat generalist, being found in grasslands, shrubs, and a variety of forest types, but it is generally found in deciduous forests with adequate leaf litter (109). Seasonality varies between regions, but immature ticks are generally active during late spring and early summer when nymphal *I. scapularis* present the greatest risk as vectors of agents of human disease. Importantly, like *I. persulcatus* in Asia, nymphs in northern areas tend to be active prior to larvae, intensifying enzootic transmission and increasing human risk (33). In the northern areas of the United States, immature black-legged ticks feed heavily on small mammals and birds. In southern areas, immature stages feed on a wider variety of hosts, including lizards, especially in southern areas of their distribution. Adults throughout their range feed on medium- and large-bodied mammals, including deer, livestock, carnivores, and people.

Rhipicephalus appendiculatus

R. appendiculatus (the African brown ear tick) is a vector of the agent causing MSF and *R. aeschlimanni* (130) as well as several important veterinary pathogens. This three-host species occurs from the southeastern corner of the Central African Republic and southern Sudan and in scattered locations throughout eastern

Democratic Republic of Congo, Uganda, Rwanda, Burundi, southwestern Kenya, Tanzania, Malawi, Zambia, Zimbabwe, southeastern Botswana, southwestern Mozambique, and the eastern half of South Africa (Color Map 4) (49, 97, 145). The patchy distribution throughout this region correlates well with moderate temperatures and precipitation (30 to 200 cm annually), adequate vegetation (including tall grass savannahs with brush or woodlands), and density of cattle (97, 130). All stages feed opportunistically on a wide variety of mammals; larvae and nymphs are found commonly on smaller antelope, hares (*Lepus* spp.), Burchell's zebra (*Equus burchellii*), warthogs (*Phacochoerus africanus*), and domestic dogs; adults are removed commonly from wild carnivores and larger ungulates, but cattle appear to be important hosts for all stages in most areas. In tropical regions, there is no discernible seasonality, and two generations may be completed during a single year. However, in southern regions, immature stages may be most common during the southern winter (April to October, with the peak in larval activity preceding that of nymphs), and adults may be most common during summer (November to March)(49, 145).

Rhipicephalus evertsi

R. evertsi is a vector of the agent causing MSF and probably CCHF. The species is widely distributed from southwestern Yemen throughout sub-Saharan Africa south of 18°N, but it is more common in the eastern half of the African continent (Color Map 2) (49, 97, 145). Larvae and nymphs of this two-host species feed on hares and ungulates, and all stages feed on large ungulates, including cattle, eland (and a variety of antelope), horses, donkeys, and zebras, as well as occasionally on people. It occurs in a variety of habitats ranging from the humid highlands of southwestern Yemen to woodlands, brushy grasslands, and rarely forests at altitudes ranging from sea level to 2,500 m. Precipitation appears to be the factor limiting its distribution to areas with >250 to 375 mm annually. However, Walker et al. (145) note a lack of understanding of factors restricting the widely tolerant species from some areas where it has not been found. In tropical regions, there is no apparent seasonality to activity, but in southern Africa the species overwinters as fed nymphs and large numbers of adults become active during spring (145).

Rhipicephalus pumilio

R. pumilio is a vector of the agents causing CCHF, Astrakhan fever, tularemia, and Q fever. The species occurs in southwestern Asia, between approximately 32

to 46°N, in Russia, Afghanistan, Turkmenistan, Uzbekistan, Kazakhstan, Tajikistan, Pakistan, Mongolia, and China (Color Map 2) (145). The species has been associated with relatively humid river valleys, oases, and foothill regions, but also with xeric desert habitats. This three-host species feeds on a wide variety of hosts, but immature stages have been recovered most commonly from gerbils (*Meriones* spp. and *Rhombomys opimus*), hedgehogs (*Hemiechinus* spp.), and hares, and adults from hares (*Lepus* spp.), canids (including jackals, wolves, and dogs of the genus *Canis* as well as red foxes [*V. vulpes*]), livestock, and people (145).

Rhipicephalus sanguineus

R. sanguineus (the brown dog tick) is a vector of the agents causing MSF, Israeli tick typhus (*R. conorii* sensu lato), NATT, RMSF (in Mexico), and tularemia. It is considered an important vector of MSF, and it is the most widespread tick in the world with a nearly global distribution between latitudes of 50°N and 30°S wherever dogs are common (49, 145). The known distribution includes the Americas from southern Canada South to Southern Brazil and central Argentina, all of Europe, the central latitudes of Russia, most of Africa (except for desert regions of the Sahel), the Middle East, South and Southeast Asia, coastal regions of northern and eastern Australia, and most oceanic islands large enough to have people and dogs; because of its ubiquity, we have not shown a distribution map for this species. Habitat associations of *R. sanguineus* are relatively less important than for most ticks because a large portion of most populations survive in homes, dog beds, barns, and other structures in which dogs sleep or spend considerable time. In tropical and subtropical regions, populations are active throughout the year, but in northern and southern regions, all stages may be inactive during colder months of winter. The brown dog tick feeds primarily on domestic dogs, but it will feed on wild carnivores and people opportunistically (49, 145).

Rhipicephalus simus

R. simus is a vector of *R. conorii*, the agent causing MSF. This three-host African species occurs south of approximately 9°S (Color Map 3) (145). Larvae and nymphs are collected most commonly from burrowing small mammals, including murid rodents and scrub hares (*Lepus saxatilis*). Adults feed on wild and domestic carnivores, antelope, warthogs (*P. africanus*), livestock, and people. This species is commonly associated with woodlands, wooded grasslands, and scrub habitats in areas receiving 45 to 140 cm of rain annually. It ranges from sea level to over 2,000 m (145). The species probably completes only a single life cycle

annually. Seasonality varies with latitude; adults are active from midspring through midautumn in northern regions, but from midwinter to midsummer in southern Africa.

Rhipicephalus turanicus

R. turanicus is a vector of the agents causing Israeli tick typhus, NATT, and Q fever. This species is widely distributed through Mediterranean Africa from Morocco to Tunisia, northeastern Egypt, Sicily, Crete, Syria, Lebanon, Israel, Jordan, Iraq, Iran, India, throughout sub-Saharan East Africa and southern Africa, and in scattered locations in West Africa from Nigeria south (Color Map 8) (145). It has a broad host range encompassing hedgehogs (*Erinaceus* spp. and *Hemiechinus* spp.), gerbils (*Meriones* spp.), hares (*Lepus* spp.), wild carnivores, wild ungulates, livestock, dogs, and people. Habitats associated with this species vary from semidesert steppe to tropical savannas and scrublands and from elevations ranging to 2,000 m (145). As expected of a species with such a broad geographic range, seasonality varies considerably among regions. However, Walker et al. (145) generalize that adults are typically most active from the late rainy season through early months of the dry season.

Argasidae

Carios rudis

C. rudis (= *O. rudis*) is a vector of TBRF caused by *Borrelia venezuelensi*. The species occurs from Panama, Colombia, Ecuador, Peru, Bolivia, Paraguay, Venezuela, and Brazil (Color Map 8) (13). It is found in rodent nests, chicken coops, and wooden buildings, and it has been recovered from beds of RMSF patients in Colombia (13).

Carios talaje

C. talaje (= *O. talaje*) is a vector of TBRF caused by *Borrelia mazzottii*. The species occurs in the southern United States, Mexico, Central America, and South America south to Argentina (Color Map 4). This species is generally a parasite of rodents and is closely associated with rodent burrows, but it is also associated with old rodent-infested buildings. *B. mazzottii* has been isolated from these ticks from Florida, Texas, Arizona, Mexico, and Panama, but no human cases have been reported north of Mexico (13).

Ornithodoros asperus

O. asperus (= *Ornithodoros verrucosus*) is a vector of TBRF caused by *Borrelia caucasica*. This species occurs in extreme southwestern Russia, Chechnya, Georgia, Azerbaijan, Armenia, Kazakhstan, and Iraq (Color Map 8), where it dwells in the caves or burrows of rodents (e.g., *R. opimus* and *Allactaga* spp.) in habitats ranging from semidesert zones to dry agricultural areas (2, 13).

Ornithodoros erraticus sensu lato

O. erraticus sensu lato is a species complex in need of taxonomic revision. This group includes *Ornithodoros macrocanus*, the vector of *Borrelia hispanica* on the Iberian Peninsula (Portugal and Spain), Greece, Cyprus, and in Mediterranean North Africa (Morocco, Algeria, Tunisia, Libya, and Egypt). Additionally, there are "small variety" *O. erraticus* sensu lato ticks that transmit TBRF caused by *Borrelia crocidurae*, *Borrelia dipodilli*, and *Borrelia merionesi* in West Africa (e.g., Senegal and likely much of rural West Africa), North Africa (Algeria and Egypt), Kenya, Turkey, Iraq, and Iran (Color Map 11). Small variety *O. erraticus* sensu lato ticks comprise *O. erraticus* sensu stricto in Africa, *O. sonrai* in Senegal, *Ornithodoros graingeri* (which transmits *Borrelia graingeri* among porcupines and possibly people in coastal areas of Kenya), *Ornithodoros grenieri* from Madagascar, and *Ornithodoros alactagalis* from Armenia, Azerbaijan, and Turkmenistan (58), but the phylogenetic relationships among these species remain unknown. Species within this group vary in terms of host preference. *O. macrocanus* is associated with pigsties in Spain where it is an important vector of African swine fever virus. Most other species within the group are associated with rodents, rodent burrows, or caves with rodent nests. All stages of these species feed quickly (~30 min), and although longevity may be prolonged, two generations are possible per year (58).

Ornithodoros hermsi

O. hermsi is a vector of TBRF caused by *B. hermsii* in western North America (Color Map 11) where it is found most commonly at middle elevations (450 to 2,500 m) of the Rocky Mountains, Cascades, Sierra Nevada Range, and the San Bernardino Mountains (46, 49, 54). *O. hermsi* is associated with coniferous forests and typically lives in nests or cracks in logs or trees near nests, where it is thought to feed primarily on chipmunks (*Tamias* spp.), ground squirrels (*Spermophilus* spp.), and woodrats (*Neotoma* spp.) (13, 32) but also opportunistically on birds and even toads (46, 54). Sometimes, such nests are built in the structures of mountain cabins or homes. When people occupy such cabins and especially when they remove rodent occupants, they expose themselves to these

vectors (130). *O. hermsi* feeds swiftly and painlessly at night, and people generally remain unaware of being bitten in their beds or sleeping bags. Ticks leave the host once they feed but have sometimes been found wandering in bedding (13, 32).

Ornithodoros moubata sensu lato

O. moubata sensu lato (African tampans) is a vector of TBRF caused by *B. duttonii* in central, eastern, and southern Africa and on Madagascar (Color Map 11). This species complex includes *Ornithodoros apertus* in Kenya, Ghana, and Botswana; *Ornithodoros porcinus* in Kenya south to South Africa and Mozambique; *Ornithodoros compactus* (which is a parasite of tortoises) in southern Africa; and *O. moubata* sensu stricto in East and South Africa, and it deserves further study to describe fully the ecological and genetic relationships (58). *O. moubata* and *Ornithodoros porcinus domesticus* are adapted to coexist with people and are responsible for most TBRF in Africa. *O. moubata* sensu stricto is "perhaps the best example of tick-human specificity" (130). At elevations above 1,500 m in the Jombeni Mountains of Kenya, this species thrives in mud and grass huts that are heated by central cooking fires surrounded by platform beds of mud or clay. The central cooking fires not only heat the hut but also dry and crack the mud of platform beds, and the cracks provide excellent cover for resting ticks. Mud platforms built farther than 3 m from fires or in unheated huts do not crack, and these situations do not support populations of *O. moubata* sensu stricto. Most other ticks within this group live in burrows of warthogs (*Phacochoerus aethiopicus*), porcupines (*Hystrix africaeaustralis*), and aardvarks (*Orycteropus afer*), as well as in cracks in hollow trees (130). Trans-ovarial transmission is well documented in this species (13), but population-level specificity in other species combinations suggests that efficiency of transovarial transmission, as with other aspects of vector competence, should be expected to vary among the different combinations of *B. duttonii* strains and the complex of subspecies comprising *O. moubata* sensu lato.

Ornithodoros parkeri

O. parkeri is a potential vector of TBRF caused by *B. parkeri* throughout western North America. Although the geographic distribution broadly overlaps that of *O. hermsi*, *O. parkeri* occurs at lower elevations (23). It is associated with burrows of ground squirrels (*Spermophilus* spp.), prairie dogs (*Cynomys* spp.), and burrowing owls (*Athene cunicularia*), and specimens also have been collected from rodent nests and caves (58). In California, this species occurs along the lower foothills and the Central Valley, while *O. hermsi* occurs in the Sierra Nevada Range and the San Bernardino Mountains. As a result of these ticks living in burrows as opposed to trees or wooden buildings, people rarely enter the microhabitat of this tick, and transmission of *B. parkeri* to people has been documented only once (13, 32).

Ornithodoros tartakovskyi

O. tartakovskyi is a vector of TBRF caused by *Borrelia latyschewii* and Q fever. This tick occurs in the Central Asian republics east of the Caspian Sea (including Kazakhstan, Uzbekistan, Turkmenistan, Kyrgyzstan, and Tajikistan), Iran, Afghanistan, and Sinkiang in northwestern China (Color Map 11) where it ranges from sea level to 2,660 m in areas of relatively high humidity (58). This species has been collected from the burrows of rodents and small carnivores, tortoise burrows, bird nests, and livestock. In southern Tajikistan, the species survives in rodent burrows along irrigation ditches where it is closely associated with Libyan jirds (*Meriones libycus*). Transovarial transmission of *B. latyschewii* is known to occur (13). *O. tartakovskyi* is somewhat unique among soft ticks in that nymphs and adults may stay on a host for several hours, days, or even months (58).

Ornithodoros tholozani

O. tholozani (= *Ornithodoros papillipes*) is a vector of TBRF caused by *Borrelia persica* and ranges from northwestern Egypt, northeastern Libya, Greece, Cyprus, and other Mediterranean islands, southern Russia, southwestern China, the Middle East, western India, Iran, and Iraq (Color Map 11). Regional specificity of strains of *B. persica* for local populations of *O. tholozani* appear common; ticks from one region may not be able to transmit *B. persica* from other regions, and transovarial transmission has been documented (13). This species thrives in homes, barns, stables, clay and stone fences used to confine livestock, caves, and rock outcrops in semidesert, steppe, and Mediterranean habitats. It is a host generalist, commonly feeding on people, livestock (cattle, camels, goats, and sheep), foxes (*Vulpes* spp.), jackals (*Canis* spp.), porcupines (*Hystrix* spp.), small rodents (*Rhombomys* spp., *Meriones* spp., *Pallasiomys* spp., and *Mesocricetus* spp.), hedgehogs (*Hemiechinus* spp. and *Paraechinus* spp.), and birds (including chickens) (58, 130).

Ornithodoros turicata

O. turicata is a vector of TBRF caused by *B. turicatae* in the western United States and Mexico. The species occurs in lowland xeric habitats from southern Kansas, Florida, and central California in the north through central Mexico (Color Map 8). Hoogstraal considered that reports from Canada and Central America were likely incorrect (58). *O. turicata* is most often associated with burrows of rodents (*Spermophilus* and *Cynomys* spp.) and reptiles (e.g., gopher tortoises, *Gopherus* spp., and snakes), woodrat (*Neotoma* spp.) nests, or rodent-infested limestone caves; however, they also infest pigsties, slaughterhouses, stables, barns, and homes (13, 32). As with most of these tick and spirochete combinations, borreliae persist for prolonged periods in tick tissues; transmission has been reported following 7 years of starvation (13, 32).

REFERENCES

1. **Acha, P. N., and B. Szyfres.** 2001. *Zoonoses and Communicable Diseases Common to Man and Animals*, 3rd ed., vol. 1. *Bacterioses and Mycoses.* Pan American Health Organization, Washington, D.C.
2. **Anastos, G.** 1957. *The Ticks, or Ixodides, of the USSR: A Review of the Literature.* Public Health Service publication 548. U.S. Department of Health, Education, and Welfare, Public Health Service, National Institutes of Health, Washington, D.C.
3. **Babalis, T., Y. Tselentis, V. Roux, A. Psaroulaki, and D. Raoult.** 1994. Isolation and identification of a rickettsial strain related to *Rickettsia massiliae* in Greek ticks. *Am. J. Trop. Med. Hyg.* 50:365–372.
4. **Bacellar, F., M. S. Núncio, M. J. Alves, and A. R. Filipe.** 1995. *Rickettsia slovaca*: un agente del grupo de las fiebres exantemáticas, en Portugal. *Enferm. Infecc. Microbiol. Clin.* 13:218–223.
5. **Bacellar, F., R. L. Regnery, M. S. Núncio, and A. R. Filipe.** 1995. Genotypic evaluation of rickettsial isolates recovered from various species of ticks in Portugal. *Epidemiol. Infect.* 114:169–178.
6. **Balayeva, N. M., M. E. Eremeeva, and D. Raoult.** 1994. Genomic identification of *Rickettsia slovaca* among spotted fever group rickettsia isolates from *Dermacentor marginatus* in Armenia. *Acta Virol.* 38:321–325.
7. **Beati, L., J. P. Finidori, and D. Raoult.** 1993. First isolation of *Rickettsia slovaca* from *Dermacentor marginatus* in France. *Am. J. Trop. Med. Hyg.* 48:257–268.
8. **Blanco, J. R., and J. A. Oteo.** 2002. Human granulocytic ehrlichiosis in Europe. *Clin. Microbiol. Infect.* 8:763–772.
9. **Bowen, G. S.** 1988. Colorado tick fever, p. 159–166. *In* T. P. Monath (ed.), *The Arboviruses: Epidemiology and Ecology*, vol. 2. CRC Press, Boca Raton, Fla.
10. **Bown, K. J., M. Begon, M. Bennett, Z. Woldehiwet, and N. H. Ogden.** 2003. Seasonal dynamics of *Anaplasma phagocytophila* in a rodent-tick (*Ixodes trianguliceps*) system, United Kingdom. *Emerg. Infect. Dis.* 9:63–70.
11. **Brown, R. N., and R. S. Lane.** 1992. Lyme disease in California: a novel enzootic transmission cycle of *Borrelia burgdorferi*. *Science* 256:1439–1442.
12. **Brown, R. N., and R. S. Lane.** 1996. Reservoir competence of four chaparral-dwelling rodents for Borrelia burgdorferi in California. *Am. J. Trop. Med. Hyg.* 54:84–91.
13. **Burgdorfer, W., and T. G. Schwan.** 1991. Borrrelia, p. 560–566. *In* W. J. H. A. Balows, Jr., K. L. Herrman, H. D. Isenberg,

and H. J. Shadomy (ed.), *Manual of Clinical Microbiology*, 5th ed. American Society for Microbiology, Washington, D.C.

14. **Cao, W. C., Y. M. Gao, P. H. Zhang, X. T. Zhang, Q. H. Dai, J. S. Dumler, L. Q. Fang, and H. Yang.** 2000. Identification of *Ehrlichia chaffeensis* by nested PCR in ticks from Southern China. *J. Clin. Microbiol.* **38:**2778–2780.

15. **Cao, W. C., Q. M. Zhao, P. H. Zhang, H. Yang, X. M. Wu, B. H. Wen, X. T. Zhang, and J. D. Habbema.** 2003. Prevalence of *Anaplasma phagocytophila* and *Borrelia burgdorferi* in *Ixodes persulcatus* ticks from northeastern China. *Am. J. Trop. Med. Hyg.* **68:**547–550.

16. **Cardeñosa, N., V. Roux, B. Font, I. Sanfeliu, D. Raoult, and F. Segura.** 2000. Short report: isolation and identification of two spotted fever group rickettsial strains from patients in Catalonia, Spain. *Am. J. Trop. Med. Hyg.* **62:**142–144.

17. **Centers for Disease Control and Prevention.** 2002. Lyme disease—United States, 2000. *Morbid. Mortal. Wkly. Rep.* **51:**29–31.

18. **Centers for Disease Control and Prevention.** 2002. Tularemia—United States, 1990–2000. *Morbid. Mortal. Wkly. Rep.* **51:**181–184.

19. **Chen, M., M. Y. Fan, D. Z. Bi, J. Z. Zhang, and Y. P. Huang.** 1998. Detection of *Rickettsia sibirica* in ticks and small mammals collected in three different regions of China. *Acta Virol.* **42:**61–64.

20. **Childs, J. E., B. A. Ellis, W. L. Nicholson, M. Kosoy, and J. W. Summer.** 1999. Shared vector-borne zoonoses of the Old World and New World: home grown or translocated? *Schweiz. Med. Wochenschr.* **129:**1099–1105.

21. **Childs, J. E., and C. D. Paddock.** 2003. The ascendancy of *Amblyomma americanum* as a vector of pathogens affecting humans in the United States. *Annu. Rev. Entomol.* **48:**307–337.

22. **Clover, J. R., and R. S. Lane.** 1995. Evidence implicating nymphal *Ixodes pacificus* (Acari: Ixodidae) in the epidemiology of Lyme disease in California. *Am. J. Trop. Med. Hyg.* **53:**237–240.

23. **Cooley, R. A., and G. M. Kohls.** 1944. *The Argasidae of North America, Central America and Cuba*, vol. 1. The University Press, Notre Dame, Ind.

24. **de Lemos, E. R., H. H. Melles, S. Colombo, R. D. Machado, J. R. Coura, M. A. Guimarães, S. R. Sanseverino, and A. Moura.** 1996. Primary isolation of spotted fever group rickettsiae from *Amblyomma cooperi* collected from *Hydrochaeris hydrochaeris* in Brazil. *Mem. Inst. Oswaldo Cruz* **91:**273–275.

25. **Dennis, D. T.** 2004. Tularemia, p. 1446–1451. *In* S. L. Gorbach, J. G. Bartlett, and N. R. Blacklow (ed.), *Infectious Diseases*, 3rd ed. Lippincott, Williams & Wilkins, Philadelphia, Pa.

26. **Dennis, D. T., and E. B. Hayes.** 2004. Relapsing fever, p. 991–995. *In* D. L. Kasper, E. Braunwald, A. Fauci, S. L. Hauser, D. L. Longo, and J. L. Jameson (ed.), *Harrison's Principles of Internal Medicine*, 16th ed. McGraw Hill, New York, N.Y.

27. **Dennis, D. T., and E. B. Hayes.** 2002. Epidemiology of Lyme borreliosis, p. 251–280. *In* J. S. Gray, O. Kahl, R. S. Lane, and G. Stanek (ed.), *Lyme Borreliosis: Biology, Epidemiology, and Control*. CABI Publishing, New York, N.Y.

28. **Dennis, D. T., T. V. Inglesby, D. A. Henderson, J. G. Bartlett, M. S. Ascher, E. Eitzen, A. D. Fine, A. M. Friedlander, J. Hauer, M. Layton, S. R. Lillibridge, J. E. McDade, M. T. Osterholm, T. O'Toole, G. Parker, T. M. Perl, P. K. Russell, and K. Tonat.** 2001. Tularemia as a biological weapon: medical and public health management. *JAMA* **285:**2763–2773.

29. **Díaz, I. A.** 2003. Rickettsiosis caused by *Rickettsia conorii* in Uruguay. *Ann. N. Y. Acad. Sci.* **990:**264–266.

30. **Dumler, J. S.** 2004. Rocky Mountain spotted fever, p. 1473–1480. *In* S. L. Gorbach, J. G. Bartlett, and N. R. Blacklow (ed.), *Infectious Diseases*, 3rd ed. Lippincott, Williams & Wilkins, Philadelphia, Pa.

31. **Dupont, H. T., J. P. Cornet, and D. Raoult.** 1994. Identification of rickettsiae from ticks collected in the Central African Republic using the polymerase chain reaction. *Am. J. Trop. Med. Hyg.* **50:**373–380.

32. **Dworkin, M. S., T. G. Schwan, and D. E. Anderson, Jr.** 2002. Tick-borne relapsing fever in North America. *Med. Clin. North Am.* **86:**417–433.

33. **Eisen, L., and R. S. Lane.** 2002. Vectors of *Borrelia burgdorferi* sensu lato, p. 91–116. *In* J. S. Gray, O. Kahl, R. S. Lane, and G. Stanek (ed.), *Lyme Borreliosis: Biology, Epidemiology, and Control*. CABI Publishing, New York, N.Y.

34. **Eldridge, B. F., T. W. Scott, J. F. Day, and W. J. Tabachnick.** 2000. Arbovirus diseases, p. 415–460. *In* B. F. Eldridge and J. D. Edman (ed.), *Medical Entomology: A Textbook on Public Health and Veterinary Problems Caused by Arthropods*. Kluwer Academic Publishers, Boston, Mass.

35. **Ellis, J., P.C. F. Oyston, M. Green, and R.W. Titball.** 2002. Tularemia. *Clin. Microbiol. Rev.* **15:**631–646.

36. **Emmons, R. W.** 1988. Ecology of Colorado tick fever. *Annu. Rev. Microbiol.* **42:**49–64.

37. **Eremeeva, M. E., L. Beati, V. A. Makarova, N. F. Fetisova, I. V. Tarasevich, N. M. Balayeva, and D. Raoult.** 1994. Astrakhan fever rickettsiae: antigenic and genotypic analysis of isolates obtained from human and *Rhipicephalus pumilio* ticks. *Am. J. Trop. Med. Hyg.* **51:**697–706.

38. **Fairchild, G. B., G. M. Kohls, and V. J. Tipton.** 1966. The ticks of Panama, p. 167–219. *In* R. L. Wenzel and V. J. Tipton (ed.), *Ectoparasites of Panama*. Field Museum of Natural History, Chicago, Ill.

39. **Feldman, K. A., R. E. Enscore, S. L. Lathrop, B. T. Matyas, M. McGuill, M. E. Schriefer, D. Stiles-Enos, D. T. Dennis, L. R. Petersen, and E. B. Hayes.** 2001. An outbreak of primary pneumonic tularemia on Martha's Vineyard. *N. Engl. J. Med.* **345:**1601–1606.

40. **Fernández-Soto, P., A. Encinas-Grandes, and R. Pérez-Sánchez.** 2003. *Rickettsia aeschlimannii* in Spain: molecular evidence in *Hyalomma marginatum* and five other tick species that feed on humans. *Emerg. Infect. Dis.* **9:**889–890.

41. **Foley, J. E., P. Foley, R. N. Brown, R. S. Lane, J. S. Dumler, and J. E. Madigan.** 2004. Ecology of granulocytic ehrlichiosis in the western United States. *J. Vector Ecol.* **29:**41–50.

42. **Fournier, P. E., J. P. Durand, J. M. Rolain, J. L. Camicas, H. Tolou, and D. Raoult.** 2003. Detection of Astrakhan fever rickettsia from ticks in Kosovo. *Ann. N. Y. Acad. Sci.* **990:**158–161.

43. **Fournier, P. E., H. Fujita, N. Takada, and D. Raoult.** 2002. Genetic identification of rickettsiae isolated from ticks in Japan. *J. Clin. Microbiol.* **40:**2176–2181.

44. **Fournier, P. E., H. Tissot-Dupont, H. Gallais, and D. R. Raoult.** 2000. *Rickettsia mongolotimonae*: a rare pathogen in France. *Emerg. Infect. Dis.* **6:**290–292.

45. **Fuentes, L., A. Calderon, and L. Hun.** 1985. Isolation and identification of *Rickettsia rickettsii* from the rabbit tick (*Haemaphysalis leporispalustris*) in the Atlantic zone of Costa Rica. *Am. J. Trop. Med. Hyg.* **34:**564–567.

46. **Furman, D. P., and E. C. Loomis.** 1984. *The Ticks of California (Acari: Ixodida)*. Bulletin of the California Insect Survey, vol. 25. University of California Press, Berkeley, Calif.

47. **Gao, G. F., P. M. Zanotto, E. C. Holmes, H. W. Reid, and E. A. Gould.** 1997. Molecular variation, evolution and geo-

graphical distribution of louping ill virus. *Acta Virol.* **41:** 259–268.

48. **Gern, L., and P.-F. Humair.** 2002. Ecology of *Borrelia burgdorferi* sensu lato in Europe, p. 149–174. *In* J. S. Gray, O. Kahl, R. S. Lane, and G. Stanek (ed.), *Lyme Borreliosis: Biology, Epidemiology, and Control.* CABI Publishing, New York, N.Y.

49. **Goddard, J.** 1989. *Ticks and Tickborne Diseases Affecting Military Personnel.* U.S. Air Force School of Aerospace Medicine, Brooks Air Force Base, Tex.

50. **Gorenflot, A., K. Moubri, E. Precigout, B. Carcy, and T. P. Schetters.** 1998. Human babesiosis. *Ann. Trop. Med. Parasitol.* **92:**489–501.

51. **Graves, S., and J. Stenos.** 2003. *Rickettsia honei*: a spotted fever group *Rickettsia* on three continents. *Ann. N. Y. Acad. Sci.* **990:**62–66.

52. **Graves, S. R., L. Stewart, J. Stenos, R. S. Stewart, E. Schmidt, S. Hudson, J. Banks, Z. Huang, and B. Dwyer.** 1993. Spotted fever group rickettsial infection in south-eastern Australia: isolation of rickettsiae. *Comp. Immunol. Microbiol. Infect. Dis.* **16:**223–233.

53. **Gray, J. S.** 2002. Biology of Ixodes species ticks in relation to tick-borne zoonoses. *Wien. Klin. Wochenschr.* **114:**473–478.

54. **Gregson, J. D.** 1956. *The Ixodoidea of Canada.* Canadian Department of Agriculture, publ. 930. Canada Department of Agriculture, Ottawa, Canada.

55. **Guglielmonte, A. A., A. Mangold, and A. E. Vinabal.** 1991. Ticks (Ixodidae) parasitizing people in four provinces of north-western Argentina. *Ann. Trop. Med. Parasitol.* **85:** 539–542.

56. **Hellenbrand, W., T. Breuer, and L. Petersen.** 2001. Changing epidemiology of Q fever in Germany, 1947–1999. *Emerg. Infect. Dis.* **7:**789–796.

57. **Herwaldt, B. L., P. C. McGovern, Michal P. Gerwel, Rachael M. Easton, and Rob Roy MacGregor.** 2003. Endemic babesiosis in another eastern state: New Jersey. *Emerg. Infect. Dis.* **9:**184–188.

58. **Hoogstraal, H.** 1985. Argasid and nuttalliellid ticks as parasites and vectors. *Adv. Parasitol.* **24:**136–238.

59. **Hornick, R.** 2001. Tularemia revisited. *N. Engl. J. Med.* **345:**1637–1639.

60. **Hubalek, Z., F. Treml, J. Halouzka, Z. Juricova, M. Hunady, and V. Janik.** 1996. Frequent isolation of *Francisella tularensis* from *Dermacentor reticulatus* ticks in an enzootic focus of tularaemia. *Med. Vet. Entomol.* **10:**241–246.

61. **Ishikura, M., H. Fujita, S. Ando, K. Matsuura, and M. Watanabe.** 2002. Phylogenetic analysis of spotted fever group rickettsiae isolated from ticks in Japan. *Microbiol. Immunol.* **46:**241–247.

62. **Jones, C. G., R. S. Ostfeld, M. P. Richard, E. M. Schauber, and J. O. Wolff.** 1998. Chain reactions linking acorns to gypsy moth outbreaks and Lyme disease risk. *Science* **279:** 1023–1026.

63. **Jongen, V. H., J. van Roosmalen, J. Tiems, J. Van Holten, and J. C. Wetsteyn.** 1997. Tick-borne relapsing fever and pregnancy outcome in rural Tanzania. *Acta Obstet. Gynecol. Scand.* **76:**834–838.

64. **Kaiser, J.** 1998. Of mice and moths—and Lyme disease? *Science* **279:**984–985.

65. **Katayama, T., Y. Furuya, Y. Yoshida, and I. Kaiho.** 1996. Spotted fever group rickettsiosis and vectors in Kanagawa prefecture. *Kansenshogaku Zasshi* **70:**561–568. (In Japanese.)

66. **Kelly, P. J.** 2001. *Amblyomma hebraeum* is a vector of *Rickettsia africae* and not *R. conorii*. *J. S. Afr. Vet. Assoc.* **72:**182.

67. **Kim, C. M., M. S. Kim, M. S. Park, J. H. Park, and J. S. Chae.** 2003. Identification of *Ehrlichia chaffeensis*, *Anaplasma*

phagocytophilum, and *A. bovis* in *Haemaphysalis longicornis* and *Ixodes persulcatus* ticks from Korea. *Vector-Borne Zoonotic Dis.* **3:**17–26.

68. **Kjemtrup, A. M., and P. A. Conrad.** 2000. Human babesiosis: an emerging tick-borne disease. *Int. J. Parasitol.* **30:** 1323–1337.

69. **Klasco, R.** 2002. Colorado tick fever. *Med. Clin. North Am.* **86:**435–440.

70. **Klompen, J. S. H., and J. H. Oliver, Jr.** 1993. Systematic relationships in the soft ticks (Acari: Ixodida: Argasidae). *Syst. Entomol.* **18:**313–331.

71. **Kollars, T. M., Jr., B. Tippayachai, and D. Bodhidatta.** 2001. Short report: Thai tick typhus, *Rickettsia honei*, and a unique rickettsia detected in *Ixodes granulatus* (Ixodidae: Acari) from Thailand. *Am. J. Trop. Med. Hyg.* **65:**535–537.

72. **Korenberg, E. I., N. B. Gorelova, and Y. V. Kovalevskii.** 2002. Ecology of *Borrelia burgdorferi* sensu lato in Russia, p. 175–200. *In* J. S. Gray, O. Kahl, R. S. Lane, and G. Stanek (ed.), *Lyme Borreliosis: Biology, Epidemiology, and Control.* CABI Publishing, New York, N.Y.

73. **Kramer, V. L., M. P. Randolph, L. T. Hui, W. E. Irwin, A. G. Gutierrez, and D. J. Vugia.** 1999. Detection of the agents of human ehrlichioses in ixodid ticks from California. *Am. J. Trop. Med. Hyg.* **60:**62–65.

74. **Kuo, M. M., R. S. Lane, and P. C. Giclas.** 2000. A comparative study of mammalian and reptilian alternative pathway of complement-mediated killing of the Lyme disease spirochete (*Borrelia burgdorferi*). *J. Parasitol.* **86:**1223–1228.

75. **Lane, R. S., R. W. Emmons, V. Devlin, D. V. Dondero, and B. C. Nelson.** 1982. Survey for evidence of Colorado tick fever virus outside of the known endemic area in California. *Am. J. Trop. Med. Hyg.* **31:**837–843.

76. **Lane, R. S., J. E. Foley, L. Eisen, E. T. Lennette, and M. A. Peot.** 2001. Acarologic risk of exposure to emerging tick-borne bacterial pathogens in a semirural community in northern California. *Vector Borne Zoonotic Dis.* **1:**197–210.

77. **Lane, R. S., and J. E. Loye.** 1989. Lyme disease in California: interrelationship of *Ixodes pacificus* (Acari: Ixodidae), the western fence lizard (*Sceloporus occidentalis*), and *Borrelia burgdorferi*. *J. Med. Entomol.* **26:**272–278.

78. **Lane, R. S., and J. E. Loye.** 1991. Lyme disease in California: interrelationship of ixodid ticks (Acari), rodents, and *Borrelia burgdorferi*. *J. Med. Entomol.* **28:**719–725.

79. **Lane, R. S., and S. A. Manweiler.** 1988. *Borrelia coriaceae* in its tick vector, *Ornithodoros coriaceus* (Acari: Argasidae), with emphasis on transstadial and transovarial infection. *J. Med. Entomol.* **25:**172–177.

80. **Lane, R. S., C. A. Peavey, K. A. Padgett, and M. Hendson.** 1999. Life history of *Ixodes* (*Ixodes*) *jellisoni* (Acari: Ixodidae) and its vector competence for *Borrelia burgdorferi* sensu lato. *J. Med. Entomol.* **36:**329–340.

81. **Lane, R. S., and G. B. Quistad.** 1998. Borreliacidal factor in the blood of the western fence lizard (*Sceloporus occidentalis*). *J. Parasitol.* **84:**29–34.

82. **LeDuc, J. W.** 1998. Diseases transmitted primarily by arthropod vectors: viral hemorrhagic fevers, p. 296–304. *In* R. B. Wallace (ed.), *Public Health and Preventive Medicine.* Appleton & Lange, Stamford, Conn.

83. **Lee, J. H., H. S. Park, K. D. Jung, W. J. Jang, S. E. Koh, S. S. Kang, I. Y. Lee, W. J. Lee, B. J. Kim, Y. H. Kook, K. H. Park, and S. H. Lee.** 2003. Identification of the spotted fever group rickettsiae detected from *Haemaphysalis longicornis* in Korea. *Microbiol. Immunol.* **47:**301–304.

84. **Levin, M. L., W. L. Nicholson, R. F. Massung, J. W. Sumner, and D. Fish.** 2002. Comparison of the reservoir competence of medium-sized mammals and *Peromyscus leucopus* for

Anaplasma phagocytophilum in Connecticut. *Vector Borne Zoonotic Dis.* 2:125–136.

85. **Linthicum, K. J., and C. L. Bailey.** 1994. Ecology of Crimean-Congo hemorrhagic fever, p. 392–437. *In* D. E. Sonenshine and T. N. Mather (ed.), *Ecological Dynamics of Tick-Borne Zoonoses.* Oxford University Press, New York, N.Y.

86. **Liu, Q. H., G. Y. Chen, Y. Jin, M. Te, L. C. Niu, S. P. Dong, and D. H. Walker.** 1995. Evidence for a high prevalence of spotted fever group rickettsial infections in diverse ecologic zones of Inner Mongolia. *Epidemiol. Infect.* 115:177–183.

87. **Macaluso, K. R., J. Davis, U. Alam, A. Korman, J. S. Rutherford, R. Rosenberg, and A. F. Azad.** 2003. Spotted fever group rickettsiae in ticks from the Masai Mara region of Kenya. *Am. J. Trop. Med. Hyg.* 68:551–553.

88. **Mahara, F.** 1997. Japanese spotted fever: report of 31 cases and review of the literature. *Emerg. Infect. Dis.* 3:105–111.

89. **Matthysse, J. G., and M. H. Colbo.** 1987. *The Ixodid Ticks of Uganda.* Entomological Society of America, College Park, Md.

90. **Maupin, G. O., K. L. Gage, J. Piesman, J. Montenieri, S. L. Sviat, L. VanderZanden, C. M. Happ, M. Dolan, and B. J. Johnson.** 1994. Discovery of an enzootic cycle of *Borrelia burgdorferi* in *Neotoma mexicana* and *Ixodes spinipalpis* from northern Colorado, an area where Lyme disease is non-endemic. *J. Infect. Dis.* 170:636–643.

91. **McQuiston, J. H., J. E. Childs, M. E. Chamberland, and E. Tabor.** 2000. Transmission of tick-borne agents of disease by blood transfusion: a review of known and potential risks in the United States. *Transfusion* 40:274–284.

92. **McQuiston, J. H., C. D. Paddock, R. C. Holman, and J. E. Childs.** 1999. The human ehrlichioses in the United States. *Emerg. Infect. Dis.* 5:635–642.

93. **Miyamoto, K., and T. Masusawa.** 2002. Ecology of *Borrelia burgdorferi* sensu lato in Japan and East Asia, p. 201–222. *In* J. S. Gray, O. Kahl, R. S. Lane, and G. Stanek (ed.), *Lyme Borreliosis: Biology, Epidemiology, and Control.* CABI Publishing, New York, N.Y.

94. **Mount, G. A., D. G. Haile, D. R. Barnard, and E. Daniels.** 1993. New version of LSTSIM for computer simulation of *Amblyomma americanum* (Acari: Ixodidae) population dynamics. *J. Med. Entomol.* 30:843–857.

95. **Niebylski, M. L., M. G. Peacock, and T. G. Schwan.** 1999. Lethal effect of *Rickettsia rickettsii* on its tick vector (*Dermacentor andersoni*). *Appl. Environ. Microbiol.* 65:773–778.

96. **Norval, R. A. I., and B. D. Perry.** 1994. Dynamic associations of tick-borne diseases affecting domestic animal health, p. 283–313. *In* D. E. Sonenshine and T. N. Mather (ed.), *Ecological Dynamics of Tick-Borne Zoonoses.* Oxford University Press, New York, N.Y.

97. **Norval, R. A. I., B. D. Perry, and A. S. Young.** 1992. *The Epidemiology of Theileriosis in Africa.* Academic Press Limited, San Diego, Calif.

98. **Nuttall, P. A., and M. Labuda.** 1994. Tick-borne encephalitis subgroup, p. 351–391. *In* D. E. Sonenshine and T. N. Mather (ed.), *Ecological Dynamics of Tick-Borne Zoonoses.* Oxford University Press, New York, N.Y.

99. **Padgett, K. A., and R. S. Lane.** 2001. Life cycle of *Ixodes pacificus* (Acari: Ixodidae): timing of developmental processes under field and laboratory conditions. *J. Med. Entomol.* 38:684–693.

100. **Parola, P., J. P. Cornet, Y. O. Sanogo, R. S. Miller, H. V. Thien, J. P. Gonzalez, D. Raoult, S. R. Telford III, and C. Wongsrichanalai.** 2003. Detection of *Ehrlichia* spp., *Anaplasma* spp., *Rickettsia* spp., and other eubacteria in ticks from the Thai-Myanmar border and Vietnam. *J. Clin. Microbiol.* 41:1600–1608.

101. **Parola, P., H. Inokuma, J. L. Camicas, P. Brouqui, and D. Raoult.** 2001. Detection and identification of spotted fever group Rickettsiae and Ehrlichiae in African ticks. *Emerg. Infect. Dis.* 7:1014–1017.

102. **Parola, P., J. Jourdan, and D. Raoult.** 1998. Tick-borne infection caused by *Rickettsia africae* in the West Indies. *N. Engl. J. Med.* 338:1391.

103. **Parola, P., R. S. Miller, P. McDaniel, S. R. Telford III, J.-M. Rolain, C. Wongsrichanalai, and Didier Raoult.** 2003. Emerging rickettsioses of the Thai-Myanmar border. *Emerg. Infect. Dis.* 9:592–595.

104. **Parola, P., G. Vestris, D. Martinez, B. Brochier, V. Roux, and D. Raoult.** 1999. Tick-borne rickettsiosis in Guadeloupe, the French West Indies: isolation of *Rickettsia africae* from *Amblyomma variegatum* ticks and serosurvey in humans, cattle, and goats. *Am. J. Trop. Med. Hyg.* 60:888–893.

105. **Paul, W. S., G. Maupin, A. O. Scott-Wright, R. B. Craven, and D. T. Dennis.** 2002. Outbreak of tick-borne relapsing fever at the north rim of the Grand Canyon: evidence for effectiveness of preventive measures. *Am. J. Trop. Med. Hyg.* 66:71–75.

106. **Peavey, C. A., R. S. Lane, and T. Damrow.** 2000. Vector competence of *Ixodes angustus* (Acari: Ixodidae) for *Borrelia burgdorferi* sensu stricto. *Exp. Appl. Acarol.* 24:77–84.

107. **Peavey, C. A., R. S. Lane, and J. E. Kleinjan.** 1997. Role of small mammals in the ecology of *Borrelia burgdorferi* in a peri-urban park in north coastal California. *Exp. Appl. Acarol.* 21:569–584.

108. **Philip, R. N., R. S. Lane, and E. A. Casper.** 1981. Serotypes of tick-borne spotted fever group rickettsiae from western California. *Am. J. Trop. Med. Hyg.* 30:722–727.

109. **Piesman, J.** 2002. Ecology of *Borrelia burgdorferi* sensu lato in North America, p. 223–250. *In* J. S. Gray, O. Kahl, R. S. Lane, and G. Stanek (ed.), *Lyme Borreliosis: Biology, Epidemiology, and Control.* CABI Publishing, New York, N.Y.

110. **Pretorius, A. M., and R. J. Birtles.** 2002. *Rickettsia aeschlimannii*: a new pathogenic spotted fever group rickettsia, South Africa. *Emerg. Infect. Dis.* 8:874.

111. **Psaroulaki, A., I. Spyridaki, A. Ioannidis, T. Babalis, A. Gikas, and Y. Tselentis.** 2003. First isolation and identification of *Rickettsia conorii* from ticks collected in the region of Fokida in Central Greece. *J. Clin. Microbiol.* 41:3317–3319.

112. **Randolph, S.** 2001. Tick-borne encephalitis in Europe. *Lancet* 358:1731–1732.

113. **Randolph, S. E., R. M. Green, M. F. Peacey, and D. J. Rogers.** 2000. Seasonal synchrony: the key to tick-borne encephalitis foci identified by satellite data. *Parasitology* 121:15–23.

114. **Randolph, S. E., D. Miklisová, J. Lysy, D. J. Rogers, and M. Labuda.** 1999. Incidence from coincidence: patterns of tick infestations on rodents facilitate transmission of tick-borne encephalitis virus. *Parasitology* 118:177–186.

115. **Raoult, D., P. E. Fournier, P. Abboud, and F. Caron.** 2002. First documented human *Rickettsia aeschlimannii* infection. *Emerg. Infect. Dis.* 8:748–749.

116. **Raoult, D., P. E. Fournier, F. Fenollar, M. Jensenius, T. Prioe, J. J. de Pina, G. Caruso, N. Jones, H. Laferl, J. E. Rosenblatt, and T. J. Marrie.** 2001. *Rickettsia africae*, a tick-borne pathogen in travelers to sub-Saharan Africa. *N. Engl. J. Med.* 344:1504–1510.

117. **Raoult, D., and V. Roux.** 1997. Rickettsioses as paradigms of new or emerging infectious diseases. *Clin. Microbiol. Rev.* 10:694–719.

118. **Ravyn, M. D., E. I. Korenberg, J. A. Oeding, Y. V. Kovalevskii, and R. C. Johnson.** 1999. Monocytic *Ehrlichia* in *Ixodes persulcatus* ticks from Perm, Russia. *Lancet* 353:722–723.

119. Rehácek, J. 1993. Rickettsiae and their ecology in the Alpine region. *Acta Virol.* **37:**290–301.

120. Roberts, F. H. S. 1970. *Australian Ticks.* Commonwealth Scientific and Industrial Research Organization (CSIRO), Melbourne, Australia.

121. Russell, R. C. 1998. Vectors vs. humans in Australia—who is on top down under? An update on vector-borne disease and research on vectors in Australia. *J. Vector Ecol.* **23:**1–46.

122. Rydkina, E., V. Roux, N. Rudakov, M. Gafarova, I. Tarasevich, and D. Raoult. 1999. New *Rickettsiae* in ticks collected in territories of the former Soviet Union. *Emerg. Infect. Dis.* **5:**811–814.

123. Sanogo, Y. O., B. Davoust, P. Parola, J. L. Camicas, P. Brouqui, and D. Raoult. 2003. Prevalence of *Rickettsia* spp. in *Dermacentor marginatus* ticks removed from game pigs (*Sus scrofa*) in southern France. *Ann. N. Y. Acad. Sci.* **990:**191–195.

124. Sanogo, Y. O., P. Parola, S. Shpynov, J. L. Camicas, P. Brouqui, G. Caruso, and D. Raoult. 2003. Genetic diversity of bacterial agents detected in ticks removed from asymptomatic patients in northeastern Italy. *Ann. N. Y. Acad. Sci.* **990:**182–190.

125. Satoh, H., Y. Motoi, G. A. Camer, H. Inokuma, M. Izawa, T. Kiyuuna, N. Kumazawa, Y. Muramatsu, H. Ueno, and C. Morita. 2002. Characterization of spotted fever group rickettsiae detected in dogs and ticks in Okinawa, Japan. *Microbiol. Immunol.* **46:**257–263.

126. Schriefer, M. E., and A. F. Azud. 1994. Changing ecology of Rocky-Mountain spotted fever, p. 314–326. *In* D. E. Sonenshine and T. N. Mather (ed.), *Ecological Dynamics of Tick-Borne Zoonoses.* Oxford University Press, New York, N.Y.

127. Shibata, S., M. Kawahara, Y. Rikihisa, H. Fujita, Y. Watanabe, C. Suto, and T. Ito. 2000. New *Ehrlichia* species closely related to *Ehrlichia chaffeensis* isolated from *Ixodes ovatus* ticks in Japan. *J. Clin. Microbiol.* **38:**1331–1338.

128. Shope, R. E., and T. F. Tsai. 1998. Diseases transmitted primarily by arthropod vectors: viral infections, p. 281–295. *In* R. B. Wallace (ed.), *Public Health and Preventive Medicine.* Appleton & Lange, Stamford, Conn.

129. Silverman, M., B. Law, and J. Carson. 1991. A case of insect borne tularemia above the tree line. *Arctic Med. Res.* **Suppl.:**377–379.

130. Sonenshine, D. E. 1993. *Biology of Ticks,* vol. 2. Oxford University Press, New York, N.Y.

131. Sonenshine, D. E. 1994. Introduction, p. 139–197. *In* D. E. Sonenshine and T. N. Mather (ed.), *Ecological Dynamics of Tick-Borne Zoonoses.* Oxford University Press, New York, N.Y.

132. Sonenshine, D. E., R. S. Lane, and W. L. Nicholson. 2002. Ticks (Ixodida), p. 517–558. *In* G. Mullen and L. Durden (ed.), *Medical and Veterinary Entomology.* Academic Press, Boston, Mass.

133. Spielman, A., M. L. Wilson, J. F. Levine, and J. Piesman. 1985. Ecology of *Ixodes dammini*-borne human babesiosis and Lyme disease. *Annu. Rev. Entomol.* **30:**439–460.

134. Takeda, T., T. Ito, M. Chiba, K. Takahashi, T. Niioka, and I. Takashima. 1998. Isolation of tick-borne encephalitis virus from *Ixodes ovatus* (Acari: Ixodidae) in Japan. *J. Med. Entomol.* **35:**227–231.

135. Talleklint-Eisen, L., and R. S. Lane. 1999. Variation in the density of questing *Ixodes pacificus* (Acari: Ixodidae) nymphs infected with *Borrelia burgdorferi* at different spatial scales in California. *J. Parasitol.* **85:**824–831.

136. Tandon, S. K. 1991. *The Ixodid Ticks of Zambia (Acarina: Ixodidae).* Zoological Survey of India, Calcutta, India.

137. Turrel, M. J., and L. A. Durden. 1994. Experimental transmission of Langat (tick-borne encephalitis virus complex) virus to the soft tick *Ornithodoros sonrai* (Acari: Argasidae). *J. Med. Entomol.* **31:**148–151.

138. Uchida, T., T. Uchiyama, K. Kumano, and D. H. Walker. 1992. *Rickettsia japonica* sp. nov., the etiological agent of spotted fever group rickettsiosis in Japan. *Int. J. Syst. Bacteriol.* **42:**303–305.

139. Uchida, T., Y. Yan, and S. Kitaoka. 1995. Detection of *Rickettsia japonica* in *Haemaphysalis longicornis* ticks by restriction fragment length polymorphism of PCR product. *J. Clin. Microbiol.* **33:**824–828.

140. Uspensky, I., and I. Ioffe-Uspensky. 2002. The dog factor in brown dog tick *Rhipicephalus sanguineus* (Acari: Ixodidae) infestations in and near human dwellings. *Int. J. Med. Microbiol.* **291:**156–163.

141. Varma, M. G. R. 1989. *Geographical Distribution of Arthropod-Borne Diseases and Their Principal Vectors.* Unpublished document WHO/VBC/89.967. World Health Organization, Geneva, Switzerland.

142. Walker, D. H. 1998. Tick-transmitted infectious diseases in the United States. *Annu. Rev. Public Health* **19:**237–269.

143. Walker, D. H., and J. S. Dumler. 1996. Emergence of the ehrlichioses as human health problems. *Emerg. Infect. Dis.* **2:**18–29.

144. Walker, J. B. 1974. *The Ixodid Ticks of Kenya.* Commonwealth Institute of Entomology, London, England.

145. Walker, J. B., J. E. Keirans, and A. G. Horak. 2000. *The Genus Rhipicephalus (Acari: Ixodidae): A Guide to the Brown Ticks of the World.* Cambridge University Press, Cambridge, England.

146. Wen, B., W. Cao, and H. Pan. 2003. Ehrlichiae and ehrlichial diseases in China. *Ann. N. Y. Acad. Sci.* **990:**45–53.

147. Williams, W. J., S. Radulovic, G. A. Dasch, J. Lindstrom, D. J. Kelly, C. N. Oster, and D. H. Walker. 1994. Identification of *Rickettsia conorii* infection by polymerase chain reaction in a soldier returning from Somalia. *Clin. Infect. Dis.* **19:**93–99.

148. Yabsley, M. J., A. S. Varela, C. M. Tate, V. G. Dugan, D. E. Stallknecht, S. E. Little, and W. R. Davidson. 2002. *Ehrlichia ewingii* infection in white-tailed deer (*Odocoileus virginianus*). *Emerg. Infect. Dis.* **8:**668–671.

149. Yamaguti, N., V. J. Tipton, H. L. Keegan, and S. Toshioka. 1971. Ticks of Japan, Korea, and Ryukyu Islands. *Brigham Young Univ. Sci. Bull. Biol. Ser.* **15:**142–148.

INDEX

Note: CP indicates a page on which a Color Plate concerning the subject is cited; CM indicates a page on which a Color Map is cited.